Impacts and Treatment of Hypothyroidism

Impacts and Treatment of Hypothyroidism

Edited by **Benjamin Copes**

FOSTER ACADEMICS

New Jersey

Published by Foster Academics,
61 Van Reypen Street,
Jersey City, NJ 07306, USA
www.fosteracademics.com

Impacts and Treatment of Hypothyroidism
Edited by Benjamin Copes

International Standard Book Number: 978-1-63242-242-2 (Hardback)

Printed in China.

Contents

Preface

Every book is initially just a concept; it takes months of research and hard work to give it the final shape in which the readers receive it. In its early stages, this book also went through rigorous reviewing. The notable contributions made by experts from across the globe were first molded into patterned chapters and then arranged in a sensibly sequential manner to bring out the best results.

In this book, information regarding the impacts as well as treatment of the disease of hypothyroidism has been provided. The disease hypothyroidism poses a much bigger challenge to mankind than estimated in studies and reports. It is the most prevalent thyroid disorder and many people remain affected by it without even being aware. The most common symptom of this disease is slow metabolism. This disorder's estimates in its subclinical manifestation vary from 3 to 8%, and it increases with age. It has been commonly observed that it affects women more than men with its rate as high as 10%. Hypothyroidism affects lipid metabolism, neurological disorders or other medical situations. This book encompasses researches on the evolution in diagnosis, regulation and exchange treatment, thyroid ultrasonography and radioiodine therapy for hypothyroidism. The book comprises of a lot of significant characterizations, end results of analytic researches and innovative strategies for endocrine practice.

It has been my immense pleasure to be a part of this project and to contribute my years of learning in such a meaningful form. I would like to take this opportunity to thank all the people who have been associated with the completion of this book at any step.

Editor

Part 1

Hypothyroidism in Conjuction with Other Diseases

1

Hypothyroidism and Obstructive Sleep Apnea

Suhaila E. Al-Jawder[1,2] and Ahmed S. BaHammam[1]
[1]*University Sleep Disorders Center, King Saud University, Riyadh,*
[2]*Department of Medicine, Salmaniya Medical Complex, Manama*
[1]*Saudi Arabia*
[2]*Kingdom of Bahrain*

1. Introduction

Hypothyroidism is relatively a common disease worldwide. Overall prevalence in adults in the United States is 4.6%. (Golden et al., 2009) It can present as mild/subclinical form or overt hypothyroidism with a prevalence of 4.3% and 0.3% of adult populations, respectively. (Golden et al., 2009) Thyroid hormone deficiency has been linked to increased risk of cardiovascular morbidities and mortalities. (McQuade et al., 2011, Resta et al., 2004) Respiratory system like other body systems and organs is affected by hypothyroidism. The spectrum of diseases involvement can range from mild dyspnea to more severe and life-threatening respiratory failure. Several pathophysiological mechanisms are responsible for the compromise in the respiratory system including reduction in central respiratory drive, respiratory muscle weakness and sleep-related breathing disorders (SBD). (Duranti et al., 1993, Saaresranta and Polo, 2002, Curnock et al., 1999) Hypothyroidism is characterized by mucopolysaccharides accumulation in the dermis, hypopharynx, tongue and other tissues. (Skatrud et al., 1981, Orr et al., 1981) In its most severe form (myxedema), patients typically present with hypothermia, hypercapnia, hypotension and bradycardia. Both hypothyroidism and obstructive sleep apnea (OSA) share common signs and symptoms. Increased fatigue and sleepiness, decreased cognitive function, decreased libido, obesity and depressed mood are common findings in both disorders. (Grunstein et al., 1993, Misiolek M and 2007, Chan et al., 2010) Periorbital edema and pedal edema are other common findings in patients with either disorder. Nevertheless, snoring which is a hallmark of OSA is also reported in hypothyroid cases. (Misiolek M and 2007, Georgalas, 2011) The overlap between the two disorders may create a problem for the treating physician in differentiating both disorders and may result in a misdiagnosis or under-recognition of one of the disorders. Therefore, it is essential to consider both diseases in high risk patients and initiate the proper therapeutic plan accordingly. This chapter discusses how hypothyroidism interferes with respiratory physiology and then discusses the relationship between hypothyroidism and sleep disordered breathing.

2. Obstructive Sleep Apnea (OSA)

OSA is a disease characterized by repeated partial (hypopnea) or complete (apnea) collapse of the upper airway while asleep accompanied by surges in the sympathetic activity, cortical arousals and episodes of hypoxia. (Chan et al., 2010) Patients usually present with complaints of excessive daytime sleepiness, un-refreshing sleep, fatigue or insomnia. Patients might have nocturnal awakenings with breathe holding, gasping, or choking. (Park et al., 2011, Madani and Madani, 2009) Very frequently, the bed partner report breathing interruptions, loud snoring or both during patient's sleep. The main risk factors for OSA are obesity, older age, family history, increasing neck circumference and male gender. (BaHammam et al., 2008, Tsara et al., 2010) Menopause is the main risk factor for women even after adjustment for age and body mass index (BMI). (Ancoli-Israel et al., 1989, Block et al., 1980) Other predisposing factors include craniofacial features, maxillomandibular malformation or adenotonsillar enlargements. (Johns et al., 1998, Moser and Rajagopal, 1987, Orr and Martin, 1981) The prevalence of OSA syndrome (AHI> 5/hour and excessive daytime sleepiness) is estimated to be 2% to 4% of adults. (Young et al., 2002, Punjabi, 2008) Epidemiologic data suggest that roughly 1 of every 5 adults has at least mild OSA and 1 of every 15 adults has at least moderate OSA. (Young et al., 2002) The National Sleep Foundation survey found that 26% of the population has a high probability of OSA. (Hiestand et al., 2006) It is always essential to identify and treat persons with OSA because of its strong association with several medical conditions, occupational and social consequences. Untreated OSA can result in increased risk of cardiovascular morbidities such as myocardial infarction, congestive heart failure, stroke, refractory hypertension, and cardiac arrhythmia. (Guilleminault et al., 1983, Logan and Bradley, 2010, Somers et al., 2008, Ehrmann et al., 2011) Furthermore, cognitive dysfunction, depression, impaired glucose tolerance, occupational and increased motor vehicle accidents are the other consequences. (Sateia, 2003, Kaplan, 1992, Horne and Reyner, 1999, Radun and Summala, 2004) Treatment with continuous positive airway pressure (CPAP) can help in restoring the airway and reversing the majority of the associated morbidities. (Jean-Louis et al., 2010, Ferini-Strambi et al., 2003)

3. Hypothyroidism and the respiratory system

Respiratory system components (respiratory center, upper airway and lower respiratory system) can be affected by deficiencies in body hormones as well as excess hormonal secretion. (Saaresranta and Polo, 2002, Saaresranta and Polo, 2003, Behan et al., 2003, Takasaki and Hayashi, 1985) Thyroid hormone is one of the major body hormones. Its deficiency has been associated with multiple cardiovascular complications, respiratory failure and coma. (McQuade et al., 2011, Takamura et al., 2010, Behnia et al., 2000, Hall and Scanlon, 1979) The involvement of the respiratory system has resulted in a spectrum of clinical disorders including SBD, pulmonary hypertension, hypoventilation and severe respiratory failure. The following section explains the mechanisms through which hypothyroidism affect the respiratory system.

Ventilatory drive

Hypothyroidism is associated with diminished ventilatory drive for both hypoxia and hypercapnia. In animal models of induced hypothyroidism, a decrease in peripheral chemoreceptor response to hypoxia and hypercapnia has been observed. (Simsek et al., 2004) In humans, approximately, one third of the hypothyroid patients have a blunted ventilatory response to hypoxia/hypercapnia. (Zwillich et al., 1975, Duranti et al., 1993, Massumi RA, 1964) Predictors of blunted ventilatory response in hypothyroidism have been identified as female gender and very high levels of thyrotropin (>90 mIU/l). (Ladenson et al., 1988) It is the severe form of hypothyroidism that is associated with diminished ventilatory control. Cases of myxedema and severe hypothyroidism (thyroid ablation) were found to have a diminished hypoxic ventilatory drive that was reversible with hormonal replacement therapy. (Zwillich et al., 1975) However, diminished hypercapnic ventilator drive was only seen in myxedema cases and was not responsive to hormonal therapy. (Zwillich et al., 1975) In a case report of a patient with hypothyroidism, central sleep apnea with blunted ventilatory response to hypoxia but normal hypercapnic ventilatory response, treatment with thyroxine therapy have resolved the central apneas and restored the hypoxic drive. The normal hypercapnic ventilatory drive has doubled with thyroxine therapy. (Millman et al., 1983) Hypoxic ventilatory drive has a rapid response to thyroxine replacement than hypercapnic ventilator drive. It might be that the central chemoreceptors require longer duration of therapy or they sustain a long-term impairment. The use of intravenous thyroxine therapy was shown to improve both hypoxic and hypercapnic ventilatory drive within one week of therapy. (Duranti et al., 1993) Severe degrees of alveolar hypoventilation and coma have also been reported in cases of severe hypothyroidism (myxedema). (Behnia et al., 2000, Orr et al., 1981, Wall, 2000, Jordan, 1995)

Hypothyroidism is reported in 3% of difficult to wean mechanically ventilated patients. (Datta and Scalise, 2004) Despite this low rate, it is a potentially treatable cause and should be considered when evaluating patients who fail to wean. Successful weaning from ventilator following correction of hypothyroidism has been reported. (Pandya et al., 1989) Difficulty in weaning can be multifactorial in hypothyroid patients due to the multiple effects exerted by the hormone deficiency on different levels of the respiratory system.

Upper respiratory tract

- **Mechanical Obstruction:** Enlargement of the thyroid gland (goiter) in the presence of hypothyroidism or euthyroid state can create a mass effect on the upper airway,(Deegan PC, 1997, De Felice et al., 2006, Eloy et al., 2007) particularly when resuming the supine position. Such mechanical obstruction becomes prominent and can be associated with severe apneas. (Teramoto et al., 1995) Progressive enlargement of the thyroid goiter can further lead to stridor and an emergency intervention might be required in such severe cases. (Deegan PC, 1997) Reports have showed improvement of OSA with thyroidectomy. (Agrama, 2011)
- **Soft Tissue Infiltration:** As a part of the generalized skin and soft tissue infiltration in hypothyroidism, the upper airway and particularly the pharynx gets narrowed. In hypothyroidism, mucopolysaccharides and proteins infiltrate the skin causing skin thickening, infiltrate the tongue causing enlargement and infiltrate the neck soft tissue resulting in variable degrees of upper airway obstruction. (Devdhar et al., 2007, Batniji RK, 2006 , Watson and Pearce, 1949) Hypothyroidism also alters the myosin heavy chain profile specifically in the main dilator muscle the genioglossus muscle, which

results in compromising the muscle function. (Petrof et al., 1992) Despite these changes in upper airway structure and function, hypothyroidism per se is not an independent risk factor for OSA if other known risk factors as male gender and obesity are not present. (Pelttari et al., 1994) Upper airway obstruction in hypothyroid patients might not be very evident initially. During stressful situations, occult hypothyroidism can result in devastating outcomes such as in post-extubation upper airway obstruction following emergency intubation or post-operatively. Cases of severe emergency obstruction in undiagnosed hypothyroidism have been reported. (Sherry and Hutchinson, 1984, Stahl N, 1988)

Lower respiratory tract

As with upper respiratory tract, the different structures of the lower respiratory tract can be affected to a variable degree with alterations in thyroid hormone levels.

- **Airways:** Very few studies have investigated airway diseases in hypothyroidism. In one study, patients with treated hypothyroidism were found to have more symptoms of breathlessness and wheeze. (Birring et al., 2003) And when evaluated by Methacholine challenge test, patients with treated hypothyroidism had more airways hyperreactivity than normal healthy individuals. Induced sputum showed higher levels of inflammatory cells, absolute neutrophil count, absolute lymphocyte count and increased levels of sputum interleukin-8 suggesting increased airway inflammation compared to control. (Birring et al., 2005)
- **The lung parenchyma**: The interstitium can also be affected in hypothyroidism; two cases of lung fibrosis have been reported in patients with severe hypothyroidism. Initiating therapy for hypothyroidism was associated with significant clinical and radiological improvement in lung fibrosis. (George et al., 2009)
- **Respiratory Muscles**: Both inspiratory and expiratory respiratory muscles are weakened in hypothyroidism in a direct linear relationship to the thyroid hormone level and it is reversible with thyroxine therapy. (Siafakas et al., 1992) Furthermore, thyroid deficient muscles have impaired free fatty acid utilization, which enhances their glycogen consumption, thereby reducing skeletal muscle endurance. (Baldwin et al., 1980) One of the major inspiratory muscles that are involved in hypothyroidism is the diaphragm. Diaphragm weakness can be very severe and associated with hypoventilation. (Martinez et al., 1989, Laroche et al., 1988)
- **Pulmonary Vasculature**: Both hyper/hypothyroidism has been associated with pulmonary arterial hypertension (PAH). (Li et al., 2007, Arroliga et al., 2000) A prevalence of 22-24% of hypothyroidism is reported in patients with PAH. (Curnock et al., 1999, Silva et al., 2009) It is thought that hypoxia/hypercapnia in hypothyroid patients is responsible for causing and worsening PAH. It is also known that both disorders are associated with autoimmune diseases, which raises the possibility of an immune pathyphysiological mechanism. (Badesch et al., 1993, Chu et al., 2002)

4. Prevalence studies of hypothyroidism in OSA

The first case reporting an apneic episode in a patient with myxedema was published in 1964. (Massumi RA, 1964) Following that, studies have investigated further the prevalence of OSA in hypothyroidism population and vice versa (Table 1). Overall, the prevalence of clinical hypothyroidism in patients diagnosed with OSA or referred to sleep centers with a clinical suspicion of OSA is not higher than the prevalence in the general population. The prevalence in patients evaluated by polysomnography for OSA is 0.7 3.4%, depending on the upper limit set for normal TSH, gender and age distribution of the studied samples. (Lin CC, 1992, Meslier et al., 1992, Winkelman JW, 1996, Kapur VK and BM, 1998, Winkelman et al., 1996) Kapur et al, reported a prevalence of 1.4% of subclinical hypothyroidism in OSA patients and this association was greater in females and those less than 50 years of age. (Kapur VK and BM, 1998) In a group of Taiwanese patients with OSA, a prevalence of 3.1% was reported despite using higher TSH level (>25 mIU/l) to define hypothyroidism. (Lin et al., 1992) The prevalence is also not significantly different in patients highly suspected to have OSA (1.5%) than those already diagnosed to have OSA by overnight sleep study (2.4%). (Skjodt et al., 1999) This is similar to Winkelman and co-workers who reported a prevalence of 1.6% in patients suspected to have OSA and 2.9% in those confirmed to have OSA. (Winkelman et al., 1996) Other studies have reported a much higher prevalence. In a study of 78 overweight and obese adult patients referred to a sleep clinic, a prevalence rate of 11.5% was reported. (Resta O, 2004) The studied population was characterized by higher BMI, older age and more females. All these three variables are known risk factors for hypothyroidism, which might have resulted in a higher rate. (Sawin CT, 1979, Bilous and Tunbridge, 1988, Fox et al., 2008) Females with OSA have been reported to have higher rates of undiagnosed and diagnosed hypothyroidism. (Winkelman et al., 1996, Alotair and Bahammam, 2008) In clinical practice, these variables are important to consider when assessing the risk of hypothyroidism in patients with suspected or diagnosed OSA. Female gender, increased BMI and older age are also well established risk factors for hypothyroidism. (Sawin CT, 1979) This might explain the higher prevalence of hypothyroidism reported in some studies. (Resta O, 2004) Nevertheless, increased age and BMI are the main risk factors for OSA. (Punjabi, 2008, Hiestand et al., 2006) Thus, the co-existence of both diseases is expected and a high index of suspension is required in high risk patients.

Some of the previous studies defined hypothyroidism as the presence of a high serum thyroid-stimulating hormone (TSH) level without commenting on thyroxine hormone level. This means that some of the patients thought to have hypothyroidism may actually have had subclinical hypothyroidism, which carries different therapeutic and prognostic implications (Miller and Husain, 2003, Winkelman et al., 1996, Pham and Shaughnessy, 2008). In a recent study, Bahammam et al. reported the prevalence of newly diagnosed clinical hypothyroidism as 0.4%, and the prevalence of newly diagnosed subclinical hypothyroidism as 11.1%. (Bahammam et al., 2011) In the non-OSA patients, the prevalence of newly diagnosed clinical hypothyroidism was reported as 1.4%, and the prevalence of newly diagnosed subclinical hypothyroidism as 4%. (Bahammam et al., 2011) The authors concluded that the prevalence of newly diagnosed clinical hypothyroidism was low; however, subclinical hypothyroidism was common among patients with OSA. In lieu of the uncertainty of the benefit achieved by treating subclinical hypothyroidism, the authors recommended not to perform routine thyroid function testing for OSA patients. (Bahammam et al., 2011)

	Number of OSA patients	Measurements used for diagnosing hypothyroidism	Mean age (year)	Mean BMI	Mean AHI	Previously diagnosed hypothyroidism	Newly diagnosed clinical hypothyroidism	Newly diagnosed subclinical hypothyroidism
Kapur et al (Kapur et al., 1998)	284	TSH and FT4	50.2			17 (5.1)	0	4 (1.41%)
†Miller et al (Miller and Husain, 2003)	75	TSH	49.8	36.2	36.4	0	7 (9.3%)	0 (FT4 not measured)
Lin et al (Lin et al., 1992)	65	TSH and FT4	49.7	--	37.9	0	2 (3.1)	0
Skjodt et al (Skjodt et al., 1999)	124	TSH and FT4	--	--	--	0	3 (2.4)	0
Winkelman et al (Winkelman et al., 1996)	103	TSH	43.9	--	20.1±29	1 (0.9)	2 (1.9)	0 (FT4 not measured)
Resta et al (Resta et al., 2004)	78	TSH and FT4	49.4	37.6	38.3	Excluded	--	9 (11.5%)
BaHammam (Bahammam et al., 2011)	271	TSH and FT4	48.7	37.7	55.2	26 (9.6%)	1 (0.4)	27 (11.1%)
AlOtair et al (Alotair and Bahammam, 2008)	191 females 193 males	--	F 53.9 M 43	F 41.8 M37.2	F 51.4 M 61.4	F 23.6% M 6.2%	--	--

† Female only

Table 1. Summary of the studies that assessed the prevalence of hypothyroidism in OSA patients.

5. Prevalence studies of OSA in hypothyroidism

Limited data are available about the prevalence of OSA in hypothyroid patients (Table 2). The incidence is estimated to range from 25-82%. Most of the obtained data are from case reports and case series and their findings are variable. In a study of 50 patients with primary hypothyroidism, 30% where found to have OSA (AHI ≥5/hour). (Jha et al., 2006) These patients had overt severe hypothyroidism as manifested by TSH levels and symptoms. For milder cases and subclinical cases, the prevalence might be less. The variability in the results is influenced by the characteristics of the studied group. Predominance of male gender can result in a higher prevalence of OSA as it is one of the main risk factors for OSA. In smaller studies, a higher prevalence has been reported. (Rajagopal et al., 1984)

	No. of Patients	OSA Citeria	No. of OSA (%)	Patients Characteristics
Jha A, et al (Jha et al., 2006)	50	AHI≥ 5/hour	15 (30%) Mild OSA 8, Moderate 1, Severe 6	Females 58%, Mean Age 34±11 years, Overweight 36%, Obese 16%
Rajagopal et al (Rajagopal et al., 1984)	11	--	9 (82%) Mean AHI (71.8/hour)	6 patients obese (AHI 99/hour) 3 non-obese (AHI 16.3/hour)
Misiolek et al (Misiolek M and 2007)	15	RDI> 10/hour	5 (33%)	11 Females, Mean Age 50.3 (30-70) years, Mean BMI 29.2 (21.3-41)kg/m2
Lin et al (Lin et al., 1992)	20	AHI≥ 5/hour	5 (25%) 3 mild OSA, 2 severe OSA	4 Females, Mean Age 49.4±7.3 years, IBW 134.6±23.2%
Hira et al (Hira HS, 1999)	20		9 (45%)	-----
Mikelson et al (Mickelson et al., 1999)	10	RDI> 10/hour	4 (40%)	----

RDI: Respiratory Disturbance Index, IBW: Ideal Body Weight

Table 2. Prevalence Studies of OSA in Hypothyroidism

6. The clinical effects of treating hypothyroidism in OSA patients

Theoretically, replacing thyroid hormone should reverse most if not all the complications associated with the state of deficiency. However, in real clinical practice, this is not absolutely correct. Changes such as respiratory muscle weakness can be reversible with thyroxine therapy. Difficult weaning in hypothyroid patients can be facilitated with thyroxine therapy too and mechanical obstruction due to thyroid goiter can be reverted with thyroidectomy. However, OSA response to thyroxine therapy is variable. In a case series of 10 hypothyroid patients with OSA, treatment with thyroxine was associated with nocturnal angina and arrhythmia in two patients. Initiation of CPAP therapy prevented angina and arrhythmia. Eight of these patients were followed after achieving euthyroid state and six of them had persistent sleep apnea requiring CPAP therapy. (Grunstein and Sullivan, 1988) Thereby, treatment of hypothyroidism in the presence of OSA can be potentially hazardous and lead to cardiovascular complications even with small doses of thyroxine as thyroxine therapy may increase metabolic rate in the presence of significant hypoxia. Combination therapy (CPAP + Thyroxine) can be helpful in such situation. In another series of nine hypothyroid patients with OSA (AHI range 17-176/hour), thyroxine therapy improved outcome. Six of them were obese and had the higher range of AHI and showed significant improvement in AHI after 3-12 months of thyroxine therapy despite no improvement in weight. (Rajagopal et al., 1984) Another series of 5 patients with OSA who received thyroxine therapy showed significant reduction in AHI after 4 months of therapy; however, snoring persisted and required longer duration of therapy to improve. (Lin et al., 1992) Snoring refers to upper airway resistance and the longer duration required to improve it is basically related to the duration needed to resolve or improve upper airway changes induced by hypothyroidism. In a larger group of patients, Resta and co-workers divided patients into 3 groups: group A: 63 patients with normal thyroid function, group B: 30 patients affected with subclinical hypothyroidism and treated with levothyroxine for at least 2 years and group C: 15 patients with TSH >4mIU/l and not treated with levothyroxine. (Resta et al., 2005) The prevalence and severity of OSA did not differ between the three groups and levothyroxine therapy did not influence OSA outcome in patients with subclinical hypothyroidism. It was also noticed that levothyroxine therapy in patients with subclinical hypothyroidism and OSA was associated with less daytime sleepiness as measured by the Epworth sleepiness scale when compared to the untreated group. (Resta et al., 2005) Untreated subclinical hypothyroidism by itself is a known cause of excessive daytime sleepiness measured both subjectively and objectively, which improved with thyroxine therapy. (Shinno et al., 2009) On the other hand, the outcome of treating primary hypothyroidism with levothyroxine in patients with OSA has resulted in a significant improvement in AHI within 7-11 months of therapy. This improvement was accompanied by significant reduction in BMI, skinfold thickness, pedal edema and other biochemical markers. (Jha et al., 2006) However, in the same study, two patients have lost follow-up and both failed to show any improvement in OSA following levothyroxine therapy. One is thought to be due to his overweight that did not reduce with therapy. (Jha et al., 2006) Failure to improve OSA by achieving euthyroid state suggests that hypothyroidism is not the only factor and other factors play a role in causing OSA. It is also thought that thyroid hormone deficiency results in long term changes in the upper airway and thus improvement in OSA lags behind achieving the euthyroid state. (Grunstein et al., 1993) Furthermore, it is the treatment of the severe forms of hypothyroidism (myxedema) that improves the concomitant OSA. (Orr et al., 1981) Based on the available evidence, thyroxine cannot be considered as the only therapeutic option for OSA in patients with hypothyroidism especially in elderlies and those with cardiovascular diseases. (Veasey et al., 2006) The degree of hypoxia accompanying apneas may worsen with initiation of thyroxine therapy. In the hypothyroid state and as a result of the low metabolic rate, oxygen consumption by several body organs is less than usual, which can help to maintain a reasonable oxygen level compared to the duration and severity of apneas. With the increment in basal metabolic rate seen with the commencement of thyroxine therapy, oxygen consumption is increased by body organs and short-duration apneas/hypopneas can result in dramatic oxygen desaturation. Therefore, CPAP therapy should not be delayed for months awaiting the results of thyroxine use. The lack of response to thyroxine suggests that either there is no casual association between hypothyroidism and OSA or those alterations in breathing mechanics and upper airways require longer duration of therapy to reverse them and that longer duration of follow up might show a beneficial effect of thyroxine therapy.

	No. of Patients	Mean Duration of Therapy	Clinical Outcome of OSA	Other Outcomes
Jha A, et al (Jha et al., 2006)	12	9 months	Significant improvement of AHI (14.3 (7.4–33.6) to 2.1 (0.8–4.6))	Significant improvement of BMI and skinfold thickness
Rajagopal et al (Rajagopal et al., 1984)	9	3-12 months	AHI decreased 71.8 ± 18.0 to 12.7 ± 6.1	No change in BMI
Misiolek et al (Misiolek M and 2007)	5	5-6 months	RDI persisted in two patients, increased in one, two patients showed insignificant reduction in RDI	BMI and loud snoring improved
Lin et al (Lin et al., 1992)	5	One year	Improved AI after 4months of therapy	Improved snoring after one year of therapy Improved hypoxic/ hypercapnic ventilator response after 4 months
Hara et al, (Hira HS, 1999)	9	3 months	6 complete recovery, partial recovery in two and no recovery in one	

Table 3. Summary of outcome studies of thyroxine therapy in OSA patients

7. Evaluating thyroid function in OSA patients

It is important when ordering a laboratory investigation for any disease to consider the prevalence of the problem, the associated complications, cost-effectiveness and the effectiveness of treating the disease. Blood tests TSH, thyroxine (T4) are not clinically indicated in patients with OSA. Hypothyroidism can be associated with severe cases of OSA +/- hypoventilation but it is not an independent risk factor. Nocturnal upper airway obstruction has been evaluated in both hypothyroid and euthyroid subjects. The incidence of upper airway obstruction is higher in hypothyroid 7.7% compared to euthyroid 1.5% but after controlling for weight, age and gender, hypothyroidism does not significantly predict upper airway obstruction. (Pelttari et al., 1994) Thus, upper airway obstruction is related to obesity and male gender and not to hypothyroidism per se. The prevalence of clinical hypothyroidism, as mentioned above, is not higher than the general population. Furthermore, there is no strong evidence to support the resolution of OSA with thyroxine therapy. However, thyroxine therapy should be initiated in hypothyroid patients to manage the other co-morbidities associated with hypothyroidism but not as a medical therapy for OSA. Thyroxine therapy can not abandon the need for CPAP therapy and should not delay its initiation. The recommended practice is to be selective when ordering TSH/T4 test to high risk population (females, morbidly obese and older age), persistent symptoms of fatigue and sleepiness despite proper CPAP therapy and in those with secondary causes for hypothyroidism (thyroid ablation, thyroidectomy, panpituitarism).

8. Conclusion

For OSA patients, the prevalence of clinical hypothyroidism is not higher than the general population. It is essential to consider the risk factors for hypothyroidism when evaluating patients for sleep apnea as well as considering OSA risk factors when evaluating hypothyroid cases. Routine blood testing for TSH and T4 should be saved for OSA patients with severe obesity, persistent sleepiness despite adequate CPAP therapy and with overt hypothyroid symptoms and signs. For hypothyroid patients with symptoms suggestive of OSA, a diagnostic sleep study is warranted and CPAP therapy should be commenced prior to thyroxine therapy especially in the elderly and patients with cardiovascular diseases. Re-evaluating OSA patients after achieving euthyroid state can be done, especially if accompanied by weight reduction. Some of OSA cases might resolve but the majority seems to persist. Long-term studies might be able to explore better the impact of thyroxine therapy and help in understanding time-course of the problem.

9. References

Agrama, M. T. 2011. Thyroidectomy for goiter relieves obstructive sleep apnea: Results of 8 cases. *Ear Nose Throat J*, 90, 315-7.

Alotair, H. & Bahammam, A. 2008. Gender differences in Saudi patients with obstructive sleep apnea. *Sleep Breath*, 12, 323-9.

Ancoli-Israel, S., Klauber, M. R., Kripke, D. F., Parker, L. & Cobarrubias, M. 1989. Sleep apnea in female patients in a nursing home. Increased risk of mortality. *Chest*, 96, 1054-8.

Arroliga, A. C., Dweik, R. A. & Rafanan, A. L. 2000. Primary pulmonary hypertension and thyroid disease. *Chest*, 118, 1224-5.

Badesch, D. B., Wynne, K. M., Bonvallet, S., Voelkel, N. F., Ridgway, C. & Groves, B. M. 1993. Hypothyroidism and primary pulmonary hypertension: an autoimmune pathogenetic link? *Ann Intern Med*, 119, 44-6.

Bahammam, A. S., Alrajeh, M. S., Al-Jahdali, H. H. & Binsaeed, A. A. 2008. Prevalence of symptoms and risk of sleep apnea in middle-aged Saudi males in primary care. *Saudi Med J*, 29, 423-6.

Bahammam, S. A., Sharif, M. M., Jammah, A. A. & Bahammam, A. S. 2011. Prevalence of thyroid disease in patients with obstructive sleep apnea. *Respir Med*, 105, 1755-1760.

Baldwin, K. M., Hooker, A. M., Herrick, R. E. & Schrader, L. F. 1980. Respiratory capacity and glycogen depletion in thyroid-deficient muscle. *J Appl Physiol,* 49, 102-6.

Batniji Rk, B. H. R., Cevera Jj, Gavin Jp, Seymour Pe, Parnes Sm 2006 Supraglottic myxedema presenting as acute upper airway obstruction. *Otolaryngol Head Neck Surg,* 134, 348-50.

Behan, M., Zabka, A. G., Thomas, C. F. & Mitchell, G. S. 2003. Sex steroid hormones and the neural control of breathing. *Respir Physiol Neurobiol,* 136, 249-63.

Behnia, M., Clay, A. S. & Farber, M. O. 2000. Management of myxedematous respiratory failure: review of ventilation and weaning principles. *Am J Med Sci,* 320, 368-73.

Bilous, R. W. & Tunbridge, W. M. 1988. The epidemiology of hypothyroidism--an update. *Baillieres Clin Endocrinol Metab,* 2, 531-40.

Birring, S. S., Morgan, A. J., Prudon, B., Mckeever, T. M., Lewis, S. A., Falconer Smith, J. F., Robinson, R. J., Britton, J. R. & Pavord, I. D. 2003. Respiratory symptoms in patients with treated hypothyroidism and inflammatory bowel disease. *Thorax,* 58, 533-6.

Birring, S. S., Patel, R. B., Parker, D., Mckenna, S., Hargadon, B., Monteiro, W. R., Falconer Smith, J. F. & Pavord, I. D. 2005. Airway function and markers of airway inflammation in patients with treated hypothyroidism. *Thorax,* 60, 249-53.

Block, A. J., Wynne, J. W. & Boysen, P. G. 1980. Sleep-disordered breathing and nocturnal oxygen desaturation in postmenopausal women. *Am J Med,* 69, 75-9.

Chan, A. S., Phillips, C. L. & Cistulli, P. A. 2010. Obstructive sleep apnoea--an update. *Intern Med J,* 40, 102-6.

Chu, J. W., Kao, P. N., Faul, J. L. & Doyle, R. L. 2002. High prevalence of autoimmune thyroid disease in pulmonary arterial hypertension. *Chest,* 122, 1668-73.

Curnock, A. L., Dweik, R. A., Higgins, B. H., Saadi, H. F. & Arroliga, A. C. 1999. High prevalence of hypothyroidism in patients with primary pulmonary hypertension. *Am J Med Sci,* 318, 289-92.

Datta, D. & Scalise, P. 2004. Hypothyroidism and failure to wean in patients receiving prolonged mechanical ventilation at a regional weaning center. *Chest,* 126, 1307-12.

De Felice, A., Fuschillo, S., Martucci, M., De Angelis, E. & Balzano, G. 2006. Euthyroid goitre and sleep apnea. *Monaldi Arch Chest Dis,* 65, 52-5.

Deegan Pc, M. V., Morgan We 1997. Goitre: a cause of obstructive sleep apnoea in euthyroid patients *Eur Respir J* 10, 500-502.

Devdhar, M., Ousman, Y. H. & Burman, K. D. 2007. Hypothyroidism. *Endocrinol Metab Clin North Am,* 36, 595-615, v.

Duranti, R., Gheri, R. G., Gorini, M., Gigliotti, F., Spinelli, A., Fanelli, A. & Scano, G. 1993. Control of breathing in patients with severe hypothyroidism. *Am J Med,* 95, 29-37.

Ehrmann, D. E., Deldin, P. J. & Pitt, B. 2011. Is sleep apnea a potential link between major depressive disorder and cardiovascular disease? *Int J Cardiol,* 147, 1-3.

Eloy, J. A., Omerhodzic, S., Som, P. M. & Genden, E. M. 2007. Goitrous Hashimoto's thyroiditis presenting as obstructive sleep apnea. *Thyroid,* 17, 691-2.

Ferini-Strambi, L., Baietto, C., Di Gioia, M. R., Castaldi, P., Castronovo, C., Zucconi, M. & Cappa, S. F. 2003. Cognitive dysfunction in patients with obstructive sleep apnea (OSA): partial reversibility after continuous positive airway pressure (CPAP). *Brain Res Bull,* 61, 87-92.

Fox, C. S., Pencina, M. J., D'agostino, R. B., Murabito, J. M., Seely, E. W., Pearce, E. N. & Vasan, R. S. 2008. Relations of thyroid function to body weight: cross-sectional and longitudinal observations in a community-based sample. *Arch Intern Med,* 168, 587-92.

Georgalas, C. 2011. The role of the nose in snoring and obstructive sleep apnoea: an update. *Eur Arch Otorhinolaryngol,* 268, 1365-73.

George, J. T., Thow, J. C., Rodger, K. A., Mannion, R. & Jayagopal, V. 2009. Reversibility of fibrotic appearance of lungs with thyroxine replacement therapy in patients with severe hypothyroidism. *Endocr Pract,* 15, 720-4.

Golden, S. H., Robinson, K. A., Saldanha, I., Anton, B. & Ladenson, P. W. 2009. Clinical review: Prevalence and incidence of endocrine and metabolic disorders in the United States: a comprehensive review. *J Clin Endocrinol Metab,* 94, 1853-78.

Grunstein, R., Wilcox, I., Yang, T. S., Gould, Y. & Hedner, J. 1993. Snoring and sleep apnoea in men: association with central obesity and hypertension. *Int J Obes Relat Metab Disord,* 17, 533-40.

Grunstein, R. R. & Sullivan, C. E. 1988. Sleep apnea and hypothyroidism: mechanisms and management. *Am J Med,* 85, 775-9.

Guilleminault, C., Connolly, S. J. & Winkle, R. A. 1983. Cardiac arrhythmia and conduction disturbances during sleep in 400 patients with sleep apnea syndrome. *Am J Cardiol,* 52, 490-4.

Hall, R. & Scanlon, M. F. 1979. Hypothyroidism: clinical features and complications. *Clin Endocrinol Metab,* 8, 29-38.

Hiestand, D. M., Britz, P., Goldman, M. & Phillips, B. 2006. Prevalence of symptoms and risk of sleep apnea in the US population: Results from the national sleep foundation sleep in America 2005 poll. *Chest,* 130, 780-6.

Hira Hs, S. L. 1999. Sleep apnea syndrome among patients with hypothyroidism. *J Assoc Physicians India,* 47, 615-618.

Horne, J. & Reyner, L. 1999. Vehicle accidents related to sleep: a review. *Occup Environ Med,* 56, 289-94.

Jean-Louis, G., Brown, C. D., Zizi, F., Ogedegbe, G., Boutin-Foster, C., Gorga, J. & Mcfarlane, S. I. 2010. Cardiovascular disease risk reduction with sleep apnea treatment. *Expert Rev Cardiovasc Ther,* 8, 995-1005.

Jha, A., Sharma, S. K., Tandon, N., Lakshmy, R., Kadhiravan, T., Handa, K. K., Gupta, R., Pandey, R. M. & Chaturvedi, P. K. 2006. Thyroxine replacement therapy reverses sleep-disordered breathing in patients with primary hypothyroidism. *Sleep Med,* 7, 55-61.

Johns, F. R., Strollo, P. J., Jr., Buckley, M. & Constantino, J. 1998. The influence of craniofacial structure on obstructive sleep apnea in young adults. *J Oral Maxillofac Surg,* 56, 596-602; discussion 602-3.

Jordan, R. M. 1995. Myxedema coma. Pathophysiology, therapy, and factors affecting prognosis. *Med Clin North Am,* 79, 185-94.

Kaplan, R. 1992. Obstructive sleep apnoea and depression--diagnostic and treatment implications. *Aust N Z J Psychiatry,* 26, 586-91.

Kapur, V. K., Koepsell, T. D., Demaine, J., Hert, R., Sandblom, R. E. & Psaty, B. M. 1998. Association of hypothyroidism and obstructive sleep apnea. *Am J Respir Crit Care Med*, 158, 1379-83.

Kapur Vk, K. T., Demaine J, Hert R, Sandblom Re, Psaty & Bm 1998 Association of hypothyroidism and obstructive sleep apnea. *Am J Respir Crit Care Med*, 158, 1379-1383.

Ladenson, P. W., Goldenheim, P. D. & Ridgway, E. C. 1988. Prediction and reversal of blunted ventilatory responsiveness in patients with hypothyroidism. *Am J Med*, 84, 877-83.

Laroche, C. M., Cairns, T., Moxham, J. & Green, M. 1988. Hypothyroidism presenting with respiratory muscle weakness. *Am Rev Respir Dis*, 138, 472-4.

Li, J. H., Safford, R. E., Aduen, J. F., Heckman, M. G., Crook, J. E. & Burger, C. D. 2007. Pulmonary hypertension and thyroid disease. *Chest*, 132, 793-7.

Lin Cc, T. K., Chen Pj 1992. The relationship between sleep apnea syndrome and hypothyroidism. *Chest*, 102, 1663-1667.

Lin, C. C., Tsan, K. W. & Chen, P. J. 1992. The relationship between sleep apnea syndrome and hypothyroidism. *Chest*, 102, 1663-7.

Logan, A. G. & Bradley, T. D. 2010. Sleep apnea and cardiovascular disease. *Curr Hypertens Rep*, 12, 182-8.

Madani, M. & Madani, F. 2009. Epidemiology, pathophysiology, and clinical features of obstructive sleep apnea. *Oral Maxillofac Surg Clin North Am*, 21, 369-75.

Martinez, F. J., Bermudez-Gomez, M. & Celli, B. R. 1989. Hypothyroidism. A reversible cause of diaphragmatic dysfunction. *Chest*, 96, 1059-63.

Massumi Ra, W. J. 1964. Severe depression of the respiratory center in myxedema. *Am J Med*, 36, 876-882.

Mcquade, C., Skugor, M., Brennan, D. M., Hoar, B., Stevenson, C. & Hoogwerf, B. J. 2011. Hypothyroidism and Moderate Subclinical Hypothyroidism Are Associated with Increased All-Cause Mortality Independent of Coronary Heart Disease Risk Factors: A PreCIS Database Study. *Thyroid*, 21, 837-43.

Meslier, N., Giraud, P., Person, C., Badatcheff, A. & Racineux, J. L. 1992. Prevalence of hypothyroidism in sleep apnoea syndrome. *Eur J Med*, 1, 437-8.

Mickelson, S. A., Lian, T. & Rosenthal, L. 1999. Thyroid testing and thyroid hormone replacement in patients with sleep disordered breathing. *Ear Nose Throat J*, 78, 768-71, 774-5.

Miller, C. M. & Husain, A. M. 2003. Should women with obstructive sleep apnea syndrome be screened for hypothyroidism? *Sleep Breath*, 7, 185-8.

Millman, R. P., Bevilacqua, J., Peterson, D. D. & Pack, A. I. 1983. Central sleep apnea in hypothyroidism. *Am Rev Respir Dis*, 127, 504-7.

Misiolek M, M. B., Namyslowski G, Scierski W, Zwirska- Korczala K, Kazmierczak-Zagorska Z, Kajdaniuk D, Misiolek H & 2007. Sleep apnea syndrome and snoring in patients with hypothyroidism with relation to overweight *J Physiol Pharmacol*, 58(Suppl 1) 77-85.

Moser, R. J., 3rd & Rajagopal, K. R. 1987. Obstructive sleep apnea in adults with tonsillar hypertrophy. *Arch Intern Med*, 147, 1265-7.

Orr, W. C., Males, J. L. & Imes, N. K. 1981. Myxedema and obstructive sleep apnea. *Am J Med,* 70, 1061-6.

Orr, W. C. & Martin, R. J. 1981. Obstructive sleep apnea associated with tonsillar hypertrophy in adults. *Arch Intern Med,* 141, 990-2.

Pandya, K., Lal, C., Scheinhorn, D., Day, I. K. & Sharma, O. P. 1989. Hypothyroidism and ventilator dependency. *Arch Intern Med,* 149, 2115-6.

Park, J. G., Ramar, K. & Olson, E. J. 2011. Updates on definition, consequences, and management of obstructive sleep apnea. *Mayo Clin Proc,* 86, 549-54; quiz 554-5.

Pelttari, L., Rauhala, E., Polo, O., Hyyppa, M. T., Kronholm, E., Viikari, J. & Kantola, I. 1994. Upper airway obstruction in hypothyroidism. *J Intern Med,* 236, 177-81.

Petrof, B. J., Kelly, A. M., Rubinstein, N. A. & Pack, A. I. 1992. Effect of hypothyroidism on myosin heavy chain expression in rat pharyngeal dilator muscles. *J Appl Physiol,* 73, 179-87.

Pham, C. B. & Shaughnessy, A. F. 2008. Should we treat subclinical hypothyroidism? *BMJ,* 337, 290-291.

Punjabi, N. M. 2008. The epidemiology of adult obstructive sleep apnea. *Proc Am Thorac Soc,* 5, 136-43.

Radun, I. & Summala, H. 2004. Sleep-related fatal vehicle accidents: characteristics of decisions made by multidisciplinary investigation teams. *Sleep,* 27, 224-7.

Rajagopal, K. R., Abbrecht, P. H., Derderian, S. S., Pickett, C., Hofeldt, F., Tellis, C. J. & Zwillich, C. W. 1984. Obstructive sleep apnea in hypothyroidism. *Ann Intern Med,* 101, 491-4.

Resta, O., Carratu, P., Carpagnano, G. E., Maniscalco, M., Di Gioia, G., Lacedonia, D., Giorgino, R. & De Pergola, G. 2005. Influence of subclinical hypothyroidism and T4 treatment on the prevalence and severity of obstructive sleep apnoea syndrome (OSAS). *J Endocrinol Invest,* 28, 893-8.

Resta, O., Pannacciulli, N., Di Gioia, G., Stefano, A., Barbaro, M. P. & De Pergola, G. 2004. High prevalence of previously unknown subclinical hypothyroidism in obese patients referred to a sleep clinic for sleep disordered breathing. *Nutr Metab Cardiovasc Dis,* 14, 248-53.

Resta O, P. N., Di Gioia G, Stefano A, Barbaro Mp, De Pergola G 2004. High prevalence of previously unknown subclinical hypothyroidism in obese patients referred to a sleep clinic for sleep disordered breathing. *Nutr Metab Cardiovasc Dis,* 14, 248-53.

Saaresranta, T. & Polo, O. 2002. Hormones and breathing. *Chest,* 122, 2165-82.

Saaresranta, T. & Polo, O. 2003. Sleep-disordered breathing and hormones. *Eur Respir J,* 22, 161-72.

Sateia, M. J. 2003. Neuropsychological impairment and quality of life in obstructive sleep apnea. *Clin Chest Med,* 24, 249-59.

Sawin Ct, C. D., Azizi F, Mannix Je, Bachaeach P 1979. The Aging Thyroid: Increased Prevalence of Elevated Serum Thyrotropin Levels in the Elderly *J Am Med Assoc,* 242, 247-50.

Sherry, K. M. & Hutchinson, I. L. 1984. Postoperative myxoedema. A report of coma and upper airway obstruction. *Anaesthesia,* 39, 1112-4.

Shinno, H., Inami, Y., Inagaki, T., Kawamukai, T., Utani, E., Nakamura, Y. & Horiguchi, J. 2009. Successful treatment with levothyroxine for idiopathic hypersomnia patients with subclinical hypothyroidism. *Gen Hosp Psychiatry,* 31, 190-3.

Siafakas, N. M., Salesiotou, V., Filaditaki, V., Tzanakis, N., Thalassinos, N. & Bouros, D. 1992. Respiratory muscle strength in hypothyroidism. *Chest,* 102, 189-94.

Silva, D. R., Gazzana, M. B., John, A. B., Siqueira, D. R., Maia, A. L. & Barreto, S. S. 2009. Pulmonary arterial hypertension and thyroid disease. *J Bras Pneumol,* 35, 179-85.

Simsek, G., Yelmen, N. K., Guner, I., Sahin, G., Oruc, T. & Karter, Y. 2004. The role of peripheral chemoreceptor activity on the respiratory responses to hypoxia and hypercapnia in anaesthetised rabbits with induced hypothyroidism. *Chin J Physiol,* 47, 153-9.

Skatrud, J., Iber, C., Ewart, R., Thomas, G., Rasmussen, H. & Schultze, B. 1981. Disordered breathing during sleep in hypothyroidism. *Am Rev Respir Dis,* 124, 325-9.

Skjodt, N. M., Atkar, R. & Easton, P. A. 1999. Screening for hypothyroidism in sleep apnea. *Am J Respir Crit Care Med,* 160, 732-5.

Somers, V. K., White, D. P., Amin, R., Abraham, W. T., Costa, F., Culebras, A., Daniels, S., Floras, J. S., Hunt, C. E., Olson, L. J., Pickering, T. G., Russell, R., Woo, M. & Young, T. 2008. Sleep apnea and cardiovascular disease: an American Heart Association/american College Of Cardiology Foundation Scientific Statement from the American Heart Association Council for High Blood Pressure Research Professional Education Committee, Council on Clinical Cardiology, Stroke Council, and Council On Cardiovascular Nursing. In collaboration with the National Heart, Lung, and Blood Institute National Center on Sleep Disorders Research (National Institutes of Health). *Circulation,* 118, 1080-111.

Stahl N, L. A. 1988. Acute upper airway obstruction due to myxoedema and upper airway abnormalities. *J Laryngol Otol,* 102, 733-4.

Takamura, N., Hayashida, N. & Maeda, T. 2010. Risk of coronary heart disease and mortality for adults with subclinical hypothyroidism. *JAMA,* 304, 2481-2; author reply 2482.

Takasaki, Y. & Hayashi, Y. 1985. [Effects of sex hormones on breathing during waking and sleep]. *Nihon Kyobu Shikkan Gakkai Zasshi,* 23, 286-95.

Teramoto, S., Nagase, T. & Fukuchi, Y. 1995. Nocturnal upper airway obstruction in hypothyroidism. *J Intern Med,* 238, 473-4.

Tsara, V., Amfilochiou, A., Papagrigorakis, J. M., Georgopoulos, D., Liolios, E., Kadiths, A., Koudoumnakis, E., Aulonitou, E., Emporiadou, M., Tsakanikos, M., Chatzis, A., Choulakis, M. & Chrousos, G. 2010. Guidelines for diagnosing and treating sleep related breathing disorders in adults and children (Part 3: obstructive sleep apnea in children, diagnosis and treatment). *Hippokratia,* 14, 57-62.

Veasey, S. C., Guilleminault, C., Strohl, K. P., Sanders, M. H., Ballard, R. D. & Magalang, U. J. 2006. Medical therapy for obstructive sleep apnea: a review by the Medical Therapy for Obstructive Sleep Apnea Task Force of the Standards of Practice Committee of the American Academy of Sleep Medicine. *Sleep,* 29, 1036-44.

Wall, C. R. 2000. Myxedema coma: diagnosis and treatment. *Am Fam Physician,* 62, 2485-90.

Watson, E. M. & Pearce, R. H. 1949. The mucopolysaccharide content of the skin in localized (pretibial) myxedema. *Am J Clin Pathol,* 19, 442-7.

Winkelman Jw, G. H., Piscatelli N, Lukas Se, Dorsey Cm, Cunningham S 1996. Are thyroid function tests necessary in patients with suspected sleep apnea? *Sleep* 19, 790-793.

Winkelman, J. W., Goldman, H., Piscatelli, N., Lukas, S. E., Dorsey, C. M. & Cunningham, S. 1996. Are thyroid function tests necessary in patients with suspected sleep apnea? *Sleep,* 19, 790-3.

Young, T., Peppard, P. E. & Gottlieb, D. J. 2002. Epidemiology of obstructive sleep apnea: a population health perspective. *Am J Respir Crit Care Med,* 165, 1217-39.

Zwillich, C. W., Pierson, D. J., Hofeldt, F. D., Lufkin, E. G. & Weil, J. V. 1975. Ventilatory control in myxedema and hypothyroidism. *N Engl J Med,* 292, 662-5.

2

Hypothyroidism on Lipid Metabolism

J. Coria Mariela*, V. Carmona Yamila*,
B. Oliveros Liliana** and S. Giménez Maria**
Instituto Multidisciplinario de Investigaciones Biológicas-CONICET, San Luis. Universidad Nacional de San Luis. Argentina

1. Introduction

The thyroid gland is important in the human body because of its ability to produce the hormones triiodothyronine (T3) and tetraiodothyronine (T4), necessaries for appropriate energy levels and an active life. It has long been known that thyroid hormones are of vital importance in maintaining the initial level of phospholipids in cell membranes and fatty acids composition of the lipids (Prasad & Kumar, 2005). T3 plays a critical role in lipid metabolism by regulating genes involved in lipogenesis and lipolysis (Zhu & Chang, 2010). The underlying mechanisms, however, have only begun to be unraveled in recent years. Hypothyroidism, characterized by low serum thyroid hormone levels, is associated with reduced metabolism, reduced lipolysis, weight gain, reduced cholesterol clearance, and elevated serum cholesterol. It is known that thyroid hormone has genomic and nongenomic effects (Davis et al., 2008). Thyroid hormones exert their effects by stimulation of thyroid hormone receptors (TRs) that have different tissue distribution and metabolic targets. Thyroid hormone receptors possess two isoforms, TRα and TRβ (Nr1a1 and Nr1a2) encoded by the TRα (*NR1A1*) and TRβ (*NR1A2*) genes, and each isoform exists as two or three subtypes, respectively (α1, α 2, β1, β2, and β3). TRα plays a key role in postnatal development, adipose tissue and cardiac metabolism, whereas TRβ regulates multiple steps in hepatic metabolism as well as thyroid hormone levels (Oetting & Yen, 2007). Nuclear mechanisms of thyroid hormone action have been extensively described but an increasing number of nongenomic effects of the hormone at the cellular level have been recognized in the past 10 years (Cheng et al. 2010). Nongenomic actions of thyroid hormone are by definition independent on nuclear receptors for the hormone and have been described at the plasma membrane, various organelles, the cytoskeleton, and in cytoplasm. The actions include alterations in the transport of solutes like Ca^{++}, Na^{+} and glucose, changes in activities of several kinases, including protein kinase C, cAMP-dependent protein kinase and mitogen-activated protein kinase. Iodothyronines also can regulate nongenomically through a protein kinase C activation of neutral lipids, phospholipids and phosphatidylinositol 4, 5-bisphosphate [PtdIns (4, 5) P2] (Axelband et al., 2011).

---

* Both authors contributed equally to this work
** Corresponding Authors

The objective of this review is to provide a current overview of the impact of hypothyroidism on lipid content, distribution and metabolism in serum, erytrocytes and different tissues of human and experimental animals. The molecular mechanisms involved in lipids regulation, with emphasis on the effect of hypothyroidism on liver, which is a fundamental organ responsible for controlling cholesterol metabolism, and on adipose tissue, where the role of thyroid hormone in regulating adipogenesis and lipolysis is complex and controversial, are discused. Finally, an overview of hipothyroidism and its correlation with lipid homeostasis in the liver and mammary gland during pregnancy and lactation is also given.

2. Hypothyroidism and circulating lipids

Thyroid dysfunctions are frequent (Benseñor et al., 2001). Abnormal serum thyrotropin (TSH) values and thyroid dysfunction are more prevalent in women than men and increase with age (Valeix et al., 2004). Hypothyroidism has been defined as those conditions which result from suboptimal circulating levels of thyroid hormones (Castieiras Lacambra et al., 1998). It affects 0.5-2.4% of the general population (Sawin et al., 1985). The term myxedema was formerly used as a synonym for hypothyroidism. It is now well kown that hypothyroidism is a graded phenomenon, including presentations with clinical manifestations (overt hypothyroidism) to asymptomatic states known as subclinical hypothyroidism (Evered & Hall, 1972). Subclinical thyroid dysfunction may be defined as an elevated TSH concentration in an asymptomatic patient with a normal serum free thyroxine concentration (Woeber, 1997). It is a common condition affecting 6-17% of the general population (Helfand, 2004). Moreover, subclinical hypothyroidism may progress to overt hypothyroidism. The rate of progression is higher with the concomitant presence of thyroperoxidase antibodies or higher levels of TSH (Vanderpump et al., 1995).

In 1952, Robertson & Kirkpatrick showed very high level of cholesterol in serum of patients with overt hypothyroidism which decreased after adequate hypothyroidism treatment. In 1972, Nikkilä & Kekki observed a moderate increase of serum triglycerides in hypothyroid patients, associated with a decrease in efficiency of triglyceride removal from plasma, which was attributed to a low lipoprotein lipase (LPL) activity. Fowler, in 1973, mentioned that serum cholesterol and triglycerides were increased in patients with "preclinical" hypothyroidism, condition equivalent to the actual subclinical hypothyroidism. Furthermore the author also suggested that the abnormal lipid pattern is the first change to occur as hypothyroidism develops and the last to disappear after treatment. It is now widely recognized that hypothyroidism is one of the most common causes of secondary dyslipidemia. The most common abnormalities of lipoprotein metabolism associated with hypothyroidism are elevated levels of total cholesterol and low-density-lipoprotein cholesterol (LDL-C), which are attributable to the effect of thyroid hormone on lipoprotein lipase activity (Lithell et al., 1981) and the expression of the LDL- receptor (Staels et al., 1990). These changes probably play an important role in atherogenesis.

2.1 Lipid profile in overt hypothyroidism

It is known that overt hypothyroidism is associated with increased fasting plasma cholesterol and triglyceride levels (Tulloch, 1974). Hypothyroid patients also usually have increased lipoprotein a, Lp(a), levels (Tzotzas et al., 2000), a low-density lipoprotein (LDL)-like particle synthesized by the liver that has been reported to promote thrombosis, inflammation, and foam cell formation (Erqou et al., 2009). Trials evaluating the effects of overt hypothyroidism on LDL subfractions have shown conflicting results. A study in newly-diagnosed hypothyroid patients (n=60) showed that hypothyroidism was associated with higher prevalence of atherogenic small and dense LDL (sdLDL) (Abbas et al., 2008). By contrast, Roscini et al. (1999) found no significant differences between overt hypothyroid patients and healthy controls regarding sdLDL levels. In addition, Pearce et al. (2008) has evaluated the effects of short-term overt hypothyroidism on LDL subfractions. Patients exhibited an increase in LDL-C that was found to be primarily due to increases in the large LDL particles, while sdLDL did not significantly change (Pearce et al., 2008). A possible explanation for these dissimilar results could be the different methodology used for the measurement of LDL subparticles. Hypothyroid patients may also exhibit elevated levels of high-density lipoprotein cholesterol (HDL-C), mainly due to increased concentration of cholesterol- and phospholipid-enriched HDL-2 particles (Pearce et al., 2008). A decreased HDL_2 catabolism and cholesteryl ester transfer protein activity has been observed. This decrease leads to a reduced transfer of cholesteryl esters from HDL to very-low-density lipoprotein (VLDL), thus increasing HDL-C levels (Dullaart et al., 1990).

Hypothyroidism correction results in a decrease of serum total cholesterol, LDL-C, apolipoprotein (apo) A1, apo B and apo E. Hypothyroidism treatment may also decrease serum triglycerides (Stockigt, 2002). The apoB/apoA-1 ratio is highly valuable for detecting atherogenic risk (Millán et al., 2009). In addition, elevated levels of LDL-C have been consistently associated with an increased risk for development of cardiovascular disease (Pekkanen et al., 1990). Recently, non-HDL-C, a measure of total cholesterol minus HDL-C, has emerged as a predictor of cardiovascular disease. After levo-thyroxine replacement, a decrease in non-HDL-C has been observed in patients with overt hypothyroidism (Ito et al., 2007). The altered serum concentrations of non-HDL-C in hypothyroidism may be related to the disturbed metabolism of LDL, remnant lipoprotein, and Apo B (Ito et al., 2007).

2.2 Lipid profile in subclinical hypothyroidism

Unlike the relationship established between overt hypothyroidism and lipid alterations, the relationship between subclinical hypothyroidism and dyslipidemia is still controversial. Despite the fact that the Colorado study of over 25.000 subjects (Caneris et al., 2000) showed a continuous graded increase in serum cholesterol over a range of serum TSH values from <0.3 to >60mU/l, there is no consensus whether mild thyroid failure has an adverse effect on plasma lipids, or whether its T4 treatment, sufficient to normalize TSH, has a beneficial effect (Stockigt, 2002).

A recent study made in 1534 Chinese subjects shows that patients with subclinical hypothyroidism (TSH > 4,8mIU/L) have higher serum triglyceride levels and lower serum HDL-C levels than euthyroid subjects (Lai et al., 2011). Similar results were found by Iqbal et al. (2006), after performing a follow-up study in subclinical hypothyroidism male patients. Subclinical hypothyroidism was also associated to a high serum total cholesterol, LDL-C and apo B levels in the female patients, and to significantly lower apo A-1 levels when males and females were analysed together. After an appropriate treatment with thyroxine, patients showed a significant reduction in the serum total cholesterol, LDL-C and apo B levels (Iqbal et al., 2006).

On the other hand, from a study of patients with Hashimoto thyroiditis it has been shown that subjects with subclinical hypothyroidism have significantly higher LDL-C and LDL-C to HDL-C ratio compared with euthyroid subjects. After treatment with small doses of levo-thyroxine there was a significant decrease of total cholesterol, non-HDL-C, LDL-C, and LDL-C to HDL-C values (Iqbal et al., 2006). Recent evidence also shows that T4 replacement therapy may improve lipid profile in the cases of subclinical hypothyroidism with Hashimoto thyroiditis. A marked total cholesterol reduction was inversely correlated with an increase in free T4 levels, but not correlated with changes in TSH levels (Tagami et al., 2010). However, properly controlled prospective studies with a larger sample size are neccesary to demonstrate whether replacement therapy alters several cardiovascular markers in patients with subclinical hypothyroidism and Hashimoto thyroiditis.

Ito et al. (2007) found that patients with subclinical hypothyroidism had serum concentrations of total cholesterol, non-HDL-C, remnant-like particle cholesterol, and apo B significantly decreased, without significant changes in the serum concentrations of LDL-C, HDL-C, triglycerides, apolipoprotein A-I, and Lp(a) after levo-thyroxine replacement. They also did not find changes in the serum levels of triglycerides, HDL-C, apo A-1, and Lp(a). On the other hand, in a randomized, double-blind, crossover study, it found that after levo-thyroxine therapy (100 μg/day), patients with subclinical hypothyroidism showed a decrease in total cholesterol, LDL-C, HDL-C, apo B, apo A-1, and apo B to apo A-1 ratio, but only total cholesterol and LDL-C decrease were significantly reduced (5,5% and 7,3% reduction respectively). The total cholesterol reduction was inversely correlated with an increase in free T4 levels, but was not correlated with changes in TSH levels. This would indicate that a significant increase in free T4, although within the normal reference range, may be a better marker for risk factors for cardiovascular disease in monitoring response to treatment in subclinical hypothyroidism than TSH level alone (Razvi et al., 2007). This last result contradicts what was observed by Asvold et al. (2007), who found that there is a linear increase in total cholesterol, LDL-C and triglyceride, and a linear decrease in HDL-C levels with increasing TSH, but this correlation was obtained with TSH values within the normal range. In opposition, a population-based study of 1350 participants did not show changes in mean levels of total cholesterol, triglycerides and LDL-C in both female and male subjects with subclinical hypothyroidism and euthyroid. Women with subclinical hypothyroidism had significantly lower HDL-C than those who were euthyroid. The differences remained significant after adjustment for age, sex, and body mass index. The HDL-C was not different between patients with subclinical hypothyroidism and euthyroid men. However, in this study it was also observed that the mean TSH levels were higher in subjects with dyslipidemia, indicating a relationship between TSH-total cholesterol, and TSH-LDL-C levels mainly in overweight women (Lu et al., 2011).

On the other hand, in a study conducted in patients with subclinical hypothyroidism, with normocholesterolemie and normotriglyceridemie, a decreased triglycerides and phospholipids transference to HDL, which was corrected with appropriate levo-thyroxine therapy, were observed. These results, evaluated using an artificial triglyceride-rich emulsion labeled with radioactive triglycerides, also showed abnormalities in plasma lipid metabolism, even when these are not detected in routine laboratory tests, in patients with subclinical hypothyroidims (Sigal et al., 2011). Moreover, contradictory results may be due to patient diversity. Mild thyroid failure may be present in two types of patients: patients with untreated mild thyroid failure and patients with a history of overt hypothyroidism, whose T4 dose are not sufficient to normalize the serum TSH level. It has been observed that the change in serum total cholesterol concentration, after an appropriate T4 treatment, is much higher in the second group of patients (Danese et al., 2000). On the other hand, the TSH influence on lipids is different in the overweight and normal weight populations, as well as in men and women. The combination of serum TSH, sex, and body mass index has important effects on serum lipid parameters (Lu et al., 2011).

Hormone thyroid influences on atherogenic serum lipoproteins are attractive metabolic actions that could hypothetically be exploited to treat obesity (Danese et al., 2000) and dyslipidemia (Aronne & Thornton-Jones, 2007). However, using supraphysiological doses of the endogenous thyroid hormones, T4 and T3, for these purposes is predictably associated with risk of thyrotoxic adverse effects in other organ systems, particularly the heart (Morkin et al., 2004) and skeleton (Biondi & Cooper, 2008). A large number of hormone thyroid analogs have been synthesized and tested in experimental animal models for their lipid-lowering activity (Johansson et al., 2005). In all case of thyromimetics therapy use, potential side-effects occur in a dose-dependent fashion; therefore dosing regimens in humans will need to be tightly controlled (Tancevski et al., 2009). Further prospective studies should be carried out to stablish that patients with subclinical hypothyroidism should receive levo-thyroxine replacement.

3. Hypothyroidism and erythrocytes

There are many results indicating that thyroid hormones stimulate erythropoiesis, and also increase erythrocyte 2, 3-diphosphoglycerate concentrations, which serve to enhance the delivery of oxygen to tissues and affect steady-state levels of circulating erythropoietin, playing a major role in abrupt adjustments of erythropoietin production. Thus, hypothyroidism has been generally associated with anemia (Fein & Rivlin, 1975; Antonijević et al., 1999; Shevtsova et al., 1994). The anemia- hypothyroidism relation has even been observed in infants with congenital hypothyroidism, in who anemia has been found to be depended on the degree of neonatal hypothyroidism (Franzese et al., 1996). This anemia may be normocytic, hypochromic-microcytic, or macrocytic, although normocytic and macrocytic anaemia are the most frequent (Fein & Rivlin, 1975; Omar et al., 2010). Macrocytosis (found in up to 55% of patients) and normocytic anemia may result from the insufficiency of the thyroid hormones themselves without nutritive deficit (Antonijević et al., 1999).

A case report of haemolytic anemia induced by hypothyroidism has been described in the literature (Nomura et al., 1991). An increased osmotic fragility is generally associated with haemolytic anemia (Schröter & Eber, 1989). In erythrocytes from streptozocin diabetic rats, an increase in red cell volume and osmotic fragility was accompanied by a defect in the ouabain-sensitive Na^+ K^+-ATPase (Kowluru et al., 1989). In hyperthyroidism it has been found that there are alterations in the number and the activity of Na^+ K^+-ATPase pump in circulating erythrocytes (Gasawara & Ishikawa, 1993). Also, under this condition, an alteration in osmotic fragility has been observed (Asl et al., 2009). In erythrocytes of hypothyroid rats, it was observed that there is an increase in osmotic fragility, demonstrated by a right shift of hemolysis curve (Dariyerli et al., 2004). However, in hypothyroid subjects these alterations have not been found (Asl et al., 2009).

On the other hand, hypothyroidism causes alterations in the lipid composition of red blood cells (Ishii & Nakao, 1968). In hypothyroid rats a 22% cholesterol and 30% phospholipid level reduction has been found, without change in fatty acid composition, in erythrocyte membranes. The simultaneous decrease in cholesterol and phospholipid levels did not alter the cholesterol/phospholipid molar ratio, thus avoiding the erythrocyte membrane abnormal function (Ruggiero et al., 1987). In a study realized in 38 patients with hypothyroidism, it was found that the level of arachidonate in erythrocyte membrane was significantly decreased both before the treatment and within the course of replacing hormonal therapy. The content of omega-3 fatty acids decreased in the course of conventional therapy (Serebriakova et al., 2008). Erythrocytes lipid changes are also found in patients with haemolytic anemia and hypothyroidism. In the red cell membrane, phosphatidylcholine and free cholesterol were increased, and the free cholesterol to phospholipid ratio was elevated. After levo-thyroxine therapy, the derangement of lipid levels was normalized with improvement of the hemolytic anemia (Nomura et al., 1991). In a hypothyroid patients group who were athyreotic as a consequence of ablation treatment for well-differentiated thyroid cancer, it was observed that the relative amounts of 18:2 omega 6 rose and those of 20:3 omega 6 fell, while the levels of all monounsaturated fatty acids increased in erythrocytes. The nature of these alterations suggests a disturbance in the delta-6 desaturase activity. The cholesterol/phospholipids ratio, polyunsaturated fatty acids content, increased intracellular Ca^{++}, protein phosphorylation, membrane protein cross-linking and membrane lipid peroxidation, among other factors, may alter the red blood cell membrane deformability (Pescarmona et al., 1983). However, in an experimental model of hypothyroidism induced in rats by methimazole addition (75 mg/100 g) to the fodder, there was no change in the erythrocyte rigidity index between control and experimental groups (Toplan et al., 2005).

Alteration in oxidative status has been observed in thyroid pathologies. Moderate hypothyroid state induced in female rabbits resulted in a significant decrease in the serum concentration of the lipid peroxidation end-product malondialdehyde. The erythrocytes of hypothyroid animals exhibited higher resistance to oxidative stress and lesser oxidative lipids damage characterized by measurement of compounds reacting with thiobarbituric acid (Brzezińska-Slebodzińska, 2003; Kowalczyk et al., 2001). Hypothyroidism induced by lithium-treatment, provoked a significant decrease in the glutathione content without change in superoxide dismutase activities, in red blood cells. This imbalance might render the erythrocytes vulnerability to oxidative stress and ultimately haemolysis (Engin et al., 2005). Alterations in the activities of catalase and glucose-6-phosphate dehydrogenase activities have been found in erythrocytes of hypothyroid patients (Sal'nikova et al., 1983; Hübner et al., 1979).

Acanthocytes are erythrocytes with several (usually 3 to 7) irregularly spaced blunted projections from the margin of the cells. These cells have increased cholesterol but normal content of phospholipids. Acanthocytes are the principal morphological abnormality in abetalipoproteinemia and in the "spur cell anemia" associated with severe alcoholic liver disease (Horton et al., 1976; Lynch, 1990). Acanthocytosis findings in cytologic blood smear suggest hypothyroidism in about 90% of cases. Other diseases related to acanthocytes are very rare, hence hypothyroidism must be excluded in all cases where acanthocytes are observed on the blood film (Antonijević et al., 1999; Betticher & Pugin, 1991). There appears to be no correlation between any of the clinical features of the hypothyroid state and the shape red cell change but patients lacking the misshapen red cells may have a less severe disturbance of serum lipids. The abnormal red cells slowly disappear by treating the hypothyroidism (Wardrop & Hutchison, 1970).

4. Hypotyroidism and liver lipids

4.1 Cholesterol

Cholesterol is an essential constituent of most biological membranes and is also a precursor of bile acids, steroid hormones, and certain vitamins. Animals rely on two mechanisms to maintain a pool of cholesterol sufficient to meet these requirements; *de novo* cholesterol synthesis from acetyl coenzyme A and absorption of cholesterol from dietary sources (Angelin, 1995). The liver is central in cholesterol metabolism, balancing hepatic cholesterol synthesis and hepatic uptake of plasma lipoproteins from the circulation against the excretion of hepatic cholesterol and bile acids in the bile. Thyroid hormone is an important regulator of cholesterol metabolism. T3 can influence the metabolism of cholesterol at several critical steps in the liver: 1- the low-density lipoprotein receptor (LDL-R), which mediates cholesterol uptake from the circulation, 2,3-hydroxy-3-methylglutaryl coenzyme A reductase, controlling cholesterol biosynthesis, and 3-cholesterol 7α-hydroxylase (CYP7A1), the rate-limiting enzyme in the synthesis of bile acids where cholesterol is used as substrate (Gullberg, 2002). To monitor the level of membrane sterols, cells employ two sterol-sensing domain (SSD)-containing proteins, sterol regulatory element-binding protein (SREBP), cleavage-activating protein (SCAP) and 2-3-hydroxy-3-methylglutaryl coenzyme A reductase that are localized within the endoplasmic reticulum. Under low sterol conditions, SCAP binds to SREBPs to escort them from the endoplasmic reticulum to the Golgi apparatus where they are processed into functional transcription factors that activate the expression of genes involved in the synthesis of cholesterol. When sterols accumulate, the 2-3-hydroxy-3-methylglutaryl coenzyme A reductase is rapidly degraded, resulting in the termination of sterol synthesis (Eberlé, 2004; Dong & Tang, 2010).

It is known that TRβ is a major mediator of T3 effects on serum cholesterol and that it is involved in the transcriptional regulation of the CYP7A1 gene. The dependence on TRβ for T3 regulation of serum cholesterol levels was supported by the fact that TRβ-selective agonist GC-1 was is as efficient as T3 in decreasing serum cholesterol in hypothyroid mice (Trost, 2000). The molecular mechanisms controlling CYP7A1 regulation by bile acids and cholesterol metabolites have been widely studied. Liver X receptor-β (LXRβ) and farnesoid X receptor are two ligand dependent transcription factors that are receptors for derivatives of cholesterol and bile acids in the control of CYP7A1 expression (Henkel, 2011). LXRβ, an oxysterol binding transcription factor, directly activates CYP7A1 transcription in response to challenge with dietary cholesterol to mice; thus LXRβ -/- mice fed cholesterol-rich diets fail to induce enzyme activity and therefore accumulate toxic levels of cholesterol in the liver (Alberti, 2001). In addition to T3, it has been recognized that growth hormone is required for normal CYP7A1 regulation in rats and mice. Experiments showed that in the absence of TRs (TRβ1-/- mice), neither cholesterol nor T3 stimulated CYP7A1 expression and activity. CYP7A1 mRNA expression and enzymatic activity remained on a high level in these mice regardless of the T3 status and irrespective of whether cholesterol was added to the diet or not. The blunted CYP7A1 stimulation in response to T3 confirms the importance of TRβ (Pramfalk et al., 2011). The absence of up-regulation in response to dietary cholesterol was at first unexpected, but is likely due to the critical dependence of normal CYP7A1 regulation on growth hormone and to the fact that TRβ1-/- mice have severely reduced growth hormone levels. TRβ also appears to be of major importance for the regulation of 2,3-hydroxy-3-methylglutaryl coenzyme A reductase transcription by T3 (Gullberg, 2000).

Reduced binding activity of hepatic LDL receptors is generally considered as a major mechanism of hyperlipidemia in hypothyroidism. There were clearly effects of T3 on LDL receptor mRNA, but they could not be distinctly ascribed to TRα1 or TRβ. Although T3 rapidly regulates the transcription of the LDL receptor gene no specific TRE (thyroid response element) has so far been described in the LDL receptor gene promoter. The suppression of CYP7A activity would lead to down-regulation of LDL receptor mRNA, however, it cannot be concluded that T3 directly regulates the LDL receptor transcription (Lopez et al., 2007).

4.2 LXR transcription factor

The liver X receptors, LXRα (NR1H3) and LXRβ (NR1H2), are ligand-activated transcription factors that belong to the nuclear hormone receptor superfamily. LXRs play a critical role in cholesterol homeostasis, bile acid metabolism and carbohydrate metabolism. The oral administration of LXR agonists to mice results in elevated hepatic fatty acid synthesis and steatosis and increased secretion of triglyceride-rich very low density lipoprotein resulting in hypertriglyceridemia. This increased hepatic lipogenesis has been largely attributed to the LXR-dependent upregulation of sterol regulatory element-binding protein 1c (SREBP-1c) expression. However, it has been reported that treating *Srebp-1c* null mice with the synthetic LXR agonist T0901317 still results in enhanced expression of many lipogenic genes, suggesting additional mechanisms by which LXR can enhance hepatic lipogenesis (Cha & Repa, 2007; Talukdar & Hillgartner, 2006).

LXR exists in two isoforms, LXRα and -β (also referred to as Nr1h3 and Nr1h2, respectively. LXRα is highly expressed in the liver, and expressed at lower levels in the adrenal glands, intestine, adipose tissue, macrophages, lung, and kidney, whereas LXRβ is ubiquitously expressed. The LXRs form heterodimers with the retinoid X receptor (RXR). The RXR/LXR heterodimers bind to LXR responsive elements (LXREs) consisting of direct repeats (DRs) of the core sequence AGGTCA separated by four nucleotides (DR-4). Although, the LXRs and TRs belong to two distinct receptor subgroups with respect to ligand-binding affinity, the two receptor systems show similarity with respect to molecular mechanisms, target genes, and physiological roles. Both TR and LXRs form heterodimers with RXR, and bind to DR-4 with identical geometry and polarity. Recently it has been shown that TRβ and LXRα interact on the mouse CYP7A1 gene promoter, suggesting the possibility of cross talk between the two receptors at the transcription level in the liver. There are structural similarity between LXRs and TRs. The mouse LXRα mRNA expression is positively regulated by TR at the transcriptional level, and a cross-talk pathway between LXRα and TRβ exists in the autoregulation of the LXRα gene. The human LXRα mRNA expression and promoter activity are also positively regulated by thyroid hormone.A cross talk between TRβ and LXRα could be a therapeutic target against dyslipidemia and atherosclerosis (Hashimoto et al., 2007). LXRα plays a pivotal role in hepatic cholesterol metabolism, whereas LXRβ has not a comparable role. LXRα is inducible by thyroid hormone, whereas LXRβ is not.

There are several possible models for explaining the molecular mechanism behind the dependence or independence on TRβ for T3 regulation of target genes. One possibility is that the promoter context determines the TR isoform that regulates expression of the target gene. This implies that TRα1 and TRβ bind certain T3 response elements with different affinities. TRα1 and TRβ, respectively, govern which TR regulates a target gene in a specific cell; this assumes that the spatial expression patterns are distinct for different TRs in the liver. This would be analogous to the metabolic zonation in the liver where different metabolic processes are spatially separated along the porto-central axis of the liver units .In fact, several of the aforementioned genes are known to be zonally expressed in the liver. The CYP7A gene is expressed in a narrow zone around the central vein. It has been reported that TRβ is expressed preferentially around the central vein in the rat (Zandieh-Doulabi et al., 2004). This has supported the idea that hepatic target gene specificity by TRs may be preferentially governed by distinct zonal expression of TRs and their respective target genes, and less by promoter selection (Gullberg et al., 2000).

4.3 Sterol regulatory element-binding proteins

Sterol regulatory element-binding proteins (SREBPs) are transcription factors that belong to the basic helix-loop-helix leucine zipper family. The mammalian genome encodes three SREBP isoforms, designated SREBP-1a, SREBP-1c, and SREBP-2. SREBP-2 is encoded by a gene on human chromosome 22q13. Both SREBP-1a and -1c are derived from a single gene on human chromosome 17p11.2 through the use of alternative transcription starts sites that produce alternate forms of exon 1, designated 1a and 1c (Tarling et al., 2004). SREBP-1a is a potent activator of all SREBP-responsive genes, including those that mediate the synthesis of cholesterol, fatty acids, and triglycerides. High-level transcriptional activation is dependent on exon 1a, which encodes a longer acidic transactivation segment than does the first exon of SREBP-1c. SREBP-1c preferentially enhances the transcription of genes required for fatty acid synthesis but not cholesterol synthesis. LXRs bind to an LXR-binding site in the SREBP-1c promoter and activate SREBP-1c transcription in the presence of LXR agonists such as oxysterol (Quack et al., 2002).

There is evidence that T3 represses mouse SREBP-1c expression at the transcriptional level. The mouse SREBP-1c promoter is negatively regulated by thyroid hormone in the Hepa1–6 cells. DNA binding of TR (RXR-TR heterodimer) is required for negative regulation of the mouse SREBP-1c gene promoter. In addition, SREBP-1c mRNA levels were increased in the hypothyroid status by about 1.5-fold compared with the control, and thyrotoxic treatment reduced the mRNA levels by about 50% compared with the control level. Thus mouse SREBP-1c gene expression in the liver is negatively regulated by thyroid hormone (Berkenstam et al., 2004).

4.4 Lipid β-oxidation in TRβ$^{PV/PV}$ mice

The PV mutation has been identified in a patient with resistance to thyroid hormone. PV exhibits potent dominant-negative activity. It is due to a C-insertion at codon 448 of the TRβ1 that leads to a mutant that has complete loss of T3 binding and transcription activity (Parrilla et al., 1991). To understand the role of TRs in lipid homeostasis *in vivo,* it has been adopted the loss-of-function approach by creating knock-in mutant mice with targeted mutation in the TRα gene (TRα1PV mouse) or TRβ gene (TRβPVmouse).

The decreased β-oxidation could also contribute to lipid accumulation in the liver of wild-type and TRβ$^{PV/PV}$ mice. The β-oxidation activity in the primary hepatocytes of TRβ$^{PV/PV}$ mice was found significantly lower (24-37%) than that of wild-type mice. Simultaneously it was observed that the expression of carnitine palmitoyl-transferase Iα (Cpt1a), a rate-controlling enzyme regulating the import of fatty acids into mitochondria, was lower (37%) in the liver of TRβ$^{PV/PV}$ mice than in wild-type mice and the expression of cytochrome P450 family 4 subfamily A polypeptide 10 (Cyp4a10) involved in microsomal ω-oxidation was significantly increased in TRβ$^{PV/PV}$ mice, 40-fold higher than wild-type. These data suggest that the reduction of β-oxidation activity and the fatty liver phenotype is mainly mediated by the decreased expression of rate-determining step regulator, Cpt1a, in TRβ$^{PV/PV}$ mice. Evidence indicates that the liver of the TRα1$^{PV/+}$ mice, is smaller than the wild-type mice with paucity in hepatic fat accumulation. Further molecular analyses have indicated that the expression and activity of PPARγ are increased in the liver of TRβ$^{PV/PV}$ mice, whereas the expression of PPAR is repressed in the liver of TRα1$^{PV/+}$ mice (Araki et al., 2009).

Differential regulation of lipogenic genes by apo-TRβ and apo-TRα1, in accord with the lipid phenotype, has also been observed in the liver of these two mutant mice.TRβ is known to be the major TR isoform in the liver, and many TR-mediated T_3 effects are believed to act via TRβ in this target tissue. Therefore, it is reasonable to expect that the mutation of the TRβ isoform would lead to observable phenotypic abnormalities. However, it has been shown that mutation of TRα1, which is a less abundant TR isoform in the liver, led to the repression of PPARγ and manifestation of abnormality in lipid metabolism in TRα1$^{PV/+}$ mice. The dominant-negative activity of TRβ is stronger in tissues where TRβ is the predominantly expressed isoform. Possibly, abnormal gene regulatory activity of the less abundantly expressed TRα1PV would be compensated by the predominantly expressed w-TRβ in the liver (Cheng, 2005). Thyroid hormone stimulates lipogenesis in the liver. Hepatic production of malonyl-CoA is the rate-limiting step in the synthesis of fatty acids and it is catalyzed by both acetyl-CoA carboxylase (ACC) 1 and 2. ACC1 is enriched in the liver and other lipogenic tissues and is regulated by TR, LXR and SREBP-1 at the transcriptional level through the ACC1 promoter II. SREBP-1 enhances ACC1 mRNA expression by forming a tetrameric complex with TR/RXR, which stabilizes SREBP-1 on its binding site. A PPARα agonist stimulates *ACC1* gene expression by enhancing the expression of SREBP-1c processing enzymes, which increases nuclear SREBP-1c activity .LXR directly stimulates *ACC1* gene expression (Grefhorst et al., 2005). In hypothyroidism all these processes are decreased. These findings indicate that apo-TRβ and apo-TRα1 have different effects on lipid metabolism and that both TR isoforms contribute to the pathogenesis of lipid metabolism changes in hypothyroidism.

4.5 Mitochondrial lipids

The hepatic mitochondrial lipid composition is altered significantly in hypothyroid rats. The total cholesterol increases, the phospholipids decrease and the cholesterol/phospholipid molar ratio increases (around 40%). Among the phospholipids, cardiolipin shows the greatest alteration (30% decreases in the hypothyroid rats). The phosphatidylethanolamine/ phosphatidylcholine ratio also decreases. Alterations were also found in the pattern of fatty acids. These changes in lipid composition may be responsible, at least in part, for the depression of the phosphate carrier activity in the liver mitochondria from hypothyroid rats (Hoch et al., 1981). In addition, hypothyroidism and thyroxin substitution affect the n-3 fatty acid composition of rat liver mitochondria. The n-6 and n-3 polyunsaturated fatty acids are affected differently by the hypothyroid state. The levels of linoleic (18:2n-6), gamma-linolenic (18:3n-6) and dihomo-gamma-linolenic acids (20:3n-6) have been found to be higher in hypothyroid rats than in controls, while the level of arachidonic acid (20:4n-6) was lower, which suggests an impairment of the elongase and desaturase activities. The n-3 polyunsaturated fatty acids, eicosapentaenoic (20:5n-3) and docosapentaenoic (22:5n-3) acids, were higher in hypothyroid rats, whereas the linolenic acid (18:3n-3) content remained constant. The level of docosahexaenoic acid 22:6n-3 was dramatically decreased in hypothyroid rats, while the levels of C22 n-6 fatty acids were unchanged. The differences were probably due to the competition between n-3 and n-6 polyunsaturated fatty acids for desaturases, elongases and acyltransferases. When hypothyroid rats were treated with thyroxin, the changes induced by hypothyroidism in the proportions of n-6 fatty acids were rapidly reversed, while the changes in the n-3 fatty acids were only partially reversed. After 21 days of thyroxin treatments, the 22:6n-3 content in liver mitochondria was only half as high in hypothyroid rats than in euthyroid rats. These results suggest that the conversion of 18:2n-6 to 20:4n-6 is suppressed in the hypothyroid state which favors the transformation of 18:3n-3 to 20:5n-3 (Raederstorff, 1991). The content of individual fatty acid component in mitochondria of livers from thyroidectomized and streptozotocin -induced diabetic rats has been measured to investigate how different hormones are interrelated to control the amount of a particular fatty acid in mitochondria. The results showed diabetes, in general, affected fatty acid contents more severely than hypothyroidism, regardless of the direction of the changes. Hypothyroidism and diabetes affected antagonistically the contents of C16 species and C18:1, which belong to a de novo synthesis (oleate series). However, the two pathological conditions affected synergistically those of higher unsaturated species, eg. C18:2, C20:3 and C20:4, which belong to a dietary-dependent synthesis (linoleate series). These findings strongly indicated that each desaturation site and elongation site is affected in a preferential order by either thyroid hormone or insulin, and that hypothyroidism and diabetes have their effects differently on the process of *de novo* synthesis and the pathways initiated from an essential fatty acid in mitochondria (Nishida et al., 1991).

The phospholipid composition and the in vitro incorporation of radioactive cytidine diphosphate-choline into phosphatidylcholine were studied in mitochondria and microsomal fraction obtained from liver and brain of 20 day old hyperthyroid or hypothyroid rats. The chemical composition of the subcellular membranes isolated from brain differed markedly in both conditions. In hyperthyroidism the microsomal fraction was slightly affected while the mitochondria were also affected, but not as severely as in hypothyroidism, in which the microsomal fraction showed no alterations. The incorporation of the radioactive precursor into brain mitochondria isolated from hyperthyroid rats was markedly decreased, while no changes were observed in microsomes. However, incorporation into brain microsomal fraction obtained from hypothyroid rats was increased, while no changes were observed in mitochondria. Similar results were obtained in the studies performed with liver subcellular membranes from hyperthyroid animals while no changes were found in those from hypothyroid rats. Thus, it seems possible that both experimental conditions affect in a different way the structure and function of brain mitochondria and microsomal fractions. These findings also give further support to authors' hypothesis that mitochondria have a certain degree of autonomy for the synthesis of phosphatidylcholine (Faryna de Raveglia et al., 1982).

5. Hypothyroidism and adipose tissue

Recent evidence shows that during the adipogenesis of 3T3-L1 cells, TRα1 mRNA is constitutively expressed in preadipocytes. Its expression continues to increase during adipogenesis, concurrent with the appearance of lipid droplets. In contrast, very little, if any, TRβ1 mRNA is detectable in either preadipocytes or adipocytes. These findings suggest a critical role of TRα1 during adipogenesis of 3T3-L1 cells (Zhu et al., 2011). It is known that that thyroid hormone could also act via nongenomic action through a plasma membrane receptor. The plasma membrane receptor is located on integrin αvβ3 at the arginine-glycine-aspartic acid (RGD) recognition site important to binding by the integrin of extracellular matrix proteins. Interestingly, snake venom-derived RGD-containing disintegrin was found to inhibit adipogenesis of primary cultured fibroblastic preadipocytes (Lin et al., 2005). These cell-based studies further expanded the complexity of understanding the regulation of adipogenesis by thyroid hormone.

5.1 Peroxisome Proliferator-Activated Receptors (PPARs)

Thyroid hormone receptors regulate adipogenesis via crosstalk signaling with PPARs. Both PPARs and TRs are ligand dependent transcription receptors of the subfamily 1 (NR1) in the nuclear receptor superfamily. The NR1 group also includes retinoic acid receptors (RARs), Rev-erb, RAR-related orphan receptors (RORs), LXRs, vitamin D3 receptors (VDRs), and the nuclear xenobiotic receptor (constitutive androstane receptor (CAR). PPARs and TRs share a conserved DNA-binding domain (DBD) and exert their activity partly by heterodimerization with a common partner, the RXR, to regulate the transcription of target genes (Liu & Brent, 2010; Hunter et al., 1996).

TRs play important roles, as do PPARs, in lipid mobilization, lipid degradation, FA oxidation, and glucose metabolism. By direct or indirect effect, thyroid status influences the expression of a number of genes involved in lipid and glucose metabolism. For example, TR isoform-specific regulation of hepatic genes involved in lipogenesis and fatty acid-oxidation has been implicated by the cDNA array analysis of TRβ knockout mice treated with or without thyroid hormone (Flores-Morales et al., 2002). Among more than 200 hepatic genes responding to T3 treatment, ~60% of them are regulated by TRβ and the remaining 40% are regulated through TRα. PPARα is one of the T3-regulated genes (Flores-Morales et al., 2002).

PPARs have been shown to affect the thyroid hormone functions in thermogenesis in vivo. Administration of the PPARγ agonist rosiglitazone to male rats shifts the energy usage to an anabolic state and markedly reduces plasma thyroid hormones. Rosiglitazone also decreases mRNA levels of the TRα1and TRβ in brown adipose tissue, and the TRα1 and TRα2 in retroperitoneal white adipose tissue (WAT). These findings explain the functions of PPARγ in up-regulating thermogenesis-related genes in WAT and brown adipose tissue, while balancing the whole body thermogenesis by down-regulating the transcription activity of TRs in these processes (Festuccia et al., 2008). PPARδ exerts an inhibitory effect on T3-induced transcription activation by TRβ on the TRE-CAT reporter gene even in the presence of overexpressed RXRα protein in cells. PPARδ could inhibit the transcriptional activity of TR action by competing for the heterodimerized partner RXR in the nucleus (Meier-Heusler et al., 1995).

5.2 Leptin

Leptin, a recently discovered protein produced in adipocytes, regulates body weight by suppressing food intake and/or increasing energy expenditure. Thyroid hormones, which increase the basal metabolic rate and thermogenesis, have been reported to be one of leptin's regulating factors because alternations in thyroid status might lead to compensatory changes in circulating leptin. Plasma leptin is significantly elevated in hypothyroid subjects, to levels similar to those seen in obese euthyroid subjects. Treatment of hypothyroidism results in a reduction in the raised plasma leptin levels. The data are consistent with the hypothesis that leptin and the pituitary-thyroid axis interact in the euthyroid state, and that hypothyroidism reversibly increases leptin concentrations. Thyroid status modifies leptin secretion independently of adiposity and noradrenaline. The data suggest leptin-thyroid interactions at hypothalamic and adipocyte level (Pinkney et al., 2000).

Hypothyroidism is clearly related to body weight gain and greater adiposity, but the range of hormonal change in serum TSH concentration associated with weight gain remains a focus of debate. It has been shown that in hypothyroidism: 1) glucose uptake in muscle and adipose tissue is resistant to insulin; 2) the suppression of lipolysis by insulin is not impaired; 3) plasma levels of triglycerides are elevated due to decreased clearance by the adipose tissue; 4) a major finding to explain most of the metabolic defects is the decrease in adipose tissue blood flow rates. These findings, taken together with published data on hyperthyroidism suggest that thyroid hormone excess and deprivation do not make a consistent story: in hypothyroidism the decrease of blood flow in adipose tissue and muscle may be considered as part of the pathogenetic mechanism of insulin resistance explaining most of the metabolic defects in these tissues; in contrast, in hyperthyroidism the increase of blood flow seems to correct the intrinsic metabolic defects in muscle and adipose tissue (Dimitriadis et al., 2006). Moreover, in hypothyroidism the targets of insulin action are not uniformly impaired: glucose uptake and proteolysis are resistant to insulin, but lipolysis is not; the latter may be necessary to relieve tissues from the burden of unsatured fatty acids surplus after meals. Low normal free T4 levels were significantly associated with increased insulin resistance. These findings are consistent with an increased cardiovascular risk in subjects with low normal thyroid function (Ross et al., 2007). In female patients with primary hypothyroidism, plasma levels of leptin were found to be increased (Hsieh et al., 2002; Teixeira et al., 2009). Thyroid hormone plays a relevant role in regulating leptin metabolism independent of body mass index and body fat (Hsieh et al., 2002). These results may explain, at least in part, low blood flow rates and insulin resistance in the forearm and adipose tissue in overt hipothyroidism.

5.3 Lipoprotein lipase

LPL is a central enzyme in lipid metabolism, and adipose LPL activity is increased in rats that are deficient in thyroid hormone. LPL is synthesized and secreted by adipocytes, and is important for the transfer of triacylglycerol fatty acids from the circulating blood into adipocytes. The cellular regulation of LPL is complex. Previous studies have described the effects of numerous hormones and physiologic conditions on the level of LPL catalytic activity, and more recent studies have identified a number of different mechanisms of LPL cellular regulation (Wang & Eckel, 2009). Among the hormonal regulators of LPL is thyroid hormone. Adipose tissue levels of LPL have consistently been increased in hypothyroid rats, although plasma triglycerides have been either decreased or unchanged during hypothyroidism. Triglyceride-derived fatty acid uptake was found to be increased in WAT in association with increased LPL activity but unaffected in oxidative tissues and decreased in liver (Klieverik et al., 2009).

Studies by Saffari et al. (1992) have shown that WAT LPL is increased in hypothyroidism via a postranslational mechanism. This finding was amply confirmed by Klieverik et al. (2009) that in three WAT depots, fatty acid uptake from VLDL particles was increased in proportion to the LPL activity. The WAT fatty acid uptake in hypothyroidism is quite significant, amounting to approximately 3 nmol/mg tissue in 2 h, comparable to the combined (VLDL plus albumin) uptake by thyrotoxic muscle. The biological meaning of these observations is also intriguing. WAT only stores triglycerides so the fat is there to stay. Then, some questions have been raised ¿is the stimulation of lipoprotein lipase in WAT of hypothyroid animals a way to protect the liver from massive steatosis? Or do these depots contribute to the thermal insulation of these thermogenic deficient mice? After all, fat is an excellent thermal insulator. However, the hypothyroid rat does not obese, even after months of hypothyroidism. It is possible that as hypothyroidism extends, lipogenesis is progressively reduced and a new steady state with only moderate obesity is reached (Silva, 2010). In adipose tissue, hypothyroidism results in a decreased responsiveness of lipolysis to catecholamines even though there is no change in beta adrenergic receptor levels. This impairment in lipolytic responsiveness is reflected in decreased cellular cAMP levels due to an increase in cAMP phosphodiesterase, which degrades cAMP. In addition, some studies have suggested some impairment in adenylate cyclase activity in hypothyroid adipose tissue. Thus, the decreased responsiveness of LPL to epinephrine in cells from hypothyroid rats is consistent with previous data on adipocyte lipolysis, and suggests that a second messenger common to both hormones, such as cAMP, is important for LPL translation (Carvalho et al., 1996; Germack et al., 2000).

5.4 Adipose tissue of TR knockout mice

Studies using TR subtype knockout mice have shown that TRα1 is essential for maintaining proper thermogenesis and that TRβ is important in regulating cholesterol metabolism. These findings suggest tissue-dependent T3-mediated TR isoform action in the maintenance of metabolic homeostasis. In hypothyroidism, however, TRs function as aporeceptors. Studies of mice deficient in all TRs (TRα1$^{-/-}$ and TRβ$^{-/-}$ mice) have shown that they exhibit a milder overall phenotype than the debilitating symptoms of severe hypothyroidism, highlighting the important role of apo-TRs in the pathogenesis of hypothyroidism. Indeed, knock-in mutant mice harboring different mutations in the TRα gene exhibit abnormalities in lipid metabolism. The TRα1PV mouse that harbors a frameshift mutation in the C-terminal 16 amino acids displays a lean phenotype, partly due to the reduction in white fat mass. The TRα1R384C knock-in mutant mouse also exhibits a lean phenotype with reduction in fat mass. The TRα1P398H knock-in mutant mouse, interestingly, has increased body fat accumulation and elevated serum levels of leptin, glucose, and insulin. These results indicate that apo-TRα1 severely perturbs lipid metabolism and energy balance but in a mutation-site-dependent manner (Liu et al., 2003).

The creation of knock-in mutant mice with an identical mutation in the TRβ (TRβPV mouse) or TRα gene (TRα1PV mouse) at the same corresponding C terminus of receptors allowed to clarify whether apo-TRβ with the same mutation as the TRα1 mutant could lead to a similar or a distinct impairment in lipid metabolism. The TRβPV mouse faithfully reproduces human RTH with dysregulation of the pituitary-thyroid axis, whereas the TRα1PV mouse has normal thyroid-pituitary functions (Kaneshige et al., 2000). Although both the homozygous (TRβ$^{PV/PV}$) and heterozygous (TRβ$^{PV/+}$) mice are viable with no severe fertility defects, homozygous TRα1$^{PV/PV}$ mice die shortly after birth, and heterozygous TRα1$^{PV/+}$ mice are dwarfs with reduced fertility (Kaneshige et al., 2001). Recently, it has been found that the reduction in the WAT contributes to the dwarfism of TRα1$^{PV/+}$ mice and that apo-TRα1 (TRα1PV) acts to repress adipogenesis of WAT by inhibition of the expression and by repression of the transcriptional activity of PPARγ. It has been found that in contrast to TRα1$^{PV/+}$ mice, no abnormality in the WAT of TRβPV mice was detected. The transcription activity of PPAR γ was repressed by TRα1PV. The dual repression effects of TRα1PV reduce the expression of several PPARγ downstream target genes involved in adipogenesis, resulting in reduced fat mass. In addition to these *in vivo* findings, it has been shown that the overexpression of TRα1PV blocked the T3-dependent adipogenesis of 3T3-L1 cells (Ying et al., 2007).

Obesity and disorders of lipid metabolism are major health issues. The findings that the apo-TR isoforms act differentially in a target-tissue-dependent manner, could help direct the design and development of T3 analogs to treat these disorders. One could envision that if fatty liver were detected in patients with hypothyroidism, it would be more beneficial to treat them with a TRβ-specific analog such as GC-1 without a major undesirable effect in other organs such as the heart. As additional advances are made in better understanding the actions of TR isoforms in lipid metabolism, novel T3 analogs for improved treatment strategies would certainly be forthcoming. The finding that TRα1PV was more effective than TRβ1PV in blocking adipogenesis suggests that TRα1 could be considered as a potential therapeutic target for decreasing adipose tissue and reducing serum fatty acids. Moreover, 3T3-L1 cells stably expressing *TRa1PV* or *TRβ1PV* could be used as model cell lines to further elucidate the role of T3 via TR in adipogenesis (Baxter & Webb, 2009).

5.5 Fatty acid-beta oxidation

The role of thyroid hormone in regulating lipolysis is also complex and controversial. It has been shown that in the fed state adipocytes from hypothyroid rats had markedly reduced sensitivity to catecholamine-induced lipolysis, whereas there was no change in catecholamine-induced lipolysis in adipocytes from hyperthyroid rats (Ben Cheikh et al., 1994). Thyroid hormones play a major role in regulating oxygen metabolism. Thyroid hormones increase both coupled and uncoupled respiration, and thyroid dysfunction impacts resting energy expenditure (REE). The underlying mechanisms are not clear, but uncoupling proteins (UCP) that produce heat instead of ATP may be involved. A positive correlation between thyroid hormones and UCP2 mRNA expression has been shown by Barbe et al. (2009). In addition, increased UCP2 mRNA expression has been demonstrated in fat biopsies from hyperthyroid patients (Hoffstedt et al., 2000). UCP2 levels in adipose tissue have been found to be significantly lower in patients in the hypothyroid state compared with the euthyroid state. The levels increased during treatment and became similar to those of healthy controls. The precise function of UCP2 in adipose tissue is not settled, but several theories exist. UCP2 may be involved in fatty acid metabolism, and UCP2 expression has been shown to be regulated by free fatty acids. UCP2 has also been suggested to be involved in the production of reactive oxygen species. Finally, UCP2 has been suggested to function as a genuine uncoupling protein, involved in lipid metabolism, since a positive association between basal free fatty acids and UCP2 expression has been demonstrated (Davis et al., 2008). The gene expression of other mitochondrial proteins participating in lipid oxidation, namely ACC and carnitine palmitoiltransferase-1, has not shown any significant changes in patients before and after treatment nor in healthy controls (Gjedde et al., 2010). These findings support the notion of UCP2 as a specific target for T3- mediated gene regulation in human adipose tissue.

6. Hypothyroidism and lipid during pregnancy and lactation

Pregnancy is a state of significant dynamic changes in metabolism, with accumulation of lipids and nutrients during about the first half; whereas during late pregnancy and lactation, these accumulated reserves are used for fetal growth and subsequently for milk synthesis (Hapon et al., 2003). The regulation and coordination of lipid metabolism on pregnancy and lactation are very important because of the sudden and profound physiological changes occuring during these physiological states (Hapon et al., 2003, 2005). It is known that undiagnosed hypothyroidism during pregnancy will lead to irreparable central nervous system defects in the newborn because the development of the child *in utero* is critically affected by the mother's thyroid status (Gartner, 2009). The prevalence of subclinical hypothyroidism in women of childbearing ages is 4-5% (Glinoer, 1997). Furthermore, at least in two population-based surveys carried out in areas with different iodine intake, suggest a 2.5% overall prevalence of compensated or uncompensated hypothyroidism during pregnancy (Parrot et al., 1960), making it a significant risk for gestational outcome.

6.1 Liver and mammary lipids in pregnancy

During the last decade there has been an increasing appreciation for the incidence of thyroid dysfunction during pregnancy as well as the resultant adverse maternal and fetal effects (Okosieme & Lazarus, 2010; Lazarous, 2011). Pregnancy is accompanied by profound alterations in thyroidal economy, resulting from a complex combination of factors that are specific to the pregnant state: the rise in T4-binding globulin concentrations as a result of estrogenic stimulation, the effects of chorionic gonadotropin on the maternal thyroid, alterations in the requirement for iodine, modifications in autoimmune regulation, and the role of the placenta in deiodination of iodothyronines (Glinoer, 1997, 2004). In rats, hypothyroidism has been associated with delayed paturition, subnormal number of fetuses, increased pup mortality, decreased pup growth, altered circulating hormones (Parrot et al., 1960, Hapon et al., 2003) and also, altered functioning of the mammary gland during lactation (Hapon et al., 2003). A clinical state of hypothyroidism during late pregnancy may limit the capacity of the maternal organism to sustain itself and the fetus adequately and to prepare the mammary tissue for the subsequent lactation, thus compromising delivery and nutrition of the newborn (Hapon et al., 2003). A linear correlation between maternal and fetal plasma triglycerides has been described to have an important implication in newborn weight (Herrera, 2002). It contributes to provide circulating triglycerides in the form of lipoprotein to the mammary gland for milk lipid synthesis (Ramos & Herrera, 1996).

Fatty acid synthesis is an important metabolic pathway that is controlled by nutrients and hormones. Thyroid hormones are involved in the regulation of hepatic lipogenesis by altering levels of fatty acid synthase and acetyl-CoA carboxylase mRNAs, and their activities (Radenne et al., 2008; Kim et al., 2005). It is known that pregnancy stimulates fatty acid synthase and glycerol-3-phosphate acyltransferase expressions in the rat liver, while a state of clinical hypothyroidism during pregnancy shows decreased hepatic triglyceride synthesis in terms of ^{14}C[glucose] incorporation and subsequently, decreases in triglycerides and enhanced cholesterol in the circulation (Bonet & Herrera, 1991; Lopez Luna & Morales, 1985). A decrease in the liver lipid synthesis has been also evidenced by the diminished incorporation of $^{3}H[H_2O]$ into triglycerides and by the expression and activity of fatty acid synthase and acetyl-CoA carboxylase in pregnant hypothyroid rats, which may be responsible for the decrease in circulating triglycerides (Hapon et al., 2005). Congenitally hypothyroid mice show alterations in apoB RNA editing that switch hepatic production from apoB-100 to apoB-48 isoform (Mukhopadhyay et al., 2003), and whose conformational competence directs the assembly of hepatic VLDL more effectively.

The liver also plays a central role in the maintenance of whole body cholesterol homeostasis by integrating the regulation of a group of hepatic enzymes, receptors, and other proteins that are important for cholesterol, lipoprotein, and biliary metabolism (Smith et al., 1998). Changes in thyroid state indirectly modify the biosynthesis of cholesterol by its effects on metabolism and on the coefficient of intestinal absorption of cholesterol (Mathe & Chevallier, 1976). The mRNA levels of 3-hydroxy-3-methylglutaryl-coenzyme A reductase, which is the rate-limiting enzyme for de novo cholesterol biosynthesis, is increased in the liver during late gestation, but the change of 3-hydroxy-3-methylglutaryl-coenzyme A reductase is not modified by hypothyroidism (Hapon et al., 2005). The mRNA levels of 7α-hydroxylase are not modified by pregnancy or by hypothyroidism. In addition, the LDL receptor mRNA, a factor involved in cholesterol uptake that is increased during late gestation, is decreased in the pregnant hypothyroid rats, contributing to the increased circulating (LDL+VLDL)-C (Hapon et al., 2005). It is well known that hypothyroidism increases cholesterol through an enhancement of LDL.

Degradation of lipids is affected by altered thyroid state. Regulation of fatty acid oxidation is mainly through key rate limiting enzymes such as carnitine palmitoyltransferase 1α and acyl-CoA oxidase. Carnitine palmitoyltransferase 1α catalyzes the transport of long chain fatty acids from cytosol into mitochondria for β-oxidation and acyl-CoA oxidase catalyzes the first rate limiting reaction in peroxisome oxidation. Thyroid hormones modulate carnitine palmitoyltransferase 1α and acyl-CoA oxidase gene transcription (Liu & Brent, 2010). It has been observed that hypothyroid rats on the 21th day of pregnancy decreased liver acyl-CoA oxidase mRNA levels but did not modify mitochondrial (carnitine palmitoyltransferase 1α) fatty acid β-oxidation. Because carnitine palmitoyltransferase 1 is regulated by the availability of malonyl-CoA, the diminished ACC activity may result in a decrease in malonyl CoA that may compensate for the effects of the hypothyroid state, resulting in no overall change in expression (Hapon et al., 2005). This is in accord with what is has was observed in vitro by Muller et al. (1981).

Experimental evidence indicates that pregnancy does not alter mammary lipogenesis, but that PTU treatment has a negative effect in the pregnant mammary gland. Glycerol-3-phosphate acyltransferase mRNA abundance, and that of LPL, is not modified by either gestation or PTU treatment (Hapon et al., 2005). Late pregnancy increases mammary acyl-CoA oxidase mRNA levels, suggesting a stimulation of fatty acid oxidation, while hypothyroidism produces a diminution of acyl-CoA oxidase. In addition, it has been found in pregnant rats that hypothyroidism increases triglycerides and total lipid content and decreases phospholipids, without modifying cholesterol in mammary gland. These findings have been associated to a lower proportion of mammary lobuloalveolar epithelial tissue in the hypothyroid pregnant rats (Hapon et al., 2005). Those effects may be a consequence of the hypothyroid state per se and not direct consequences of the increase of circulating prolactin (Hapon et al., 2003), since in mammary tissue, the increased prolactin should have stimulated lipid synthesis.

6.2 Lipids during lactation

Lactation is characterized by low levels of plasma thyroid hormone, triglyceride and VLDL, and elevated levels of plasma cholesterol (Denis et al., 2003; Smith et al., 1998). Triglyceride-rich particles are rapidly cleared from the circulation during the lactating phase, likely by conversion to IDL/LDL-size particles through the action of LPL in the mammary gland to supply lipids for milk production (Smith et al., 1998). Experiments in rats indicate that hypothyroidism in mothers produces a diminution in hepatic lipid synthesis due to a decrease in $^{3}H[H_2O]$ incorporation to triglycerides, and a decrease of ACC expression and activity (Hapon et al., 2007). In addition, PTU-induced hypothyroid during lactation reduces mammary ACC activity (on days 15 and 20 of lactation) and ACC and LPL mRNA on day 20. It is well known that ACC and milk synthesis are induced during lactogenesis (Martyn & Falconer, 1983). These findings suggest less secretion of triglycerides-rich particles into circulation during mid to late lactation, compromising the fulfillment of lactational triglyceride requirements (Hapon et al., 2007). Also, a drastic diminution in milk quality has been found in PTU-induced hypothyroid during lactation. A decrease in triglycerides in mid and late lactation along with a decrease of milk lactose on mid lactation, may contribute significantly to the severe growth deficit previously observed in the litters born from hypothyroid mothers (Hapon et al., 2003). Thyroid hormones also modulate the expression of various mammary proteins involved in cellular proliferation (de Launoit & Kiss, 1989; González-Sancho et al.,

1999). Administration of a moderate oral dose of T3 to lactating rats and mice dams induces a higher growth rate in the pups; this positive effect seems to be mainly due to augmented secretion of milk that, in addition, contains an elevated proportion of triglycerides (Quevedo-Corona et al., 2000; Capuco et al., 1999). The impaired growth of the litters of hypothyroid mothers can be largely attributed to the low milk quality along with the impaired milk ejection. In accordance with a reduced capacity to eject milk, the PTU-treated mothers show significantly lower circulating oxytocin concentrations after suckling compared with control mothers (Hapon et al., 2003). Because mammary gland physiology is similar across species, biological concepts developed for lactating rat model may be instructive for human lactation (Hapon et al., 2007). It can be concluded that a state of clinical or subclinical hypothyroidism may well be aggravated by the pregnant state, and that the adequate function of the mammary glands may be compromised. In particular, the availability of triglycerides to the fetus and to the mammary gland that is preparing for lactation is affected (Hapon et al., 2003). This, along with the decrease in the proportion of epithelial mammary tissue and in lipid synthesis, at the time when the initiation of milk synthesis is about to proceed, may contribute to the future lactation deficit of hypothyroid mothers.

7. Conclusion

The experimental and epidemiological evidences presented in this review indicate that hypothyroidism severely disturbs the lipid homeostasis in liver and adipose tissue contributing to the alteration of circulating lipids. Lipid metabolism of liver and mammary gland are also markedly altered during pregnancy and lactation by hypothyroidism. Therefore monitoring thyroid status and adjusting the T4 dose during pregnancy is very important due to changes in T4 metabolism throughout pregnancy. Thus both maternal and neonatal alterations can easily be prevented. Further understanding of the molecular mechanisms behind the dependence or independence on thyroid receptors for T3 regulation of target genes involved in the lipid homeostasis will entail therapeutic potentials not only for the prevention and treatment of thyroid disorders but also for prevalent diseases in the world, such as obesity and cardiovascular disease.

8. References

Abbas, J.M.; Chakraborty, J.; Akanji, A.O. & Dói, S.A. (2008). Hypothyroidism results in small dense LDL independent of IRS traits and hypertriglyceridemia. *Endocrine Journal*, Vol.55, No.2, (May, 2008), pp. 381–389, ISSN: 0918-8959

Angelin, B. (1995). Studies on the regulation of hepatic cholesterol metabolism in humans. *The European Journal of Clinical Investigation,* Vol .25, No.4, (April, 1995), pp. 215-224, ISSN: 0014-2972

Antonijević, N.; Nesović, M.; Trbojević, B. & Milosević, R. (1999). Anemia in hypothyroidism. *Medicinski Pregled,* Vol.52, No.3-5, (March-May, 1999), pp. 136-140, ISSN: 0025-8105

Alberti, S.; Schuster, G.; Parini, P.; Feltkamp, D.; Diczfalusy, U.; Rudling, M.; Angelin, B.; Björkhem , I.; Pettersson, S. & Gustafsson, J.A. (2001). Hepatic cholesterol metabolism and resistance to dietary cholesterol in LXRbeta-deficient mice. *The*

Journal of Clinical Investigation, Vol.107, No.5, (March, 2001), pp. 565-573, ISSN: 0021-9738

Araki, O.; Ying, H.; Zhu, X.G.; Willingham, M.C. & Cheng ,S.Y. (2009). Distinct dysregulation of lipid metabolism by unliganded thyroid hormone receptor isoforms. *Molecular Endocrinology,* Vol.23, No.3, (March, 2009), pp. 308-315, ISSN: 0888-8809

Aronne, L.J. & Thornton-Jones, Z.D. (2007). New targets for obesity pharmacotherapy. *Clinical Pharmacology Therapy,* Vol.81, No.5, (May, 2007), pp. 748-752, ISSN: 0009-9236

Asl, S.Z.; Brojeni, N.K.; Ghasemi, A.; Faraji, F.; Hedayati, M. & Azizi, F. (2009). Alterations in osmotic fragility of the red blood cells in hypo- and hyperthyroid patients. *Journal Endocrinology Investigation,* Vol.32, No.1, (January, 2009), pp. 28-32, ISSN: 0391-4097

Asvold, B.; Vatten, L.J.; Nilsen, T.I. & Bjoro, T. (2007). The association between TSH within the reference range and serum lipid concentrations in a population-based study. The HUNT Study. *The European Journal of Endocrinology,* Vol.156, No.2, (February, 2007), pp. 181-186, ISSN: 0804-4643

Axelband, F.; Dias, J.; Ferrão, F.M. & Einicker-Lamas, M. (2011). Nongenomic signaling pathways triggered by thyroid hormones and their metabolite 3-iodothyronamine on the cardiovascular system. *Journal of Cellular Physiology,* Vol. 226, No.1, (January, 2011), pp. 21-28, ISSN: 0021-9541

Barbe, P.; Larrouy D.; Boulanger, C.; Chevillotte, E.; Viguerie, N.; Thalamas, C.; Trastoy, M.O.; Roques, M.; Vidal, H. & Lnagin, D. (2001). Triiodothyronine- mediated up-regulation of UCP2 and UCP3 mRNA expression in human skeletal muscle without coordinated induction of mitochondrial respiratory chain genes. *FASEB Journal,* Vol.15, No.1, (January 2001), pp. 13-15, ISSN: 0892-6638

Baxter, J.D. & Webb, P. (2009). Thyroid hormone mimetics: potential applications in atherosclerosis, obesity and type 2 diabetes. *Nature Reviews Drug Discovy,* Vol.8, No.4, (April, 2009), pp. 308-320, ISSN: 1474-1776

Ben Cheikh, R.; Chomard, P.; Dumas, P. & Autissier, N. (1994). Influence of prolonged fasting on thyroid hormone modulation of lipolysis in isolated epididymal adipocytes of Wistar rats. *European Journal Endocrinoly,* Vol.131, No.5, (Nov, 1994), pp. 516-521, ISSN: 0804-4643

Benseñor, I.M.; Goulart, A.C.; Lotufo, P.A.; Menezes, P.R. & Scazufca, M. (2011). Prevalence of thyroid disorders among older people: results from the São Paulo Ageing & Health Study. *Cad Saude Publica,* Vol.27, No.1, (January, 2011), pp. 155-161, ISSN: 0102-311X

Berkenstam, A.; Farnegardh, M. & Gustafsson, J.A. (2004). Convergence of lipid homeostasis through liver X and thyroid hormone receptors. *Mechanism Aging Development,* Vol.125, No.10-11, (October-November, 2004), pp. 707-717, ISSN: 0047-6374

Betticher, D.C. & Pugin, P. (1991). Hypothyroidism and acanthocytes: diagnostic significance of blood smear. *Schweiz Medical Wochenschr,* Vol.121, No.31-32, (August, 1991), pp. 1127-1132, ISSN: 0036-7672

Biondi, B. & Cooper, D.S. (2008). The clinical significance of subclinical thyroid dysfunction. *Endocronology Reviews,* Vol.29, No.1, (February, 2008), pp. 76-131, ISSN: 0163-769X

Brzezińska-Slebodzińska, E. (2003). Influence of hypothyroidism on lipid peroxidation, erythrocyte resistance and antioxidant plasma properties in rabbits. *Acta Veterinary Hungaric,* Vol.51, No.3, (July, 2003), pp. 343-351, ISSN: 0236-6290

Bonet, B. & Herrera, E. (1991). Maternal hypothyroidism during the first half of gestation compromises normal catabolic adaptations of late gestation in the rat. *Endocrinology,* Vol.129, No.1, (July, 1991), pp. 210-216, ISSN: 0013-7227

Canaris, G.J.; Manowitz, N.R.; Maayor, G. & Riggway, C. (2000). The Colorado thyroid disease prevalence study. *Archives of Internal Medicine,* Vol.160, No.4, (February, 2000), pp. 526-534, ISSN: 0003-9926

Capuco, A.V.; Kahl, S.; Jack, L.J.; Bishop, J.O. & Wallace, H. (1999). Prolactin and growth hormone stimulation of lactation in mice requires thyroid hormones. *Proceedings of the Society for Experimental Biology and Meodicine,* Vol.221, No.4, (September, 1999), pp. 345-351, ISSN: 0037-9737

Carvalho, S.D.; Bianco, A.C. & Silva, J.E. (1996). Effects of hypothyroidism on brown adipose tissue adenylyl cyclase activity. *Endocrinology,* Vol.137, No.12, (December, 1996), pp. 5519-5529, ISSN: 0013-7227

Castieiras Lacambra, M.J.; Fuentes Arderiu, X. & Queraltó Compañó, J.M. Bioquímica Clínica y patología molecular Volumen 2, Ed Reverte, España. ISBN: 8429118551

Cha, J.Y; Repa, J.J. (2007). The liver X receptor (LXR) and hepatic lipogenesis. The carbohydrate-response element-binding protein is a target gene of LXR. *Journal Biologycal Chemistry,* Vol. 282, No.1, (January, 2007), pp. 743-751, ISSN: 1067-8816

Cheng, S.Y. (2005).Thyroid hormone receptor mutations and disease: beyond thyroid hormone resistance. *Trends Endocrinology Metabolism,* Vol.16, No 4, (May-June, 2005), pp. 176-182, ISSN: 1043-2760

Cheng, S.Y.; Leonard, J.L. & Davis, P.J. (2010). Molecular aspects of thyroid hormone actions. *Endocrine Reviews,* Vol.31, No.2, (April, 2010), pp. 139-170, ISSN: 0163-769X

Danese, M.D.; Ladenson, P.W.; Meinert, C.L. & Powe, N.R. (2000). Effect of Thyroxine Therapy on Serum Lipoproteins in Patients with Mild Thyroid Failure: A Quantitative Review of the Literature. *Jounal of Clinical Endocrinoly Metabolism,* Vol.85, No.9, (September, 2000), pp. 2993-3001 ISNN: 0021-972X

Dariyerli, N.; Toplan, S.; Akyolcu, M.C.; Hatemi, H. & Yigit, G. (2004). Erythrocyte osmotic fragility and oxidative stress in experimental hypothyroidism. *Endocrine,* Vol.25, No.1, (October, 2004), pp. 1-5 ISSN: 1355-008X

Davis, L.M.; Rho, J.M. & Sullivan, P.G. (2008). UCP-mediated free fatty acid uncoupling of isolated cortical mitochondria from fasted animals: correlations to dietary modulations. *Epilepsia,* Vol.1, No.8, (November, 2008), pp. 117-119, ISSN: 0013-9580

de Launoit, Y. & Kiss, R. (1989). Influence of L-thyroxine, L-triiodothyronine, thyroid stimulating hormone, or estradiol on the cell kinetics of cultured mammary cancer cells. *In Vitro Cell Developmental Biology,* Vol.25, No.7, (July, 1989), pp. 585-591, ISSN: 0883-8364

Denis, R.G.; Williams, G. & Vernon, R.G. (2003). Regulation of serum leptin and its role in the hyperphagia of lactation in the rat. *Journal of Endocrinology,* Vol.176, No.2, (February, 2003), pp. 193–203, ISSN: 0022-0795

Dimitriadis, G.; Mitrou, P.; Lambadiari, V.; Boutati, E.; Maratou, E.; Koukkou, E.; Tzanela, M.; Thalassinos, N. & Raptis, S.A. 2006. Glucose and lipid fluxes in the adipose tissue after meal ingestion in hyperthyroidism. *The Journal of Clinical Endocrinology and Metabolism,* Vol. 91, No.12, (December, 2006), pp. 1112–1118, ISSN: 0021-972X

Dimitriadis, G.; Mitrou, P.; Lambadiari, V.; Boutati, E.; Maratou, E.; Koukkou, E.; Tzanela, M.; Thalassinos, N. & Raptis, S.A. 2006. Insulin action in adipose tissue and muscle in hypothyroidism. *The Journal of Clinical Endocrinology and Metabolism,* Vol. 91, No.12, (December, 2006), pp. 4930-4937, ISSN: 0021-972X

Dong, X.Y. & Tang, S.Q. (2010). Insulin-induced gene: a new regulator in lipid metabolism.*Peptides* Vol.31, No.11, (November, 2004), pp. 2145-50, ISSN: 0196-9781

Dullaart, R.P.; Hoogenberg, K.; Groener, J.E.; Dikkeschei, L.D.; Erkelens, D.W. & Doorenbos, H. (1990). The activity of cholesteryl ester transfer protein is decreased in hypothyroidism: a possible contribution to alterations in high-density lipoproteins. *European Journal Clinical Investigation,* Vol.20, No.6 (December, 1990), pp. 581-587, ISSN: 0014-2972

Eberlé, D.; Hegarty, B.; Bossard, P.; Ferré, P. & Foufelle, F. (2004). SREBP transcription factors: master regulators of lipid homeostasis. *Biochimie.* Vol.86, No 11, (November, 2004), pp. 839-48.ISSN: 0300-9084

Engin, A.; Altan, N. & Isik, E. (2005). Erythrocyte glutathione levels in lithium-induced hypothyroidism. *Drugs in R& D,* Vol.6, No.1, (2005), pp. 35-40. ISSN: 1174-5886

Erqou, S.; Kaptoge, S.; Perry, P.L.; Di Angelantonio, E.; Thompson, A.; White I.R., Marcovina S.M., Collins R., Thompson S.G. & Danesh J. (2009). Lipoprotein(a) concentration and the risk of coronary heart disease, stroke, and nonvascular mortality. *JAMA,* Vol.302, No.4, (July, 2009), pp. 412-423, ISSN: 0098-7484

Evered, D. & Hall, R. (1972). Hypothyroidism. *British Medical J,* Vol.1, (Jan 1972), pp. 290-293. ISSN: 0007-1447.

Faryna de Raveglia, I.A.; Pasquini, J.M. & Soto, E.F. (1982). Effect of thyroid dysfunction upon phospholipid composition and CDP-choline incorporation in mitochondria and microsomal fraction isolated from liver and brain of suckling rats. *Neurochemical Research,* Vol.7, No.1, (January, 1982), pp. 37-47, ISSN: 0364-3190

Fein, H.G. & Rivlin, R.S. (1975). Anemia in thyroid diseases. *The Medical Clinics of North American,* Vol.59, No.5, (September, 1975), pp. 1133-1145, ISSN: 0025-7125

Festuccia, W.T.; Oztezcan, S.; Laplante, M.; Berthiaume, M.; Michel, C.; Dohgu, S.; Denis, R.G.; Brito, M.N.; Brito, N.A.; Miller, D.S.; Banks, W.A.; Bartness, T.J.; Richard, D.& Deshaies, Y. (2008). Peroxisome proliferator-activated receptor-gamma-mediated positive energy balance in the rat is associated with reduced sympathetic drive to adipose tissues and thyroid status. *Endocrinology,* Vol.149, No.5, (May, 2008), pp. 2121-2130, ISSN: 0013-7227

Flores-Morales, A.; Gullberg, H.; Fernandez, L.; Ståhlberg N.; Lee, N.H.; Vennström, B. & Norstedt G. (2002). Patterns of liver gene expression governed by TRbeta. *Molecular endocrinology,* Vol.16, No.6, (June, 2002), pp. 1257-1268, ISSN: 0888-8809

Fowler, P.B. (1973). Treatment of hypothyroidism. *British Medical Journal,* Vol.3, (August, 1973), pp. 352-353, ISSN: 0007-1447

Franzese, A.; Salerno, M.; Argenziano, A.; Buongiovanni, C.; Limauro, R. & Tenore, A. (1996). Anemia in infants with congenital hypothyroidism diagnosed by neonatal screening. *Journal of Endocrinoly Investigation,* Vol.19, No.9, (October, 1996), pp. 613-619. ISSN: 0391-4097

Gärtner, R. (2009). Thyroid diseases in pregnancy. *Current Opinion in Obstetric Gynecology,* Vol.21, No.6, (December, 2009), pp. 501-507, ISSN: 1040-872X

Gasawara, H. & Ishikawa, M. (1993). Evaluation of Peripheral Metabolic Status by Determination of Na-K ATPase Pump Activity in Circulating Erythrocytes in Patients with Thyroid Diseases and Nonthyroidal Illnesses. *Endocrine Journal,* Vol.40, No.1, (February 1993), pp. 27-33, ISSN: 0918-8959

Germack, R.; Starzec, A. & Perret, G.Y. (2000). Regulation of β1- and β3-adrenergic agonist-stimulated lipolytic response in hyperthyroid and hypothyroid rat white adipocytes. *British Journal of Pharmacology,* Vol.129, No.3, (January, 2009), pp. 448-456, ISSN: 1476-5381

Gjedde, S.; Gormsen, L.C.; Riis, A.L.; Jørgensen, J.O.; Rungby, J.; Møller, N.; Weeke, J. & Pedersen, S.B. (2010). Reduced expression of uncoupling protein 2 in adipose tissue in patients with hypothyroidism. *Clinical Endocrinology of Metabolism,* Vol.95, No.7, (July, 2010), pp. 3537-3541, ISSN: 0021-972X

Glinoer, D. (1997). The Regulation of thyroid function in pregnancy:pathways of endocrine adaptation from physiologyto pathology. *Endocrine Reviews,* Vol.18, No.3, (June, 1997), pp. 404-433, ISSN: 0163-769X

Glinoer, D. (2004). The regulation of thyroid function during normal pregnancy: importance of the iodine nutrition status. *Best Practice & Research Clinical Endocrinology & Metabolism,* Vol.18, No.2, (June, 2004), pp. 133-152, ISSN: 1521-690X

Grefhorst, A.; van Dijk, T.H.; Hammer, A.; van der Sluijs, F.H.; Havinga, R.; Havekes, L.M.; Romijn, J.A.; Groot, P.H.; Reijngoud, D.J. & Kuipers, F. (2005). Differential effects of pharmacological liver X receptor activation on hepatic and peripheral insulin sensitivity in lean and ob/ob mice. *American Journal of Physiology, Endocrinology and Metabolism,* Vol.298, No.5, (November, 2005), pp. 829-838, ISSN: 0193-1849

González-Sancho, J.M.; Alvarez-Dolado, M.; Caelles, C. & Muñoz, A. (1999). Inhibition of tenascin-C expression in mammary epithelial cells by thyroid hormone. *Molecular Carcinogenesis,* Vol.24, No.2, (February, 1999), pp.99-107, ISSN: 0899-1987

Gullberg, H.; Rudling ,M.; Forrest ,D.; Angelin ,B.; Vennström B.(2000). Thyroid hormone receptor beta-deficient mice show complete loss of the normal cholesterol 7alpha-hydroxylase (CYP7A) response to thyroid hormone but display enhanced resistance to dietary cholesterol. *Molecular Endocrinology,* Vol.14, No.11, (November, 2000), pp. 1739-49, ISSN: 0888-8809

Gullberg, H.; Rudling, M.; Saltó, C.; Forrest, D.; Angelin, B. & Vennström, B. (2002). Requirement for thyroid hormone receptor beta in T3 regulation of cholesterol metabolism in mice. *Molecular Endocrinology,* Vol.16, No.8, (August, 2002), pp. 1767-1777, ISSN: 0888-8809

Hapon, M.B.; Simoncini, M.; Via, G. & Jahn, G.A. (2003). Effect of hypothyroidism on hormone profiles in virgin, pregnant and lactating rats, and on lactation. *Reproduction,* Vol.126, No.3, (September, 2003), pp. 371-382, ISSN: 1470-1626

Hapon, M.B.; Varas, S.M.; Jahn, G.A. & Gimenez, M.S. (2005). Effects of hypothyroidism on mammary and liver lipid metabolism in virgin and late-pregnant rats. *Journal of Lipid Research,* Vol.46, No.6, (June, 2005), pp. 1320-1330, ISSN: 0022-2275

Hapon, M.B.; Varas, S.M.; Gimenez, M.S. & Jahn, G.A. (2007). Reduction of mammary and liver lipogenesis and alteration of milk composition during lactation in rats by hypothyroidism. *Thyroid,* Vol.17, No.1, (January, 2007), pp. 11-18, ISSN: 1050-7256

Hashimoto, K.; Matsumoto, S.; Yamada, M.; Satoh, T. & Mori, M. (2007). Liver X Receptor-β Gene Expression Is Positively Regulated by Thyroid Hormone. *Endocrinology,* Vol.148, No 10, (October, 2007) pp. 4667–4675, ISSN:0013-7227

Helfand, M. (2004). Screening for subclinical thyroid dysfunction in nonpregnant adults: a summary of the evidence for the U.S. Preventive Services Task Force. *Annals of International Medicine,* Vol.140, No.2, (January, 2004), pp. 128-141, ISSN: 0003-4819

Henkel, A.S.; Anderson, K.A.; Dewey, A.M.; Kavesh, M.H.& Green RM. (2011) A chronic high-cholesterol diet paradoxically suppresses hepatic CYP7A1 expression in FVB/NJ mice. *Journal of Lipid Research,* Vol.52, No.2 (February, 2011), pp. 289-298, ISSN: 0022-2275

Herrera, E. (2002). Lipid metabolism in pregnancy and its consequences in the fetus and newborn. *Endocrine,* Vol.19, No.1, (October, 2002), pp. 43-55, ISSN: 1355-008X

Hoch, F.L.; Subramanian, C.; Dhopeshwarkar, G.A. & Mead, J.F. (1981). Thyroid control over biomembranes: VI. Lipids in liver mitochondria and microsomes of hypothyroid rats. *Lipids,* Vol.16, No.5, (May, 1981), pp. 328-335, ISSN: 0024-4201

Hoffstedt J., Folkesson R., Wahrenberg H., Wennlund A., van Harmelen V. & Arner P. (2000). A marked upregulation of uncoupling protein 2 gene expression in adipose tissue of hyperthyroid subjects. *Hormone and Metabolic Research,* Vol.32, No.11-12, (November-December 2000), pp. 475-479, ISSN: 0018-5043

Horton, L.; Coburn, R.J.; England, J.M. & Himsworth, R.L. (1976). The haematology of hypothyroidism. The *Quaterly Journal of Medicine,* Vol.45, No.177, (January, 1976), pp. 101-123. ISSN: 1460-2725

Hsieh, C.J.; Wang, P.W.; Wang, S.T.; Liu, R.T.; Tung, S.C.; Chien, W.Y.; Lu, Y.C.; Chen. J.F.; Chen, C.H. & Kuo, M.C. (2002). Serum leptin concentrations of patients with sequential thyroid function changes. *Clinical Endocrinology,* Vol.57, No.1, (July, 2002), pp. 29-34, ISSN: 0300-0664

Hübner, G.; Meng, W.; Meisel, P.; Ventz, M.; Hampel, R. & Bleyer, H. (1979). Behavior of the erythrocyte glucose-6-phosphate dehydrogenase in patients with functional thyroid disorders and in hyperthyroxinemic rats. *Zeitscrift Für die Gesamte Innere Medizin,* Vol.34, No.14, (July, 1979), pp. 386-389, ISSN: 0044-2542

Hunter, J.; Kassam, A.; Winrow, C.J.; Rachubinskib, R.A. & Capone, J.P. (1996). Crosstalk between the thyroid hormone and peroxisome proliferator-activated receptors in regulating peroxisome proliferator-responsive genes. *Molecular and Cellular Endocrinology,* Vol.116, No.2, (February, 1996), pp. 213-221, ISSN: 0303-7207

Iqbal, A; Jorde, R. & Figenschau, Y. (2006). Serum lipid levels in relation to serum thyroid-stimulating hormone and the effect of thyroxine treatment on serum lipid levels in subjects with subclinical hypothyroidism: the Tromsø Study. *Journal of International Medicine*, Vol.260, No.1, (July, 2006), pp. 53-61, ISSN: 0954-6820

Ishi,i J. & Nakao, K. (1968). Analysis of the human erythrocyte lipid in various functional conditions of the thyroid. *Tohoku Journal Experiment of Medicine,* Vol. 94, No.2, (February, 1968), pp. 169-175, ISSN: 0040-8727

Ito, M.; Arishima, T.; Kudo, T.; Nishihara, E.; Ohye, H.; Kubota, S.; Fukata, S. & Amino, N. (2007). Effect of Levo-Thyroxine Replacement on Non-High-Density Lipoprotein Cholesterol in Hypothyroid Patients. *The Journal of Clinical Endocrinology and Metabolism,* Vol.92, No.2, (February, 2007), pp. 608-611, ISSN: 0021-972X

Johansson, L.; Rudling, M.; Scanlan, T.S.; Lundåsen, T.; Webb, P.; Baxter, J.; Angelin, B. & Parini, P. (2005). Selective thyroid receptor modulation by GC-1 reduces serum lipids and stimulates steps of reverse cholesterol transport in euthyroid mice. *Proceeding of the National Academy of Sciences,* Vol.102, No.29 (July, 2005), pp. 10297-10302, ISSN: 0027-8424

Kaneshige, M.; Kaneshige, K.; Zhu, X.; Dace, A.; Garrett, L.; Carter, T.A.; Kazlauskaite, R.; Pankratz, D.G.; Wynshaw-Boris, A.; Refetoff, S.; Weintraub, B.; Willingham, M.C.; Barlow, C. & Cheng, S. (2000). Mice with a targeted mutation in the thyroid hormone beta receptor gene exhibit impaired growth and resistance to thyroid hormone. *Proceeding of the National Academia of Sciences,* Vol.97, No.24, (November, 2000), pp. 13209-13214, ISSN: 0087-8424

Kaneshige, M.; Suzuki, H.; Kaneshige, K.; Cheng, J.; Wimbrow, H.; Barlow, C.; Willigham, M.C. & Chang, S. (2001). A targeted dominant negative mutation of the thyroid hormone alpha 1 receptor causes increased mortality, infertility, and dwarfism in mice. *Proceeding of the National Academia of Sciences,* Vol.98, No.26, (December, 2001), pp. 15095-15100, ISSN: 0087-8424

Kim, Y.J.; Lee, M.S.; Lee, H.J.; Wu, Y.; Freake, H.C.; Chun, H.S. & Kim, Y. (2005). Hormones and nutrients regulate acetyl-CoA carboxylase promoter I in rat primary hepatocytes. *Journal of Nutritional Science and Vitaminolog,* Vol.51, No.2, (April, 2005), pp. 124-128, ISSN: 0301-4800

Klieveri, L.P.; Coomans, C.P.; Endert, E.; Sauerwein, H.P.; Havekes, L.M.; Voshol, P.J.; Rensen, P.C.; Romijn J.A.; Kalsbeek, A. & Fliers, E. (2009). Thyroid hormone effects on whole-body energy homeostasis and tissue-specific fatty acid uptake in vivo. *Endocrinology,* Vol.150, No.12, (December, 2009), pp. 5639-5648, ISSN: 0013-7227

Kowalczyk, E.; Urbanowicz, J.; Kopff, M.; Ciećwierz, J. & Andryskowski, G. (2011). Elements of oxidation/reduction balance in experimental hypothyroidism. *Endokrynol Poskal,* Vol.62, No.3, (2011), pp. 220-223, ISSN: 0423-104X

Kowluru, R.; Bitensky, M.W.; Kowluru, A.; Dembo, M.; Keaton, P.A. & Buican, T. (1989). Reversible sodium pump defect and swelling in the diabetic rat erythrocyte: effects on filterability and implications for microangiopathy. *Proceeding of the National Academy of Sciences,* Vol.86, No.9, (May, 1989), pp. 3327-3331, ISSN: 0027-8424

Lai, Y.; Wang, J.; Jiang, F.; Wang, B.; Chen, Y.; Li, M.; Liu, H.; Li, C.; Xue, H.; Li, N.; Yu, J.; Shi, L.; Bai, X.; Hou, X.; Zhu, L.; Lu, L.; Wang, S.; Xing, Q.; Teng, X.; Teng, W &

Shan, Z. (2011). The relationship between serum thyrotropin and components of metabolic syndrome. *Endocrine Journal,* Vol.58, No.1, (November, 2010), pp. 23-30, ISSN: 0918-8959

Lazarus, J.H. (2011). Screening for Thyroid Dysfunction in Pregnancy: Is It Worthwhile? *Journal of Thyroid Research,* (Jun 2011), ID397012, ISSN: 2042-0072

Lin, Y.T.; Tang, C.H.; Chuang, W.J.; Wang, S.M.; Huang, T.F.; Fu, W.M. (2005). Inhibition of adipogenesis by RGD-dependent disintegrin. *Biochemical Pharmacology,* Vol.70, No.10, (November, 2005), pp. 1469-1478, ISSN: 0006-2952

Lithell, H.; Boberg, J.; Hellsing, K.; Ljunghall, S.; Lundqvist, G.; Vessby, B. & Wide, L. (1981). Serum lipoprotein and apolipoprotein concentrations and tissue lipoprotein-lipase activity in overt and subclinical hypothyroidism: the effect of substitution therapy. *European Journal of Clinical Investigation,* Vol.11, No.1, (February, 1981), pp. 3-10, ISSN: 0014-2972

Liu, Y.Y.; Schultz, J.J. & Brent, GA. (2003). A thyroid hormone receptor alpha gene mutation (P398H) is associated with visceral adiposity and impaired catecholamine-stimulated lipolysis in mice. *Journal of Biological Chemistry,* Vol.278, No.40, (October, 2003), pp. 38913–38920, ISSN: 0021-9258

Liu, Y.Y. & Brent, G.A. (2010). Thyroid hormone crosstalk with nuclear receptor signaling in metabolic regulation. *Trends in Endocrinology and Metabolism,* Vol.21, No.3, (March, 2010), pp. 166-173, ISSN: 1043-2760

Lopez, D.; Abisambra Socarrás, J.F.; Bedi, M.; Ness, G.C. (2007). Activation of the hepatic LDL receptor promoter by thyroid hormone. *Biochimica Biophysica Acta,* Vol.1771, No.9, (September, 2007), pp. 1216-1225, ISSN: 0006-3002

López-Luna, P. & Morales, S. (1985). Effect of the hypothyroidism on the levels of different metabolites in pregnant rats. *Revista Española de Fisiologia,* Vol.41, No.3, (September, 1985), pp. 311-316, ISSN: 0034-9402

Lu, L.; Wang, B.; Shan, Z.; Jiang, F.; Teng, X.; Chen, Y.; Lai, Y.; Wang, J.; Xue, H.; Wang, S.; Li, C.; Liu, H.; Li, N.; Yu, J.; Shi, L.; Hou, X.; Xing, Q.; Bai, X. & Teng W. (2011). The correlation between thyrotropin and dyslipidemia in a population-based study. *Journal of Korean Medical Science,* Vol.26, No.2, (February, 2011), pp. 243-249, ISSN: 1011-8934

Lynch, E.C. (1990). Chapter 155 Peripheral Blood Smear, In: *Clinical Methods: The History, Physical, and Laboratory Examinations,* Walker HK, Hall WD, Hurst JW, editors. 3rd edition, Butterworths, Boston. ISBN-10: 0-409-90077-X

Martyn, P. & Falconer, I.R. (1985). The effect of progesterone on prolactin stimulation of fatty acid synthesis, glycerolipid synthesis and lipogenic enzyme activities in mammary glands of pseudopregnant rabbits, after explant culture or intraductal injection. *The Biochemical Journal,* Vol.231, No.2, (October, 1985), pp. 321-328, ISSN: 0264-6021

Mathe, D. & Chevallier, F. (1976). Effects of the thyroid state on cholesterol metabolism in the rat. *Biochimica Biophysica Acta,* Vol.441, No.1, (July, 1976), pp.155-164, ISSN: 0006-3002

Meier-Heusler S.C.; Zhu X.; Juge-Aubry, C.; Pernin, A.; Burger, A.G.; Cheng, S.Y. & Meier, C.A.. (1995). Modulation of thyroid hormone action by mutant thyroid hormone receptors, c-erbA alpha 2 and peroxisome proliferator-activated receptor: evidence for different mechanisms of inhibition. *Molecular and cellular endocrinology*, Vol.107, No.1, (January, 1995), pp. 55-66, ISSN: 0303-7207

Millán, J.; Pintó, X.; Muñoz, A.; Zúñiga, M.; Rubiés-Prat, J.; Pallardo, L.F.; Masana, L.; Mangas, A.; Hernández-Mijares, A., González-Santos, P.; Ascaso, J.F. & Pedro-Botet, J. (2009). Lipoprotein ratios: Physiological significance and clinical usefulness in cardiovascular prevention. *Vascular Health Risk Management*, Vol.5, (September, 2009), pp. 757-765, ISSN: 1176-6344

Morkin, E., Ladenson, P.; Goldman, S. & Adamson, C. (2004). Thyroid hormone analogs for treatment of hypercholesterolemia and heart failure: past, present and future prospects. *Journal of Molecular and Cellular Cardiology*, Vol.37, No.6, (December, 2004), pp. 1137-1146, ISSN: 0022-2828

Mukhopadhyay, D.; Plateroti, M., Anant, S.; Nassir, F.; Samarut, J. & Davidson, N.O. (2003).Thyroid hormone regulates hepatic triglyceride mobilization and apolipoprotein B messenger ribonucleic Acid editing in a murine model of congenital hypothyroidism. *Endocrinology*, Vol.144, No.2, (febrero, 2003), pp. 711-719, ISSN: 0013-7227

Müller, M.J.; Köster, H. & Seitz, H.J. (1981). Effect of thyroid state on ketogenic capacity of the isolated perfused liver of starved rats. *Biochimica Biophysica Acta*, Vol.666, No.3, (December, 1981), pp. 475-481, ISSN: 0006-3002

Nikkilä, E.A. & Kekki, M. (1972). Plasma Triglyceride Metabolism in Thyroid Disease. *Journal of Clinical Investigation*, Vol.51, No.8, (August, 1972), pp. 2103-2114, ISSN: 0021-9738

Nishida, M., Sasaki, T.; Terada, H. & Kawada, J. (1991). Synergistic and antagonistic effects on fatty acid composition in the liver mitochondria of rats by thyroidectomy and streptozotocin-administration. *Research Communication in Chemical Pathology and Pharmacology*, Vol.74, No.3, (December, 1991), pp. 317-326, ISSN: 0034-5164

Nomura, S.; Eimoto, T.; Osawa, G.; Yawata, Y. & Horino, M. (1991). Case report: hypothyroidism as a possible cause of an acquired reversible hemolytic anemia. *The American Journal of Medical Sciences*, Vol.302, No.1, (July, 1991), pp. 23-27, ISSN: 0002-9629

Oetting, A. & Yen, P.M. (2007). New insights into thyroid hormone action. *Best Practice & Research. Clinical Endocrinology and Metabetabolism*, Vol.21, No.2, (June, 2007), pp. 193-208, ISSN: 1521-690X

Okosieme, O.E. & Lazarus, J.H. (2010). Thyroid dysfunction in pregnancy: optimizing fetal and maternal outcomes. *Expert Review of Endocrinology and Metabolism*, Vol.5, No.4, (July, 2010), pp. 521–529, ISSN: 1744-6651

Omar, S.; Hadj Taeib, S.; Kanoun, F.; Hammami, M.B.; Kamoun, S.; Ben Romdhane, N.; Feki, M.; Slimane, H. & Kaabachi N. (2010). Erythrocyte abnormalities in thyroid dysfunction. La *Tunisie Médicale*, Vol.88, No.11, (November, 2010), pp. 783-788, ISSN: 0041-4131

Parrilla, R.J.; Mixson, A.J.; McPherson, J.A.; McClaskey, J.H. & Weintraub, B.D. (1991). Characterization of seven novel mutations of the c-erbA beta gene in unrelated kindreds with generalized thyroid hormone resistance. Evidence for two "hot spot" regions of the ligand binding domain. *The Journal of Clinical Investigation*, Vol.88, No.6, (December, 1991), pp. 2123-2130, ISSN: 0021-9738

Parrot, M.W.; Johnston, M.E. & Durbin, P.W. (1960). The effects of thyroid and parathyroid deficiency on reproduction in the rat. *Endocrinology*, Vol.67 (October, 1960), pp. 467-483, ISSN: 0013-7227

Pearce, E.N.; Wilson, P.W.; Yang, Q.; Vasan, R.S. & Braverman, L.E. (2008). Thyroid function and lipid subparticle sizes in patients with short-term hypothyroidism and a population-based cohort. *Journal of Clinical Endocrinology and Metabolism, Vol.93*, No.3, (March, 2008), pp. 888-894, ISSN: 0021-972X

Pekkanen, J.; Linn, S.; Heiss, G.; Suchindran, C.M.; Leon, A.; Rifkind, B.M. & Tyroler, H.A. (1990). Ten-year mortality from cardiovascular disease in relation to cholesterol level among men with and without preexisting cardiovascular disease. *The New England Journal of Medicine*, Vol.322, No.24, (June, 1990), pp. 1700-1777, ISSN: 0028-4793

Pescarmona, G.P.; Ghigo, D. & Bosia, A. (1983). The molecular basis for increased rigidity of the erythrocyte membrane. *La Ricerca in Clinical e in Laboratorio*, Vol.13, No.3, (1983), pp. 141-147, ISSN: 0390-5748

Pinkney, J.H.; Goodrick, S.J.; Katz, J.R.; Johnson, A.B.; Lightman, S.L.; Coppack, S.W.; Medbak, S. & Mohamed-Ali, V. (2000).Thyroid and sympathetic influences on plasma leptin in hypothyroidism and hyperthyroidism. *International Journal of Obesity and Related Metabolic Disorders*, Vol.24, No.2, (June, 2000), pp. 165-166, ISSN: 0307-0565

Pramfalk, C.; Pedrelli, M. & Parini P. (2011). Role of thyroid receptor β in lipid metabolism. *Biochimistry Biophysical Acta*, Vol.1812, No.8, (August, 2011), pp. 929-937, ISSN: 0006-3002

Prasad, R. & Kumar, V. (2005). Thyroid hormones increase Na+-Pi co-transport activity in intestinal brush border membrane: role of membrane lipid composition and fluidity. *Molecular and Cellular Biochemistry*, Vol. 278, No.1-2, (October, 2005), pp. 195-202, ISSN: 0.800-8177

Prast, J.M. (2009). Effect of treatment with levothyroxine in the lipid profile of the patients with subclinical hypothyroidism. *Endocrinologia y Nutrición*, Vol.56, No.1, (March, 2009), pp. 13-17, ISSN: 1575-0922

Quack, M.; Frank, C. & Carlberg, C. (2002). Differential nuclear receptor signaling from DR4-type response elements. *Journal Cell Biochemistry*, Vol.86, No.3, (July, 2002), pp. 601-612, ISSN: 0739-2312

Quevedo-Corona, L.; Franco-Colin, M.; Caudillo-Romero, M.; Pacheco-Rosado, J.; Zamudio-Hernandez, S. & Racotta, R. (2000). 3,5,3'-Triiodothyronine administered to rat dams during lactation increases milk yield and triglyceride concentration and hastens pups growth. *Life Sciences*, Vol.66, No.21, (April, 2000), pp. 2013-2021, ISSN: 0024-3205

Raederstorff, D.; Meier, C.A.; Moser, U. & Walter, P. (1991). Hypothyroidism and thyroxin substitution affect the n-3 fatty acid composition of rat liver mitochondria. *Lipids*, Vol.26, No.10, (October, 1991), pp. 781-787, ISSN: 0024-4201

Radenne, A.; Akpa, M.; Martel, C.; Sawadogo, S.; Mauvoisin, D. & Mounier, C. (2008). Hepatic regulation of fatty acid synthase by insulin and T3: evidence for T3 genomic and nongenomic actions. *American Journal of Physiology, Endocrinology and Metabolism*, Vol.295, No.4, (October, 2008), pp. 884-894, ISSN: 0193-1849

Ramos, P. & Herrera, E. (1996). Comparative responsiveness to prolonged hyperinsulinemia between adipose-tissue and mammary gland lipoprotein lipase activities in pregnant rats. *Early Pregnancy,* Vol.2, No.1, (March, 1996), pp. 29-35, ISSN: 1354-4195

Razvi, S.; Ingoe, L.; Keeka, G.; Oates, C.; McMillan, C. & Weaver, J.U. (2007). The beneficial effect of L-thyroxine on cardiovascular risk factors, endothelial function, and quality of life in subclinical hypothyroidism: randomized, crossover trial. *The Journal of Clinical Endocrinology and Metabolism,* Vol.92, No.5, (May, 2007), pp. 1715-1723, ISSN: 0021-972X

Robertson, J.D. & Kirkpatrick, H.F. (1952). Changes in basal metabolism, serumprotein-bound iodine, and cholesterol during treatment of hypothyroidism with oral thyroid and L-thyroxine sodium. *British Medical Journal*, Vol.1, No.4750, (March, 1952), pp. 624-628, ISSN: 007-1474

Roos, A.; Bakker, S.J.; Links, T.P.; Gans, R.O. & Wolffenbuttel, B.H. (2007). Thyroid function is associated with components of the metabolic syndrome in euthyroid subjects. *Clinical Endocrinology Metabolis,* Vol.92, No2, (February, 2007), pp. 491-496, ISSN: 0021-972X

Roscini, A.R.; Lupattelli, G.; Siepi, D.; Pagliaricci, S.; Pirro, M. & Mannarino, E. (1999). Low-density lipoprotein size in primary hypothyroidism. Effects of hormone replacement therapy. *Annals of Nutrition and Metabolism*, Vol.43, No.6, (September, 1999), pp. 374-379, ISSN: 0250-6807

Ruggiero, F.M.; Gnoni, G.V. & Quagliariello, E. (1987). Effect of hypothyroidism on the lipid composition of rat plasma and erythrocyte membranes. *Lipids*, Vol.22, No.3, (March, 1987), pp. 148-151, ISSN: 0024-4201

Saffari, B.;Ong,J.M. & Kern, P.A.(1992). Regulation of adipose tissue lipoprotein lipase gene expression by thyroid hormone in rats. *Journal Lipid Research,* Vol.33, No.2, (February, 1992), pp. 241–249, ISSN: 0022-2275

Sal'nikova, L.A.; Nikolaeva, L.V. & Lopatina, N.I. (1983). Methemoglobin and catalase activity in erythrocytes of children with hypothyroidism. *Voprosy Meditsinkoï Khimii*, Vol.29, No.2, (March-April, 1983), pp. 101-104, ISSN: 0042-8809

Sawin, C.T.; Bigos, S.T.; Land, S. & Bacharach P. (1985). The aging thyroid. Relationship between elevated serum thyrotropin level and thyroid antibodies in elderly patients. *The American Journal of Medicene*, Vol.79, No.5, (November, 1985), pp. 591-595, ISSN: 0002-9343

Sawin, C.T.; Castelli,W.P.; Hershman, J.M.; McNamara, P. & Bacharach, P. (1985). The aging thyroid: thyroid deficiency in the Framingham study. *Archives of Internal Medicine,* Vol.145, No.8, (August, 1985), pp. 1386-1388, ISSN: 0003-9926

Serebriakova, O.V.; Govorin, A.V.; Prosianik, V.I. & Baksheeva, E.V. (2008). Fatty acid composition of the blood serum and erythrocyte membrane lipids in patients with hypothyroidism and left ventricular diastolic dysfunction. *Klinichescaia Meditsina,*Vol.86, No.2, (2008), pp. 40-43, ISSN: 0023-2149

Schröter, W. & Eber, S.W. (1989). Molecular pathology of the erythrocyte membrane. Erythrocyte membrane defects as a cause of congenital hemolytic anemia. *Monatsschr Kinderheilkd,* Vol.137, No.7, (July, 1989), pp. 368-379, ISSN: 0026-9298

Shevtsova, N.M.; Kozlov, I. & Novitskiĭ, V.V. (1994). Mechanism of hematopoietic disorders in primary experimental hypothyroidism. *Patologichescaia Fiziologiia i Ekpserimental'naia Terapiia,* Vol.1, (January-March, 1994), pp. 14-16, ISSN: 0031-2991

Sigal, G.A.; Medeiros-Neto, G.; Vinagre, J.C.; Diament, J. & Maranhão, R.C. (2011). Lipid metabolism in subclinical hypothyroidism: plasma kinetics of triglyceride-rich lipoproteins and lipid transfers to high-density lipoprotein before and after levothyroxine treatment. *Thyroid,* Vol.21, No.4, (April, 2011), pp. 347-353, ISSN:1050-7256

Silva, J.E. (2010). Fat and energy economy in hypo- and hyperthyroidism are not the mirror image of one another. *Endocrinology,* Vol.151, No.1, (January, 2010), pp. 4-6, ISSN: 0013-7227

Smith, J.L.; Lear, S.R.; Forte, T.M.; Ko, W.; Massimi, M. & Erickson, S.K. (1998). Effect of pregnancy and lactation on lipoprotein and cholesterol metabolism in the rat. *Journal of Lipid Research,* Vol.39, No.11, (November, 1998), pp. 2237-2249, ISSN: 0022-2275

Staels, B.; Van Tol, A.; Chan, L.; Will, H.; Verhoeven, G. & Auwerx, J. (1990). Alterations in thyroid status modulate apolipoprotein, hepatic triglyceride lipase, and low density lipoprotein receptor in rats. *Endocrinology,* Vol.127, No.3, (September, 1990), pp. 1144-1152, ISSN: 0013-7227

Stockigt, J.R. (2002). Case finding and screening strategies for thyroid dysfunction. *Clinica Chimica Acta,* Vol.315, No. 1-2, (January, 2002), pp.111-124, ISSN: 0009-8981

Tagami, T.; Tamanaha, T.; Shimazu, S.; Honda, K.; Nanba, K.; Nomura, H.; Yoriko, S.U.; Usui, T.; Shimatsu A. & Naruse, M. (2010). Lipid profiles in the untreated patients with Hashimoto thyroiditis and the effects of thyroxine treatment on subclinical hypothyroidism with Hashimoto thyroiditis. *Endocrine Journal,* Vol.57, No.3, (December, 2010), pp. 253-258, ISSN: 0918-8959

Tancevski, I.; Eller, P. ; Patsch, J.R. & Ritsch, A. (2009). The resurgence of thyromimetics as lipid-modifying agents. *Current Opinion in Investigational Drugs,* Vol.10, No.9, (September, 2009), pp. 912-918, ISSN: 1472-4472

Talukdar, S. & Hillgartner, F.B. (2006).The mechanism mediating the activation of acetyl-coenzyme A carboxylase-alpha gene transcription by the liver X receptor agonist T0-901317. *Journal Research,* Vol.47, No.11, (November, 2006), pp. 2451-2461, ISSN: 0022-2275.

Tarling, E.; Salter, A. & Bennett, A. (2004).Transcriptional regulation of human SREBP-1c (sterol-regulatory-element-binding protein-1c): a key regulator of lipogenesis. *Biochemical Society Transaction,* Vol.32, No.1, (February, 2004), pp. 107-109, ISSN: 0300-5127

Teixeira, P.F.; Cabral, M.D.; Silva, N.A.; Soares, D.V.; Braulio, V.B.; Couto, A.P.; Henriques, J.L.; Costa, A.J.; Buescu, A & Vaisman, M. (2009). Serum leptin in overt and subclinical hypothyroidism: effect of levothyroxine treatment and relationship to menopausal status and body composition. *Thyroid,* Vol.19, No.5, (May, 2009), pp. 443-50, ISSN: 1050-7256

Trost, S.U.; Swanson, E.; Gloss, B.; Wang-Iverson, D.B.; Zhang, H.; Volodarsky, T.; Grover, G.J.; Baxter, J.D.; Chiellini, G.; Scanlan,T.S.; et al. (2000) .The thyroid hormone receptor-beta-selective agonist GC-1 differentially affects plasma lipids and cardiac activity. *Endocrinology.* Vol.141, No.9, (September, 2000), pp. 3057-3064, ISSN: 0013-7227

Toplan, S.; Dariyerli, N.; Ozdemir, S.; Akyolcu, M.C.; Hatemi, H. & Yigit, G. (2005). The effects of experimental hypothyroidism on hemorheology and plasma fibrinogen concentration. *Endocrine,* Vol.28, No.2, (November, 2005), pp. 153-156, ISSN: 1355-008X

Tulloch, B.R. (1974). Lipid Changes in Thyroid Disease: The Effect of Thyroxine and Analogues. *Proceeding of the Royal Society of Medice,* Vol.67, No.7, (July, 1974), pp. 670-671, ISSN: 0035-9157

Tzotzas, T.; Krassas, G.E.; Konstantinidis, T. & Bougoulia, M. (2000). Changes in lipoprotein(a) levels in overt and subclinical hypothyroidism before and during treatment. *Thyroid,* Vol.10, No.9, (September, 2000), pp. 803-808, ISSN: 1050-7256

Valeix, P.; Dos Santos, C.; Castetbon, K.; Bertrais, S.; Cousty, C. & Hercberg, S. (2004). Thyroid hormone levels and thyroid dysfunction of French adults participating in the SU.VI.MAX study.*Annales d´Endocrinologie,* Vol.65, No.6, (December, 2004), pp. 477-486, ISSN: 003-4266

Vanderpump, M.P.; Tunbridge, W.M.; French, J.M. & et al. (1995). The incidence of thyroid disorders in the community: a twenty-year follow-up of the Whickham Survey.*Clinical Endocrinology,* Vol.43, No.1, (July, 1995), pp. 55-68, ISSN: 0300-0664

van Doormaal, J.J.; Muskiet, F.A.; Jansen, G.; Wolthers, B.G.; Sluiter, W.J. & Doorenbos, H. (1986). Increase of plasma and red cell cholesterol sulfate levels in induced hypothyroidism in man. *Clinica Chimica Acta,* Vol.155, No.3, (March, 1986), pp. 195-200, ISSN: 0009-8981

Wang, H. & Eckel, R.H. (2009).Lipoprotein lipase: from gene to obesity. *American Journal Physiology Endocrinology Metabolism,* Vol.297, No.2, (August, 2009), pp. 271-288, ISSN: 0193-1849

Wardrop, C.A. & Hutchison, H.E. (1969). Red cell shape in hypothyroidism. *Lancet,* Vol.1, No.7608, (June, 1969), pp. 1243. ISSN: 0140-6736

Woeber, K.A. (1997). Subclinical thyroid dysfunction. *Archives of Internal Medicene,* Vol.157, No.10, (May, 1997), pp. 1065-1068, ISSN: 0003-9926

Ying, H.; Araki, O.; Furuya, F.; Kato, Y. & Cheng, S.Y. (2007). Impaired adipogenesis caused by a mutated thyroid hormone alpha 1 receptor. *Molecular and Cellular Biology,* Vol.27, No.6, (March, 2007), pp. 2359–2371, ISSN: 0270-7306

Zandieh-Doulabi, B.; Platvoet-ter Schiphorst, M.; Kalsbeek, A.; Wiersinga, W.M. & Bakker, O. (2004). Hyper and hypothyroidism change the expression and diurnal variation of thyroid hormone receptor isoforms in rat liver without major changes in their zonal distribution. *Molecular Cellular Endocrinology,* Vol.219, No.1-2, (April, 2004), pp. 69-75, ISSN:0300-8177.

Zhu, X. & Cheng, S.Y. (2010). New insights into regulation of lipid metabolism by thyroid hormone. Current Opinion in Endocrinology, Diabetes and Obesity, Vol.17, No.5, (October, 2010), pp. 408-413, ISSN: 1752-296X

Zhu, X.G.; Kim, D.W.; Goodson, M.L.; Privalsky, M.L. & Cheng, S.Y. (2011). NCoR1 regulates thyroid hormone receptor isoform-dependent adipogenesis. *Journal of Molecular Endocrinology,* Vol.46, No.3, (June, 2011), pp. 233-244, ISSN: 0952-5041

3

Differential Adaptations of the Hypothalamus-Pituitary-Thyroid Axis Between Food Restriction and Anorexia

P. de Gortari, E. Alvarez-Salas,
M. Morales-Mulia and V. Alcántara-Alonso
Dirección de Investigaciones en Neurociencias /Instituto Nacional de Psiquiatría Ramón de la Fuente M.
México

1. Introduction

The hypothalamic-pituitary thyroid (HPT) axis plays a critical role in mediating changes in metabolism and thermogenesis. Its regulation is mainly determined by thyrotropin-releasing hormone (TRH), which is a tripeptide (pGlu-His-ProNH$_2$) synthesized in the paraventricular nucleus (PVN) of the hypothalamus. TRH-containing-neurons of medial and periventricular parvocellular compartments of the PVN are essential for HPT axis regulation since they are the only ones with hypophysiotrophic properties (Lechan & Fekete, 2006). Axon terminals of TRHergic neurons are highly dense in the median eminence (ME), in close apposition to capillaries of the hypophysial-portal system (Toni & Lechan, 1993), where TRH is released and able to stimulate the synthesis and release of thyrotropin (TSH) and prolactin from anterior pituitary (Bowers et al., 1968; Harris et al., 1978). TSH then stimulates thyroxine (T_4) and triiodothyronine (T_3) synthesis in the thyroid gland as well as their release into the peripheral circulation. Under normal conditions only a small fraction of T_3 is generated by the thyroid gland, the remainder of T_3, which is available for binding sites in the plasma and body cells, is produced by monodeiodination of T_4 (Danforth, 1983). This action is catalyzed by both type 1 (D1) or type 2 (D2) iodothyronine deiodinases, the first is abundant in liver, kidney and pituitary (Araujo et al., 2008) whereas the latter is mainly present in brown adipose tissue (BAT), pituitary and Central Nervous System (CNS) (Diano et al., 1998). The enzyme activity of the liver and kidney is responsive to the nutritional status of an organism and is found to be more active during states of accelerated glucose metabolism (Danforth, 1983).

Thyroid hormones (TH) are highly active in the metabolism and necessary for most bodily functions such as growth, development and maintenance of homeostasis; they are able to increase metabolic rate by accelerating fuel oxidation in nearly all tissues: TH activate lipolysis, glucose metabolism and protein synthesis (Yen, 2001).

Hypothalamic TRH expression in the PVN and TSH release from the anterior pituitary are inhibited by T_3, performing a negative feedback loop that regulates HPT axis function

(Ching & Utiger, 1983; Lechan & Hollenberg, 2003; Reichlin et al., 1978). TRH synthesis is negatively controlled by T_3 that acts through its binding to thyroid hormone receptor (TR); TRs are derived from two genes (TRα and TRβ) encoding different T_3-binding TR active isoforms (Yen, 2001). TRs are DNA binding transcription factors able to recognize specific DNA sequences in the promoter regions of T_3 target genes; in fact, T_3 regulates DNA-dependent RNA polymerase enzyme activity increasing or decreasing content of several mRNAs. Pro-TRH gene promoter contains a consensus region for the thyroid-hormone response element (TRE) (Segerson et al., 1987). Hyperthyroidism facilitates that TR sites are occupied by its ligand, which in turn are translocated to the nucleus and by binding to the TRE region in the DNA, inhibit TRH transcription. In contrast, when a decreased T_3 tissue concentration is present, un-liganded TR is bound to a co-activator protein, increasing pro-TRH transcription (Lechan & Kakucska, 1992; Perello et al., 2006).

Besides its regulation at the transcription level, THs are also involved in the processing of the large inactive precursor (pre-pro-TRH): once proTRH is transported from the endoplasmic reticulum (ER) to the trans-Golgi network (TGN), a proteolytic processing occurs. Those processes are conducted by two prohormone convertases (PCs), PC1/3 and PC2, which cleave proTRH at basic residues flanking TRH sequence (Nillni et al., 1995, 1996; Schaner et al., 1997). PCs activity may also be regulated by TH (Espinosa et al., 2007; Perello et al., 2006). During hypothyroidism, end products of proTRH processing increase (Perello et al., 2006), while a decreased post-translational processing of proTRH is observed in T_4 treatment-induced hyperthyroidism (Segerson et al., 1987) rendering an accumulation of TRH unprocessed intermediate forms combined with a down-regulation of PCs (Perello et al., 2006). Several studies suggest that thyroid hormones negatively regulate the PC expression through the binding of its receptors to a consensus region localized in PC genes promoters (Li et al., 1999, 2000; Shen et al., 2005). Therefore, HPT axis regulation by thyroid status in the PVN may lead to an altered hormonal biosynthesis.

Besides TH control of proTRH transcription, corticosterone is also able to regulate it. Rat TRH gene promoter also contains a consensus region for glucocorticoids; it is a composite GRE element (cGRE) that is located at -218, -197 bp. It has been studied the effect of corticosterone or the synthetic corticosteroid dexamethasone under different conditions: it is observed *in vivo* that adrenalectomized animals present an increased TRH expression in the PVN, while administering rats with glucocorticoids on their drinking water, it is induced a decrease in peptide mRNA levels. Moreover, hypothalamic primary cultured cells added with dexamethasone present a reduced TRH synthesis. Furthermore, although nuclear extracts of hypothalamic cells incubated with 8Br-cAMP, present an increased transcription rate of TRH, the combined effect of glucocorticoids and cAMP pathway activators, is unable to elevate peptide synthesis (Diaz-Gallardo et al., 2010).

Degradation of the released peptide is achieved by the pyroglutamyl peptidase II (PPII, EC 3.4.19.6). It is a highly specific membrane-bound metallopeptidase that exclusively hydrolyzes the pyroglutamyl-histidyl peptide bond of TRH (Charli et al., 1998) in the extracellular space. PPII is widely distributed in the CNS and in some peripheral tissues (Heuer et al., 2000; Vargas et al., 1987). Its soluble form is named thyroliberinase present in serum, which is thought to be synthesized in the liver and derived from the same gene than PPII.

Anterior pituitary PPII enzyme is regulated by different factors and hormones: low serum TH levels decrease its activity and mRNA content, while hyperthyroidism increases both, suggesting that PPII regulation participates in the negative feedback of the TH that controls the HPT axis function (Bauer, 1988; Ponce et al., 1988; Schomburg & Bauer, 1995). Estrogens in contrast, affect PPII activity negatively, which may allow TRH to increase the duration of its effect in the anterior pituitary (Bauer, 1988). On the other hand, the addition of TRH to pituitary cultured cells induces a down-regulation of both PPII mRNA levels and activity (Vargas et al., 1994, 1998); furthermore, incubation with activators of cAMP pathway may mimic TRH effect on PPII (Vargas et al., 1998).

Body weight changes in obesity, fasting or food restriction are associated to alterations in circulating TH content. *In vivo* studies have shown that inhibition of pituitary PPII, increases the duration of TRH-induced release of TSH (Scalabrino et al., 2007), thus it is likely that PPII regulation might contribute to the reestablishment of the HPT axis homeostasis. The activity in serum of the soluble enzyme thyroliberinase, is known to be modified by body weight changes in obese humans independently of their thyroid hormone levels (Friedman et al., 1995). Thus, all those data support that TRH degradation plays a regulating role in the HPT axis function.

2. Adaptive hypothyroidism

Adaptive function of HPT axis allows animals to respond to changes in energy demands during growth, gestation, lactation or sickness periods. Nutrient availability that is modified with seasons or changing weather, triggers adaptive changes in the HPT function leading organisms to enlarge fat and glycogen deposits or to slow its degradation, depending on energy needs.

Main function of the thyroid gland is to maintain the basal metabolic rate in all cells. Thyroid hormone levels are challenged during the transition from fed to a starvation state; during starvation a reduced metabolic rate helps to preserve energy stores. This response is considered as the major evolutionary mechanism designed to ensure survival when food is scarce, although nowadays it may represent a risk to become obese during times of great food availability (Levin, 2006; Ogden et al., 2007a, 2007b).

During food restriction and starvation the feedback mechanism exerted by TH on hypothalamus and pituitary, is altered. Low body weight accompanied by decreased leptin serum levels induce a decrease in TH serum concentration (Ahima et al., 1996). In spite of the induced hypothyroidism, food deprivation for 3 days reduces the hypothalamic proTRH mRNA content, the amount of proTRH-derived peptides in the PVN, TRH release into hypophysial portal blood (Rondeel et al., 1992), pituitary levels of TSHβ mRNA and TSH plasma levels; it also induces a marked increase in plasma corticosterone content (van Haasteren et al., 1995). Re-feeding of starved male rats normalizes T_4 serum levels within 3 days, while T_3 and TSH content increases above the values observed before starvation.

Both male and female rats respond to a 4 day food deprivation with a body weight loss however, females have a better adaptation to energy deficit than males: they present decreased T_4 and T_3 levels together with reduced TSH serum levels after starvation (Rondeel et al., 1992), also their basal hypothalamic TRH release is lower than in males (Rondeel et al.,

1992). HPT axis adaptation depends on the age of animals: fasted weaning rats do not decelerate the HPT axis function; in spite of its 30% loss of weight compared to non fasted animals, TRH release remains active, TSH serum levels do not decay and PPII enzymatic activity is reduced, presumably allowing the peptide to exert its effects on the pituitary for a longer time (de Gortari et al., 2000). In contrast, adult animals after 72 h of fasting show a decreased TRH content in the ME, reduced TSH serum levels and no change in PPII activity (de Gortari et al., 2000). The fact that TSH does not change or is reduced when T_3 and T_4 serum levels are low is probably due to a decreased expression of the thyroid receptors in thyrotrophes induced by starvation (Bavli, 1980; St Germain & Galton, 1985; van Doom et al., 1984). A more recent explanation involves a central deregulation of deiodinases activities causing the fasting-associated changes in thyroid function.

Food deprivation is a stressful situation that enhances adrenal release of corticosteroids (Garcia-Belenguer et al., 1993; Mitev et al., 1993; Woodward et al., 1991). Starvation-induced corticosterone secretion reduces TRH and TSH-β synthesis and release; dexamethasone treatment also reduces the hypothalamic TRH secretion into hypophysial portal blood (van Haasteren et al., 1995). Thus, corticosterone is a factor that may be participating in the HPT adaptive changes to nutrient deficit.

2.1 Underlying factors of negative energy balance-associated hypothyroidism

Some factors have been studied as contributors to decreased synthesis of TRH in the PVN during fasting or food restriction, such as the activity of deiodinases. Type 2 deiodinase (D2) enzyme activity and its mRNA content in the tanycytes of the medial basal hypothalamus, increases with fasting (Lechan & Fekete, 2005); D2 converts T_4 to T_3 and therefore is responsible for the maintenance of the medial basal hypothalamic (MBH) local T_3 concentration (Diano et al., 1998), thus the inhibition of TRH expression observed in the medial PVN of starved rats may be a consequence of a higher production of local T_3 (Coppola et al., 2005).

Besides corticosterone and deiodinase activity, leptin peripheral administration can prevent the fall of TH in starved rodents, and the reduced expression of proTRH in the PVN after fasting (Ahima et al., 1996; Legradi et al., 1997). In other words, fasting-induced decrease of serum leptin content is able to reduce proTRH expression in the PVN, also to facilitate the high secretion of corticosterone that contributes to elevate D2 activity (Coppola et al., 2005) around the third ventricle. Thus, starvation and food restriction create a state of tertiary hypothyroidism and of reduced metabolic rate in the whole body that might serve as an important energy-conserving mechanism until re-feeding occurs.

Leptin is not only modified in situations of negative energy balance; patients with primary hypothyroidism due to autoimmune thyroid disease, present an increase in body weight, decreased appetite and low leptin serum levels, so it is suggested that changes in leptin levels do not explain the alterations in appetite usually found in these patients; but as mentioned, lower leptin serum levels could contribute to the decrease in energy expenditure in hypothyroidism (Valcavi et al., 1997).

At the central level, the hypothalamus is the primary component in the nervous system that interprets adiposity or nutrient related inputs; it finally directs hormonal and behavioral responses to regulate energy intake. Neurons in the hypothalamic arcuate nucleus (ARC) receive circulating adiposity levels and relay their responses to second-order neurons in the PVN and lateral hypothalamus to mediate effects on food intake and energy homeostasis; TRHergic neurons are among those second-order neurons stimulated by the melanocortin system (Nillni, 2010).

Hypophysiotrophic TRH neurons receive inputs from other regions of the brain as well as from the circulation. The most important afferent connections to PVN TRHergic cells include catecholamine neurons from the brainstem (Sawchenko & Swanson, 1982) and from the ARC, a nucleus with a prominent role in energy homeostasis.

Two are the main populations of neurons arising from ARC that send their axons to PVN TRHergic cells: those co-expressing neuropeptide Y and agouti-related protein (NPY/AgRP) (Broberger et al., 1998) and those co-expressing cocaine and amphetamine regulated transcript and α-melanocyte stimulating hormone (CART/α-MSH) (Vrang et al., 1999). Both NPY and AgRP stimulate food intake, whereas CART/ α-MSH reduce it. Hypothalamic T_3 production, catalyzed by D2, triggers the synthesis of mitochondrial uncoupling protein 2, which is critical for the activation of NPY/AgRP neurons during fasting (Coppola et al., 2007). NPY and AgRP inhibit TRH gene expression on hypophysiotrophic TRH neurons (Fekete et al., 2001, 2002), in contrast, CART/α-MSH stimulate TRH gene expression in the PVN, and this effect is enhanced by leptin (Fekete et al., 2000a, 2000b); both neuronal populations of ARC express leptin receptors and are inversely regulated by circulating leptin concentrations (Ahima et al., 2000).

Neuropeptides derived from the ARC play a significant role in the response of thyroid axis to both starvation and illness. Physiologically, the interaction of the ARC inputs on hypophysiotropic TRH neurons may be the primary mechanism for the development of central hypothyroidism associated with fasting, initiated by leptin (Ahima et al., 1996; Lechan & Fekete, 2004; Legradi et al., 1997). Serum leptin concentrations drop dramatically during fasting, and leptin replacement partly prevents starvation-induced decrease in serum T_4 levels and increases serum corticosterone in mice (Ahima et al., 1996). In general, leptin has a central physiologic role in providing information about energy stores and energy balance to brain centers that regulate appetite, energy expenditure and neuroendocrine functions (Campfield et al., 1995; Pelleymounter et al., 1995).The fall in circulating levels of leptin is sensed by the hypothalamus, which triggers increased appetite, decreased energy expenditure and a changed neuroendocrine function in a direction that favors survival.

Although the hypothalamic effects of leptin are mediated via the melanocortin system, which plays a role in feeding behavior, evidence exists about a direct role of leptin on PVN TRHergic cells (Harris et al., 2001; Nillni et al., 2000); nevertheless, ARC-derived neuropeptides still play the most significant role in the regulation of proTRH neurons, via synaptic input from leptin-responsive POMC and NPY/AgRP neurons located in the ARC (Fekete et al., 2000; Legradi & Lechan, 1998; Schwartz et al., 1996).

As a consequence of negative energy balance, the normal feedback mechanism for the regulation of hypophysiotrophic TRH neurons is overridden and a state of central hypothyroidism is induced, commonly referred to as "nonthyroidal illness" or the "sick euthyroid syndrome" (Wiersinga & Boelen, 1996).

2.2 Non-thyroidal illness syndrome

Alterations in neuroendocrine axis develop secondary to illness. An activation of the hypothalamic-pituitary-adrenal (HPA) axis is well documented (Vermes & Beishuizen, 2001). Although acute or chronic sickness can cause alterations on TSH and/or T_4 concentrations in plasma (Fliers et al., 2001), low circulating T_3 levels are the most common consequence of HPT axis adaptations. The main accepted term to make reference to these changes on HPT axis is the non-thyroidal illness syndrome (NTIS) (Warner & Beckett, 2010), given that not primary alterations in the thyroid gland are involved and that patients are considered clinically euthyroid. Probably this reduction on HPT axis function is a beneficial adaptive response in order to reduce energy expenditure in a sick organism.

There are many factors involved in the hormonal changes that result in the NTIS; these include modifications to the hypothalamic-pituitary axis, altered binding of thyroid hormone to circulating binding proteins, a modified entry of thyroid hormones into tissues, changes in thyroid hormone metabolism or alterations that are due to a modified expression of deiodinase enzymes (Warner & Beckett, 2010).

It seems that the low TSH levels associated with critical illness (or failure of TSH to increase in the presence of low T_3 and T_4) arise from a central hypothyroidism caused by alterations in the set point of the HPT axis regulation. This idea is supported by the fact that the administration of TRH to patients with prolonged critical illness at least partially restores serum T_3, TSH and T_4 content (Van den Berghe et al., 1998, 1999). The underlying mechanisms for the decreased TRH in hypothalamic neurons in patients who died with serum biochemistry of the NTIS may include the secretion of pro-inflammatory cytokines (Fliers et al., 1997); a different cause may be the chronic low food intake.

As mentioned previously, activation and inactivation of TH are carried out by a group of three iodotiroinine deiodinases. Changes on peripheral deiodinase enzymes' activity during illness are known to be an effect rather than the cause of alterations on circulating T_3 and T_4 in the NTIS (Debaveye et al., 2008; O'Mara et al., 1993). The rapid fall in T_3 seen in acute illness is more likely due to either impaired thyroidal production of T_3 (induced by a central hypothyroidism) and/or the result of the acute phase response leading to a decrease in serum thyroid hormone-binding protein (Warner & Beckett, 2010).

Administration of bacterial lipopolysaccharide (LPS) is a manner to study acute infection and immune activation. It has been shown that after 12 h of LPS administration, type 2 deiodinase mRNA synthesis increases in tanycytes lining the third ventricle. The ensuing local thyrotoxicosis may suppress the HPT axis by local feedback inhibition of hypophysiotrophic TRH synthesis and contribute to the mechanism of central hypothyroidism associated to infection (Fekete et al., 2004), which as previously mentioned, is probably an homeostatic response to preserve energy deposits during illness (De Groot, 1999). Contrary to the mechanism of central hypothyroidism associated to fasting (Legradi et al., 1997; Rondeel et al., 1992; van Haasteren et al., 1995), infection increases the gene expression of pro-opiomelanocortin (POMC) (the precursor molecule of α-MSH) and CART in the ARC, it does not increase NPY expression (Sergeyev et al., 2001) and elevates circulating levels of leptin (Grunfeld et al., 1996). These changes should elevate TRH expression; nevertheless during infection, stimulation of D2 synthesis by the increased LPS-induced pro-inflammatory cytokines concentration, is a more powerful stimulus that maintains low PVN TRH expression (Fekete et al., 2004). As happens during starvation, the increase in hypothalamic T_3 content may suppress the synthesis of TRH in hypophysiotrophic neurons either by local feedback inhibition through the release of T_3 from tanycytes' apical processes into the cerebrospinal fluid (CSF), or by its uptake from hypophysiotrophic TRH axonal processes in the median eminence and by its retrograde transport to the hypothalamic PVN. T_3 may also be released into the portal capillary system for conveyance to the anterior pituitary and exerts a direct effect on the thyrotrophes of the anterior pituitary where, it inhibits TSH secretion (Lechan & Fekete, 2005).

3. Dehydration-induced anorexia

There is a balance between food intake and energy utilization: an increased feeding behavior in animals compensates high energy waste. However, this equilibrium may be altered by different psychological and physiological stimuli that may induce the display of an aberrant behavior such as anorexia. Anorexia is defined as a loss of appetite despite of a low body weight and of an energy deficit. It may result during illness, after stress exposure, or as a response to homeostatic challenges such as cellular dehydration (Siegfried et al., 2003). In contrast to food restricted or dieting individuals, anorexic patients present normal or subnormal serum levels of T_4 and TSH (Stoving et al., 2001); also, a blunted TSH release form the pituitary after TRH administration (Tamai et al., 1986). Alterations of the HPT axis in anorexia nervosa have most likely a central origin, due to the reduced hypothalamic TRH secretion, and resemble those of the NTIS.

Besides its hypophysiotrophic role, TRH is implicated with neuromodulating effects in the CNS. As an icv injection of TRH in different animal species, reduces their food and liquid intake (Choi et al., 2002; Karydis & Tolis, 1998; Vijayan & McCann, 1977; Vogel et al., 1979), it has been proposed as an anorexigenic factor, which has been tested in *ad libitum* feeding animals, in those subjected to stress-induced eating models, and also in fasted and hungry animals during the re-feeding period (Horita, 1998; Morley & Levine, 1980; Steward et al., 2003; Suzuki et al., 1982; Vijayan & McCann, 1977). As mentioned, PVN TRHergic neurons express receptors for different feeding-regulating peptides synthesized in the ARC, such as NPY, AgRP, CART and α-MSH; also for leptin (Ob-Rb) which suggests that the hormone has an indirect effect on TRH expression by acting on feeding-related synthesizing neurons of the ARC, but also has a direct action on PVN TRHergic cells (Wittmann et al., 2009). As TRHergic neurons of the anterior part of the PVN are known to have projections to the ARC, to dorsomedial and to ventromedial hypothalamic nuclei, it is likely that besides its role in energy homeostasis, motivational aspects related to food intake might also be under TRH control.

To investigate TRH participation in feeding motivation we have used the dehydration-induced anorexia (DIA) model. Male and female adult animals subjected to this paradigm ingest a hyperosmolar solution of NaCl (2.5%) during 7 days, which reduces its food intake and body weight since day 1. Analysis of the expression of feeding-regulating peptides in the ARC of males after 5 days has shown a decreased synthesis of POMC and increased NPY mRNA levels (Watts et al., 1999), which have anorexigenic and orexigenic effects, respectively. All those changes are signals that should be increasing appetite and food ingestion in animals, however feeding is suppressed in dehydrated rats, which suggests that inhibitory control networks, other than those of the ARC, are activated (Watts, 2001, 2007).

The involvement of some hypothalamic peptides in feeding motivation may be identified using this paradigm, since changes in their synthesis due to dehydration in DIA animals are compared to those of a forced food-restricted group (pair-fed, FFR) that eat the exact amount of food ingested by DIA

Studies from other laboratories and ours have shown that when sacrificed either after 5 or 7 days (Jaimes-Hoy et al., 2008; Watts et al., 1999), both experimental animals from DIA and FFR groups present reduced leptin serum levels and high corticosterone concentrations (Table 1). Thus, both groups have a negative energy balance that only in FFR animals, activates feeding.

	TSH	T_3	T_4	Leptin	Corticosterone	Prolactin
Control	100 ± 13	100 ± 4	100 ± 2.5	100 ± 8	100 ± 7	100 ± 9
DIA	151 ± 21*+	64 ± 3*	99 ± 16	37 ± 5*	218 ± 17*	101 ± 9+
FFR	73 ± 12*	74 ± 9*	75 ± 9	33 ± 4*	263 ± 23*	20 ± 4*

Table 1. Serum hormones content in female rats after 7 days of dehydration or food restriction. Values are expressed as the mean ± SEM in percentage of difference vs C= 100%, n= 8 animals/group). Control values of TSH: 2.1 ± 0.22 ng/ml; T_3: 74 ± 2.7 ng/dl; T_4: 1.58 ± 0.09 µg/dl; leptin: 425 ± 33 pg/ml; corticosterone: 151 ± 15 ng/ml; prolactin: 0.97 ± 0.09 ng/ml) *p<0.05 vs C, +p<0.05 vs FFR. Modified from Jaimes-Hoy et al., 2008.

In order to identify changes in HPT axis function during those metabolic alterations, and with the notion that an icv injection of TRH has an anorectic role, female and male Wistar rats have been subjected to DIA paradigm for 7 days; their body weight and food intake is registered daily and is compared to that of FFR animals and to those of a control (C) group that is offered food *ad libitum* and tap water along the experiment. When compared food ingestion of animals from the same group by gender, results show that males eat more than females: dehydration induces a drastic decrease in food intake of males during the first four days, and a steady intake thereafter (Table 2); in contrast, females continuously decrease their food consumption up to day 6. DIA group of males have a dramatic weight loss since the first day, achieving a reduction of 32% of body weight by the 7th day when compared to controls (C=100%, FFR =73%, DIA = 68%). Females do not have such a drastic decrease, by the end of the experiment they lose 25% of controls' weight (C=100%, FFR =82.4%, DIA = 75%). Despite FFR group is pair-fed to dehydrated animals their body weight loss is less pronounced than in DIA rats (Figure 1).

	Day 0	1	2	3	4	5	6	7
Females								
Control	100 ± 1	100 ± 3	100 ± 7	100 ± 6	100 ± 5	100± 11	100± 10	100 ± 4
DIA	100 ± 1	48 ± 3**	25 ± 5**	15 ± 4**	12 ± 3**	6 ± 2**	3 ± 2**	5 ± 3**
Males								
Control	100 ± 1	100 ± 6	100 ± 8	100 ± 5	100 ± 5	100± 10	100± 10	100 ± 7
DIA	100 ± 1	55 ± 2*	22 ± 2*	12 ± 2*	11 ± 3*	9 ± 3**	9.4 ± 4**	10 ± 4*

Table 2. Food intake of female and male adult rats subjected to dehydration-induced anorexia model during 7 days. Values are expressed as the mean ± SEM as percentage of controls (C=100%) (n= 6 animals/group). *p<0.001, **p<0.0001 vs. control values.

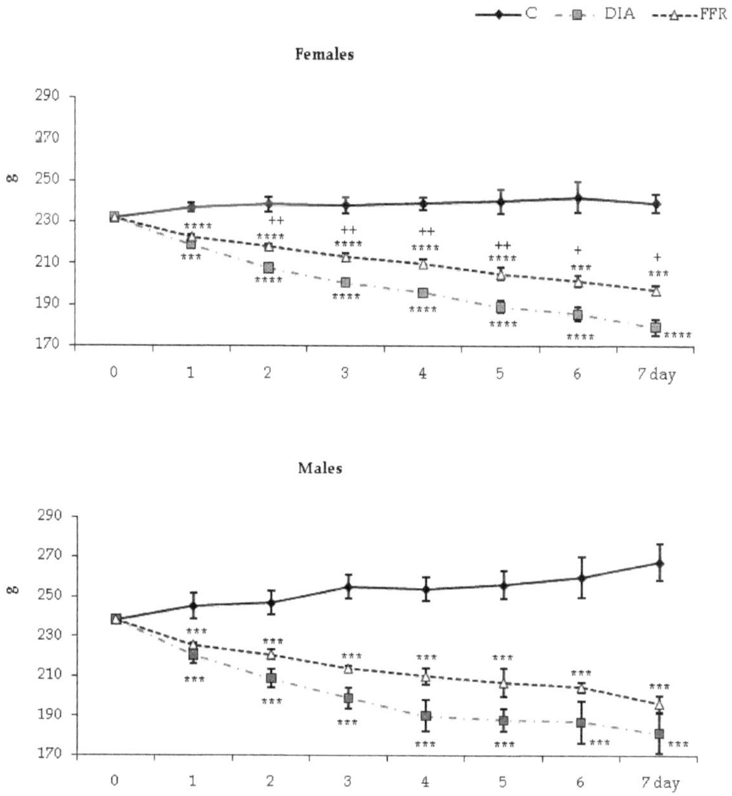

Fig. 1. Body weight of female and male adult rats subjected to dehydration-induced anorexia model or to forced-food restriction during 7 days. Controls: C, dehydrated-induced anorexic: DIA, forced-food restricted animals FFR. Values are expressed as the mean ± SEM in grams (n= 6/group). Modified from de Gortari et al., 2009. ***$p<0.001$, ****$p<0.0001$ vs. control group; +$p<0.05$, ++$p<0.01$ vs FFR.

We have also analyzed weight changes in white and brown adipose tissue of females affected by dehydration or food restriction, but there is no change. Thus, dehydration seems to contribute to the greater body weight loss of DIA animals. Different analysis of muscle hormonal content, such as T_3 local levels produced by deiodinases activity, would be necessary to identify a specific high catabolic rate of dehydrated animals in that tissue.

Measuring the content of TRH (by radioimmunoassay) in the ME of dehydrated and FFR animals, it is observed that DIA group of both sexes has reduced peptide content. Analysis of some other parameters of the HPT axis function, such as TSH, T_4 and T_3 serum levels have been described; also, TRH mRNA levels in the PVN and expression of TRH-R1 and of PPII in the anterior pituitary. As TSH levels increase after 7 days of dehydration, and TRH content in the ME is low (and is high in FFR), we have inferred an active peptide release from the hypothalamus in dehydrated animals that maintains elevated TSH serum content (Table 1). Knowing that at least in cultured cells, TRH addition down-regulates synthesis of its receptor (Yang & Tashjian, Jr., 1993), the reduced expression of anterior pituitary TRH-R1 of male and female DIA animals (Table 3) have supported that TRH is being released only after dehydration.

	PVN pro-TRH mRNA	ME TRH content	Pituitary TRH-R1 mRNA
Control	100 ± 4.8	100 ± 11	100 ± 16
DIA	130 ± 9*+	76 ± 4*+	77 ± 10*+
FFR	62 ± 5*	148 ± 10*	138 ± 22*

Table 3. PVN proTRH expression, peptide content in the ME, and TRH-R1 mRNA levels in the pituitary of female rats exposed to dehydration for 7 days. Expression changes are measured by RT-PCR. Values are expressed as the mean ± SEM as percentage of controls (C=100%) (n= 6 animals/group). *p<0.05 vs. control; +p<0.05 vs. FFR. (Jaimes-Hoy et al., 2008)

The low expression of TRH-R1 in the pituitary of anorexic animals resembles the delayed response of TSH to a TRH injection in anorexic patients (Tamai et al., 1986). The down-regulation of TRH-R1 receptors is most likely a result of the high release of TRH from the ME of DIA animals that in a long term may alter the function of the pituitary.

In spite of the high TSH serum levels observed in DIA, a low T_3 serum content is present when compared to C and FFR groups. It is possible that in the thyroid gland of dehydrated animals, the TSH receptor is internalized as is observed in hypothyroid conditions using both *in vivo* and *in vitro* studies (Baratti-Elbaz et al., 1999; Denereaz & Lemarchand-Beraud, 1995) when TSH content is elevated; results suggest a low binding of TSH to its receptor that is observed (up to 70%) in the hypothyroid condition when compared to euthyroid subjects but only when T_3 levels decrease (Denereaz & Lemarchand-Beraud, 1995).

An elevation of pro-TRH expression, analyzed by RT-PCR is observed in both males and in female dehydrated animals when compared to C and to FFR (Table 3). As expected, FFR of both gender present reduced TRH mRNA levels in the PVN (Table 3). Among the factors that are known to affect PVN TRH expression, we can mention the decreased leptin and increased corticosterone serum levels. However, since the concentration of those hormones is similarly changed in both experimental animals, the differential mRNA levels of TRH between DIA and FFR cannot be attributed to their hypothalamic effects. It would be possible, that D2 activity in the medial basal hypothalamus is decreased in DIA animals. As previously stated, D2 converts T_4 in the active hormone T_3 controlling its hypothalamic levels that may differ from those in the peripheral content. If dehydration causes a decrease on D2 activity, this would lead to a low T_3 local content that may stimulate TRH synthesis. The opposite has been shown in fasted animals: an increased D2 expression and activity seems responsible for the low TRH mRNA levels in the PVN during a negative energy balance.

All changes in the HPT axis of DIA group are representative of a primary hypothyroidism that is paradoxical since animals are under a negative energy balance and is contrasting to the tertiary hypothyroidism developed in fasting or food restriction.

However, it is still un-known which TRHergic neurons of the PVN are activated during dehydration.

TRHergic cells of the anterior part of the PVN (aPVN) do not project to the median eminence (Ishikawa et al., 1988; Kawano et al., 1991; Merchenthaler & Liposits, 1994) thus, they are neither hypophysiotropic nor under negative feedback by TH (Nishiyama et al., 1985; Segerson et al., 1987). Two of the major projection fields of aPVN TRH neurons are the ARC and the dorsomedial hypothalamus (DMH) (Morton et al., 2006; Wittmann et al., 2009) thus, it is possible that the observed anorectic effect of the icv administered TRH is mediated by neurons of that subdivision (Wittmann et al., 2009), but it awaits to be elucidated. Feeding-regulating role of TRH from the anterior part of the PVN TRH is also supported by studies showing an unaltered expression of the peptide in suckling rats (Sanchez et al., 2001) that are known to develop hyperphagia during lactation periods (Xu et al., 2009). It is likely that the lack of increase in TRH synthesis only in the aPVN of suckling rats would allow them to increase their food intake. Moreover, NPY from DMH is responsible for the hyperphagic drive during lactation, a major projection field of TRHergic neurons from the aPVN (Wittmann et al., 2009).

TRH from the aPVN may also have different roles to those related to food intake. Through its connections with the preoptic area, TRH from that subdivision of the PVN may regulate thermogenesis by activating the sympathetic nervous system (Morrison et al., 2008). This idea is supported by the fact that DIA female animals exposed to cold do not have a further increase on TRH expression than those maintained at room temperature (Jaimes-Hoy et al., 2008).

Activation of TRHergic neurons of the aPVN during dehydration, would be explaining the lack of decrease prolactin serum levels present in female rats subjected to DIA (Jaimes-Hoy et al., 2008) when compared to FFR rats (Table 1); besides its direct effect on prolactin secretion from pituitary lactotrophs (Grosvenor & Mena, 1980), TRH from the aPVN is able to inhibit the tuberoinfundibular dopaminergic system (Goldstein et al., 2007) increasing hormone release from the anterior pituitary to the blood. The main projection of aPVN TRH neurons is the dorsomedial part of the ARC (Wittmann et al., 2009), a region involved in the regulation of prolactin secretion (Freeman et al., 2000), suggests that aPVN subdivision may be involved in changes induced by dehydration, however, speculations may be confirmed by in situ hybridization analysis that would allow the identification of PVN TRHergic neurons activated in DIA.

Different signals that regulate food intake may be responsible for the paradoxical HPT function and the increased TRH mRNA levels of the PVN in dehydrated rats. One of them is the orexinergic system. During fasting, pre-pro-orexin-synthesizing cells in the lateral hypothalamic area (LHA) are activated; its derived peptides, orexin A and B, are factors that stimulate feeding (Sakurai et al., 1998). Orexins-containing neurons from LHA project to the PVN (Peyron et al., 1998) where its receptors have been identified (Backberg et al., 2002). Those are findings that support orexins participation in energy homeostasis (Yamamoto et al., 1999) and thermoregulation (Jaszberenyi et al., 2002). Orexin A is the peptide involved in activation of food intake, its injection increases feeding and decreases body temperature (Jaszberenyi et al., 2002). Those effects of orexin A are mediated through its interaction with the NPY system (Muroya et al., 2004). In contrast, orexin B is implicated in arousal and with wakefulness effects (Lin et al., 1999; Siegel, 1999).

Besides information arriving from LHA orexinergic neurons, PVN also receives connections from the ARC including NPY-synthesizing neurons. In the PVN, some of the target cells of NPY are those that synthesize TRH that contain NPY-Y1 receptors (Broberger et al., 1999); NPY-Y1 receptors are activated during fasting or food restriction by the increased release of NPY, which in turn inhibits TRH synthesis (Fekete et al., 2001, 2002).

Thus, changes in the LHA pre-pro-orexin (Ox) mRNA levels and PVN orexin (Ox-1R) and NPY (Y1, Y5) receptors of male rats subjected to DIA paradigm for seven days, have been analyzed and compared to those of animals that are food-restricted. As PVN receives direct information from circulating leptin levels concerning size and volume of adiposities and TRHergic neurons of that hypothalamic region contain Ob-Rb receptors, thus studies have been made to analyze alterations in the expression of PVN leptin receptor that would account for the differential expression of TRH between DIA and FFR male animals.

LHA of dehydrated animals, present unchanged expression of the pre-pro-orexin mRNA content, in contrast to that of FFR rats that have increased synthesis of the orexigenic peptide (Figure 2), supporting that this area is responsive to the negative energy balance. It has been previously described that *c-fos* expression is not activated in LHA orexinergic cells in DIA paradigm (Watts et al., 2007). Furthermore, non-responding orexinergic neurons have been observed in animals where an anorexic behavior is induced by a LPS injection (Becskei et al., 2008). Results support that the anorexic behavior presented by DIA animals may be due to an inactivation of the orexinergic system in the LHA that should be stimulating energy intake through its connections to the PVN (Peyron et al., 1998). It is known that orexins act directly on NPYergic projections coming from the ARC and afferent to the PVN through its orexin receptors expressed in NPY-synthesizing neurons. Thus, it would be possible that TRH expression in the PVN is increased in DIA animals by the impaired inhibiting effect of the orexinergic system during dehydration.

In the PVN of FFR animals, the expression of the orexin-receptor is lower than in DIA and C groups; this may be due to the inferred increased orexins release in the PVN that as for other receptors induces a desensitization mechanism that leads to a protein down-regulation. DIA animals present a higher synthesis of Ox-R1 than that of FFR, which may be interpreted as a compensatory increase due to poor peptide release in those animals, and also as an impaired receptor signaling; it has been observed in other models of anorexia (Ballinger et al., 2001). It is likely that orexins released in the PVN or food-restricted rats inhibit TRH release, and in consequence, TSH serum levels also are low, as has been observed by an icv injection of orexins (Mitsuma et al., 1999). Using the DIA paradigm it is evident that anorexic animals do not have that pathway activated thus, the differential change in Ox-R1 mRNA levels between FFR and DIA groups could be an additional responsible factor for the enhanced expression of proTRH in the PVN of dehydrated rats. Since LHA orexin-containing neurons send projections to magnocellular and also to parvocellular neurons of the PVN (Backberg et al., 2002), it is possible that orexins may be affecting energy homeostasis, but also that they may be participating in regulation of water balance or blood pressure, processes in which TRH has also been implicated.

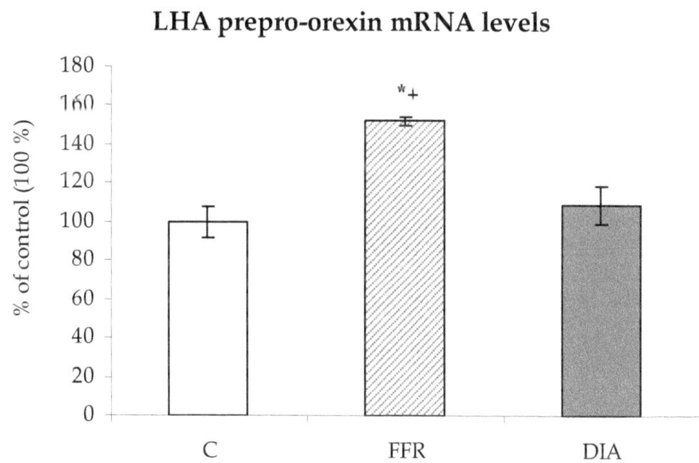

Fig. 2. Prepro-orexin mRNA levels in the lateral hypothalamic area (LHA), mRNA levels were semi-quantified by RT-PCR. Values (in percentage) are the ratio of prepro-orexin cDNA/cyclophilin cDNA expressed as the mean ± SEM calculated as % of naïve values (C= 100 %), n=8. *$p<0.01$ vs naïve, +$p<0.001$ FFR vs.DIA. Modified from García-Luna et al., 2010.

Besides orexins in the LHA, TRH expression is also differentially altered in this nucleus between anorexic and food restricted animals. Synthesis of TRH is reduced only in the FFR rats, while it increases after 7 days of DIA. LHA TRHergic cells send projections to the septum, an area involved in arousal (Ishikawa et al., 1986; Prokai, 2002), thus, it is not unlikely that the peptide synthesized in LHA has functions related to maintain an alertness state in food restricted animals.

As both DIA and FFR groups have increased synthesis of NPY in the ARC (Watts et al., 1999), and leptin serum levels are similarly low, it is not possible to think that behavioral differences in feeding motivation of those groups are due to an impaired response of ARC NPYergic neurons to the decreased leptin serum content. However, an alteration in the downstream pathway of leptin signaling in the PVN of DIA animals, may contribute to the development of anorexia after dehydration. We have found an increased expression of the Ob-Rb in the PVN of FFR group only when compared to DIA. This suggests that leptin receptors in dehydrated animals are at least, slightly activated vs FFR; this difference could be compensating the low leptin levels and may increase PVN TRH synthesis. In FFR, Ob-Rb seems not to be functional, thus TRH expression remains low. Reduced serum leptin content may not be correlating with hormonal levels in the cerebrospinal fluid of dehydrated animals due to alterations in the peptide transport to the brain that has been proposed in anorexic and in obese patients (Schwartz et al., 1996). It is not unlikely either, that dehydration is increasing sensitivity and affinity of Ob-Rb receptors for their ligand, which is overcoming the low leptin serum levels and is contributing to the development of anorexia in DIA animals.

By the analysis of the expression of NPY receptors in the PVN, we have observed that only FFR animals present decreased Y1 mRNA levels, when compared to DIA animals that have similar values to the control group. This suggests that NPY in FFR is able to activate Y1 and to favor food-seeking behavior; the unchanged synthesis in anorexic animals may be related to a failed inhibition of their PVN TRH synthesis. A similar NPY release than a control group and a differential expression of NPY-Y1 occurs in another model of anorexia (Ballinger et al., 2001); furthermore, an Y1 agonist injection facilitates a positive energy balance. Thus, an impaired function of the Y1 receptor in the PVN may also be participating in the anorexic behavior of dehydrated animals.

3.1 CRH actions on the regulation of HPT axis in anorexic animals

CRH and its receptors regulate in concert, the autonomic, behavioral, immunologic and endocrine responses of the organism allowing it to face a changing environment. Starvation, body weight loss and negative energy balance are some of the stressful conditions that induce differential changes in the hypothalamus-pituitary adrenal axis (HPA) axis, as well as in central CRH metabolism, enabling the organism to adapt to situations of nutrient deficit. CRH also participates in the regulation of energy intake and utilization through its actions on the sympathetic nervous system, activating thermogenesis in the BAT (Arase et al., 1988; LeFeuvre et al., 1987).

In DIA paradigm (Jaimes-Hoy et al., 2008; Watts et al., 1999), CRH expression in the PVN decreases in a greater extent than in food restricted rats (Brady et al., 1990; Isse et al., 1999) after 7 days. Although expression of CRH-R1 receptor in the PVN is up-regulated in several stressful conditions supposedly by CRH release into the PVN which in turn, up-regulates CRH expression (Imaki et al., 1996; Mansi et al., 1996; Turnbull & Rivier, 1997), CRH-R1 mRNA levels are unchanged in DIA animals. In contrast, the expression of CRH-R2 decreases only in the PVN of DIA group. The lack of response of FFR animals is coincident with that reported after starvation (Makino et al., 1998). CRH-R2 is the receptor involved in the anorexigenic effects of administered CRH (Arase et al., 1988; Krahn et al., 1990; Morley & Levine, 1982) since, the knockdown of CRH-R2, but not of CRH-R1, attenuates CRH-induced appetite and food intake reduction (Smagin et al., 1998).

CRH synthesis in the LHA of DIA animals is increased when compared to those of food-restricted and control groups (Watts et al., 1999). LHA CRHergic neurons have projections directly to the PVN, and are proposed as important targets for osmosensitive afferents from the forebrain, the middle preoptic nucleus and subfornical organ and from the fusiform nucleus of the bed nucleus of the *stria terminallis,* which are projections that mediate part of the response of peptidergic mRNAs in the LHA during dehydration (Kelly & Watts, 1996). It is possible that an increased release of CRH from the LHA impinges on CRH-R2 receptors of the PVN, causing a receptor down-regulation, as shown in the pituitary for CRH-R1 (Rabadan-Diehl et al., 1996).

Using *in vitro* studies with cultured hypothalamic cells, it is observed that the addition of CRH (10 nM) increases TRH mRNA levels after 1 h, analyzed by RT-PCR (de Gortari et al., 2009). Thus, it has been performed an injection in the PVN of a specific antagonist of CRH-R2 receptors to dehydration-subjected animals. Three different doses of antisauvagine-30 (ASG-30) have been administered since the first day of DIA paradigm. Anorexic animals injected with the middle dose (30 nM= MD) increase their food intake on day 4 to 288 ± 25%

compared to the control group (saline injected and also subjected to DIA, 100 ± 26%). Weight loss of those animals does not change in saline-injected DIA animals (S-DIA), in contrast, changes of the HPT axis induced by dehydration are antagonized by the intra-PVN injections of ASG-30: pro-TRH mRNA levels decrease when compared to saline-injected DIA group (Figure 3); TRH-R1 expression in anterior pituitary increases and serum levels of TSH and T_4 decrease with the administration of the medial and high doses of the CRH-R2 antagonist. Antagonizing CRH-R2 in the PVN of animals subjected to DIA paradigm, the anorexigenic effects of dehydration are attenuated and the ability of the HPT axis to adjust to the negative energy balance condition is restored. These results together with the *in vitro* stimulation of CRH on pro-TRH expression of hypothalamic cultured cells, suggest that the DIA-induced activation of HPT axis is affected at the PVN level by CRH through CRH-R2 activation. It however remains to be shown that the DIA-activated CRHergic neurons of the lateral hypothalamus, which project to the PVN, target TRH synthesizing cells and that those cells express CRH-R2. The negative correlation found between PVN-pro-TRH mRNA levels and food intake gives further support for TRH anorectic effects (Choi et al., 2002; Schuhler et al., 2007).

The failure of HPT adaptation during anorexia becomes deleterious to the subject as greater body weight loss is observed; it is possible that the use of CRH-R2 antagonists in anorexic patients ameliorates its reduced appetite.

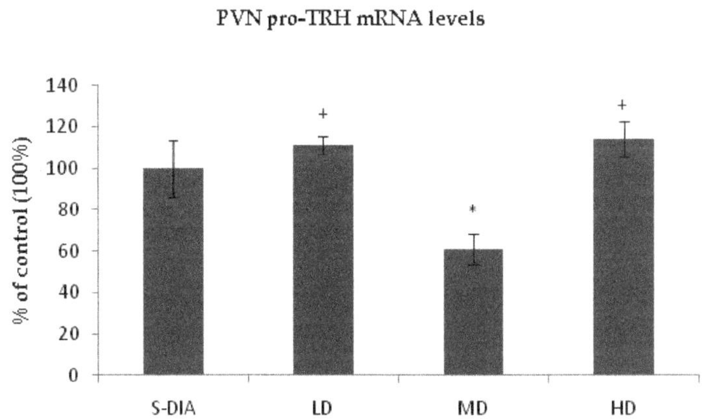

Fig. 3. Expression changes of pro-TRH mRNA levels in the PVN of dehydrated male animals injected with a specific antagonist of CRH-R2 (antisauvagina-30, ASG-30) directly in the PVN during seven days. S-DIA: saline injected dehydrated animals; LD, low-dose group of dehydrated animals and injected with 15 nM of ASG-30; MD, medium-dose group of dehydrated animals injected with 30 nM of ASG-30; HD, high dose group of dehydrated animals injected with 60 nM of ASG-30. Values are the means ± SEM of the ratio of proTRH cDNA/cyclophilin signal cDNA (arbitrary units); data is expressed as % of S-DIA values, considered as 100% (n=3 for LD, HD, n=6 for S-DIA and MD). $+p<0.05$ vs. MD group, $*p<0.05$ vs. S-DIA. Modified from de Gortari et al., 2009.

4. Developed hypothyroidism during zinc deficiency

Zinc is a mineral with a relevant role in growing, cell differentiation and regulation of metabolism. It participates in different biological functions such as DNA synthesis and genes expression (Vallee, 1977). It is also crucial to several enzymatic processes (Vallee & Falchuk, 1993), that in turn influence hormonal and neural transmissions (Xie & Smart, 1991).

There are both saturated a non-saturated mechanisms of Zn absorption (Seal & Mathers, 1989; Tacnet et al., 1990). Two main protein families are in charge of Zn transport: 1) at least 15 members of the ZIP (i.e., Zn-regulated metal transporter, Iron-regulated metal transporter-like protein) family (Eide, 2004) and 2) ten members of the ZnT (Zn Transporter) family (Liuzzi & Cousins, 2004). Absorption rate is able to adjust to Zn availability, i.e., there is an increase on the maximum Zn absorption rate in rat enterocytes cell cultures, following a reduction on dietary Zn (Hoadley et al., 1987), just as there is an increase on trans-epithelial Zn flux on CACO-2 cells after treatment with 5 μM when compared to one of 25 μM Zn (Reeves et al., 2001).

Zinc widespread functions impinge on several aspects of organism physiology, best demonstrated by the variety of symptoms associated with zinc-deficiency (Prasad, 1984). Clinic manifestations comprehend anorexia, growth retardation, dermatitis, diarrhea, weight loss and impaired immune responses. Among mineral deficiency causes we can mention malnutrition, alcoholism, absorption alterations, chronic renal insufficiency, etc.

In most studies, Zn deficiency results in an overall 40% to 50% decrease in food intake (Gaetke et al., 2002; Rains et al., 1998). However, in severe Zn deficiency, food intake can be reduced by as much as 70% (Essatara et al., 1984; Kasarskis et al., 1996). Although severe Zn deficiency is considered to be rare, mild or moderate deficiency is believed to be widespread throughout the world (Caulfield et al., 1998). In rodents, the most striking feature of experimental Zn deficiency is the cyclic feeding behavior that develops during Zn deprivation. Early studies report that this behavior is characterized by both a reduction of mean food intake, and periodic cyclic changes in daily food intake that disappear as soon as Zn is reintroduced in the diet (Chesters & Quarterman, 1970; Williams & Mills, 1970); an underlying alteration in hypothalamic galanin and NPY gene expression may be responsible for the altered feeding patterns in Zn deficient rats (Selvais et al., 1997).

Zinc deficient rats weight less than rats that consume the same amount of Zn-adequate food (Gaetke et al., 2002). This observation suggests that Zn deficiency has an impact on metabolic rate that is independent on food intake; however, it seems that the most profound effect of Zn status on metabolic rate and substrate utilization is the result of Zn deficiency-induced anorexia (Evans et al., 2004).

Both caloric restriction and Zn deficiency are known to reduce T_3 serum levels when compared to *ad libitum* fed animals, in addition, T_3 concentration is lower in Zn deficient vs. caloric restricted rats. In adult Zn deficient rats, a reduced hypothalamic TRH content and inhibited release from ME are observed, also T_4 and TSH levels are diminished. Because Zn deficiency causes a major decrease in serum free (fT_3) and fT_4 levels than caloric restriction, it seems that lack of Zn impairs the extra-thyroidal T_3 synthesis (Morley et al., 1980). In fact, there is a decrease in D1 liver activity secondary to Zn deficiency. Also Pekary et al., (Pekary et al., 1991) have shown that processing of the pro-TRH is altered, since the convertases are

Zn-dependent enzymes, moreover, T_3 receptors, in common with other members of the nuclear receptor family, are thought to be included among the nuclear zinc-binding proteins. They all contain nine invariant cysteine residues in the DNA-binding region (Evans, 1988). If Zn is removed through chelating processes, T_3 receptors produced from a bacterial expression system lose their ability to bind to DNA (Miyamoto et al., 1991), thus it is clear that Zn deficiency affects TH metabolism (Kralik et al., 1996).

Since during gestation and lactation periods metal demand increases, Zn requirements are also greater. In fact, it is recognized that around 80% of pregnant women world-wide are likely to have inadequate zinc intakes (Shah & Sachdev, 2001). The increased requirements need to be fulfilled by an enhanced ingestion or by adjusting metal homeostasis. One of these adjustments involves an increase on intestinal Zn absorption during both pregnancy and lactation (Davies & Williams, 1977; Moser-Veillon, 1995). Moreover, during lactation in humans and rodents, milk Zn concentration is maintained over a wide range of dietary Zn intake, and decreases only after plasma Zn concentration is reduced (Krebs, 1998; Moore et al., 1984). Zn transporters in the rat mammary gland respond to marginal Zn intake during lactation, when there is a reduced Zn-T1 protein level, thus allowing the mammary gland to reduce serosal Zn export through this ubiquitous transporter during Zn deficiency, also a higher ZnT-4 mRNA expression and protein levels is observed in order to maintain milk Zn concentration (Kelleher & Lonnerdal, 2002); this is due to the fact that vesicular ZnT-4 participates in the import of Zn into endocytotic or secretory vesicles, which ultimately releases Zn into milk (Murgia et al., 1999). Gestational Zn deficiency affects different processes where TRH has an active role: thyroid axis function, energetic homeostasis, body weight regulation, stress responses and growth. Offspring may present increases in T_4 content in the umbilical cord, decreased T_3 concentration, impaired TR function and a reduced body weight (Mahajan et al., 2005) as a result of intrauterine under nutrition. As pituitary PPII is a metalloenzyme and its activity depends on Zn, it might be affected during intrauterine Zn deficiency, leading to HPT alterations, although this remains to be studied.

It is possible that HPT axis adapts during Zn deficiency differently than in response to fast and malnutrition. This would be important, since animals with a Zn deficient diet have a reduction in the amount of food intake, thus it would be possible that some changes in the HPT axis function are due to an associated malnutrition however, there might be alterations that are only due to Zn deficiency.

5. Conclusions

Trying to identify if the degradation of TRH in the portal blood by the ectoenzyme pyroglutamyl aminopeptidase II (PPII) is an event involved in the adaptive regulation of the HPT axis during fasting, we evaluated PPII activity changes in the anterior pituitary of adults and young fasted animals and found a differential enzyme regulation that depends on the age of animals. While adults show the expected deceleration of the HPT axis function, the reduced TRH release and TSH serum content, weaning rats have a decreased PPII activity that may facilitate TRH effects on the thyrotrophes, which maintain elevated their TSH blood concentration, impairing adaptation of young animals to the negative energy balance. It supports that PPII-induced TRH degradation in the anterior pituitary may be a regulatory site of the HPT axis function that depends on the age of animals and on the etiology of hypothyroidism.

Using the model of DIA, we have been able to analyze the expression changes of peptides involved in feeding motivation, and to discriminate from those that decelerate energy utilization. DIA animals lose weight since day one of dehydration and develop an anorexic behavior.

We have found that a primary hypothyroidism is induced in anorexic rats, in contrast to the tertiary hypothyroidism of the pair-fed animals, despite of the negative energy balance developed in both groups. Dehydration impairs the adaptation of the HPT axis to the nutrient deficit: TRH expression is increased in the PVN, its release from the median eminence is active and TSH serum content is higher than in pair-fed and control animals. We also have found a reduced expression of the TRH receptors in the pituitary of anorexic animals that may be the result of the increased release of the peptide, as a desensitization mechanism. This resembles the blocked response of the pituitary to TRH administration in anorexic patients. Thus, we have been able to induce with this paradigm, changes of the HPT axis similar to those that are developed in anorexia nervosa.

The increased mRNA levels of TRH found in the PVN of anorexic animals and not in the pair-fed group support that the peptide of that hypothalamic region participates not only in energy homeostasis but in feeding motivation and anorexic behavior.

Given that TRHergic PVN neurons receive orexinergic input from LHA and NPYergic afferents from ARC, we analyzed changes in the LHA pre-pro-orexin (Ox) mRNA levels and PVN orexin (Ox-1R) and NPY (Y1, Y5) receptors of male rats. LHA prepro-orexinergic cells are activated in forced food restricted animals; Ox1-R and Y1 expression is reduced in food restricted vs. controls and anorexic group. Thus, compensatory changes in PVN receptor expression of some feeding-related peptides in anorexic rats may alter TRHergic neural response to energy demands.

CRH is another likely responsible factor for the increased TRH mRNA levels of the PVN of anorexic animals. Injection of a specific CRH-R2 antagonist in the PVN of dehydrated animals reduces TRH expression, the TSH blood concentration, and is able to attenuate anorexic behavior of DIA animals. Thus, specific antagonists of the CRHergic pathway may be potential therapeutic agents for anorexic patients.

6. Acknowledgements

We thank the participation of MC Cinthia García Luna in studies of expression of leptin and NPY receptors in anorexic animals; also the technical assistance of Ma. Isabel Amaya. Some of these data have been obtained with the support of CONACyT 61410 and 128316.

7. References

Ahima, R.S.; Prabakaran, D.; Mantzoros, C.; Qu, D.; Lowell, B.; Maratos-Flier, E. & Flier, J.S. (1996). Role of leptin in the neuroendocrine response to fasting. *Nature*, Vol. 382, No. 6588, (July 1996), pp. (250-252).

Ahima, R.S.; Saper, C.B.; Flier, J.S. & Elmquist, J.K. (2000). Leptin regulation of neuroendocrine systems. *Front Neuroendocrinol*, Vol. 21, No. 3, (July 2000), pp. (263-307).

Arase, K.; York, D.A.; Shimizu, H.; Shargill, N. & Bray, G.A. (1988). Effects of corticotropin-releasing factor on food intake and brown adipose tissue thermogenesis in rats. *Am J Physiol*, Vol. 255, No. 3 Pt 1, (September 1988), pp. (E255-E259).

Araujo, R.L.; de Andrade, B.M.; de Figueiredo, A.S.; da Silva, M.L.; Marassi, M.P.; Pereira, V.S.; Bouskela, E. & Carvalho, D.P. (2008). Low replacement doses of thyroxine during food restriction restores type 1 deiodinase activity in rats and promotes body protein loss. *J Endocrinol*, Vol. 198, No. 1, (July 2008), pp. (119-125).

Backberg, M.; Hervieu, G.; Wilson, S. & Meister, B. (2002). Orexin receptor-1 (OX-R1) immunoreactivity in chemically identified neurons of the hypothalamus: focus on orexin targets involved in control of food and water intake. *Eur J Neurosci*, Vol. 15, No. 2, (January 2002), pp. (315-328).

Ballinger, A.B.; Williams, G.; Corder, R.; El-Haj, T. & Farthing, M.J. (2001). Role of hypothalamic neuropeptide Y and orexigenic peptides in anorexia associated with experimental colitis in the rat. *Clin Sci (Lond)*, Vol. 100, No. 2, (February 2001), pp. (221-229).

Baratti-Elbaz, C.; Ghinea, N.; Lahuna, O.; Loosfelt, H.; Pichon, C. & Milgrom, E. (1999). Internalization and recycling pathways of the thyrotropin receptor. *Mol Endocrinol*, Vol. 13, No. 10, (October 1999), pp. (1751-1765).

Bauer, K. (1988). Degradation and biological inactivation of thyrotropin releasing hormone (TRH): regulation of the membrane-bound TRH-degrading enzyme from rat anterior pituitary by estrogens and thyroid hormones. *Biochimie*, Vol. 70, No. 1, (January 1988), pp. (69-74).

Bavli, S.Z. (1980). Fasting, but not glucagon administration, decreases anterior pituitary nuclear thyroid hormone receptors in rats. *Metabolism*, Vol. 29, No. 7, (July 1980), pp. (636-642).

Becskei, C.; Riediger, T.; Hernadfalvy, N.; Arsenijevic, D.; Lutz, T.A. & Langhans, W. (2008). Inhibitory effects of lipopolysaccharide on hypothalamic nuclei implicated in the control of food intake. *Brain Behav Immun*, Vol. 22, No. 1, (January 2008), pp. (56-64).

Bowers, C.Y.; Lee, K.L. & Schally, A.V. (1968). A study on the interaction of the thyrotropin-releasing factor and L-triiodothyronine: effects of puromycin and cycloheximide. *Endocrinology*, Vol. 82, No. 1, (January 1968), pp. (75-82).

Brady, L.S.; Smith, M.A.; Gold, P.W. & Herkenham, M. (1990). Altered expression of hypothalamic neuropeptide mRNAs in food-restricted and food-deprived rats. *Neuroendocrinology*, Vol. 52, No. 5, (November 1990), pp. (441-447).

Broberger, C.; Johansen, J.; Johansson, C.; Schalling, M. & Hokfelt, T. (1998). The neuropeptide Y/agouti gene-related protein (AGRP) brain circuitry in normal, anorectic, and monosodium glutamate-treated mice. *Proc Natl Acad Sci U S A*, Vol. 95, No. 25, (December 1998), pp. (15043-15048).

Broberger, C.; Visser, T.J.; Kuhar, M.J. & Hokfelt, T. (1999). Neuropeptide Y innervation and neuropeptide-Y-Y1-receptor-expressing neurons in the paraventricular hypothalamic nucleus of the mouse. *Neuroendocrinology*, Vol. 70, No. 5, (November 1999), pp. (295-305).

Campfield, L.A.; Smith, F.J.; Guisez, Y.; Devos, R. & Burn, P. (July 1995). Recombinant mouse OB protein: evidence for a peripheral signal linking adiposity and central neural networks. *Science*, Vol. 269, No. 5223, (July 1995), pp. (546-549).

Caulfield, L.E.; Zavaleta, N.; Shankar, A.H. & Merialdi, M. (1998). Potential contribution of maternal zinc supplementation during pregnancy to maternal and child survival. *Am J Clin Nutr*, Vol. 68, No. 2 Suppl, (August 1998), pp. (499S-508S).

Charli, J.L.; Vargas, M.A.; Cisneros, M.; de, G.P.; Baeza, M.A.; Jasso, P.; Bourdais, J.; Perez, L.; Uribe, R.M. & Joseph-Bravo, P. (1998). TRH inactivation in the extracellular compartment: role of pyroglutamyl peptidase II. *Neurobiology (Bp)*, Vol. 6, No. 1, (1998), pp. (45-57).

Chesters, J.K. & Quarterman, J. (December 1970). Effects of zinc deficiency on food intake and feeding patterns of rats. *Br J Nutr*, Vol. 24, No. 4, (1970), pp. (1061-1069).

Ching, M.C. & Utiger, R.D. (1983). Hypothalamic portal blood immunoreactive TRH in the rat: lack of effect of hypothyroidism and thyroid hormone treatment. *J Endocrinol Invest*, Vol. 6, No. 5, (October 1983), pp. (347-352).

Choi, Y.H.; Hartzell, D.; Azain, M.J. & Baile, C.A. (2002). TRH decreases food intake and increases water intake and body temperature in rats. *Physiol Behav*, Vol. 77, No. 1, (September 2002), pp. (1-4).

Coppola, A.; Hughes, J.; Esposito, E.; Schiavo, L.; Meli, R. & Diano, S. (2005). Suppression of hypothalamic deiodinase type II activity blunts TRH mRNA decline during fasting. *FEBS Lett*, Vol. 579, No. 21, (August 2005), pp. (4654-4658).

Coppola, A.; Liu, Z.W.; Andrews, Z.B.; Paradis, E.; Roy, M.C.; Friedman, J.M.; Ricquier, D.; Richard, D.; Horvath, T.L.; Gao, X.B. and others (2007). A central thermogenic-like mechanism in feeding regulation: an interplay between arcuate nucleus T3 and UCP2. *Cell Metab*, Vol. 5, No. 1, (January 2007), pp. (21-33).

Coppola, A.; Meli, R. & Diano, S. (2005). Inverse shift in circulating corticosterone and leptin levels elevates hypothalamic deiodinase type 2 in fasted rats. *Endocrinology*, Vol. 146, No. 6, (June 2005), pp. (2827-2833).

Danforth E Jr (1983). The role of thyroid hormones and insulin in the regulation of energy metabolism. *Am J Clin Nutr*, Vol. 38, No. 6, (December 1983), pp. (1006-1017).

Davies, N.T. & Williams, R.B. (1977). The effect of pregnancy and lactation on the absorption of zinc and lysine by the rat duodenum in situ. *Br J Nutr*, Vol. 38, No. 3, (November 1977), pp. (417-423).

De Groot, L.J. (1999). Dangerous dogmas in medicine: the nonthyroidal illness syndrome. *J Clin Endocrinol Metab*, Vol. 84, No. 1, (January 1999), pp. (151-164).

de Gortari, P.; González-Alzati, M.E.; Cisneros, M.; Joseph-Bravo P. (2000). Effect of fasting on the content of thyrotropin-releasing hormone and its RNAm in the central nervous system and pyroglutamyl peptidase II activity in the anterior pituitary of post-weaned and adult rats. *Neuroscience*, Vol. 3, pp. (255-65).

de, Gortari, P.; Mancera, K.; Cote-Velez, A.; Amaya, M.I.; Martinez, A.; Jaimes-Hoy, L. & Joseph-Bravo, P. (2009). Involvement of CRH-R2 receptor in eating behavior and in the response of the HPT axis in rats subjected to dehydration-induced anorexia. *Psychoneuroendocrinology*, Vol. 34, No. 2, (February 2009), pp. (259-272).

Debaveye, Y.; Ellger, B.; Mebis, L.; Darras, V.M. & Van den Berghe, G. (2008). Regulation of tissue iodothyronine deiodinase activity in a model of prolonged critical illness. *Thyroid*, Vol. 18, No. 5, (May 2008), pp. (551-560).

Denereaz, N. & Lemarchand-Beraud, T. (1995). Severe but not mild alterations of thyroid function modulate the density of thyroid-stimulating hormone receptors in the rat thyroid gland. *Endocrinology*, Vol. 136, No. 4, (April 1995), pp. (1694-1700).

Diano, S.; Naftolin, F.; Goglia, F. & Horvath, T.L. (1998). Fasting-induced increase in type II iodothyronine deiodinase activity and messenger ribonucleic acid levels is not reversed by thyroxine in the rat hypothalamus. *Endocrinology*, Vol. 139, No. 6, (June 1998), pp. (2879-2884).

Diaz-Gallardo, M.Y.; Cote-Velez, A., Charli, J.L. & Joseph-Bravo, P. (2010). A rapid interference between glucocorticoids and cAMP-activated signalling in hypothalamic neurones prevents binding of phosphorylated cAMP response element binding protein and glucocorticoid receptor at the CRE-Like and composite GRE sites of thyrotrophin-releasing hormone gene promoter. *J Neuroendocrinol*, Vol. 22, No. 4, (April 2010), pp. (282-293).

Eide, D.J. (2004). The SLC39 family of metal ion transporters. *Pflugers Arch*, Vol. 447, No. 5, (February 2004), pp. (796-800).

Espinosa, V.P.; Ferrini, M.; Shen, X.; Lutfy, K.; Nillni, E.A. & Friedman, T.C. (2007). Cellular colocalization and coregulation between hypothalamic pro-TRH and prohormone convertases in hypothyroidism. *Am J Physiol Endocrinol Metab*, Vol. 292, No. 1, (January 2007), pp. (E175-E186).

Essatara, M.B.; Levine, A.S.; Morley, J.E. & McClain, C.J. (1984). Zinc deficiency and anorexia in rats: normal feeding patterns and stress induced feeding. *Physiol Behav*, Vol. 32, No. 3, (March 1984), pp. (469-474).

Evans, R.M. (1988). The steroid and thyroid hormone receptor superfamily. *Science*, Vol. 240, No. 4854, (May 1988), pp. (889-895).

Evans, S.A.; Overton, J.M.; Alshingiti, A. & Levenson, C.W. (2004). Regulation of metabolic rate and substrate utilization by zinc deficiency. *Metabolism*, Vol. 53, No. 6, (June 2004), pp. (727-732).

Fekete, C.; Gereben, B.; Doleschall, M.; Harney, J.W.; Dora, J.M.; Bianco, A.C.; Sarkar, S.; Liposits, Z.; Rand, W.; Emerson, C. and others (2004). Lipopolysaccharide induces type 2 iodothyronine deiodinase in the mediobasal hypothalamus: implications for the nonthyroidal illness syndrome. *Endocrinology*, Vol. 145, No. 4, (April 2004), pp. (1649-1655).

Fekete, C.; Kelly, J.; Mihaly, E.; Sarkar, S.; Rand, W.M.; Legradi, G.; Emerson, C.H. & Lechan, R.M. (2001). Neuropeptide Y has a central inhibitory action on the hypothalamic-pituitary-thyroid axis. *Endocrinology*, Vol. 142, No. 6, (June 2001), pp. (2606-2613).

Fekete, C.; Legradi, G.; Mihaly, E.; Tatro, J.B.; Rand, W.M. & Lechan, R.M. (2000a). alpha-Melanocyte stimulating hormone prevents fasting-induced suppression of corticotropin-releasing hormone gene expression in the rat hypothalamic paraventricular nucleus. *Neurosci Lett*, Vol. 289, No. 2, (August 2000), pp. (152-156).

Fekete, C.; Mihaly, E.; Luo, L.G.; Kelly, J.; Clausen, J.T.; Mao, Q.; Rand, W.M.; Moss, L.G.; Kuhar, M.; Emerson, C.H. and others (2000b). Association of cocaine- and amphetamine-regulated transcript-immunoreactive elements with thyrotropin-releasing hormone-synthesizing neurons in the hypothalamic paraventricular nucleus and its role in the regulation of the hypothalamic-pituitary-thyroid axis during fasting. *J Neurosci*, Vol. 20, No. 24, (December 2000), pp. (9224-9234).

Fekete, C.; Sarkar, S.; Rand, W.M.; Harney, J.W.; Emerson, C.H.; Bianco, A.C. & Lechan, R.M. (2002). Agouti-related protein (AGRP) has a central inhibitory action on the hypothalamic-pituitary-thyroid (HPT) axis; comparisons between the effect of AGRP and neuropeptide Y on energy homeostasis and the HPT axis. *Endocrinology*, Vol. 143, No. 10, (October 2002), pp. (3846-3853).

Fliers, E.; Alkemade, A. & Wiersinga, W.M. (2001). The hypothalamic-pituitary-thyroid axis in critical illness. *Best Pract Res Clin Endocrinol Metab*, Vol. 15, No. 4, (December 2001), pp. (453-464).

Fliers, E.; Guldenaar, S.E.; Wiersinga, W.M. & Swaab, D.F. (1997). Decreased hypothalamic thyrotropin-releasing hormone gene expression in patients with nonthyroidal illness. *J Clin Endocrinol Metab*, Vol. 82, No. 12, (December 1997), pp. (4032-4036).

Freeman, M.E.; Kanyicska, B.; Lerant, A. & Nagy, G. (2000). Prolactin: structure, function, and regulation of secretion. *Physiol Rev*, Vol. 80, No. 4, (October 2000), pp. (1523-1631).

Friedman, T.C.; Yanovski, J.A.; Jayasvasti, V.; Yanovski, S.Z.; Koenig, R.J. & Wilk, S. (1995). Pyroglutamyl peptidase-II ("thyroliberinase") activity in human serum: influence of weight and thyroid status. *J Clin Endocrinol Metab*, Vol. 80, No. 4, (April 1995), pp. (1086-1089).

Gaetke, L.M.; Frederich, R.C.; Oz, H.S. & McClain, C.J. (2002). Decreased food intake rather than zinc deficiency is associated with changes in plasma leptin, metabolic rate, and activity levels in zinc deficient rats(small star, filled). *J Nutr Biochem*, Vol. 13, No. 4, (April 2002), pp. (237-244).

Garcia-Belenguer, S.; Oliver, C. & Mormede, P. (1993). Facilitation and feedback in the hypothalamo-pituitary-adrenal axis during food restriction in rats. *J Neuroendocrinol*, Vol. 5, No. 6, (December 1993), pp. (663-668).

García-Luna, C.; Amaya, MI.; Alvarez-Salas, E.; de Gortari, P. (2010). Prepro-orexin and feeding-related peptides receptors expression in dehydration-induced anorexia. *Regul Pept*, Vol.159, No. 1-3, (January 2010), pp. (54-60).

Grosvenor, C.E. & Mena, F. (1980). Evidence that thyrotropin-releasing hormone and a hypothalamic prolactin-releasing factor may function in the release of prolactin in the lactating rat. *Endocrinology*, Vol. 107, No. 4, (October 1980), pp. (863-868).

Grunfeld, C.; Zhao, C.; Fuller, J.; Pollack, A.; Moser, A.; Friedman, J. & Feingold, K.R. (1996). Endotoxin and cytokines induce expression of leptin, the ob gene product, in hamsters. *J Clin Invest*, Vol. 97, No. 9, (May 1996), pp. (2152-2157).

Harris, A.R.; Christianson, D.; Smith, M.S.; Fang, S.L.; Braverman, L.E. & Vagenakis, A.G. (F1978). The physiological role of thyrotropin-releasing hormone in the regulation of thyroid-stimulating hormone and prolactin secretion in the rat. *J Clin Invest*, Vol. 61, No. 2, (February 1978), pp. (441-448).

Harris, M.; Aschkenasi, C.; Elias, C.F.; Chandrankunnel, A.; Nillni, E.A.; Bjoorbaek, C.; Elmquist, J.K.; Flier, J.S. & Hollenberg, A.N. (2001). Transcriptional regulation of the thyrotropin-releasing hormone gene by leptin and melanocortin signaling. *J Clin Invest*, Vol. 107, No. 1, (January 2001), pp. (111-120).

Heuer, H.; Schafer, M.K.; O'Donnell, D.; Walker, P. & Bauer, K. (2000). Expression of thyrotropin-releasing hormone receptor 2 (TRH-R2) in the central nervous system of rats. *J Comp Neurol*, Vol. 428, No. 2, (December 2000), pp. (319-336).

Hoadley, J.E.; Leinart, A.S. & Cousins, R.J. (1987). Kinetic analysis of zinc uptake and serosal transfer by vascularly perfused rat intestine. *Am J Physiol*, Vol. 252, No. 6 Pt 1, (June 1987), pp. (G825-G831).

Horita, A. (1998). An update on the CNS actions of TRH and its analogs. *Life Sci*, Vol. 62, No. 17-18, (1998), pp. (1443-1448).

Imaki, T.; Naruse, M.; Harada, S.; Chikada, N.; Imaki, J.; Onodera, H.; Demura, H. & Vale, W. (1996). Corticotropin-releasing factor up-regulates its own receptor mRNA in the paraventricular nucleus of the hypothalamus. *Brain Res Mol Brain Res*, Vol. 38, No. 1, (May 1996), pp. (166-170).

Ishikawa, K.; Taniguchi, Y.; Inoue, K.; Kurosumi, K. & Suzuki, M. (1988). Immunocytochemical delineation of thyrotrophic area: origin of thyrotropin-releasing hormone in the median eminence. *Neuroendocrinology*, Vol. 47, No. 5, (May 1988), pp. (384-388).

Ishikawa, K.; Taniguchi, Y.; Kurosumi, K. & Suzuki, M. (1986). Origin of septal thyrotropin-releasing hormone in the rat. *Neuroendocrinology*, Vol. 44, No. 1, (1986), pp. (54-58).

Isse, T.; Ueta, Y.; Serino, R.; Noguchi, J.; Yamamoto, Y.; Nomura, M.; Shibuya, I.; Lightman, S.L. & Yamashita, H. (1999). Effects of leptin on fasting-induced inhibition of neuronal nitric oxide synthase mRNA in the paraventricular and supraoptic nuclei of rats. *Brain Res*, Vol. 846, No. 2, (November 1999), pp. (229-235).

Jaimes-Hoy, L.; Joseph-Bravo, P. & de, G.P. (2008). Differential response of TRHergic neurons of the hypothalamic paraventricular nucleus (PVN) in female animals submitted to food-restriction or dehydration-induced anorexia and cold exposure. *Horm Behav*, Vol. 53, No. 2, (February 2008), pp. (366-377).

Jaszberenyi, M.; Bujdoso, E.; Kiss, E.; Pataki, I. & Telegdy, G. (2002). The role of NPY in the mediation of orexin-induced hypothermia. *Regul Pept*, Vol. 104, No. 1-3, (March 2002), pp. (55-59).

Karydis, I. & Tolis, G. (1998). Orexis, anorexia, and thyrotropin-releasing hormone. *Thyroid*, Vol. 8, No. 10, (October 1998), pp. (947-950).

Kasarskis EJ; Sparks DL & Slevin JT (1996). Changes in hypothalamic noradrenergic systems during the anorexia of zinc deficiency. *Biological Trace Element Research*, Vol. 9, No. 1, (1996), pp. (25-35).

Kawano, H.; Tsuruo, Y.; Bando, H. & Daikoku, S. (1991). Hypophysiotrophic TRH-producing neurons identified by combining immunohistochemistry for pro-TRH and retrograde tracing. *J Comp Neurol*, Vol. 307, No. 4, (May 1991), pp. (531-538).

Kelleher, S.L. & Lonnerdal, B. (2002). Zinc transporters in the rat mammary gland respond to marginal zinc and vitamin A intakes during lactation. *J Nutr*, Vol. 132, No. 11, (November 2002), pp. (3280-3285).

Kelly, A.B. & Watts, A.G. (1996). Mediation of dehydration-induced peptidergic gene expression in the rat lateral hypothalamic area by forebrain afferent projections. *J Comp Neurol*, Vol. 370, No. 2, (June 1996), pp. (231-246).

Krahn, D.D.; Gosnell, B.A. & Majchrzak, M.J. (1990). The anorectic effects of CRH and restraint stress decrease with repeated exposures. *Biol Psychiatry*, Vol. 27, No. 10, (May 1990), pp. (1094-1102).

Kralik, A.; Eder, K. & Kirchgessner, M. (1996). Influence of zinc and selenium deficiency on parameters relating to thyroid hormone metabolism. *Horm Metab Res*, Vol. 28, No. 5, (May 1996), pp. (223-226).

Krebs, N.F. (1998). Zinc supplementation during lactation. *Am J Clin Nutr*, Vol. 68, No. 2 Suppl, (August 1998), pp. (509S-512S).

Lechan RM & Hollenberg A (2003). Thyrotropin-releasing hormone (TRH), In: *Encyclopedia of Hormones*, Henry H.L. & Norman A.W., (Ed.), pp. (510-524), Academic Press, ISBN 0-12-341103-3, San Diego, CA

Lechan, R.M. & Fekete, C. (2004). Feedback regulation of thyrotropin-releasing hormone (TRH): mechanisms for the non-thyroidal illness syndrome. *J Endocrinol Invest*, Vol. 27, No. 6 Suppl, (2004), pp. (105-119).

Lechan, R.M. & Fekete, C. (2005). Role of thyroid hormone deiodination in the hypothalamus. *Thyroid*, Vol. 15, No. 8, (August 2005), pp. (883-897).

Lechan, R.M. & Fekete, C. (2006). The TRH neuron: a hypothalamic integrator of energy metabolism. *Prog Brain Res*, Vol. 153, No. 2006), pp. (209-235).

Lechan, R.M. & Kakucska, I. (1992). Feedback regulation of thyrotropin-releasing hormone gene expression by thyroid hormone in the hypothalamic paraventricular nucleus. *Ciba Found Symp*, Vol. 168, No. 1992), pp. (144-158).

LeFeuvre, R.A.; Rothwell, N.J. & Stock, M.J. (1987). Activation of brown fat thermogenesis in response to central injection of corticotropin releasing hormone in the rat. *Neuropharmacology*, Vol. 26, No. 8, (August 1987), pp. (1217-1221).

Legradi, G.; Emerson, C.H.; Ahima, R.S.; Flier, J.S. & Lechan, R.M. (1997). Leptin prevents fasting-induced suppression of prothyrotropin-releasing hormone messenger ribonucleic acid in neurons of the hypothalamic paraventricular nucleus. *Endocrinology*, Vol. 138, No. 6, (June 1997), pp. (2569-2576).

Legradi, G. & Lechan, R.M. (1998). The arcuate nucleus is the major source for neuropeptide Y-innervation of thyrotropin-releasing hormone neurons in the hypothalamic paraventricular nucleus. *Endocrinology*, Vol. 139, No. 7, (July 1998), pp. (3262-3270).

Levin, B.E. (2006). Central regulation of energy homeostasis intelligent design: how to build the perfect survivor. *Obesity (Silver Spring)*, Vol. 14 Suppl 5, No. August 2006), pp. (192S-196S).

Li, Q.L.; Jansen, E.; Brent, G.A.; Naqvi, S.; Wilber, J.F. & Friedman, T.C. (2000). Interactions between the prohormone convertase 2 promoter and the thyroid hormone receptor. *Endocrinology*, Vol. 141, No. 9, (September 2000), pp. (3256-3266).

Li, Q.L.; Jansen, E. & Friedman, T.C. (1999). Regulation of prohormone convertase 1 (PC1) by gp130-related cytokines. *Mol Cell Endocrinol*, Vol. 158, No. 1-2, (December 1999), pp. (143-152).

Lin, L.; Faraco, J.; Li, R.; Kadotani, H.; Rogers, W.; Lin, X.; Qiu, X.; de Jong, P.J.; Nishino, S. & Mignot, E. (1999). The sleep disorder canine narcolepsy is caused by a mutation in the hypocretin (orexin) receptor 2 gene. *Cell*, Vol. 98, No. 3, (August 1999), pp. (365-376).

Liuzzi, J.P. & Cousins, R.J. (2004). Mammalian zinc transporters. *Annu Rev Nutr*, Vol. 24, No. 2004), pp. (151-172).

Mahajan, S.D.; Aalinkeel, R.; Singh, S.; Shah, P.; Gupta, N. & Kochupillai, N. (2005). Thyroid hormone dysregulation in intrauterine growth retardation associated with maternal malnutrition and/or anemia. *Horm Metab Res*, Vol. 37, No. 10, (October 2005), pp. (633-640).

Makino, S.; Nishiyama, M.; Asaba, K.; Gold, P.W. & Hashimoto, K. (1998). Altered expression of type 2 CRH receptor mRNA in the VMH by glucocorticoids and starvation. *Am J Physiol*, Vol. 275, No. 4 Pt 2, (October 1998), pp. (R1138-R1145).

Mansi, J.A.; Rivest, S. & Drolet, G. (1996). Regulation of corticotropin-releasing factor type 1 (CRF1) receptor messenger ribonucleic acid in the paraventricular nucleus of rat hypothalamus by exogenous CRF. *Endocrinology*, Vol. 137, No. 11, (November 1996), pp. (4619-4629).

Merchenthaler, I. & Liposits, Z. (1994). Mapping of thyrotropin-releasing hormone (TRH) neuronal systems of rat forebrain projecting to the median eminence and the OVLT. Immunocytochemistry combined with retrograde labeling at the light and electron microscopic levels. *Acta Biol Hung*, Vol. 45, No. 2-4, (1994), pp. (361-374).

Mitev, Y.; Almeida, O.F. & Patchev, V. (1993). Pituitary-adrenal function and hypothalamic beta-endorphin release in vitro following food deprivation. *Brain Res Bull*, Vol. 30, No. 1-2, (1993), pp. (7-10).

Mitsuma, T.; Hirooka, Y.; Mori, Y.; Kayama, M.; Adachi, K.; Rhue, N.; Ping, J. & Nogimori, T. (1999). Effects of orexin A on thyrotropin-releasing hormone and thyrotropin secretion in rats. *Horm Metab Res*, Vol. 31, No. 11, (November 1999), pp. (606-609).

Miyamoto, T.; Sakurai, A. & DeGroot, L.J. (1991). Effects of zinc and other divalent metals on deoxyribonucleic acid binding and hormone-binding activity of human alpha 1 thyroid hormone receptor expressed in Escherichia coli. *Endocrinology*, Vol. 129, No. 6, (December 1991), pp. (3027-3033).

Moore, M.E.; Moran, J.R. & Greene, H.L. (1984). Zinc supplementation in lactating women: evidence for mammary control of zinc secretion. *J Pediatr*, Vol. 105, No. 4, (October 1984), pp. (600-602).

Morley, J.E.; Gordon, J. & Hershman, J.M. (1980). Zinc deficiency, chronic starvation, and hypothalamic-pituitary-thyroid function. *Am J Clin Nutr*, Vol. 33, No. 8, (August 1980), pp. (1767-1770).

Morley, J.E. & Levine, A.S. (1980). Thyrotropin releasing hormone (TRH) suppresses stress induced eating. *Life Sci*, Vol. 27, No. 3, (July 1980), pp. (269-274).

Morley, J.E. & Levine, A.S. (1982). Corticotrophin releasing factor, grooming and ingestive behavior. *Life Sci*, Vol. 31, No. 14, (October 1982), pp. (1459-1464).

Morrison, S.F.; Nakamura, K. & Madden, C.J. (July 2008). Central control of thermogenesis in mammals. *Exp Physiol*, Vol. 93, No. 7, (July 2008), pp. (773-797).

Morton, G.J.; Cummings, D.E.; Baskin, D.G.; Barsh, G.S. & Schwartz, M.W. (2006). Central nervous system control of food intake and body weight. *Nature*, Vol. 443, No. 7109, (September 2006), pp. (289-295).

Moser-Veillon, P.B. (1995). Zinc needs and homeostasis during lactation. *Analyst*, Vol. 120, No. 3, (March 1995), pp. (895-897).

Murgia, C.; Vespignani, I.; Cerase, J.; Nobili, F. & Perozzi, G. (1999). Cloning, expression, and vesicular localization of zinc transporter Dri 27/ZnT4 in intestinal tissue and cells. *Am J Physiol*, Vol. 277, No. 6 Pt 1, (December 1999), pp. (G1231-G1239).

Muroya, S.; Funahashi, H.; Yamanaka, A.; Kohno, D.; Uramura, K.; Nambu, T.; Shibahara, M.; Kuramochi, M.; Takigawa, M.; Yanagisawa, M. and others (2004). Orexins (hypocretins) directly interact with neuropeptide Y, POMC and glucose-responsive neurons to regulate Ca 2+ signaling in a reciprocal manner to leptin: orexigenic neuronal pathways in the mediobasal hypothalamus. *Eur J Neurosci*, Vol. 19, No. 6, (March 2004), pp. (1524-1534).

Nillni, E.A. (2010). Regulation of the hypothalamic thyrotropin releasing hormone (TRH) neuron by neuronal and peripheral inputs. *Front Neuroendocrinol*, Vol. 31, No. 2, (April 2010), pp. (134-156).

Nillni, E.A.; Friedman, T.C.; Todd, R.B.; Birch, N.P.; Loh, Y.P. & Jackson, I.M. (1995). Pro-thyrotropin-releasing hormone processing by recombinant PC1. *J Neurochem*, Vol. 65, No. 6, (December 1995), pp. (2462-2472).

Nillni, E.A.; Luo, L.G.; Jackson, I.M. & McMillan, P. (1996). Identification of the thyrotropin-releasing hormone precursor, its processing products, and its coexpression with convertase 1 in primary cultures of hypothalamic neurons: anatomic distribution of PC1 and PC2. *Endocrinology*, Vol. 137, No. 12, (December 1996), pp. (5651-5661).

Nillni, E.A.; Vaslet, C.; Harris, M.; Hollenberg, A.; Bjorbak, C. & Flier, J.S. (2000). Leptin regulates prothyrotropin-releasing hormone biosynthesis. Evidence for direct and indirect pathways. *J Biol Chem*, Vol. 275, No. 46, (November 2000), pp. (36124-36133).

Nishiyama, T.; Kawano, H.; Tsuruo, Y.; Maegawa, M.; Hisano, S.; Adachi, T.; Daikoku, S. & Suzuki, M. (1985). Hypothalamic thyrotropin-releasing hormone (TRH)-containing neurons involved in the hypothalamic-hypophysial-thyroid axis. Light microscopic immunohistochemistry. *Brain Res*, Vol. 345, No. 2, (October 1985), pp. (205-218).

O'Mara, B.A.; Dittrich, W.; Lauterio, T.J. & St Germain, D.L. (1993). Pretranslational regulation of type I 5'-deiodinase by thyroid hormones and in fasted and diabetic rats. *Endocrinology*, Vol. 133, No. 4, (October 1993), pp. (1715-1723).

Ogden, C.L.; Carroll, M.D.; McDowell, M.A. & Flegal, K.M. (2007a). Obesity among adults in the United States--no statistically significant chance since 2003-2004. *NCHS Data Brief*, Vol. 1, (November 2007), pp. (1-8).

Ogden, C.L.; Yanovski, S.Z.; Carroll, M.D. & Flegal, K.M. (2007b). The epidemiology of obesity. *Gastroenterology*, Vol. 132, No. 6, (May 2007), pp. (2087-2102).

Pekary, A.E.; Lukaski, H.C.; Mena, I. & Hershman, J.M. (September 1991). Processing of TRH precursor peptides in rat brain and pituitary is zinc dependent. *Peptides*, Vol. 12, No. 5, (September 1991), pp. (1025-1032).

Pelleymounter, M.A.; Cullen, M.J.; Baker, M.B.; Hecht, R.; Winters, D.; Boone, T. & Collins, F. (1995). Effects of the obese gene product on body weight regulation in ob/ob mice. *Science*, Vol. 269, No. 5223, (July 1995), pp. (540-543).

Perello, M.; Friedman, T.; Paez-Espinosa, V.; Shen, X.; Stuart, R.C. & Nillni, E.A. (2006). Thyroid hormones selectively regulate the posttranslational processing of prothyrotropin-releasing hormone in the paraventricular nucleus of the hypothalamus. *Endocrinology*, Vol. 147, No. 6, (June 2006), pp. (2705-2716).

Peyron, C.; Tighe, D.K.; van den Pol, A.N.; de, L.L.; Heller, H.C.; Sutcliffe, J.G. & Kilduff, T.S. (1998). Neurons containing hypocretin (orexin) project to multiple neuronal systems. *J Neurosci*, Vol. 18, No. 23, (December 1998), pp. (9996-10015).

Ponce, G.; Charli, J.L.; Pasten, J.A.; Aceves, C. & Joseph-Bravo, P. (1988). Tissue-specific regulation of pyroglutamate aminopeptidase II activity by thyroid hormones. *Neuroendocrinology*, Vol. 48, No. 2, (August 1988), pp. (211-213).

Prasad, A.S. (1984). Discovery and importance of zinc in human nutrition. *Fed Proc*, Vol. 43, No. 13, (October 1984), pp. (2829-2834).

Prokai, L. (2002). Central nervous system effects of thyrotropin-releasing hormone and its analogues: opportunities and perspectives for drug discovery and development. *Prog Drug Res*, Vol. 59, No. 2002), pp. (133-169).

Rabadan-Diehl, C.; Kiss, A.; Camacho, C. & Aguilera, G. (1996). Regulation of messenger ribonucleic acid for corticotropin releasing hormone receptor in the pituitary during stress. *Endocrinology*, Vol. 137, No. 9, (September 1996), pp. (3808-3814).

Rains, T.M.; Hedrick, S.; Randall, A.C.; Lee, R.G.; Kennedy, K.J. & Shay, N.F. (1998). Food intake patterns are altered during long-term zinc deficiency in rats. *Physiol Behav*, Vol. 65, No. 3, (December 1998), pp. (473-478).

Reeves, P.G.; Briske-Anderson, M. & Johnson, L. (December 2001). Pre-treatment of Caco-2 cells with zinc during the differentiation phase alters the kinetics of zinc uptake and transport(2). *J Nutr Biochem*, Vol. 12, No. 12, (December 2001), pp. (674-684).

Reichlin S; Martin JB & Jackson IMD (1978). Regulation of thyroid-stimulating hormone (TSH) secretion., In: *The endocrine hypothalamus*, Jeffcoste AL & Hutchinson JSM, (Ed.), pp. (229-269), Academic Press Inc., ISBN 0-12-382150-9, London, UK.

Rondeel, J.M.; Heide, R.; de Greef, W.J.; van, T.H.; van Haasteren, G.A.; Klootwijk, W. & Visser, T.J. (1992). Effect of starvation and subsequent refeeding on thyroid function and release of hypothalamic thyrotropin-releasing hormone. *Neuroendocrinology*, Vol. 56, No. 3, (September 1992), pp. (348-353).

Sakurai, T.; Amemiya, A.; Ishii, M.; Matsuzaki, I.; Chemelli, R.M.; Tanaka, H.; Williams, S.C.; Richarson, J.A.; Kozlowski, G.P.; Wilson, S. and others (1998). Orexins and orexin receptors: a family of hypothalamic neuropeptides and G protein-coupled receptors that regulate feeding behavior. *Cell*, Vol. 92, No. 5, (March 1998), pp. (1-

Sanchez, E.; Uribe, R.M.; Corkidi, G.; Zoeller, R.T.; Cisneros, M.; Zacarias, M.; Morales-Chapa, C.; Charli, J.L. & Joseph-Bravo, P. (2001). Differential responses of thyrotropin-releasing hormone (TRH) neurons to cold exposure or suckling indicate functional heterogeneity of the TRH system in the paraventricular nucleus of the rat hypothalamus. *Neuroendocrinology*, Vol. 74, No. 6, (December 2001), pp. (407-422).

Sawchenko, P.E. & Swanson, L.W. (1982). The organization of noradrenergic pathways from the brainstem to the paraventricular and supraoptic nuclei in the rat. *Brain Res*, Vol. 257, No. 3, (November 1982), pp. (275-325).

Scalabrino, G.A.; Hogan, N.; O'Boyle, K.M.; Slator, G.R.; Gregg, D.J.; Fitchett, C.M.; Draper, S.M.; Bennett, G.W.; Hinkle, P.M.; Bauer, K. and others (2007). Discovery of a dual action first-in-class peptide that mimics and enhances CNS-mediated actions of thyrotropin-releasing hormone. *Neuropharmacology*, Vol. 52, No. 7, (June 2007), pp. (1472-1481).

Schaner, P.; Todd, R.B.; Seidah, N.G. & Nillni, E.A. (1997). Processing of prothyrotropin-releasing hormone by the family of prohormone convertases. *J Biol Chem*, Vol. 272, No. 32, (August 1997), pp. (19958-19968).

Schomburg, L. & Bauer, K. (1995). Thyroid hormones rapidly and stringently regulate the messenger RNA levels of the thyrotropin-releasing hormone (TRH) receptor and the TRH-degrading ectoenzyme. *Endocrinology*, Vol. 136, No. 8, (August 1995), pp. (3480-3485).

Schuhler, S.; Warner, A.; Finney, N.; Bennett, G.W.; Ebling, F.J. & Brameld, J.M. (2007). Thyrotrophin-releasing hormone decreases feeding and increases body temperature, activity and oxygen consumption in Siberian hamsters. *J Neuroendocrinol*, Vol. 19, No. 4, (April 2007), pp. (239-249).

Schwartz, M.W.; Seeley, R.J.; Campfield, L.A.; Burn, P. & Baskin, D.G. (1996). Identification of targets of leptin action in rat hypothalamus. *J Clin Invest*, Vol. 98, No. 5, (September 1996), pp. (1101-1106).

Seal, C.J. & Mathers, J.C. (1989). Intestinal zinc transfer by everted gut sacs from rats given diets containing different amounts and types of dietary fibre. *Br J Nutr*, Vol. 62, No. 1, (July 1989), pp. (151-163).

Segerson, T.P.; Kauer, J.; Wolfe, H.C.; Mobtaker, H.; Wu, P.; Jackson, I.M. & Lechan, R.M. (1987). Thyroid hormone regulates TRH biosynthesis in the paraventricular nucleus of the rat hypothalamus. *Science*, Vol. 238, No. 4823, (October 1987), pp. (78-80).

Selvais, P.L.; Labuche, C.; Nguyen, X.N.; Ketelslegers, J.M.; Denef, J.F. & Maiter, D.M. (1997). Cyclic feeding behaviour and changes in hypothalamic galanin and neuropeptide Y gene expression induced by zinc deficiency in the rat. *J Neuroendocrinol*, Vol. 9, No. 1, (January 1997), pp. (55-62).

Sergeyev, V.; Broberger, C. & Hokfelt, T. (2001). Effect of LPS administration on the expression of POMC, NPY, galanin, CART and MCH mRNAs in the rat hypothalamus. *Brain Res Mol Brain Res*, Vol. 90, No. 2, (June 2001), pp. (93-100).

Shah, D. & Sachdev, H.P. (2001). Effect of gestational zinc deficiency on pregnancy outcomes: summary of observation studies and zinc supplementation trials. *Br J Nutr*, Vol. 85 Suppl 2, No. May 2001), pp. (S101-S108).

Shen, X.; Li, Q.L.; Brent, G.A. & Friedman, T.C. (2005). Regulation of regional expression in rat brain PC2 by thyroid hormone/characterization of novel negative thyroid hormone response elements in the PC2 promoter. *Am J Physiol Endocrinol Metab*, Vol. 288, No. 1, (January 2005), pp. (E236-E245).

Siegel, J.M. (1999). Narcolepsy: a key role for hypocretins (orexins). *Cell*, Vol. 98, No. 4, (August 1999), pp. (409-412).

Siegfried, Z.; Berry, E.M.; Hao, S. & Avraham, Y. (2003). Animal models in the investigation of anorexia. *Physiol Behav*, Vol. 79, No. 1, (June 2003), pp. (39-45).

Smagin, G.N.; Howell, L.A.; Ryan, D.H.; De Souza, E.B. & Harris, R.B. (1998). The role of CRF2 receptors in corticotropin-releasing factor- and urocortin-induced anorexia. *Neuroreport*, Vol. 9, No. 7, (May 1998), pp. (1601-1606).

St Germain, D.L. & Galton, V.A. (1985). Comparative study of pituitary-thyroid hormone economy in fasting and hypothyroid rats. *J Clin Invest*, Vol. 75, No. 2, (February 1985), pp. (679-688).

Steward, C.A.; Horan, T.L.; Schuhler, S.; Bennett, G.W. & Ebling, F.J. (2003). Central administration of thyrotropin releasing hormone (TRH) and related peptides inhibits feeding behavior in the Siberian hamster. *Neuroreport*, Vol. 14, No. 5, (April 2003), pp. (687-691).

Stoving, R.K.; Hangaard, J. & Hagen, C. (2001). Update on endocrine disturbances in anorexia nervosa. *J Pediatr Endocrinol Metab*, Vol. 14, No. 5, (May 2001), pp. (459-480).

Suzuki, T.; Kohno, H.; Sakurada, T.; Tadano, T. & Kisara, K. (1982). Intracranial injection of thyrotropin releasing hormone (TRH) suppresses starvation-induced feeding and drinking in rats. *Pharmacol Biochem Behav*, Vol. 17, No. 2, (August 1982), pp. (249-253).

Tacnet, F.; Watkins, D.W. & Ripoche, P. (1990). Studies of zinc transport into brush-border membrane vesicles isolated from pig small intestine. *Biochim Biophys Acta*, Vol. 1024, No. 2, (May 1990), pp. (323-330).

Tamai, H.; Mori, K.; Matsubayashi, S.; Kiyohara, K.; Nakagawa, T.; Okimura, M.C.; Walter, R.M., Jr.; Kumagai, L.F. & Nagataki, S. (1986). Hypothalamic-pituitary-thyroidal dysfunctions in anorexia nervosa. *Psychother Psychosom*, Vol. 46, No. 3, (1986), pp. (127-131).

Toni, R. & Lechan, R.M. (1993). Neuroendocrine regulation of thyrotropin-releasing hormone (TRH) in the tuberoinfundibular system. *J Endocrinol Invest*, Vol. 16, No. 9, (October 1993), pp. (715-753).

Turnbull, A.V. & Rivier, C. (1997). Corticotropin-releasing factor (CRF) and endocrine responses to stress: CRF receptors, binding protein, and related peptides. *Proc Soc Exp Biol Med*, Vol. 215, No. 1, (May 1997), pp. (1-10).

Valcavi, R.; Zini, M.; Peino, R.; Casanueva, F.F. & Dieguez, C. (1997). Influence of thyroid status on serum immunoreactive leptin levels. *J Clin Endocrinol Metab*, Vol. 82, No. 5, (May 1997), pp. (1632-1634).

Vallee, B.L. (1977). Zinc biochemistry in normal and neoplastic growth processes. *Experientia*, Vol. 33, No. 5, (May 1977), pp. (600-601).

Vallee, B.L. & Falchuk, K.H. (1993). The biochemical basis of zinc physiology. *Physiol Rev*, Vol. 73, No. 1, (January 1993), pp. (79-118).

Van den Berghe, G.; de, Z.F.; Baxter, R.C.; Veldhuis, J.D.; Wouters, P.; Schetz, M.; Verwaest, C.; Van, d., V; Lauwers, P.; Bouillon, R. and others (1998). Neuroendocrinology of prolonged critical illness: effects of exogenous thyrotropin-releasing hormone and its combination with growth hormone secretagogues. *J Clin Endocrinol Metab*, Vol. 83, No. 2, (February 1998), pp. (309-319).

Van den Berghe, G.; Wouters, P.; Weekers, F.; Mohan, S.; Baxter, R.C.; Veldhuis, J.D.; Bowers, C.Y. & Bouillon, R. (1999). Reactivation of pituitary hormone release and metabolic improvement by infusion of growth hormone-releasing peptide and thyrotropin-releasing hormone in patients with protracted critical illness. *J Clin Endocrinol Metab*, Vol. 84, No. 4, (April 1999), pp. (1311-1323).

van Haasteren, G.A.; Linkels, E.; Klootwijk, W.; van, T.H.; Rondeel, J.M.; Themmen, A.P.; de Jong, F.H.; Valentijn, K.; Vaudry, H.; Bauer, K. and others (1995). Starvation-induced changes in the hypothalamic content of prothyrotrophin-releasing hormone (proTRH) mRNA and the hypothalamic release of proTRH-derived peptides: role of the adrenal gland. *J Endocrinol*, Vol. 145, No. 1, (April 1995), pp. (143-153).

van Doom, J.; van der Heide, D. & Roelfsema, F. (1984). The influence of partial food deprivation on the quantity and source of triiodothyronine in several tissues of athyreotic thyroxine-maintained rats. *Endocrinology*, Vol. 115, No. 2, (August 1984), pp. (705-711).

Vargas, M.; Mendez, M.; Cisneros, M.; Joseph-Bravo, P. & Charli, J.L. (1987). Regional distribution of the membrane-bound pyroglutamate amino peptidase-degrading thyrotropin-releasing hormone in rat brain. *Neurosci Lett*, Vol. 79, No. 3, (August 1987), pp. (311-314).

Vargas, M.A.; Bourdais, J.; Sanchez, S.; Uriostegui, B.; Moreno, E.; Joseph-Bravo, P. & Charli, J.L. (1998). Multiple hypothalamic factors regulate pyroglutamyl peptidase II in cultures of adenohypophyseal cells: role of the cAMP pathway. *J Neuroendocrinol*, Vol. 10, No. 3, (March 1998), pp. (199-206).

Vargas, M.A.; Joseph-Bravo, P. & Charli, J.L. (1994). Thyrotropin-releasing hormone downregulates pyroglutamyl peptidase II activity in adenohypophyseal cells. *Neuroendocrinology*, Vol. 60, No. 3, (September 1994), pp. (323-330).

Vermes, I. & Beishuizen, A. (2001). The hypothalamic-pituitary-adrenal response to critical illness. *Best Pract Res Clin Endocrinol Metab*, Vol. 15, No. 4, (December 2001), pp. (495-511).

Vijayan, E. & McCann, S.M. (1977). Suppression of feeding and drinking activity in rats following intraventricular injection of thyrotropin releasing hormone (TRH). *Endocrinology*, Vol. 100, No. 6, (June 1977), pp. (1727-1730).

Vogel, R.A.; Cooper, B.R.; Barlow, T.S.; Prange, A.J., Jr.; Mueller, R.A. & Breese, G.R. (1979). Effects of thyrotropin-releasing hormone on locomotor activity, operant performance and ingestive behavior. *J Pharmacol Exp Ther*, Vol. 208, No. 2, (February 1979), pp. (161-168).

Vrang, N.; Larsen, P.J.; Clausen, J.T. & Kristensen, P. (1999). Neurochemical characterization of hypothalamic cocaine- amphetamine-regulated transcript neurons. *J Neurosci*, Vol. 19, No. 10, (May 1999), pp. (RC5-

Warner, M.H. & Beckett, G.J. (2010). Mechanisms behind the non-thyroidal illness syndrome: an update. *J Endocrinol*, Vol. 205, No. 1, (April 2010), pp. (1-13).

Watts, A.G. (2001). Neuropeptides and the integration of motor responses to dehydration. *Annu Rev Neurosci*, Vol. 24, No. 2001), pp. (357-384).

Watts, A.G.; Salter, D.S. & Neuner, C.M. (2007). Neural network interactions and ingestive behavior control during anorexia. *Physiol Behav*, Vol. 91, No. 4, (July 2007), pp. (389-396).

Watts, A.G.; Sanchez-Watts, G. & Kelly, A.B. (1999). Distinct patterns of neuropeptide gene expression in the lateral hypothalamic area and arcuate nucleus are associated with dehydration-induced anorexia. *J Neurosci*, Vol. 19, No. 14, (July 1999), pp. (6111-6121).

Wiersinga WM & Boelen A (1996). Thyroid hormone metabolism in nonthyroidal illness. *Current Opinion in Endocrinology,Diabetes and Obesity*, Vol. 3, No. 5, (1996), pp. (422-427).

Williams, R.B. & Mills, C.F. (1970). The experimental production of zinc deficiency in the rat. *Br J Nutr*, Vol. 24, No. 4, (December 1970), pp. (989-1003).

Wittmann, G.; Fuzesi, T.; Singru, P.S.; Liposits, Z.; Lechan, R.M. & Fekete, C. (2009). Efferent projections of thyrotropin-releasing hormone-synthesizing neurons residing in the anterior parvocellular subdivision of the hypothalamic paraventricular nucleus. *J Comp Neurol*, Vol. 515, No. 3, (July 2009), pp. (313-330).

Woodward, C.J.; Hervey, G.R.; Oakey, R.E. & Whitaker, E.M. (1991). The effects of fasting on plasma corticosterone kinetics in rats. *Br J Nutr*, Vol. 66, No. 1, (July 1991), pp. (117-127).

Xie, X.M. & Smart, T.G. (1991). A physiological role for endogenous zinc in rat hippocampal synaptic neurotransmission. *Nature*, Vol. 349, No. 6309, (February 1991), pp. (521-524).

Xu, J.; Kirigiti, M.A.; Cowley, M.A.; Grove, K.L. & Smith, M.S. (2009). Suppression of basal spontaneous gonadotropin-releasing hormone neuronal activity during lactation: role of inhibitory effects of neuropeptide Y. *Endocrinology*, Vol. 150, No. 1, (January 2009), pp. (333-340).

Yamamoto, Y.; Ueta, Y.; Date, Y.; Nakazato, M.; Hara, Y.; Serino, R.; Nomura, M.; Shibuya, I.; Matsukura, S. & Yamashita, H. (1999). Down regulation of the prepro-orexin gene expression in genetically obese mice. *Brain Res Mol Brain Res*, Vol. 65, No. 1, (February 1999), pp. (14-22).

Yang, J. & Tashjian, A.H., Jr. (1993). Regulation of endogenous thyrotropin-releasing hormone (TRH) receptor messenger RNA by TRH in GH4C1 cells. *Mol Endocrinol*, Vol. 7, No. 6, (June 1993), pp. (753-758).

Yen, P.M. (2001). Physiological and molecular basis of thyroid hormone action. *Physiol Rev*, Vol. 81, No. 3, (July 2001), pp. (1097-1142).

4

Hypothyroidism After Hemithyroidectomy: Incidence, Risk Factors, Natural History and Management

Jandee Lee and Woong Youn Chung
Department of Surgery, Yonsei Univeristy College of Medicine
South Korea

1. Introduction

Thyroid lobectomy or hemithyroidectomy is considered an adequate treatment for several thyroid diseases such as large benign nodules, follicular neoplasm, and some suspected malignancies. Thyroid lobectomy theoretically preserves sufficient functioning native thyroid tissue for patients to keep euthyroid status postoperatively without the need for thyroid hormone replacement. Still, it is known that some patients who have undergone hemithyroidectomy will require thyroid hormone replacement because they have developed hypothyroidism, which is commonly diagnosed as a result of elevated levels of thyroid-stimulating hormone (TSH). Currently, the incidence and risk of hypothyroidism in patients undergoing partial thyroidectomy remains unclear. Several studies about thyroid function after hemithyroidectomy for benign thyroid disease have been published. The reported incidence of hypothyroidism ranges from 5% to 49%, with most between 15-30%. The incidence rates vary widely depending on the follow-up period and on how hypothyroidism is defined by authors. These variations have led to our interest in defining uniform criteria for diagnosis and treatment of postoperative hypothyroidism, thereby identifying patients at the greatest risk of requiring long-term thyroid hormone replacement.

Hypothyroidism after hemithyroidectomy remains an unpredictable complication. Several results have pointed to the degree of lymphocytic infiltration within the thyroid gland and the amount of thyroid remnant as possible predictors of hypothyroidism. Other reports about risk factors for hypothyroidism have indicated links to the preoperative TSH level, anti-TPO antibodies, multinodular goiter, and preoperative thyrotoxicosis. However, definite risk factors for development of hypothyroidism after hemithyroidectomy have yet to be completely characterized.

Patients with symptomatic hypothyroidism such as weight gain, fatigue, generalized edema, muscle pain and lethargy warrant treatment, as do patients with mild disease and medical comorbidities. Of late, some authors have advocated thyroxine replacement for all patients undergoing hemithyroidectomy to prevent progression of multi-nodular changes in the contralateral lobe, but others have asserted that it should not be necessary to prescribe thyroxine replacement for all patients. Patients who develop chronic hypothyroidism after hemithyroidectomy may require life-long thyroxine replacement, as well as routine laboratory tests. The side effects of long-term thyroid hormone replacement have included arrhythmias, osteopenia, changes of lipid metabolism, and mood changes. Early diagnosis of the subclinical state, followed by treatment of symptomatic hypothyroidism should be priorities.

The risk of postoperative hypothyroidism after thyroid lobectomy is not negligible and should not be overlooked. Careful monitoring for patients who may develop hypothyroidism will improve patient care. At present, there is no universal algorithm for monitoring postoperative residual thyroid function in patients who have undergone hemithyroidectomy. In most patients, the follow-up is dependent on the discretion of the physician in charge based on clinical suspicion or the development of definite symptoms. From a practical viewpoint, only select patients at risk of developing hypothyroidism after partial thyroidectomy have been followed on a regular schedule.

In this chapter, we evaluate the incidence, natural history, and risk factors for hypothyroidism in patients undergoing thyroid lobectomy, and we review postoperative thyroid hormone replacement. We also aim to clarify a uniform monitoring and follow-up protocol for patients after hemithyroidectomy.

2. Hypothyroidism after hemithyroidectomy

2.1 Definition of hypothyroidism

Thyroid hormones are essential regulators of metabolism and transport, and thyroid hormone deficiencies of any cause result in hypothyroidism. Hypothyroidism may be primary, i.e., resulting from a defect in the thyroid gland itself, or secondary, i.e., resulting from a TSH deficiency related to pituitary or hypothalamic disease. Although there is no universally accepted definition of normal thyroid function, thyroid function assays have indicated that a TSH concentration of 4.5 uIU/L is the upper limit of normal (Surks et al., 2004; Hollowell et al., 2002).

Thyroid hormone deficiency affects nearly all organs and functions in the human body (Laurberg et al., 2005). The changes induced by hypothyroidism include the slowing and lowering of processes, which may mimic the alterations associated with aging. Symptoms and signs of hypothyroidism differ according to the severity and duration of the thyroid deficiency, the age of the patient, and the occurrence of other systemic diseases. Early symptoms of hypothyroidism are often nonspecific and insidious in onset and can include fatigue, lethargy, constipation, cold intolerance, muscle stiffness and cramping, carpal tunnel syndrome, decreased libido, depression, hair loss, menstrual irregularity, menorrhagia, and infertility. With little functional thyroid reserve, the severity of hypothyroidism can progress to a clinical picture of myxedema. At this stage, patients appear bored, depressed, and hypokinetic, with a hoarse voice, dull, expressionless faces, sparse hair, and a large tongue. The skin is cool to the touch, dry, and rough, with facial and periorbital puffiness and often generalized edema. Fluid may collect in various parts of the body, and pleural effusion, pericardial effusion, and ascites are common. On physical examination or chest X-ray, the cardiac silhouette may appear enlarged, due to chamber dilatation or pericardial effusion. Constipation is common, due to slowed gastrointestinal motility, and a dynamic ileus may cause megacolon or intestinal obstruction. A psychiatric syndrome ("myxedema madness") has been described, and neurologic findings include a delayed or hung-up relaxation phase of deep tendon reflexes, muscle weakness, and ataxia (Wartofsky et al., 2006).

Hypothyroidism can be classified as subclinical or overt (clinical), with the latter defined as abnormal serum TSH and free T4 concentrations, or as the development of hypothyroidism symptoms. Subclinical hypothyroidism is a mild degree of biochemical abnormality, characterized by increased serum TSH and T4 estimates within the laboratory reference range (Wartofsky et al., 2006). Although the cause and clinical abnormalities observed in individuals with subclinical hypothyroidism do not differ from those with overt hypothyroidism, including high TSH and low T4 concentrations, the former is milder. Either form of hypothyroidism, however, is a potential consequence of hemithyroidectomy and has a substantial impact on postoperative patient outcomes and quality of life. Hypothyroidism occurring soon after thyroid surgery or radioiodine therapy may normalize spontaneously after some months. In these patients, partial substitution therapy or control for some months before therapy is appropriate. This chapter focuses only on overt or subclinical hypothyroidism following hemithyroidectomy.

2.2 Incidence

Hemithyroidectomy, defined as the complete removal of the unilateral lobe, isthmus and where present, the pyramidal lobe of the thyroid, is a relatively common procedure for a variety of thyroid pathologies. Hemithyroidectomy is commonly indicated for patients with large benign tumors causing compressive symptoms or cosmetic concerns, as well as for toxic nodules. It is also indicated for patients with follicular lesions classified as "indeterminate" thyroid nodules to exclude thyroid carcinoma, as long as these nodules do not show any clinical features of malignancy other than in fine needle aspiration cytology (FNAC) results. Thyroid lobectomy is performed in patients with indeterminate nodules because 20-30% of nodules harbor thyroid malignancy. Hemithyroidectomy and central compartment lymph node dissection (CCND) are also usually performed on patients in Korea and Japan with papillary thyroid microcarcinoma (PTMC) (Tomoda et al., 2011). The worldwide incidence of PTMC has increased significantly, probably due to more frequent use of thyroid ultrasonography (US) as an essential part of initial health examinations. Although total thyroidectomy is the most common standard operation for thyroid cancers, hemithyroidectomy rather than total thyroidectomy may be preferred for low risk patients with PTMC to eliminate the risks of permanent hypocalcemia and bilateral recurrent and superior laryngeal nerve palsy associated with total thyroidectomy. In addition, hemithyroidectomy theoretically leaves sufficient functioning native thyroid tissue for the patient to remain euthyroid without the need for thyroid hormone replacement.

Several studies have evaluated thyroid function after hemithyroidectomy for benign thyroid disease. The reported incidence of hypothyroidism after hemithyroidectomy has been found to vary from 5.0% to 49%, with most studies reporting a range of 15-30% (Wormald et al., 2008; Chu et al., 2011; Su et al, 2009; Spanheimer et al, 2011). This disparity in results is partially due to differences in their definition of hypothyroidism and to differences in length of follow-up. Hypothyroidism, both clinical and subclinical, is a potential consequence of hemithyroidectomy and has been associated with a number of adverse clinical outcomes. However, hypothyroidism after hemithyroidectomy is an under-reported or under-recognized complication, with patients most often monitored only for a short time postoperatively. Table 1 summarizes the incidence of hypothyroidism after hemithyroidectomy.

Author (year)	Patients (n)	Time for TSH measurement to determine postoperative hypothyroidism	Definition of postoperative hypothyroidism	Incidence (overt or subclinical) (%)
McHenry, et al. (2000)	71	At least 5 weeks after operation	Serum TSH>3.59μIU/L	Total: 25/71 (35%) (Overt: 9/71 (12.7%) Subclinical: 16/71 (22.5%))
Miller, et al. (2006)	90	At least 8-10 weeks after surgery	Serum TSH>6.0mIU/L	Total: 24/90 (27%)
Seiberling, et al. (2007)	58	At least 6 weeks after surgery	Serum TSH>4.0μIU/ml	Total: 14/58 (24.1%)
Koh, et al. (2008)	136	1,2, & 6 months after surgery	Serum TSH>4.0μU/ml	Total: 58/136 (42.6%) (Overt: 11/136 (8.1%) Subclinical: 47/136 (34.6%))
Wormald, et al. (2008)	82	3,6,& 12 months after surgery	Serum TSH>4.5μIU/L	Total: 15/82 (18.3%) Overt: 5/82 (6.1%) Subclinical: 10/82(12.2%)
Moon, et al. (2008)	101	2 months, and every 2-3 months (more than 1 year) after surgery	Serum TSH>4.7μIU/L	Total: 37/101 (36.6%)
De Carlucci Jr, et al. (2008)	168	4 to 8 weeks after surgery	Serum TSH>5.5mU/L	Total: 61/186 (32.8%)
Su, et al. (2009)	294	At least 3 months after surgery	Serum TSH>4.0mIU/L	Total: 32/294 (10.9%)
Stoll, et al. (2009)	547	6 to 8 weeks after surgery	Serum TSH>4.82μIU/mL	Total: 78/547 (14.3%)
Spanheimer, et al. (2011)	71	6 weeks after surgery	Serum TSH>4.20μIU/mL	Total: 24/71 (33.8%)
Tomoda, et al. (2011)	233	At least 4-6 weeks, and 3 months after surgery	Serum TSH>5.0mIU/l	Total: 57/233 (24.4%)
Johner, et al. (2011)	117	6 weeks(or 3 months), 6 months & 12 months after surgery	Serum TSH>5.5μIU/L	Total: 21.6% (Permanent: 7.8%)
Chu, et al. (2011)	263	2 weeks, 3 months, 6 months, and yearly after surgery	Serum TSH>5.5mIU/L	Total: 38/263 (14.4%)

Table 1. Incidence of posthemithyroidectomy hypothyroidism

Recently, however, Johner et al (2011) reported that the overall incidence of early postoperative hypothyroidism was 21.6%, with the incidence of permanent hypothyroidism only 7.8%. In addition to showing that the incidence of hypothyroidism following hemithyroidectomy is low, this study showed that a significant proportion of individuals who become biochemically hypothyroid (asymptomatic) demonstrate only a transient elevation in their TSH levels. The low incidence of sustained hypothyroidism supports the adoption of a watch-and-wait approach in patients with biochemical hypothyroidism after hemithyroidectomy. Previously, it was common practice to prescribe suppressive doses of thyroxine after hemithyroidectomy, but it is now thought that the remaining thyroid lobe may compensate. Since the pituitary-thyroid axis must adapt after hemithyroidectomy, serial TSH measurements after surgery will identify only those individuals who remain biochemically hypothyroid or become symptomatic and therefore require treatment with thyroid hormone. This will spare a significant number of patients the need for, and potential risks of, long-term thyroid hormone replacement therapy.

2.3 Natural history

TSH is important for pathologic thyroid growth, and elevated serum TSH may contribute to the development of recurrent nodular or diffuse thyroid enlargement. The efficacy of administering TSH-suppressive doses of thyroxine to prevent thyroid nodule recurrence after surgery has not been determined. Most studies that reported a beneficial effect of suppressive therapy in reducing recurrent nodular thyroid disease after thyroidectomy have been from areas of iodine deficiency, whereas most studies that found no benefit of suppressive therapy have been from iodine-sufficient areas (McHenry & Slusarczyk, 2000).

Hypothyroidism is now one of the most common morbidities observed after hemithyroidectomy. Most patients will continue to have normal thyroid function after hemithyroidectomy, although some will have mildly elevated TSH during the perioperative period that may normalize without pharmacologic intervention due to compensation by the remaining thyroid lobe. This may be characterized by both an increase in serum TSH concentration and an augmented release of TSH in response to TRH signaling (Lombardi et al, 1983) (Campion et al., 1995), adaptive mechanisms that may persist for 12-18 months after surgery. Animal experiments have shown that serum TSH concentration declines initially, subsequently returning to normal with compensatory hypertrophy of the remaining thyroid lobe followed by a significant elevation in serum TSH for as long as 5 months after surgery (Clark et al., 1976). Compensatory hypertrophy of the remaining thyroid lobe has been observed histologically following hemithyroidectomy (Marine et al., 1926).

Some patients with symptomatic hypothyroidism require treatment, as do patients with mild hypothyroidism and medical comorbidities. The physiological and clinical signs of hypothyroidism are generally completely reversed by appropriate thyroid hormone replacement treatment. Some physicians therefore advocate thyroxine replacement to prevent progression of multinodular changes in the contralateral lobe, whereas others prescribe thyroxine replacement for all patients after hemithyroidectomy. The possibility of compensatory hypertrophy of the residual lobe should be balanced by the need for close follow-up of patients with borderline thyroid reserves, and the potential for deterioration at times of physiological stress and progression of underlying thyroiditis. Routine thyroxine replacement may be recommended, rather than close follow-up monitoring, for some post-hemithyroidectomy patients with risk factors, such as elevated thyroid antibody concentrations or histologic evidence of autoimmune thyroiditis (Su et al., 2009). In contrast, other researchers have reported that elevated serum TSH concentration alone may not justify the initiation of thyroid hormone replacement, since nearly 70% of individuals who developed biochemical (asymptomatic) hypothyroidism during the early postoperative period after hemithyroidectomy recovered normal thyroid function without pharmacologic intervention (Johner et al., 2011). Therefore, determination of the true indication is important prior to initiating thyroid hormone replacement therapy.

A small number of patients who develop hypothyroidism after thyroid lobectomy require life-long thyroid hormone replacement, as well as routine laboratory examinations and medical adjustments. Furthermore, chronic thyroxine therapy may be associated with adverse effects, including arrhythmias (atrial fibrillation) or loss of calcium from the bones resulting in osteopenia or osteoporosis. High serum cholesterol concentrations may result in cardiac sclerosis with all its complications, suggesting that hormone replacement therapy be delayed. Thus, an increased ability to recognize which patients are most at risk for developing hypothyroidism will improve patient care. Although closer monitoring or earlier initiation of thyroid hormone replacement therapy may be advisable for these high-risk patients, no specific TSH concentration alone is indicative of increased risk of permanent or overt hypothyroidism, suggesting that transient biochemical hypothyroidism be closely monitored rather than routinely treated. Accurate detection and diagnosis of sustained hypothyroidism after thyroid surgery is also important to avoid its associated morbidity and mortality (Johner et al., 2011).

2.4 Risk factors

Among the factors found to predict hypothyroidism after hemithyroidectomy are patient age, sex, preoperative TSH concentration, the presence of anti-thyroid antibodies, autoimmune thyroiditis in the excised lobe, and volume of remnant thyroid bed. Although these factors are also important in determining treatment plans for patients with thyroid disease, the correlation between risk factors and onset of hypothyroidism remains unclear. Table 2 shows a summary of risk factors that predict hypothyroidism after hemithyroidectomy.

Author (year)	Incidence of posthemithyroidectomy hypothyroidism	Risk factors (Postoperative hypothyroidism vs. Euthyroid state)
McHenry, et al. (2000)	35%	Higher preoperative serum TSH level (μIU/L) (1.94±1.00 vs. 1.10±0.74)
Miller, et al. (2006)	27%	Hashimoto's thyroiditis, multinodular goiter, higher preoperative serum TSH level (mIU/L) (3.15±1.14 vs. 1.95±0.92)
Seiberling, et al. (2007)	24.1%	Higher preoperative serum TSH level (μIU/ml) (2.39 vs. 1.07), chronic inflammation (lymphocytic thyroiditis or Hashimoto's thyroiditis) (50.0% vs. 6.8%)

Author (year)	Incidence of posthemithyroidectomy hypothyroidism	Risk factors (Postoperative hypothyroidism vs. Euthyroid state)
Koh, et al. (2008)	42.6%	Higher preoperative serum TSH level (μU/ml) (2.15±1.30 vs. 1.29±0.9), preoperative microsomal Ab, thyroglobulin Ab, higher grade of lymphocytic infiltration of resected thyroid gland
Wormald, et al. (2008)	18.3%	Higher preoperative serum TSH level (μIU/L) (>1.6 vs. <1.6), higher grade of lymphocytic infiltration of resected thyroid gland
Moon, et al. (2008)	36.6%	Higher preoperative serum TSH level (μIU/L) (2.46±1.16 vs. 1.22±0.89), BSA-adjusted remnant thyroid volume (2.73±1.34 vs. 3.48±1.50)
De Carlucci Jr, et al. (2008)	32.8%	Higher preoperative serum TSH level (mU/L) (2.1 vs. 1.2), smaller remnant thyroid volume (mL) (3.9 vs. 6.0), right vs. left lobectomy, higher thyroperoxidase antibody serum levels
Su, et al. (2009)	10.9%	High-normal preoperaitve serum TSH level; TSH 2.5-4.0mIU/L (%) (18.8 vs. 3.8), thyroiditis in histology (%) (46.8 vs. 11.8), elevated thyroid antibodies levels (%) (47.8 vs. 11.5)
Stoll, et al. (2009)	14.3%	Higher preoperative serum TSH level (μIU/mL) (2.12 vs. 1.35), lower mean free T4 (ng/dL) (1.03 vs. 1.34), Hashimoto's thyroiditis
Spanheimer, et al. (2011)	33.8%	Thyroiditis on surgical pathology
Tomoda, et al. (2011)	24.4%	Higher preoperative serum TSH level (mIU/l) (2.73±1.36 vs. 1.24±0.82), older age (years) (56.2±13 vs. 48.97±15)
Johner, et al. (2011)	21.6%	Higher preoperative serum TSH level, high degree of lymphocytic infiltraiton, high degree of germinal center formation
Chu, et al. (2011)	14.4%	Older age, higher preoperative serum TSH level, longer follow-up period, more frequent thyroiditis on histology, lighter resected tissue weight, positive antimicrosomal antibodies. * By multivariate analysis, only resected tissue weight, and concomitant thyroiditis on histology turned out to be independent predicting factors.

Table 2. Risk factors for predicting posthemithyroidectomy hypothyroidism

Some known risk factors can be determined only after surgery, such as lymphocytic infiltration, associated thyroiditis, and the weight of the resected gland, whereas others, such as preoperative TSH concentration, age, and presence of thyroid autoantibody, are known preoperatively. In addition, the remnant thyroid volume may be easily measured from preoperative US. Because most patients scheduled for hemithyroidectomy due to thyroid nodules are evaluated by thyroid US, the remnant thyroid volume could be easily determined, allowing the surgeon to decide whether to perform a diagnostic hemithyroidectomy.

2.4.1 Elevated preoperative TSH concentration

Preoperative TSH concentration is significantly associated with postoperative hypothyroidism. In addition, studies using a TSH cutoff value, such as >1.6 or >2.0 uIU/mL, have found that patients with elevated TSH are 7-10 times more likely to develop hypothyroidism after surgery. Thus, "normally elevated" preoperative TSH >1.5 uIU/mL, especially when combined with lower preoperative T4 concentrations or specific antibodies, may indicate a potentially increased risk of hypothyroidism after hemithyroidectomy, allowing appropriate preoperative counseling of patients (Table 2).

2.4.2 Degree of chronic inflammation and autoimmune disease

2.4.2.1 Hashimoto's thyroiditis and presence of autoantibodies

Thyroiditis is also associated with postoperative hypothyroidism. Hashimoto's thyroiditis is an inflammatory disease that is the most common cause of hypothyroidism. Moreover, Hashimoto's thyroiditis has been found to significantly increase the need for thyroid hormone supplementation following hemithyroidectomy. Patients diagnosed with Hashimoto's thyroiditis were found to be almost four times more likely to develop hypothyroidism after hemithyroidectomy (Stoll et al., 2009). Hashimoto's thyroiditis is also characterized by intense lymphocytic infiltration of the thyroid and the presence of thyroid autoantibodies. Moreover, several types of autoimmune thyroiditis are closely associated with circulating thyroid autoantibodies such as microsomal Ab and thyroglobulin Ab (Seiberling et al, 2007). The presence of thyroid autoantibodies was found to strongly correlate with post-hemithyroidectomy hypothyroidism. Similar relationships have been observed among Hashimoto's thyroiditis, autoimmune thyroiditis, the degree of lymphocytic infiltration, the presence of chronic inflammation, or detectable thyroid autoantibodies and the occurrence of hypothyroidism after hemithyroidectomy. The association among Hashimoto's thyroiditis, a "normal elevated" TSH concentration, a low free T4 concentration, and thyroid autoantibodies is likely due to the underlying pathologic disease process. In addition, preoperatively measured thyroid autoantibodies may predict postoperative hypothyroidism.

2.4.2.2 Degree of lymphocytic infiltration

Lymphocytic infiltrate into the thyroid gland has been found to decrease thyroid function, and a semiquantitative analysis of this infiltrate usually reflects the risk of hypothyroidism. The degree of lymphocytic infiltration, graded on a scale of 0-IV, into the resected thyroid lobe may aid in predicting the development of hypothyroidism in post-hemithyroidectomy patients (Koh et al, 2008). An extensive review of histopathologic data, which assessed whether the degree of lymphocytic infiltration and germinal center formation within the thyroid lobe could accurately predict the development of postoperative hypothyroidism, found that when inflammation was graded based on the extent of lymphocytic infiltration (graded 0-3) and the frequency of germinal centers was qualitatively assessed as a histologic measure of immunologic activation (graded 0-3), most patients with lymphocytic infiltration or germinal center formation in the resected thyroid lobe are at increased risk for post-hemithyroidectomy hypothyroidism (Johner et al, 2011). Other studies have assessed the relationship between postoperative pathologic findings and risk of developing hypothyroidism, but, since these findings were detected after surgery, they could not be used to determine the need for postoperative thyroidectomy.

Taken together, these findings indicate that Hashimoto's thyroiditis and other risk factors, such as lymphocytic infiltration and the presence of autoantibodies, significantly increase the risks for developing postoperative hypothyroidism after thyroid lobectomy. Preoperative evaluation is therefore important in counseling patients about a possible future need for thyroid hormone replacement therapy.

2.4.3 Amount of remnant thyroid gland

One of the major risk factors for hypothyroidism after hemithyroidectomy is the amount of remnant thyroid gland. Small remnant thyroid volume has been recognized as a risk factor for hypothyroidism (De Carlucci Jr et al., 2008). Remnant thyroid volumes can be measured on preoperative US images and can be calculated using the equation (Miccoli et al., 2006):

$$\text{Volume} = \text{length X width X depth X } \pi / 6.$$

Patients who developed post-hemithyroidectomy hypothyroidism were found to have a significant smaller body surface area (BSA)-adjusted remnant thyroid volume than patients who remained euthyroid (Moon et al, 2008). Another predictive factor may be BSA-adjusted remnant thyroid volume, determined by calculating remnant thyroid volume/BSA ratio. BSA can be calculated using the Mosteller formula:

$$\text{BSA} = \sqrt{}(\text{height X weight}/3600).$$

2.4.4 Risk scoring systems

Risk-scoring systems that can predict hypothyroidism after hemithyroidectomy are summarized in Table 3.

Having a valid model predictive of postoperative hypothyroidism is also useful when making follow-up plans for patients undergoing hemithyroidectomy. Most surgeons recommend regular postoperative visits to the clinic, although some counsel their patients to visit only when surgery-related symptoms develop.

A unique risk-scoring system that can predict hypothyroidism after hemithyroidectomy was recently described (Tomoda et al, 2011). In this system, risk scores are calculated as the sum of a patient's age and preoperative TSH concentration. The rates of hypothyroidism in patients with risk scores of 0, 1, 2, and 3 were found to be 3%, 20%, 39%, and 70%, respectively, suggesting that the potential risk of postoperative hypothyroidism should be discussed with patients before surgery based on this scoring system.

Author (year)	Number of patients	Risk scoring system
Moon, et al. (2008)	101	Risk scoring system using two independent risk predictors (TSH level and BSA-adjusted remnant thyroid volume) was created based on the results of logistic regression analyses. The incidences of hypothyroidism were 5.3%, 12.1%, 51.7%, and 85.0% according to the risk scores of 0,1,2, and 3, respectively.
Stoll, et al. (2009)	547	When stratified into 3 groups based on their preoperative TSH measurement (≤1.5, 1.51-2.5, and ≥2.51μIU/mL), the rate of hypothyroidism increased significantly at each level (13.5%, 20.5%, and 41. 3%, respectively)
Tomoda, et al. (2011)	233	A risk-scoring system was calculated by summing the score of risk factors such as preoperative TSH level (<1, 1-2.49, and ≥2.5μIU/ml) and patient's age (<55, and ≥55 year). The incidences of hypothyroidism were 3, 20, 39, and 70% according to the risk scores of 0, 1, 2 and 3, respectively.
Johner, et al. (2011)	117	Assessment of the histologic scoring criteria for thyroid lymphocytic infiltration (score 0-3), and germinal centers (score 0-3) as well as classification of TSH levels (<5.5, 5.5-6.9, 7-14.9, and≥15μIU/L) can predict potential risks associated with long -term thyroid hormone replacement therapy.

Table 3. Risk scoring system in posthemithyroidectomy hypothyroidism

An alternative risk-scoring system using two factors, TSH concentration and remnant thyroid volume, was based on the results of logistic regression analyses (Moon et al, 2008). This score system was developed using independently predictive factors, with the highest score of each variable determined by its β regression coefficient. Logistic regression analysis was used to derive an equation that calculates the probability (P) of developing hypothyroidism after hemithyroidectomy:

$$P = 1/\ (1 + e\text{- } (-1.325+1.191{*}\text{preoperative TSH}-0.435{*}\text{remnant thyroid volume}).$$

The incidences of hypothyroidism in patients with risk scores of 0, 1, 2, and 3 were found to be 5.3%, 12.1%, 51.7%, and 85.0%, respectively, with the model having an overall accuracy in predicting post-hemithyroidectomy hypothyroidism of about 77. 2%.

In summary, elevated preoperative TSH concentration, Hashimoto's thyroiditis, small remnant thyroid volume, and/or advanced age are associated with increased risk of developing hypothyroidism and a greater likelihood of requiring thyroid hormone supplementation after hemithyroidectomy. Patient counseling on the need for hormone replacement should therefore be based on these factors.

2.5 Postoperative thyroid hormone replacement after hemithyroidectomy

Hypothyroidism is an underappreciated sequel of hemithyroidectomy. It is most often mild and subclinical, requiring low doses of thyroid hormone to normalize serum TSH concentrations. Hypothyroidism has been reported in up to one third of euthyroid patients who undergo hemithyroidectomy. Formerly, it was common practice to routinely start patients with nodular thyroid disease on "prophylactic" TSH-suppressive doses of thyroid hormone (L-thyroxine) following hemithyroidectomy to prevent recurrence (Gharib & Mazzaferri, 1998), based on the hypothesis that suppression of the hypothalamic-pituitary axis would reduce the risk of abnormalities developing in the contralateral thyroid remnant. Thus, routine administration of L-thyroxine to hemithyroidectomy patients could be expected to decrease the incidence of hypothyroidism. More recently, however, L-thyroxine (TSH-suppression therapy) has not been not routinely prescribed for all patients after hemithyroidectomy, largely due to its questionable efficacy in thyroid suppression and prevention of the development of nodules in the remaining contralateral thyroid lobe. In addition, thyroxine administration may cause subclinical hyperthyroidism, which has been associated with possible side effects including decreased bone mineral density, particularly in postmenopausal women, a three-fold increase in the incidence of atrial fibrillation, and aggravation of ischemic heart disease (Mchenry & Slusarczyk, 2000). Therefore, early detection of postoperative hypothyroidism and treatment with L-thyroxine may inhibit the development of overt hypothyroidism and its potential complications. Although administration of thyroid hormone to suppress serum TSH levels in euthyroid patients may not be of value, treatment of patients with elevated TSH is important for relieving the symptoms of hypothyroidism and may be important in reducing recurrent thyroid disease. Administration of thyroxine after hemithyroidectomy may also require long-term monitoring of thyroid function and it has not been determined how long these patients should continue on thyroxine. These problems encouraged us to investigate the frequency of hypothyroidism following hemithyroidectomy, as well as its potential risk factors and management.

The unfavorable side effects of TSH-suppressive doses of thyroid hormone are known, whereas replacement doses of thyroxine have not been associated with the adverse sequelae observed with TSH-suppressive doses of thyroxine. Patients with postoperatively elevated TSH concentrations may represent a subgroup at high risk for the development of recurrent nodular or diffuse thyroid enlargement. Normalization of serum TSH concentrations may help minimize the potential negative effects of elevated serum TSH concentrations without subjecting patients to the adverse sequelae associated with TSH-suppressive doses of L-thyroxine. Therefore, the selective use of L-thyroxine therapy for patients with elevated TSH after hemithyroidectomy may help prevent recurrent nodular or diffuse thyroid enlargement without the unnecessary administration of L-thyroxine to patients with a normal serum TSH level and exposing them to its harmful effects (McHenry and Slusarczyk, 2000).

In summary, hypothyroidism after hemithyroidectomy is usually mild and asymptomatic, and can be treated with lower than normal replacement doses of L-thyroxine to maintain serum TSH concentrations within their normal range.

2.6 Post-hemithyroidectomy follow-up guidelines

Theoretically, a single thyroid lobe should possess enough functioning thyrocytes for a patient to remain euthyroid. In fact, many surgeons and patients choose hemithyroidectomy owing to the belief that postoperative thyroid hormone therapy will not be required. However, patients with risk factors for hypothyroidism, such as severe preoperative thyroiditis, may not have sufficient thyroid tissue remaining after thyroid lobectomy. Thus, all patients who undergo hemithyroidectomy should be counseled regarding the potential need for lifelong thyroid hormone therapy.

There is no widely accepted guideline or algorithm for the monitoring of thyroid function after hemithyroidectomy, leaving hypothyroidism as the most common resulting complication. Follow-up guidelines vary widely and generally consist of a single postoperative measurement of TSH. Some patients may not be examined at all until the development of overt hypothyroidism. If thyroid dysfunction is detected, the decision to start thyroid hormone replacement therapy is usually based on the preference of the treating physician, patient symptoms, and the degree and duration of TSH elevation, rather than on evidence obtained from clinical trials. Therefore, it is important to identify those patients who are at risk of developing hypothyroidism soon after surgery so that they can be more attentively monitored using thyroid function tests. Additionally, it would be of benefit to identify risk factors predictive of the development of early hypothyroidism.

One of the difficulties in monitoring thyroid function other than thyroid hormone concentrations after hemithyroidectomy is that many symptoms of subclinical hypothyroidism are nonspecific. Although most physicians recommend regular postoperative visits, some recommend visits only when patients develop surgery-related symptoms. Although routine and continuous long-term monitoring of thyroid hormone concentrations after hemithyroidectomy is a possible solution, it is often ineffective and not cost effective due to unnecessary hospital visits. In contrast, unrecognized hypothyroidism after hemithyroidectomy may have an unfavorable effect on a patient's general health. This may inevitably result in overt hypothyroidism in some patients, increasing the risks of developing cardiovascular and/or neuropsychiatric diseases. To overcome this dilemma, preoperative risk factors for hypothyroidism after hemithyroidectomy have been formulated to identify high-risk patients. Table 4 summarizes several follow-up protocols followed after hemithyroidectomy.

In most patients, hypothyroidism after hemithyroidectomy manifests as an increased serum TSH concentration within 3-12 months after surgery. Moreover, hypothyroidism in most of these patients is rarely severe or progressive. Therefore, patients who are postoperatively euthyroid rarely go on to develop hypothyroidism, making yearly evaluations by measuring serum TSH concentrations sufficient. Thus, most thyroid function should be monitored once yearly for life (McHenry & Sulsarczyk, 2000; Miller et al., 2006).

The pituitary-thyroid axis undergoes adaptation following partial thyroidectomy, with most patients showing an increase in serum TSH at 1 month (Tomoda et al, 2011). Since most patients who will develop subclinical hypothyroidism will not do so within the first 3 months after surgery, it may be advisable to measure TSH concentration 4 weeks and 3 months after surgery. At 3 months, patients with subclinical hypothyroidism (>10 uIU/ml) may be prescribed L-thyroxine. TSH concentrations should again be measured at 6 and 12 months, and every 6 or 12 months thereafter, unless patients manifest overt symptoms of hypothyroidism.

Author (year)	Recommended follow-up protocol
McHenry, et al. (2000)	All symptomatic patients should be treated with L-T4 replacement. If it is elected not to treat asymptomatic patients, they should have a baseline serum fT4 and total T3 level measured and a yearly evaluation including measurement of serum fT4, T3, TSH levels to assess for progression to overt hypothyroidism.
Miller, et al. (2006)	Recommendation is to obtain a postoperative TSH measurement 8 to 12 weeks after surgery, followed by the measurement of TSH levels at 6 months and 12 months after surgery. If the TSH level is normal at 12 months, biannual to annual determination of TSH levels was encouraged unless symptoms of hypothyroidism manifest.
Koh, et al. (2008)	If preoperative risk factors (presence of microsomal Ab and thyroglobulin Ab, or higher degree of lymphocytic infiltration of resected thyroid gland) were present, these patients were to be follow up at least for 12 months with explanation of possibility of developing postsurgical hypothyroidism.
Wormald, et al. (2008)	Patients with risk factors (raised TSH level or lymphocytic infiltration) should undergo thyroid function tests at 3,6,12 months and annually thereafter postoperatively. In all other patients, testing of thyroid function once at 1-year is sufficient.
Moon, et al. (2008)	Frequent follow-up and thyroid function monitoring can be tailored to high-risk patients if a valid prediction model can be established in prospective studies.
Su, et al. (2009)	TSH monitoring at 6 months, 12 months, and then yearly for 2 years was recommended for asymptomatic patients. High-risk patients should have serial TSH for the first year, then yearly thereafter.
Tomoda, et al. (2011)	Postoperative TSH level should be checked 4 weeks after surgery and again 3 months. At 3 months after operation, the decision regarding prescription of levothyroxine to patients with subclinical hypothyroidism (more than 10μIU/ml). After 3 months after operation, the measurement of TSH levels was recommended at 6 and 12 months after surgery. If the TSH level is normal at 12 months, biannual to annual determination of TSH levels could be checked unless symptoms of hypothyroidism manifest.
Johner, et al. (2011)	To obtain a postoperative TSH measurement for all patients at 6 weeks after surgery, followed by the measurement of TSH levels at 6 and 12 months after surgery was advised. TSH level at 3 months was no longer recommended because most patients displayed marked increase in their TSH level immediately after surgery, that subsequently normalized over time.

Table 4. Recommendation protocol for follow-up after hemithyroidectomy

Another follow-up protocol recommends that all symptomatic or asymptomatic patients with hypothyroidism be treated with L-thyroxine (McHenry & Slusarczyk, 2000). If treatment of asymptomatic patients is not preferred, serum free T4 and total triiodothyronine (T3) concentrations should be measured at baseline, followed by yearly evaluations including measurements of serum free T4, T3, and TSH to assess the progression to overt hypothyroidism.

Another recommendation is to measure TSH 8 to 12 weeks after surgery, as well as at 6 and 12 months. If TSH concentration is normal at 12 months, it should be measured every 6 to 12 months thereafter, unless patients develop symptoms of hypothyroidism (Miller et al., 2006).

A recent modification of an earlier algorithm (Johner et al, 2011) recommended that TSH be measured 6 and 12 months after hemithyroidectomy, indicating that the measurement of TSH at 3 months was no longer required because most study participants displayed marked increases in serum TSH concentration immediately after surgery, which subsequently normalized over time. This new algorithm recommended that serum TSH be measured biannually in asymptomatic patients with mild biochemical hypothyroidism (TSH 5.6-6.9 uIU/L). This follow-up schedule allows for the timely detection of biochemical hypothyroidism and appropriate surveillance for individuals managed conservatively, with an expectation of eventual return to normal thyroid function.

Although it has been suggested that all hemithyroidectomy patients be monitored for as long as possible, it may be more practical to use a selective monitoring strategy in which monitoring is dependent on the presence of risk factors.

3. Conclusion

The incidence of hypothyroidism after hemithyroidectomy is not negligible and should not be overlooked. Approximately 15-30% of patients who undergo hemithyroidectomy may have this complication, and some may need thyroid hormone replacement therapy. Risk factors such as elevated preoperative TSH levels, elevated concentrations of thyroid autoimmune antibodies, degree of thyroiditis, age, and residual thyroid volume are associated with an increased risk of hypothyroidism after hemithyroidectomy. Patients at increased risk for postoperative hypothyroidism should be made aware of their risk factors and undergo more intensive follow-up.

4. Acknowledgment

All authors including Drs. Lee, and Chung have no conflicts of interest or financial ties to disclose.

5. References

Campion, L.; Gallou, G. & Ruelland, A. (1995) Lipid and thyroid changes after partial thyroidectomy: guidelines for L-thyroxine therapy? *Clin Chem,* Vol.41, No.3, pp.473-474

Chu, KK. & Lang, BH. (2011) Clinicopathologic predictors for early and late biochemical hypothyroidism after hemithyroidectomy. *Am J Surg,* Epub ahead of print. DOI:10.1016/j.amjsurg.2011.03.004

Clark, OH; Lambert, WR. & Cavalieri, RR. (1976) Compensatory thyroid hypertrophy after hemithyroidectomy in rats. *Endocrinology,* Vol.99, No.4, pp.988-995

De Carlucci Jr, D.; Tavares MR. & Obara, MT. (2008) Thyroid function after unilateral total lobectomy: risk factors for postoperative hypothyroidism. *Arch Otolarygol Head Neck Surg,* Vol.134, No.10, pp.1076-1079

Gharib, H. & Mazzaferri, EL. (1998) Thyroxine suppressive therapy in patients with nodular thyroid disease. *Ann Intern Med,* Vol.128, No.5, (March 19989), pp.386-394

Hollowell, JG.; Staehling, NW. & Flanders, WD. (2002) Serum TSH, T(4), and thyroid antibodies in the United States population (1988 to 1994): National Health and Nutrition Examination Survey (NHANES III). *J Clin Endocrinol Metab,* Vol.87, No.2, pp.489-499

Johner, A.; Griffith, OL. & Walker, B. (2011) Detection and management of hypothyroidism following thyroid lobectomy: evaluation of a clinical algorithm. *Ann Surg Oncol,* Epub ahead of print. DOI 10.1245/s10434-011-1627-1

Koh, YW.; Lee, SW. & Choi, EC. (2008) Prediction of hypothyroidism after hemithyroidectomy: a biochemical and pathological analysis. *Eur Arch Otorhinolaryngol,* Vol.265, No.4, pp.453-457

Laurberg, P.; Andersen, S. & Bülow Pederse, I. (2005) Hypothyroidism in the elderly: pathophysiology, diagnosis and treatment. *Drugs Aging,* Vol.22, No.1, pp.23-38

Lombardi, G.; Panza, N. & Lupoli, G. (1983) Study of the pituitary-thyroid axis in euthyroid goiter after partial thyroidectomy. *J Endocrinol Invest,* Vol.6, No.6, pp.485-487

Marine, D. (1926) Control of compensatory hyperplasia of the thyroid of guinea-pigs by administration of iodine. *Arch Pathol,* Vol.2, pp.829

McHenry, CR. & Slusarczyk SJ. (2000) Hypothyroidism after hemithyroidectomy: incidence, risk factors, and management. *Surgery,* Vol.128, No.6, pp.994-998

Miccoli, P.; Minuto, MN. & Orlandini, C. (2006) Ultrasonography estimated thyroid volume: a prospective study about its reliability. *Thyroid,* Vol.16, No.1, (January 2006), pp.37-39

Miller, FR.; Paulson, D. & Prihoda, TJ. (2006) Risk factors for the development of hypothyroidism after hemithyroidectomy. *Arch Otolaryngol Head Neck Surg,* Vol.132, No.1, pp.36-38

Moon, HG.; Jung, EJ. & Park, ST. (2008). Thyrotropin level and thyroid volume for prediction of hypothyroidism following hemithyroidectomy in an Asian patient cohort. *World J Surg,*Vol. 32, No.11, pp. 2503-2508

Seiberling, KA.; Dutra, JC. & Bajaramovic, S. (2007) Hypothyroidism following hemithyroidectomy for benign nontoxic thyroid disease. *Ear Nose Throat J,* Vol.86, No.5, pp.295-299

Spanheimer, PM.; Sugg, SL. & Lal, G. (2011) Surveillance and intervention after thyroid lobectomy. *Ann Surg Oncol,* Vol.18, No.6, pp.1729-1733

Stoll, SJ.; Pitt, SC. & Liu, J. (2009) Thyroid hormone replacement after thyroid lobectomy. *Surgery,* Vol.146, No.4, pp.554-558

Su, SY.; Grodski, S. & Serpell, JW. (2009) Hypothyroidism following hemithyroidectomy: a retrospective reveiw. *Ann Surg,* Vol.250, No.6, pp.991-994

Surks, MI.; Ortiz, E. & Daniels, GH. (2004) Subclinical thyroid disease: scientific review and guidelines for diagnosis and management. *JAMA,* Vol.291, No.2, pp.228-238

Tomoda, C.; Ito, Y. & Kobayashi, Y. (2011) Subclinical hypothyroidism following hemithyroidectomy: a simple risk-scoring system using age and preoperative thyrotropin level. *ORL J Otorhinolaryngol Relat Spec,* Vol.73, No.2, pp.68-71

Wartofsky, L. & Van Nostrand, D. (2006) Overt and 'subclinical' hypothyroidism in women *Obstet Gynecol Surv,* Vol.61, No.8, pp.535-4542

Wormald, R.; Sheahan, P. & Rowley, S. (2008) Hemithyroiectomy for benign thyroid disease: who needs for follow-up for hypothyroidism? *Clin Otolaryngol,* Vol.33, No.6, pp.587-591

5

Hypothyroidism in Thalassemia

Kallistheni Farmaki
General Hospital of Corinth
Greece

1. Introduction

Thalassemia major is an inherited hemoglobin disorder resulting in chronic hemolytic anemia. Chronic blood transfusion therapy caused excessive iron accumulation in different organs which was associated with high early fatalities. With the introduction of iron chelators, especially the oral ones during the last decade, rates of survival have improved (Tefler et al, 2009) but endocrine complications became more and more frequent in long-term survivors and substantially affect their quality of life. (De Sanctis et al, 2006).

The frequency of hypothyroidism in Thalassemia patients ranges from 6 to 30% among different countries depending on chelation regimens (De Sanctis et al, 2004). Lower prevalence was found in patients who had evidence of lower iron load as measured by ferritin levels (Borgna-Pignatti et al, 2004). The prognosis depends on the amount and the duration of iron overload.

Primary hypothyroidism that may affect thalassemic patients from the second decade of life is mainly due to gland infiltration by iron overload. Autoimmune thyroiditis is absent (Delvecchio & Cavallo, 2010). Central hypothyroidism caused by decreased secretion of thyrotropin stimulating hormone (TSH) from the anterior pituitary gland or by decreased secretion of thyrotropin-releasing hormone (TRH) from the hypothalamus is less common. The thyroid gland appears to fail before the thyroid-pituitary axis, which is less sensitive than the gonadal axis to iron-induced damage (Landau et al, 1993).

A wide spectrum of pathogenic mechanisms is involved. Tissue chronic hypoxia (Magro et al, 1990) and iron overload have a direct toxic effect on the thyroid gland. High concentrations of labile plasma iron and labile cell iron which are considered responsible in the formation of free radicals and the production of reactive oxygen species (ROS) may lead to cell and organ damage (Esposito et al, 2003). In severe iron overloaded thalassemia patients the anterior pituitary may be damaged and regulatory hormonal secretion (LH, FSH, TRH) may be disrupted. (Cavallo et al, 1984). Organ siderosis (liver, cardiac and skeletal muscle, kidney) may affect specific receptors, which regulate thyroid hormone action and convert T4 to the bioactive T3. Recent studies have also demonstrated the incidence of Interferon induced thyroiditis in 40% of Thalassemia patients with Hepatitis C treated with IFNα, which seems to be induced by IFNα via both immune stimulatory and direct toxic effects on the thyroid. (Menconi et al, 2011).

Hypothyroidism may create major cardiovascular changes, such as a decrease in cardiac output because of decrease in oxygen and substrate utilization, a decrease in cardiac contractility, a reduction in heart rate and an increase in peripheral vascular resistance (Klein & Danzi, 2007). Thyroid hormones may also play a critical role in brain development in infants and in modulating brain metabolic activity in adults as shown by structural changes related to myelin, studied by brain imaging techniques (Bernal, 2002). Recent research aims to combine modern brain imaging techniques with years of experience in neuropsychological and clinical evaluations of thyroid dysfunctions. It is now clear that without optimal thyroid function, mood disturbance, cognitive impairment and other psychiatric symptoms can emerge.

As the symptoms of hypothyroidism are non-specific, but the consequences affect virtually every organ system, an early systematic laboratory evaluation and control of thyroid function is recommended in all TMp annually. Iron overload induced hypothyroidism may respond to adequate chelation therapy promoting prevention or/and reversal of the disease and other associated comorbidities. In one case of hereditary hemochromatosis, reversal of hypothyroidism was reported after iron depletion (Hudec et al, 2008). Also, a long-term follow-up study of Italian TMp demonstrated that regular iron chelation may prevent thyroid dysfunction and the development of clinically significant myocardial dysfunction. In addition, therapy with L-thyroxin should be considered in hypothyroidic, moderately and severely iron overloaded TMp (De Sanctis et al, 2008a).

The newer challenges of chelation therapy include the prevention and reversal of iron related morbidities by reducing and maintaining iron and free iron to very low levels (Kolnagou et al, 2009). With adequate chelation therapy, endocrinopaties may be stable or reversible in thalassemia major patients (TMp). (Gamberini et al, 2008). Each chelator has different properties influencing the clinical management of iron overload (Kalinowski et al, 2005). Additionally, each patient has a different safety and efficacy profile with regards to their response to chelation therapy. Iron excretion is dose dependent with wide subject-to-subject variability. A negative iron balance, which ensures prevention or/and reversal of iron overload complications, is difficult to achieve with monotherapy. Combined chelation treatment may be a better approach. It results in increased iron excretion compared to monotherapy alone, probably acting by a shuttle or/and additive effect and it was proved to increase overall survival (Telfer,2009) and achieve treatment goals with manageable adverse reactions (Kontoghiorghes et al, 2010). Also with combined chelation, compliance to the daily lifelong commitment was improved as short-term results were readily evident to TMp themselves.

Our group has had significant experience with the use of combined chelation regimen in TMp regarding the reversal of endocrine complications (Farmaki, 2008; 2010a; 2010b; 2011). Our results on hypothyroidism will be highlighted throughout this chapter. Controversies about exploration of thyroid function and regular follow up in TMp, adequate chelation and arguments for and against T4 treatment will be discussed.

2. Patients and methods

This was an open label, observational, single centre study conducted in the Thalassemia Unit, of the General Hospital of Corinth, Greece, for a period of seven years. The study was approved by the hospital ethical committee and written informed consent was obtained from all patients.

2.1 All participants were transfusion-dependent thalassemia major patients (TMp), who presented with more than one iron-overload complication as defined by clinical and laboratory criteria.

2.2 Prior to initiation of this study, all patients received chelation monotherapy with DFO, 40 mg/kg; 8–12 h, subcutaneously, 3–5 days/week.

2.3 All participants were switched to an intensive combination scheme with DFO and Deferiprone (DFP) consisting of both daily oral administration of DFP 75–100 mg/kg/d in three divided doses and subcutaneous DFO (20–40 mg/kg; 8–12 h, 2–6 d/week. Individual dosing and frequency of DFO infusions were determined by patients' clinical and laboratory assessments, such as iron overload indices and comorbidities.

2.4 Although serum ferritin is not an accurate index, we estimated the trends of monthly serial measures of serum ferritin by Chemiluminescent Microparticle Immunoassay (CMIA) by Architect Abbott Diagnostics.

2.5 Quantification of heart and liver iron load was determined annually by Signa-MRI 1.5 Tesla, multi-echo T2* and liver iron concentration (LIC) in mg/gr dry weight (g dw) derived from the T2*L value by Ferriscan (St Pierre et al 2005, Wood et al, 2005).

2.6 A systematic control of thyroid function was performed annually by thyroid-stimulating hormone (TSH), free triiodothyronine (FT3) and free thyroxine (FT4) screening. At baseline and after 5-7 years a thyroid releasing hormone TRH stimulation test was conducted. Following intravenous infusion of 200 mcg TRH, blood samples were taken at 0, 30, 60, 90 and 120 min for TSH measurements. The area under the curve (AUC) was also calculated for estimating integrated response during the test. All patients on hormone replacement therapy discontinued thyroxin at least 30 days before the test.

2.7 Cardiac function was assessed annually, with tissue 1Echo-Doppler TD (Philips ie33 system). Patients were classified according to the New York Heart Association (NYHA) criteria.

2.8 Gonadal function was assessed by peripheral hormone levels: testosterone and free testosterone or oestradiol and progesterone. In addition, serum basal levels of follicle-stimulating hormone (FSH) and luteinizing hormone (LH) were assayed. Gonadotrophin response was also assayed after intravenous infusion of 200 lg gonadotrophin-releasing hormone (GnRH). Samples were taken at 0, 30, 60, 90 and 120 for the measurement of FSH and LH. All analyses were performed by CMIA technology using the automatic immuno-analyzer ARCITECT, i2000SR,

2.9 Safety was evaluated by close clinical and laboratory monitoring of adverse reactions, according to each drug SPC. A full check up of each patient was implemented at baseline before protocol initiation and patients' records were thoroughly reviewed systematically in order to determine any changes.

2.10 All statistical analyses were carried out using the statistical package for the social sciences software (SPSS release 13.0, Chicago, IL, USA). All p values were two sided; the level of significance was < 0.05.

3. Results

Fifty-two patients, 25 males and 27 females, aged 10–49 years at baseline, were followed over a period of 5–7 years. The mean age at baseline was 25.2 ± 8.9 years compared to 32.9 ± 9.8 at the end of the study. Two patients discontinued the study after experiencing repeated episodes of neutropenia and withdrew their consent.

3.1 After combined chelation (DFO & DFP) there was a statistically significant reduction of the total body iron load, as indicated by mean ferritin levels, MRI liver and heart iron quantification (T_2*L & T_2*H) and LIC calculated by Ferriscan, shown in table 1.

Parameter	Baseline studies	End of study	p-value
Ferritin (µg/L)	3421.6 ± 882.0	87 ± 25	<.001
MRI T2*H (ms)	13.8 ± 9.8	35.5 ± 8.1	<.001
MRI T2*L (ms)	1.5 ± 8.2	34.4 ± 5.4	<.001
LIC (mg/g dwt)	15.7 ± 11.1	0.9 ± 0.2	<.001

Table 1. Results (mean ± SD) of iron load assessments in Thalassemia patients

3.2 Euthyroid patients 32/50 demonstrated a significant increase in the mean FT_4 (0.80±0.09 vs. 1.10±0.09 ng/ml p<0.001) and FT_3 levels (1.6±0.2 vs. 2.9±0.5 pg/ml, p<0.001). No new cases of hypothyroidism were observed after combined chelation.

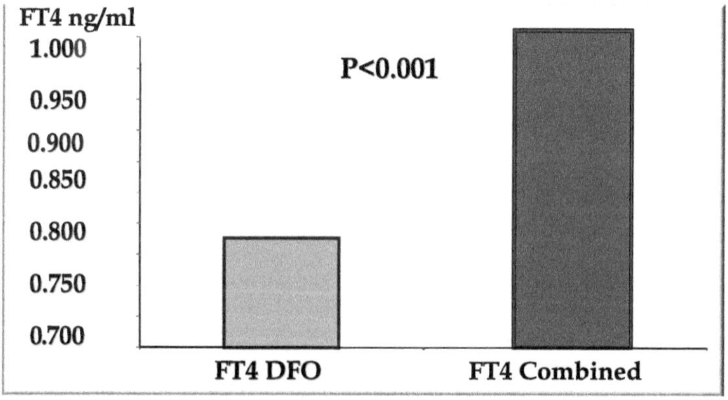

Fig. 1. FT4 levels at baseline (DFO monotherapy) and after combined chelation in euthyroid Thalassemia patients

3.3 At baseline, while on DFO monotherapy 18/50 patients were hypothyroid. After combined chelation 14/18 who had subclinical or compensated hypothyroidism presented a significant increase in mean FT4 (0.70±0.06 vs. 1.07±0.12 ng/ml, p<0.001) and mean FT3 (1.30±0.3 vs. 2.50±0.6 pg/ml, p<0.001). In addition, a significant decrease in the mean TSH (4.12±0.63 vs. 6.27±1.08µIU/ml p<0.001) and TSH quantitative secretion, calculated as the area under the curve (AUC=2231±241 vs. 1332±131 p<0.001) in response to the TRH stimulation test were observed.

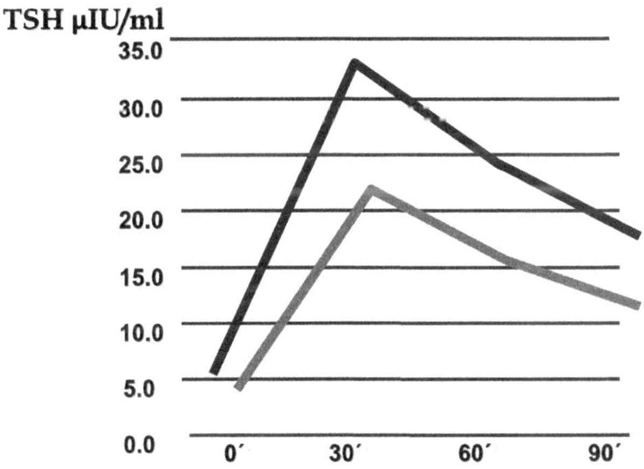

Fig. 2. TRH test at baseline (gray line) and during the reassessment (black line) after combined chelation in TMp with hypothyroidism. Basal TSH: 4.12 ± 0.63 vs. 6.27 ± 1.08, p=0.01. At 30′ mins TSH: 22.13 ± 2.18 vs. 34.06 ± 4.75, p=0.005. At 60′ mins TSH: 15.89 ± 1.13 vs. 25.69 ± 3.72, p=0.002. At 90′ mins TSH: 11.83±1.26 vs. 19.44±3.27, p=0.001.

3.4 Regarding safety, apart from the 2 patients who withdrew from the study, combined chelation was otherwise well tolerated. Adverse events like joint symptoms (5%), gastrointestinal upset (8%) were managed with symptomatic treatment and an increase in liver enzymes (11%) with a temporarily dose reduction of DFP. One case of tinnitus and one with ocular problems required a transient interruption of DFO for 1-2 months after which were reversed, in both cases.

4. Discussion

4.1 An early systematic laboratory evaluation and control of thyroid function is recommended in all TMp annually because thyroid hormones may affect the function of virtually every organ system.

4.1.1 Hypothyroidism symptoms are not typical (fatigue, cold intolerance, weight gain). Criteria for the diagnosis of subclinical hypothyroidism (SH) was an elevated basal TSH concentration (>5 TSH µIU/ml) or an increase of the TSH levels during the test more than 20 µIU/ml from the basal value or additional low levels of FT4 and FT3 respectively.

4.1.2 In case of borderline TSH and FT4 levels a TRH stimulation test has to be performed. An exaggerated TSH response (> or = 21 microIU/Ml) to TRH may occur in 20%-33% of thalassemia patients with normal FT4 levels (Zervas et al, 2002; De Sanctis et al, 2008c). Also, a 15-year longitudinal study has demonstrated that more than 30% of TMp had an abnormal response to TRH test and that 14% change from normal to uncompensated hypothyroidism (Landau et al, 1993). Moreover, TRH stimulation test can also differentiate primary from central hypothyroidism.

4.1.3 In our study, while on DFO monotherapy 18/50 (36%) patients presented with laboratory findings of hypothyroidism. Classification of hypothyroidism in TMp according to laboratory tests is shown in table 2. Among them 14/18 (78%) had subclinical or compensated hypothyroidism and 4/18 (22%), mostly older patients, had overt hypothyroidism.

	FT4	T3	TSH	TSH response to TRH Test
Subclinical Hypothyroidism	normal	normal	Increased > 5-10 mU/L	increased
Compensate Hypothyroidism	slight decrease	slight decrease	normal or increased	exaggerated
Overt Hypothyroidism	decreased	normal or decreased	Increased >10 mU/L	exaggerated

Table 2. Classification of hypothyroidism in TMp according to laboratory tests

4.1.4 Although ultrasonography is one of the techniques most frequently used to evaluate the volume and structure of thyroid gland, it is not ubiquitous in TMp as autoimmune thyroiditis is absent (Mariotti et al, 2011) and most echogenicity patterns are not specific. However, Pitrolo et al, 2004 reported a reduced echogenicity in 47% of TMp and a diffuse spotty echogenicity in 33% of them, indicative of thyroid dysfunction. Also, Filosa et al, 2006 reported features of dyshomogeneity of the parenchyma with different degrees of severity in TMp, which were in accordance with the criteria of Sostre and Reyes and also a slow worsening of thyroid function in 25% of TMp during a 12 year-period of follow up.

4.1.5 Magnetic resonance imaging (MRI) plays an adjunctive role in the further investigation of primary hypothyroidism or/and central hypothyroidism with pituitary dysfunction. Hekmatnia et al, 2010 demonstrated that signal reduction may precede pituitary volume loss and could be expected first on MRI especially in hypogonadic thalassemia patients. Additionally the use of pituitary R2, have allowed to define age-specific norms for pituitary volume allowing earlier recognition of relevant iron deposition and damage and prevention of pan-hypopituitarism (Wood et al, 2010).

4.2 Hypothyroidism & total body iron overload

4.2.1 Serum ferritin levels of approximately 3,000 ng/ml in TMp were found to correlate with hypothyroidism according to Gamberini et al, 2008. De Sanctis et al, 2008c, reported that TSH peak values correlated directly with ferritin levels, ALT, and the compliance index to chelation therapy. In our study, the intensification of chelation with combined therapy and the achievement of normal serum ferritin levels, led to an amelioration of thyroid function with significant increase in the secretion of FT_4 and FT_3 levels both in euthyroid as well as in hypothyroid TMp. While on DFO monotherapy, there were safety concerns with low ferritin levels (Piga et al, 1988), with combined chelation, no significant adverse effects associated with lowering patients' body iron load to normal levels were observed. In some TMp, thyroid impairment was transient, and their secretory capacity improved. In the elderly TMp, with a late onset of chelation therapy, the detrimental effect of iron accumulation led to a permanent impairment of thyroid function suggesting that iron-induced toxicity is mainly time dependent.

4.2.2 Liver iron concentration (LIC) has been regarded as the reference standard for estimating body iron loading and has been shown to accurately predict total body iron stores (Angelucci et al, 2000). R2 and R2* magnetic resonance imaging (MRI) relaxation time techniques allow for non-invasive estimation of LIC in patients with hemoglobinopathies. The LIC cut-off points of 7 and 15 mg Fe/g dw have been used to categorize iron overload status, predict morbidity and mortality, and tailor iron chelation therapy in TMp for the past two decades. However, LIC ≥6 mg Fe/g dw was found to be the best threshold for discriminating the presence and absence of endocrine/bone morbidity (hypothyroidism, osteoporosis, or hypogonadism). According to Musallam et al, 2011, Thalassemia patients with a LIC ≥6 mg Fe/g dw were 4.05 times more likely to have endocrine morbidity compared with patients with a LIC <6 mg Fe/g dw. Liver iron overload also seems to influence hormonal peripheral metabolism (Maggiolini et al, 1995). In our study at baseline, 98% of patients had hepatic iron overload (LIC ≥ 1.5 mg/g dw), and among them 64% had severe iron overload (LIC>12 mg/g dw). After 5 to 7 years of intensive combined chelation, TMp had a normal mean LIC: 0.9±0.2 vs. 15.7±11,1 mg/g dw and this was correlated r= -0.679 p<0.03 with a significant increase of FT4 levels in all TMp. This provides clear evidence that iron-induced tissue damage is reversible, suggesting that such reductions may prevent or reverse thyroid dysfunction.

4.2.3 Extrahepatic tissues have different kinetics of iron uptake and clearance than the liver, because they selectively, or almost selectively, load circulating non-transferrin bound iron (NTBI) (Glickstein et al, 2005). Long periods of unprotected exposure to NTBI could predispose to increased iron uptake in endocrine glands. The cellular labile iron (LIP) expansion in iron overload conditions poses a threat to cell integrity. Iron-mediated oxidative stress triggers apoptosis, volume loss, and fatty replacement in the organs leading to their dysfunction over time.

4.3 Hypothyroidism and iron chelators

4.3.1 With DFO monotherapy the incidence of primary hypothyroidism in TMp was approximately 30%. In some retrospective studies this incidence was shown to decrease over time according to compliance, but in most cases there was a progression from subclinical to overt hypothyroidism (De Sanctis, 2008c). In our study, at baseline while on DFO monotherapy, 18/50 TMp (36%), were treated with thyroxin replacement therapy. Among them 14/18 (78%) had subclinical or compensated hypothyroidism and 4/18 (22%), mostly older patients had overt hypothyroidism. The incidence was high possibly because of inadequate dosing, poor compliance, or relative poor thyroid protection from DFO-specific properties. Monotherapy usually maintains iron balance but does not decrease iron that has accumulated over an extensive period. As TMp require transfusions indefinitely, a negative iron balance is difficult to achieve. Besides, chelator efficacy depend on their availability in plasma or interstitial fluids and their membrane-crossing ability in accessing and neutralizing intracellular LIP which pose a threat to cell integrity. DFO contrary to oral chelators, is a large positively charged, lipophobic molecule with low membrane permeation abilities and thereby low cell iron extraction capacity.

4.3.2 Combined chelation with DFO and DFP because of an additive or synergistic effect on iron excretion, seems to be the treatment of choice in achieving a negative iron balance, normalizing body iron load and reversing clinical and subclinical iron overload complications. Of the 50 patients completing the study, 18 (36%) were treated with thyroxin replacement therapy at baseline while on DFO monotherapy. After combined chelation and an important decrease in total body iron overload 14/18 who had subclinical or compensated hypothyroidism presented a significant increase in mean FT4, FT3 ($p<0.001$)and an decrease in TSH (reflected by the AUC calculation). Among them, 10/18 (56%) discontinued thyroxin therapy (Fisher's exact test $p<0.001$) and 4/18 (22%) reduced their thyroxin dose. The remaining 4 (8% of the total study group) who had biochemical overt hypothyroidism, while they all improved their TRH stimulation test, only 2 converted to compensated hypothyroidism with TSH levels 5-10mIU/ml and normal FT4 & FT3 levels. The time needed to reverse hypothyroidism with combined chelation varies according to the patient age and iron load status. Besides combined chelation may prevent hypothyroidism as no new-onset nor worsening of thyroid dysfunction was observed during the study period. Whether the overall improvement in thyroid function that was achieved in our patients can be solely attributed to the intensification of chelation therapy and better compliance or if there is a tissue-specific effectiveness of DFP in iron removal from thyroid gland is debatable.

4.3.3 To our knowledge, this is the first report that documents, the beneficial effect of long-term combined therapy in normalizing total body iron load and reversing most of the cases of subclinical and compensate hypothyroidism in TMp.

4.4 Hypothyroidism & cardiac dysfunction

4.4.1 Thyroid hormones control several enzymes involved in regulating calcium fluxes in the heart including the calcium-dependent adenosine triphosphatase and phospholamban. In case of hypothyroidism, the decreases in the expression and activity of these enzymes could potentially impair systolic performance and diastolic relaxation of the ventricles, leading to a reduction in cardiac output (Klein & Danzi, 2007). Additionally thyroid hormones play a role in reducing peripheral vascular resistance by relaxing vascular smooth muscle cells. Thus, in case of hypothyroidism there is an increase in peripheral vascular resistance and a reduction in tissue perfusion and oxygen utilization. Symptoms of cardiovascular dysfunction are not common or prominent but may include dyspnea, exercise intolerance, and edema. Findings on physical examination may include bradycardia, hypertension, nonpitting edema, and pleural or pericardial effusion. Laboratory indices like dyslipidemia with high serum total and low-density-lipoprotein (LDL) cholesterol concentrations are common in hypothyroidism.

4.4.2 In a recent long-term follow-up study (De Sanctis, 2008a), was mentioned that cardiac involvement may be present in 50% of hypothyroid TMp with moderate or severe iron overload. Among them, 16,6% died during the follow-up from heart failure and arrhythmia, in a 4-year interval. The changes in cardiovascular function in hypothyroidism respond to replacement therapy with L-thyroxine and an adequate chelation regimen (De Sanctis, 2008b).

4.4.3 In our study, all hypothyroid TMp were presented at baseline with moderate to severe cardiac iron overload (mean MRI T2*H: 13.8 ± 9.8 msec) and 16/18 (88,8%) with a cardiac dysfunction (mean LVEF of $54 \pm 1.5\%$) and classified according to their symptoms 4/16

(25%) NYHA Class I, 7/16 (44%) Class II, 3/16 (19%) Class III and 2/16 (12%) Class IV. Twelve of them were on cardiac medications (angiotensin-converting enzyme [ACE] inhibitors, anti-arrhythmics, digoxin or diuretics). After combined chelation therapy, the overall change from cardiac iron loaded to non-iron loaded was significant (Fisher's exact test $p < 0.001$) with mean MRI T2*H increased to normal levels 35.5 ± 8.1ms and mean LVEF: 65 ± 2.8%, respectively. Only in 2/16 less compliant TMp, although ameliorated cardiac dysfunction (one of Class IV and one of Class III improved to Class II) kept on cardiac medication. None of our TMp died during the follow-up interval, from heart failure or arrhythmia. No new cases of cardiac dysfunction were observed suggesting that combined chelation may prevent or reverse cardiac complications. A considerable body of data now exists confirming that DFP is superior to DFO in reducing iron in the heart (Pennell et al, 2006) and reversing cardiac complications and that combined chelation (DFP–DFO) can have a more marked effect in purging cardiac iron (Anderson et al, 2002; Tanner et al, 2007, 2008), as it was observed in this study. Maggio et al, 2009 speculated that DFP had a protective effect on the heart even before cardiac iron declined significantly, most likely because of the clearance of cellular toxic labile iron. In any case, reversal of cardiac complications and discontinuation of cardiac medication, as documented here, is a significant achievement. Reversal of hypothyroidism, in the same TMp, possibly sustained cardiac amelioration.

4.5 Hypothyroidism & hypogonadism

4.5.1 Subclinical hypothyroidism may be associated with male and female gonad dysfunction and interferes with their reproductive ability (Trokoudes et al 2006). The awareness of the thyroid status in any infertile couple is crucial, because of its significant, frequent and often reversible or preventable effect on infertility.

4.5.2 Indeed, among our hypothyroid TMp one female with secondary amenorrhea, after 5 years of combined chelation, the normalization of her total body iron load and the improvement of her overall hormonal profile, gave birth to 2 healthy children after normal conception.

4.6 The decision to treat TMp with L-thyroxin

4.6.1 Although the course of thyroid disease in TMp is a slow process and it might take years to progress from normal to uncompensated hypothyroidism, the decision to treat with L-thyroxin is crucial. In the normal population, experts recommend treatment with thyroid hormone if TSH levels >10 mU/l. In thalassaemic patients more criteria are taken into consideration (Gharib et al, 2005; De Sanctis et al, 2008b). It is particularly recommended in TMp with cardiac dysfunction because of the potential for reducing the risk of cardiac problems (Biondi & Cooper, 2008). The therapeutic use of thyroid hormones in the clinical treatment of mood disorders or memory impairment is taking on a new dimension even in patients with euthyroid hormonal state (Bauer et al, 2008). Additionally, thyroxine treatment in subclinical hypothyroidism may restore ovulatory dysfunction and adverse pregnancy outcome. Trokoudes et al, 2006 underlined that awareness of the thyroid status in the infertile couple is crucial, because of its significant, frequent and often reversible or preventable effect on infertility.

4.6.2 Therefore in our group of TMp the decision to treat was individualized and based on patients' clinical history and aggravating factors (hyperlipidaemia, cardiac dysfunction, diabetes, pregnancy, depression). For this reason, the overall prevalence in our group (18/50 36%) was higher than that reported by others (Cunningham et al, 2004; Borgna-Pignatti et al, 2005). After the use of combined chelation and the reversal of cardiac, glucose metabolism abnormalities and hypogonadism and other aggravating factors, thyroxine treatment was reconsidered according to thyroid investigation of each individual patient. Thereby 56% of TMp with subclinical or compensated hypothyroidism discontinued thyroxin therapy and 22% reduced their thyroxin dose.

4.6.3 Special attention has to be paid in hypothyroid children and adolescents presenting clinical features that include declining growth velocity, short stature and pubertal delay. Replacement therapy with T4 should be installed in order to restore normal growth and development. Once growth and pubertal development are complete, thyroid hormone treatment can be discontinued and thyroid function re-evaluated. Patients and families should be aware that treatment may sometimes cause temporary behavior symptoms, poorer school achievement, and may not restore full growth potential.

4.6.4 After initiation of T4 therapy, the patient should be reevaluated and serum TSH should be measured in six weeks, and the dose adjusted accordingly. A systematic follow-up biochemical monitoring (TSH) should be performed every six months to determine if re-titration of the dose is necessary. For patients whose serum TSH is confirmed to be at the upper limits or above the normal reference range, is recommended to increase the dose of T4 with the aim of lowering the serum TSH value into the lower half of the normal range.

4.6.5 As T4 should be taken once per day, on an empty stomach (one hour before eating or two hours after), sometimes compliance is difficult to achieve, considering that TMp take many medications. Also some of them may interfere with T4 absorption and should be taken several hours after the T4 dose. Additionally a high-fiber diet or coffee uptake can interfere with the absorption of T4.

4.6.6 A close monitoring of TSH is recommended in hypothyroid TMp with cardiac dysfunction and osteoporosis, as over-replacement with T4 may cause atrial fibrillation and accelerated bone loss with risk of fractures.

5. Conclusion

This study demonstrated that hypothyroidism in Thalassemia, is a frequent iron overload complication. In most TMp there are no obvious clinical signs of hypothyroidism, so a regular follow-up for early detection and a timely replacement treatment should be implemented especially in children and adolescents with growth failure and pubertal delay. The use of intensive combined chelation and the reduction of total body iron load to normal levels may play a leading role in the prevention or/and reversal of hypothyroidism in Thalassemia. As shown in our study there was a reversal of most cases of subclinical and compensated hypothyroidism. Additionally this treatment regimen may prevent the progression from subclinical to overt hypothyroidism or may improve some cases of overt hypothyroidism, suggesting that even iron-induced damage of the thyroid pituitary axis might be reversed. Combined chelation was well tolerated and had a positive impact on patient quality of life. It remains to be established, possibly through clinical trials in the future, whether other chelation regimens, will offer comparable benefits.

6. References

Anderson LJ, Wonke B, Prescott E, Holden S, Walker JM, Pennell DJ, (2002) Comparison of effects of oral deferiprone and subcutaneous desferrioxamine on myocardial iron concentrations and ventricular function in beta-thalassaemia. Lancet, Vol. 360, pp. 516-520.

Angelucci E, Brittenham GM, McLaren CE, Ripalti M, Baronciani D, Giardini C, Galimberti M, Polchi P, Lucarelli G, (2000), Hepatic iron concentration and total body iron stores in thalassemia major. N Engl J Med. Vol. 343(5), pp. 327-31.

Bauer M, Goetz T, Glenn T, Whybrow PC, Gjessing R, (2008) The thyroid-brain interaction in thyroid disorders and mood disorders. Journal of Neuroendocrinology, Vol. 20, pp. 1101–1114.

Bernal J. (2002) Action of thyroid hormone in brain, Journal of Endocrinological Investigation, Vol. 25, pp. 268–288.

Biondi B, Cooper DS, (2008) The clinical significance of subclinical thyroid dysfunction, Endocr Rev, Vol. 29(1), pp. 76-131.

Borgna-Pignatti C, Rugolotto S, De Stefano P, Zhao H, Cappellini MD, Del Vecchio GC. (2004) Survival and complications in patients with thalassemia major treated with transfusion and deferoxamine, Haematologica, Vol. 89(10), pp. 1187-93.

Borgna-Pignatti C, Cappellini MD, De Stefano P, Del Vecchio GC, Forni GL, Gamberini MR, Ghilardi R, Piga A, Romeo MA, Zhao H, Cnaan A, (2006) Cardiac morbidity and mortality in deferoxamine- or deferiprone-treated patients with thalassemia major. Blood, Vol. 107, pp. 3733-3737.

Cavallo L, Licci D, Acquafredda A, Marranzini M, Beccasio R, Scardino ML, Altomare M, Mastro F, Sisto L, Schettini F, (1984) Endocrine involvement in children with beta-thalassaemia major. Transverse and longitudinal studies. I. Pituitary-thyroidal axis function and its correlation with serum ferritin levels, Acta Endocrinol (Copenh). Vol. 107(1), pp. 49-53.

Delvecchio, M.; Cavallo, L. (2010). Growth and endocrine function in thalassemia major in childhood and adolescence. J. Endocrinol. Invest, Vol.33, pp. 61-68.

De Sanctis V, Eleftheriou A, Malaventura C. (2004) Prevalence of endocrine complications and short stature in patients with thalassaemia major: a multicenter study by the Thalassaemia International Federation (TIF). Pediatr Endocrinol Rev, Suppl 2, pp. 249-55.

De Sanctis V, Roos M, Gasser T, Fortini M, Raiola G, Galati MC; Italian Working Group on Endocrine Complications in Non-Endocrine Diseases. (2006). Impact of long-term iron chelation therapy on growth and endocrine functions in thalassaemia. J Pediatr Endocrinol Metab, Vol.19, pp. 471-80.

De Sanctis V, De Sanctis E, Ricchieri P, Gubellini E, Gilli G, Gamberini MR. (2008a). Mild subclinical hypothyroidism in thalassaemia major: prevalence, multigated radionuclide test, clinical and laboratory long-term follow-up study, Pediatr Endocrinol Rev, Vol.6, Suppl 1, pp. 174-80.

De Sanctis V, Govoni MR, Sprocati M, Marsella M, Conti E. (2008b) Cardiomyopathy and pericardial effusion in a 7 year-old boy with beta-thalassaemia major, severe primary hypothyroidism and hypoparathyroidism due to iron overload, Pediatr Endocrinol Rev, Vol.6 Suppl 1, pp. 181-4.

De Sanctis V, Tanas R, Gamberini MR, Sprocati M, Govoni MR, Marsella M. (2008c) Exaggerated TSH response to TRH ("sub-biochemical" hypothyroidism) in prepubertal and adolescent thalassaemic patients with iron overload: prevalence and 20-year natural history, Pediatr Endocrinol Rev, Vol.6, Suppl 1, pp. 170-3.

Esposito BP, Breuer W, Sirankapracha P, Pootrakul P, Hershko C, Cabantchik ZI. (2003). Labile plasma iron in iron overload: redox activity and susceptibility to chelation. Blood, Vol.102(7), pp.2670-7.

Farmaki K., Tzoumari I., Pappa Ch. (2008). Reversal of Hypothyroidism in Well Chelated β-Thalassemia Major Patients.. Blood, Vol 112:11, pp. 1323-1324.

Farmaki K, Tzoumari I, Pappa C, Chouliaras G, Berdoukas V. (2010a). Normalisation of total body iron load with very intensive combined chelation reverses cardiac and endocrine complications of thalassaemia major. Br J Haematol, Vol. 148(3), pp. 466-75.

Farmaki K, Berdoukas V. (2010b). Reversal Of Endocrinopathies In Transfusional Iron Overload Patients - The Next Frontier In Iron Chelation - EJCMO, Vol. 2(4), pp. 59-66.

Farmaki K, Tzoumari I, Pappa C, (2011) Combining oral chelators in transfusion dependents Thalassemia major patients, may prevent or reverse iron overload complications, Blood cell Mol Dis, Vol. 47, pp. 33-40

Filosa A, Di Maio S, Aloj G, Acampora C, (2006) Longitudinal study on thyroid function in patients with thalassemia major, J Pediatr Endocrinol Metab, Vol. 19(12), pp. 1397-1404.

Gamberini MR, De Sanctis V, Gilli G. (2008). Hypogonadism, diabetes mellitus, hypothyroidism, hypoparathyroidism: incidence and prevalence related to iron overload and chelation therapy in patients with thalassaemia major followed from 1980 to 2007 in the Ferrara Centre, Pediatr Endocrinol Rev, Vol.6 Suppl 1, pp. 158-69.

Gharib, H., Tuttle, R.M., Baskin, H.J., Fish, L.H., Singer, P.A., McDermott, M.T. (2005) Consensus statement #1: subclinical thyroid dysfunction: a joint statement on management from the American Association of Clinical Endocrinologists, the American Thyroid Association, and The Endocrine Society. Thyroid, Vol. 15, pp. 24–28.

Glickstein H, El RB, Shvartsman M, Cabantchik ZI, (2005), Intracellular labile iron pools as direct targets of iron chelators: a fluorescence study of chelator action in living cells. Blood. Vol. 106(9), pp. 3242-50.

Hekmatnia A, Radmard AR, Rahmani AA, Adibi A, Khademi H, Magnetic resonance imaging signal reduction may precede volume loss in the pituitary gland of transfusion-dependent beta-thalassemic patients, Acta Radiol. 2010 Feb;51(1):71-7.

Hudec M, Grigerova M, Walsh CH. (2008) Secondary hypothyroidism in hereditary hemochromatosis: recovery after iron depletion, Thyroid, Vol.18(2), pp. 255-7.

Jain M, Sinha RS, Chellani H, Anand NK. (1995) Assessment of thyroid functions and its role in body growth in thalassemia major. Indian Pediatr, Vol.32, pp. 213-9.

Kalinowski DS, Richardson DR. (2005) The evolution of iron chelators, for the treatment of iron overload disease and cancer. Pharmacol Rev. vol. 57(4), pp.547-583.

Klein I, Danzi S. (2007) Thyroid disease and the heart. Circulation, vol. 116, pp. 1725.

Kolnagou A, Yazman D, Economides C, Eracleous E, Kontoghiorghes GJ, (2009) Uses and limitations of serum ferritin, magnetic resonance imaging T2 and T2* in the diagnosis of iron overload and in the ferrikinetics of normalization of the iron stores in thalassemia using the International Committee on Chelation deferiprone/deferoxamine combination protocol, Hemoglobin, vol. 33(5), pp. 312-322.

Kontoghiorghes GJ, Kolnagou A, Peng CT, Shah SV, Aessopos, (2010) Safety issues of iron chelation therapy in patients with normal range iron stores including thalassaemia, neurodegenerative, renal and infectious diseases, Expert Opin Drug Saf. Vol.9(2), pp. 201-6.

Landau H, Matoth I, Landau-Cordova Z, Goldfarb A, Rachmilewitz EA, Glaser B. (1993). Cross-sectional and longitudinal study of the pituitary-thyroid axis in patients with thalassaemia major, Clin Endocrinol (Oxf), Vol.38(1), pp. 55-61.

Maggio, A., Vitrano, A., Capra, M., Cuccia, L., Gagliardotto, F., Filosa, A., Magnano, C., Rizzo, M., Caruso, V., Gerardi, C., Argento, C., Campisi, S., Cantella, F., Commendatore, F., D'Ascola, D.G., Fidone, C., Ciancio, A., Galati, M.C., Giuffrida, G., Cingari, R., Giugno, G., Lombardo, T., Prossomariti, L., Malizia, R., Meo, A., Roccamo, G., Romeo, M.A., Violi, P., Cianciulli, P. & Rigano, P. (2009) Improving survival with deferiprone treatment in patients with thalassemia major: a prospective multicenter randomised clinical trial under the auspices of the Italian Society for Thalassemia and Hemoglobinopathies. Blood Cells, Molecules, and Diseases, Vol. 42, pp.247–251.

Maggiolini M, De Luca G, Bria M, Sisci D, Aquila S, Pezzi V, Lanzino M, Giorno A, Tamburrini O, Della Sala M, Corcioni E, Brancati C, Ando S. (1995) Follow-up study of thyroid function in polytransfused thalassemic patients, Endocrine, Vol.3(2), pp.91-4.

Magro S, Puzzonia P, Consarino C, Galati MC, Morgione S, Porcelli D, Grimaldi S, Tancrè D, Arcuri V, De Santis V (1990). Hypothyroidism in patients with thalassemia syndromes. Acta Haematol, Vol. 84, pp. 72-6.

Mariotti S, Pigliaru F, Cocco MC, Spiga A, Vaquer S, Lai ME, (2011), β-thalassemia and thyroid failure: is there a role for thyroid autoimmunity? Pediatr Endocrinol Rev. vol. 8 Suppl 2, pp. 307-9

Menconi F, Hasham A, Tomer Y. (2011). Environmental triggers of thyroiditis: Hepatitis C and interferon-α, J Endocrinol Invest, Vol.34(1), pp. 78-84.

Musallam KM, Cappellini MD, Wood JC, Motta I, Graziadei G, Tamim H, Taher AT, (2011) Elevated liver iron concentration is a marker of increased morbidity in patients with {beta} thalassemia intermedia, Haematologica, Jul 26.

Pennell, D.J., Berdoukas, V., Karagiorga, M., Ladis, V., Piga, A., Aessopos, A., Gotsis, E.D., Tanner, M.A., Smith, G.C., Westwood, M.A., Wonke, B. & Galanello, R. (2006) Randomized controlled trial of deferiprone or deferoxamine in beta-thalassemia major patients with asymptomatic myocardial siderosis. Blood, Vol.107, pp. 3738–3744.

Piga A, Luzzatto L, Capalbo P, Gambotto S, Tricta F, Gabutti V, (1988), High-dose desferrioxamine as a cause of growth failure in thalassemic patients. Eur J Haematol, vol. 40, pp. 380-381.

Pitrolo L, Malizia G, Lo Pinto C, Malizia V, Capra M, (2004) Ultrasound thyroid evaluation in thalassemic patients: correlation between the aspects of thyroidal stroma and function, Pediatr Endocrinol Rev, vol. 2(2), pp. 313-315.

St Pierre TG, Clark PR, Chua-anusorn W, Fleming AJ, Jeffrey GP, Olynyk JK, Pootrakul P, Robins E, Lindeman R, (2005), Noninvasive measurement and imaging of liver iron concentrations using proton magnetic resonance. Blood. Vol. 105(2), pp. 855-61

Tanner, M.A., Galanello, R., Dessi, C., Smith, G.C., Westwood, M.A., Agus, A., Roughton, M., Assomull, R., Nair, S.V., Walker, J.M. & Pennell, D.J. (2007) A randomized, placebo-controlled, doubleblind trial of the effect of combined therapy with deferoxamine and deferiprone on myocardial iron in thalassemia major using cardiovascular magnetic resonance. Circulation, Vol. 115, pp. 1876–1884.

Tanner, M.A., Galanello, R., Dessi, C., Smith, G.C., Westwood, M.A., Agus, A., Pibiri, M., Nair, S.V., Walker, J.M. & Pennell, D.J. (2008) Combined chelation therapy in thalassemia major for the treatment of severe myocardial siderosis with left ventricular dysfunction. Journal of Cardiovascular Magnetic Resonance, Vol. 10, pp. 12.

Telfer PT, Warburton F, Christou S, Hadjigavriel M, Sitarou M, Kolnagou A. (2009). Improved survival in thalassemia major patients on switching, from desferrioxamine to combined chelation therapy with desferrioxamine and deferiprone. Haematologica, Vol. 94(12), pp. 1777-8.

Trokoudes KM, Skordis N, Picolos MK, Infertility and thyroid disorders, Curr Opin Obstet Gynecol. 2006 Aug;18(4):446-51.

Wood JC, Enriquez C, Ghugre N, Tyzka JM, Carson S, Nelson MD, et al. MRI R2 and R2* mapping accurately estimates hepatic iron concentration in transfusiondependent thalassemia and sickle cell disease patients. Blood. 2005;106(4):1460-5.

Wood JC, Noetzl L, Hyderi A, Joukar M, Coates T, Mittelman S, (2010) Predicting pituitary iron and endocrine dysfunction, Ann N Y Acad Sci. Vol. 1202, pp. 123-8

Zervas A., Katapodi A., Protonotariou A., Livadas S., Karagiorga M., Politis C., Tolis G. (2002) Assessment of thyroid function in two hundred patients with beta-thalassemia major, Thyroid, Vol.12(2), pp. 151-4.

Hypothyroidism, Oxidative Stress and Reproduction

Antonio Mancini[1], Elena Giacchi[2], Sebastiano Raimondo[1], Chantal Di Segni[1], Andrea Silvestrini[3] and Elisabetta Meucci[3]
[1]*Department of Internal Medicine*
[2]*Center for Study and Research on Natural Fertility Regulation*
[3]*Institute of Biochemistry and Clinical Biochemistry*
Catholic University of the Sacred Heart, Rome
Italy

1. Introduction

It is well known that in both sexes thyroid hormones influence sexual development and reproductive function; clinical and experimental evidences suggest that the hypothalamic-pituitary-thyroid axis and the hypothalamic-pituitary-ovary axis are physiologically related and act together as unified system in a number of pathological conditions (Doufas & Mastorakos, 2000).

In women, both hyper- and hypo-thyroidism may result in menstrual disturbances. In hyperthyroidism the most common manifestations are simple oligomenorrhea and anovulatory cycles. Hypothyroidism results in changes in cycle length, amount of bleeding, and usually is associated with abnormal menstrual cycles characterized mainly by polymenorrhea and anovulatory cycles (Krassas et al., 1999). Also subclinical hypothyroxinemia can be associated with short luteal phase and insufficient progesterone secretion (Bohnet et al., 1981); similar pictures are present in a variety of situations characterized by low T3 levels (malnutrition, chronic illness, exercise), known as "non-thyroidal illness" (De Groot, 2006).

Interference between thyroid gland function and the ovary are described in three main areas: the secretion of GnRH, the peripheral metabolism of steroids and prolactin secretion. Previous studies demonstrated a direct ovarian effect: TSH possesses a luteotropic activity (Wurfel, 1992) and the expression of thyroid hormone receptors has been documented in all ovarian cell types: surface epithelial cells, oocytes, granulosa and theca cells, stromal cells (Dittrich et al., 2011). Many studies were also performed in males, both in animals and humans and extensively reviewed (Krassas et al., 2010).

Despite the clinical relevance of the association between thyroid and reproductive health, its physiopathological mechanisms are still poorly understood and no definitive trials on thyroid hormone replacement allow unequivocal conclusions. Among the new mechanisms proposed, a link could be related to oxidative stress (OS).

Oxidative stress is defined as the unbalancing between production of free radicals, molecules characterized by high reactivity due to one or more unpaired electrons in the external orbital, and antioxidant defenses in the biological systems. Nowadays, it is considered an important pathogenetic mechanism in different diseases (Halliwell & Gutteridge, 1979). Among free radicals the most important and studied are reactive oxygen species (ROS), of which most *in vivo* production occurs mainly during oxidative processes of energetic substrates in the mitochondrial respiratory chain (Littarru, 1994; Kang & Hamasaki, 2003). However, other important kinds of free radicals exist, besides ROS, among which nitrogen reactive species are the most studied (Lancaster, 1992).

An augmented ROS production can be the consequence of an augmented electronic flow in the respiratory chain, when it is activated by an increased energetic demand or contribution of substrates (Turrens & Boveris, 1980), as occurs in obesity. An uncontrolled production of free radicals is linked to many pathological events, such as rheumatoid arthritis and myocardial infarction (Littarru, 1994), and in general ROS damage occurs in inflamed tissues, characterized by cellular lysis and intracellular content release. Moreover in diabetes mellitus, oxidation accompanies glycation *in vivo*, while antioxidant capacity is decreased, finally resulting in an increased susceptibility to oxidative stress (Wolff et al., 1991).

It is possible to characterize different cellular defensive mechanisms against the free radical damage (Littarru, 1994). The first mechanism is the prevention of production or the rapid inactivation of free radicals, thanks to the action of enzymes, like catalase, peroxidase glutathion complex and superoxydedismutase (SOD), or of transition-metal binding proteins, like transferrin, ferritin and ceruloplasmin. The second mechanism interrupts propagation of the lipid peroxidation chain by a reaction with the intermediate radicals and the consequent neutralization. This mechanism is acted by molecules called "scavengers", which can be water-soluble, such as albumin, bilirubin, ascorbic acid, urates and thiols, or liposoluble, such as vitamin E and coenzyme Q_{10}, the only liposoluble antioxidant synthesized in living organisms. The mobility of scavengers, particularly the liposoluble ones and above all at membrane level, allows to intercept radicals and transform them into more stable molecules and therefore to stop radical chain. The third defensive mechanism uses processes which remove molecules damaged by oxidative attack, allowing the reconstitution of normal structures (e.g. specific phospholypases remove the peroxidized fatty acids, making possible the re-acylation of damaged molecule by an acyl-CoA and the respective enzyme) (Littarru, 1994). Different studies suggest that OS can be present in hypothyroidism and could be a factor involved in infertility associated to thyroid insufficiency.

2. Thyroid hormones and oxidative stress

Previous studies have shown that both hyperthyroidism and hypothyroidism are associated with enhanced oxidative stress involving enzymatic and non-enzymatic antioxidants (Resch et al., 2002). Besides, some complications of hyperthyroidism are due just to the oxidative stress in target tissues (Asayama & Kato, 1990). Thyroid hormones *per se* can act as oxidants and produce DNA-damage (contrasted by catalase), probably through the phenolic group, similar to that of steroidal estrogens (Dobrzynska et al., 2004). Many other mechanisms, reviewed by Venditti & Di Meo (2006), can be involved: enhanced NOS gene expression with NO overproduction; activation of hepatic nuclear factor-kB and following increase of cytokines stimulating ROS generation; uncoupling mechanisms involving UCP-2 and UCP-3, regulated by thyroid hormones; increased turnover of mitochondrial proteins; mitoptosis, regulated by peroxisome proliferator-activated receptor gamma coactivator-1, which is upregulated by T3 administration. Thyroid hormones influence lipid composition of rat tissues (Hoch, 1988) and therefore the susceptibility to oxidative stress.

However, there is a specificity in tissue response, and discrepant effects of T3 and T4 are possible. In rat liver, T3-induced hyperthyroidism was found to be associated with altered lipid-peroxidation indices, including elevated levels of TBARS and hydroperoxydes (Fernandez *et al.*, 1985; Venditti *et al.*, 1997; Huth *et al.*, 1998; Venditti *et al.*, 1999). On the contrary, no change in TBARS was found in homogenized livers from rats made hyperthyroid by administration of T4 over a 4-week period (Asayama et al., 1987). As regards testis, no significant change (TBARS or hydroperoxydes) was observed in lipid peroxidation of hyperthyroid adult rats, but hyperthyroidism promoted protein oxidation rate as indicated by an enhanced content of protein-bound carbonyls (Choudhury et al., 2003). In conclusion, we should emphasize the fact of a tissue-linked variability in the effects of hyperthyroidism on the activity of antioxidant enzymes (Mn-SOD or Cu,Zn-SOD, catalase, glutathion-peroxidase) with differential effects of the two thyroid hormones (Venditti & Di Meo, 2006).

At a systemic level, also in humans, hyperthyroidism has been associated with reduced circulating levels of alpha-tocopherol (Ademoglu *et al.*, 1998; Bianchi *et al.*, 1990) and Coenzyme Q_{10} (Bianchi et al., 1990; Mancini et al., 1991). Coenzyme Q_{10} showed a trend to increase in hypothyroidism (Mancini et al., 1991); it appeared to be a sensitive index of tissue effect of thyroid hormones, in situations in which drug interference, such as amiodarone (Mancini et al., 1989) or systemic illness inducing a low-T3 conditions (Mancini et al., 2005) complicate the interpretation of thyroid hormone levels.

However, data on hypothyroidism in humans are conflicting. Baskol et al showed in a group of 33 patients with primary hypothyroidism elevated malondialdehyde (MDA) and nitric oxide (NO) levels and low paraoxonase (PON1) activity, while superoxide dismutase (SOD) was not different from controls. Interestingly, thyroid treatment decreased MDA and increased PON1, without reaching levels observed in controls (Baskol et al., 2007). They concluded that a prooxidant environment in hypothyroidism could play a role in the pathogenesis of atherosclerosis in such patients. Elevated MDA levels were also shown in subclinical hypothyroidism (Torun et al., 2009); the increased in OS was attributed to lack of antioxidants but also to altered lipid metabolism, since MDA showed a correlation with LDL-cholesterol, total cholesterol and triglycerides. Total antioxidant status (TAS) was similar in overt hypothyroidism, subclinical hypothyroidism and controls.

Different studies confirmed the NO elevation (Coria et al., 2009; Erdamar et al., 2008). Data on other parameters are more conflicting. As PON-1 is concerned, a decreased activity was observed both in hypo- and hyperthyroidism (Azizi et al., 2003), while not significant differences with controls were shown in other studies (Coria et al., 2009).

Another study (Santi et al., 2010) showed increased levels of thiobarbituric acid reactive substances (TBARS), but also of antioxidants, such as SOD, catalase (CAT) and Vitamin E.

All these parameters correlated with T3; moreover the correlation between T3 and CAT remained significant also when corrected with total cholesterol. While TBARS elevation was also shown also in some studies (Nanda et al., 2007; Erdamar et al., 2008), other studies did not confirm the datum in overt hypothyroidism (Coria et al., 2009) and in subclinical hypothyroidism (Kebapcilar et al., 2007).

We showed low Total Antioxidant Capacity (TAC) levels in hypothyroid patients (Mancini et al., 2010a) and increased CoQ_{10} levels also in secondary hypothyroidism (mainly due to its metabolic role in mitochondrial respiratory chain and therefore underutilized in hypothyroid tissue). In the last case, hypothyroidism has a predominant effect on other conditions influencing CoQ_{10} in opposite direction, such as acromegaly and hypoadrenalism (Mancini et al., 2010a; Mancini et al., 2010b).

Finally, new perspectives concern DUOX (Dual OXidase) genes expression, which is crucial for H_2O_2 generation essential for thyroid peroxidase (TPO)-catalyzed thyroid hormone synthesis (Ohye & Sugawara, 2010). Two oxidases of such family are present in thyroid (DUOX1 and DUOX2) and work together maturation factors (DUOXA1 and DUOXA2), which allow DUOX proteins to translocate to the follicular cell membrane and exert their enzymatic activity (OHYE). Cases of hypothyroidism due to mutation of DUOX or DUOXA genes have been presented in literature (Varela et al., 2006; Ohye et al., 2008). While defects of this system interfere with thyroid hormone synthesis, another new intracellular ROS generating system has been demonstrated in the human thyroid gland: NADPH oxidase 4 (NOX4) (Weyemi et al., 2010); defects in such a system could be associated with thyroid cancer (via activation by H-Ras oncongene) and Hashimoto's thyroiditis (in such a situation increased extracellular production cause an increased ICAM-1 expression and cytokine release) (Sharma et al., 2008).

3. Hypothyroidism and male infertility

Hypothyroidism can cause interference with male fertility, both via endocrine mechanisms and direct effect on spermatogenesis, as recently reviewed (Krassas et al., 2010). The best definite alteration is the decrease in SHBG and total testosterone (T) concentrations, while free T are reduced in approximately 60% of hypothyroid male; thyroxine therapy induces an increase in free T (Donnelly & White, 2000). While in females PRL elevation in hypothyroidism is a crucial phenomenon inducing hypogonadism, in males PRL levels are not frequently augmented. Similarly, gonadotropin levels are often in the normal range, but a blunted gonadotropin (Gn) response to GnRH support the hypothesis of a reduced pituitary responsiveness to hypothalamic stimulation (Velazquez & Bellabarba Arata, 1997). The exaggerated T response to hCG also underlines the role of hypothalamic-pituitary unit rather than a primary testicular effect. A decrease has also been shown in DHEA, DHEAS, andostendiol and pregnenolone sulfate (Tagawa et al., 2001). The endocrine dysfunction partially explain the sexual symptoms complained in such patients, such as decreased libido or erectile dysfunction (Carani et al., 2005; Krassas et al., 2008).

The studies on hypothyroidism and spermatogenesis are not conclusive, since reports concerning small groups of patients are reported in literature (Krassas et al., 2010); the hypothesis that severe and prolonged thyroid deficiency occurring early in life can result in abnormal testicular biopsies is based on histological and endocrine evaluation of 6 adult hypothyroid men (De la Balze et al., 1962). Similarly, in a group of 8 hypothyroid males, various degrees of testicular atrophy were shown (Wortsman et al., 1987). Another group of 10 hypothyroid patients treated with T4 (with a discontinuation or decrease of therapy for at least a spermatogenetic cycle) presented a decrease in semen volume, progressive forward motility and cumulative percentage of mobile spermatozoa forms, but without significant changes in these parameters during the phase of reinduced hypothyroidism; it was concluded therefore that short-term postpubertal hypothyroidism does not cause severe seminal alterations (Corrales Hernàndez et al., 1990).

Another prospective, controlled study evaluated semen analysis, biochemical parameters (fructose and acid phosphatase), teratozoospermia index and acridine orange test, in 25 hypothyroid men, before and after 6-9 months T4 treatment (Krassas et al., 2008) in comparison with 15 normal fertile men. The authors concluded that hypothyroidism had an adverse effect on spermatogenesis, with sperm morphology as the only parameter that was significantly affected. These data, therefore, need to be reevaluated, considering the variations in parameters of fertile men which have been introduced by the new version of the WHO manual for semen analysis (WHO, 2010) which are remarkably different from those previously adopted as normal range (WHO, 1999).

Finally, even if the topic of autoimmune thyroid disease (AITD) is extensively studied in females (see the following paragraph), some data in males are reported. The prevalence of thyroid antibody positivity in a population of infertile men was found to be 7.5%; there was no difference in prevalence of abnormal thyroid function tests in normozoospermic vs pathozoospermic patients (11.1 vs 11.8%), but when correlating thyroid autoimmunity with semen parameters, the authors found a significantly higher presence of TPO-Abs in pathozoospermic and asthenozoospermic vs normozoospermic infertile men (6.7% and 7.2% respectively vs 1.6%) (Trummer et al., 2001). This datum was not confirmed in other studies (Krassas et al., 2010). The causal effect of thyroid autoimmunity is far to be understood; only one study showed the presence of TPO-Abs in men with serum sperm autoantibodies (Paschke et al., 1994).

The hypothesis that OS, which is well known to interfere with male fertility (Iwasaki & Gagnon, 1992; Aitken & Krausz, 2001; Agarwal & Saleh, 2002), can be related to thyroid disfunction induced us to perform a case-control study, evaluating TAC and seminal parameters in an unselected group of infertile man and controls (Mancini et al., 2009) and correlating these values with systemic hormones. TAC was measured using the system H_2O_2-metmyoglobin as source of radicals. They interact with the chromogenous compound 2,2^I,-azinobis (3-ethylbenzothiazoline-6-sulphonate) (ABTS) generating its radical cationic form ($ABTS^{\bullet +}$) which can be spectroscopically and kinetically detected (Rice-Evans & Miller, 1994; Meucci et al., 2003). This colorimetric assay was compared with the enhanced chemiluminescence one, which is the most commonly used method for measuring TAC in seminal plasma (Said et al., 2003). The colorimetric assay was found to be a reliable and accurate method, simpler and cheaper than the chemiluminescence one. Antioxidants induce a "lag time" in accumulation and appearance of $ABTS^{\bullet +}$ which is proportional to the antioxidant concentration itself, so that TAC can be expressed as Lag phase. The possible release of intracellular antioxidants from broken cells was preliminarily excluded by measuring the enzyme LDH in seminal plasma specimens (Mancini et al., 1994).

The correlation analysis between hormones and seminal parameters showed an inverse correlation between PRL and sperm motility, and a direct correlation of TAC with PRL and FT4, but not with gonadotropins or gonadal steroids. Our data suggest that systemic hormones may play a role in regulating seminal antioxidant capacity. This is interesting also because some hormones, such as thyroid and pituitary ones, are not usually tested in the first level evaluation of male patients with fertility problems.

4. Hypothyroidism and female infertility

Hypothyroidism is frequently associated with infertility, due to different reasons: altered peripheral estrogen metabolism, alterations in GnRH secretion causing abnormal pulsatile LH release, hyperprolactinemia and defects in hemostasis (Krassas, 2000).

Similarly to what observed in males, plasma SHBG is decreased, with lowering of total T and estradiol, but their ubound fractions are increased. The metabolism is profoundly affected, with decrease of metabolic clearance rate of androstendione and estrone and increase in peripheral aromatization (Redmond, 2004; Longcope et al., 1990). The 5α/β ratio of androgen metabolism is decreased and there is an augmented excretion of 2-oxygenated estrogens (Gallagher, 1966). The alterations in steroid metabolism are corrected by replacement therapy (Gordon & Southren, 1977). As in male, gonadotropin levels are usually normal (Larsen, 1998), but with blunted or delayed response to GnRH (Marino et al., 2006; Valenti et al., 1984). Hyperprolactinemia can be induced by augmented TRH secretion, also causing galactorrhea in some patients, reversible with thyroid therapy (Honbo et al., 1978). Finally, decreased levels of clotting factors VII, VIII, IX and XI have been shown and can contribute to polymenorrhea and menorrhagia (Ansell, 1996).

Many studies have been performed also in subclinical hypothyroidism (SCH); the prevalence of SCH in infertile women was 11% in one study (Bohnet et al., 1981), but not considered as an infertility factors by others (Bals-Pratsch et al., 1997). A positive correlation was found in early follicular phase between basal TSH, LH and T; moreover women with elevated TSH response to TRH had lower pregnancy rate than women with normal TSH response (Gerhard et al., 1991). In a controlled prospective study of 438 women with infertility of various origin, the median TSH levels were significantly higher than controls (Poppe et al., 2002). Moreover more frequent miscarriages were observed in women with higher basal TSH levels, irrespective of the presence of AITD (Raber et al., 2003).

We want to focuse our attention on luteal deficiency, on one side, and AITD, the most prevalent associated etiology in patients of reproductive age, on the other one.

Progesterone secreted by the corpus luteum plays an important role in the maintenance of early pregnancy. Immediately after implantation, under the influence of human chorionic gonadotropin (hCG) secreted by the trophoblast, the corpus luteum receives a signal to continue to producing 17-α-progesterone along with estradiol, estrone, and relaxin (Szlachter et al., 1980; Bigazzi et al., 1981). The corpus luteum maintains its capacity to synthesize progesterone almost throughout the pregnancy, but at approximately 7 weeks gestation, its functional ability decreases markedly at the start of the luteoplacental transition. The removal of the corpus luteum before the eighth week of gestation results in abortion, whereas after the ninth week it does not (Csapo et al., 1973). Abnormalities of the luteal phase have been reported to occur in up to 35% of women with recurrent pregnancy losses (Insler, 1992). There are several causes for luteal phase deficiency, including stress, exercise, weight loss, hyperprolactinemia, and menstrual cycles at the onset of puberty or perimenopause.

Luteal phase deficiency (LPD) presents without any significant change in menstrual cycle lenght, despite prolonged follicular phases and shortened progesterone-deficient luteal phases (De Souza et al., 1998). Clinically, LPD is associated with abnormal corpus luteal function, which includes the mentionated short luteal phases and inadequate progesterone production, and also inappropriate endometrial stimulation and maturation (Ginsburg, 1992). These luteal phase alterations cause asynchronous follicular growth, compromised oocyte maturation, and differentiated (out of phase) function of the endometrium, which is associated with low rates of cycle fecundity and high rates of embryonic loss, i.e. infertility and spontaneous abortion (Ginsburg, 1992).

As above stated, hypoactive thyroid hormone is associated with infertility, even if severe forms of hypothyroidism rarely complicate pregnancy because they are associated with anovulation. However, in mild hypothyroidism, pregnancies can occur and are associated with higher rates of pregnancy loss and maternal complications (Davis et al., 1988; Stray-Pedersen & Stray-Pedersen, 1984). Even if an association exists between low thyroid function and pregnancy loss, a direct evidence for a causal role is missing (Clifford et al., 1994). One hypothesis for this correlation is that luteal phase defect has been linked to thyroid hypofunction. In consideration that production of progesterone is a pivotal element of a successful pregnancy, it is possible that pregnancy loss could be related to a deficient corpus luteum action (Daya et al., 1988).

An important study was published by Negro et al (2006) showing, in a large cohort of women, that patients with positive thyroid autoantibodies (TPO-ab), even if euthyroid at the early stages of pregnancy, would benefit from L-thyroxine administration to improve outcome of pregnancy, and namely the rate of spontaneous miscarriage and premature delivery. Ab-positive women were significantly older than control population (suggesting that AITD could delay conception due to its relation with infertility) but exhibit a mean serum TSH, although normal, significantly higher than controls; women were randomly assigned to two groups, one without treatment, and the other with L-thyroxine treatment. In group without therapy, serum TSH progressively increased during gestation, in the meantime serum free T4 (FT4) decreased by 30%, suggesting reduced functional thyroid reserve due to AITD. On the contrary, in treated group, the miscarriage rate was reduced by 75% and frequency of premature delivery by 69%. Similar results were reported by other authors showing that age, TPO positivity and high TSH levels were independently associated with the risk of miscarriage in multivariate analysis (Sieiro Netto et al., 2004). An association between miscarriage and AITD had been previously described (Stagnaro-Green et al., 1990; Glinoer et al., 1991) and support in other population studies, confirming this association also in the case of apparent normal thyroid function (Poppe & Glinoer, 2003). A recent review separately considered association of AITD and miscarriage, AITD and recurrent miscarriage and finally AITD and early pregnancy loss after in vitro fertilization

(Stagnaro-Green & Glinoer, 2004). Finally another confirmation came from a meta-analysis of all case-controlled and longitudinal studies, with an increased risk by 3-fold. Poppe et al. performed a prospective cohort study in women undergoing the first Assisted Reproduction Technology (ART) cycle, excluding over thyroid dysfunction. The prevalence of antiTPO was 14%, without differences in TSH, FT4 and age; in this positive group, pregnancy rate was 53% vs 43%, with an odds ratio of 0.67, but in pregnant group the miscarriage rate was 53% and 23% respectively, with and odds ratio of 3.77 (Poppe et al., 2003). Autoimmune thyroiditis are clearly associated with clinically relevant events occurring before, during and after pregnancy (Muller & Berghout, 2003). The hypothesis to explain this strong association were, of course, based on the concept of a generalized autoimmune disorders or a subtle thyroid hormone deficiency.

In this sense, a light is brought by studies performed with the administration of L-thyroxine. Vaquero et al (2000) included patients with Ab positivity and two previous first-trimester miscarriage, achieving a greater pregnancy outcome than untreated patients (81% vs 55%). Negro reported a reduction of miscarriage rate after L-thyroxine treatment in Ab positive infertile women who underwent in vitro fertilization (Negro et al., 2006). Finally, Abalovich et al. (2002) underlined the importance of adequate hormone treatment, comparing patients with hypothyroidism already known before pregnancy (adequate treatment) and patients with uncompletely adjusted replacement therapy: the pregnancy ended with abortion in 60% and 71% of cases, respectively.

In conclusion we believe it is prudent to screen for thyroid disease and normalize thyroid functions, when these are found abnormal, prior to conception or to return to a "normal" menstrual cycle, moreover Ab+ women should be carefully evaluated before pregnancy for sublinical hypothyroidism.

We report here some personal data on subclinical hypothyroidism, in couples users of Billings Ovulation Method (BOM); it is based on vulvar observation of the "Mucus Symptom", whose pattern is an accurate and precise marker of the ovarian function (Bllings, 1972), validated by laboratory research and field trials (Billings, 1991; Brown et al., 1987). BOM can be useful in studying subtle abnormalities in thyroid-gonadotropin interaction; the simple identification of the mucus peak and the evaluation of luteal phase length allow to detect a precise timing to perform hormonal assays. Therefore, we used BOM to evaluated the prevalence of subclinical hypothyroidism in women, users of the method for achieving or spacing pregnancy, and whose cycle abnormalities were not referred to cervical pathology. Preliminary data, still unpublished, but presented at the World Congress on Fertility & Sterility (Giacchi et al., 2007) were collected in 42 couples consulting our Center: 22 exhibited an history of infertility (1-4 ys), with a range age of women: 26-42 ys. Criteria of exclusion were male infertility and cervical pathology. Evaluation of progesterone levels was performed on the 6th-7th day after the "peak of mucus symptom", or on the 6th-7th day before the expected menses, when no peak occurred. We evaluated basal plasma levels of FT3, FT4, TSH, PRL and performed a TRH test (200 ug iv, with TSH evaluation at 0, 30, 60 min) when TSH was normal or high normal. The presence of anti-TPO and anti-thyroglobulin autoantibodies was also evaluated. Progesterone (P), FT3 and FT4 were assayed by RIA; TSH was assayed by IRMA method. Coefficients of variation: intra-assay CV 2.6% for P, 3.8% for FT3, 4.1% for FT4, 4.5% for TSH; inter-assay CV 3.9% for P, 3.9% for FT3, 4.9% for FT4, 3.4% for TSH. Normal ranges: Progesterone: 7-30 ng/ml; FT3: 2.3-4.2

pg/ml; FT4 8.5-15.5 pg/ml; TSH 0.35-2.80 μUI/ml. TRH (Relefact 200 μg) was fournished by Hoechst, Italy. Subclinical hypothyroidism was defined as TSH peak response > 15 μg/ml, according to previous studies and comparison with age-matched controls (Giacchi et al., 2001). Women were classified in three groups according to the BOM mucus symptom different patterns: Anovulatory pattern of the mucus symptom (n=2), post-peak phases shortened and/or affected by spotting (n=22), normal lenght of luteal phase, but P in the lower range of postovulatory values (n=18); among these two presented hypermenorrhea. Mean ± levels of the studied hormones are reported in table 1. Normal PRL levels were present in this group of patients. The prevalence of subclinical hypothyroidism, as above defined, in this group was 80%; prevalence of thyroid autoantibodies: 10%. After L-thyroxine treatment, we observed a clear and significant increase in progesterone levels (evaluated 6-7 day after the "peak" of the "mucus symptom") and the resumption of ovulation in the two women with anovulatory cycles (Fig. 1), strongly supporting a pathogenetic role of hypothyroidism in anovulation or luteal failure.

		women number	P (ng/ml)	FT3 (pg/ml)	FT4 (pg/ml)	basal TSH levels μU/ml	TSH peak μU/ml	PRL (ng/ml)
No peak anovulatory cycles		2	0,3 ± 0,2	3,6 ± 1,5	9,0 ± 0,5	3,4 ± 0,8	24,5 + 1,5	19,5 ± 1,0
post peak phase lenght	< 11 g	22	10,7 ± 1,1	4,0 ± 1,0	10,1 ± 0,8	2,7 ± 0,2	21,2 ± 1,5	16,1 ± 1,6
	≥ 11 g	18	9,1 ± 0,8	3,8 ± 1.0	9,1 ± 0,8	3,0 ± 0,2	22,5 + 1,3	17,5 ± 1,2

Table 1. Mean ± SEM hormone levels in patients consulting our Center for infertility and monitored by Billings' Ovulation Method.

An hypothesis linking thyroid dysfunction and luteal deficiency is that concerning OS. Oxidative stress is associated with decreased female fertility in animals and in vitro models, but some observations in humans also reinforces this concept. Exposures associated with OS (extremes of body weight, alcohol, tobacco and caffeine intake) may induce pregnancy complications (e.g. preeclampsia) ; while intake of antioxidants nutrients, included use of multivitamins, have a beneficial role in female fertility (Ruder et al., 2009). More recently, it has been hypothesized that the exposure to environmental pollutants in fetal life may alter DNA methylation, causing altered gene expression in adult life (Li et al., 1997; Anway et al., 2005); therefore this widespread condition should be added to the factors favouring OS. A role of reduced antioxidant defence has also been hyothesized in polycystic ovary, unexplained infertility and outcome of in vitro fertilization (Ruder et al., 2008).

When specifically considering luteal function, it has been shown than the corpus luteum has a high concentrations of antioxidants, especially β-carotene, to which is related the bright yellow color (Rodgers et al., 1995); other carotenoids and vitamins C and E are also present and may contribute to ROS scavenging (Aten et al., 1992; Matzuk et al., 1998; Behrman et al., 2001. Moreover ROS are produced during luteal regression (Behrman et al., 2001), in part through cytochrome P450 enzymes involved in the first step of steroidogenesis (Rodgers et al., 1995).

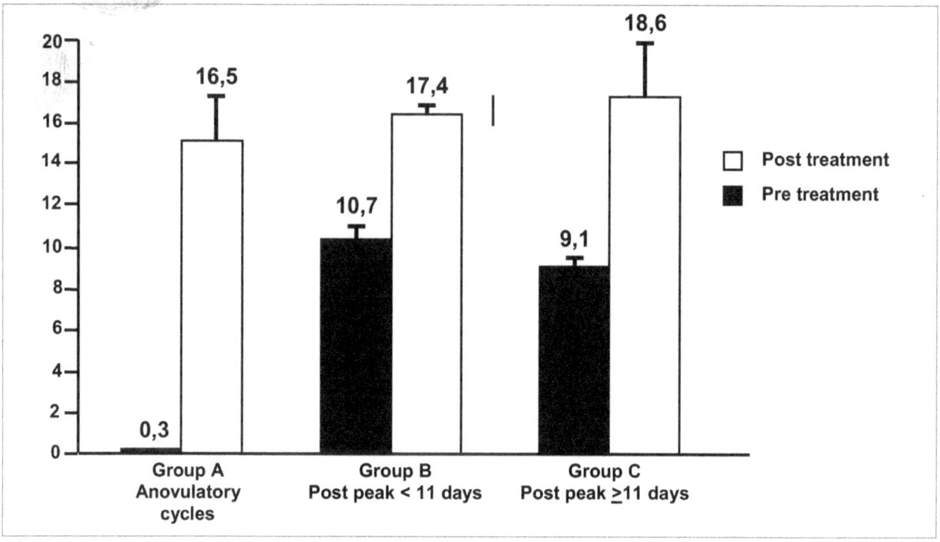

Fig. 1. Post-peak (according to BOM) Progesterone levels (ng/ml) before and after replacement l-T4 treatment .

However, the role of ROS in ovary is particularly complex. On one side, they play a physiological role: regulated ROS generation by the pre-ovulatory follicle is an important promoter of ovulatory sequence; in particular, the resumption of meiosis I (MI) induced by hormonal factor after puberty, is induced by ROS and inhibited by antioxidants (Takami et al., 1999; Kodman & Behrman, 2001). Another beneficial effects could be related to a ROS involvement in intracellular signalling between hypoxia and angiogenig response (Basini et al.,2004). Surprisingly, antioxidants are, on the contrary, beneficial for MII, which arises in response to periovulatory LH peak (Behrman et al., 2001). Follicular ROS initiate apoptosis whereas follicular glutathione (GSH), in addition to FSH, protect against apoptosis in cultured preovulatory rat follicles (Tsai-Turton & Luderer, 2006). Moreover, cyclical ROS production may contribute to oophoritis associated with autoimmune premature ovarian failure (Behrman et al., 2001). It has been suggested that ROS under moderate concentrations play a role in signal transduction processes involved in growth and protection from apoptosis (Basini et al., 2004). In rat thecal-intestitial cells, which regulate steroidogesis and follicle growth in secondary follicle, ROS induced a biphasic effect on proliferation (positive at lower and negative at higher concentrations). Therefore controlled ROS levels may be needed to maintain DNA synthesis, cell proliferation and growth of ovarian mesenchyme in such animal model (Duleba et al., 2004). Finally, epidemiologic data suggest a positive role of dietary antioxidants (Ruder et al., 2008): preconceptional multivitamin supplementation may enhance fertility, perhaps increasing menstrual cycle regularity (Czeizel et al., 1994; Dudas et al., 1995) or via prevention of ovulatory disorders (Chavarro et al., 2007). Despite all these evidences, it must be reminded the difference by in vitro models and in vivo conditions and the need of more data of antioxidants levels in hypothyroidism, which could be useful for therapeutic purposes.

5. Conclusions

Taken together, all the reported data confirm the role of thyroid hormones in human fertility; also subclinical hypothyroidism should be considered in the evaluation of an infertile couple, even if it is not routinely evaluated in the first level approach to this problem. Oxidative stress could be a phenomenon liking hypothyroidism, also in subclinical form, with altered sperm motility, in males, and luteal phase deficiency in females, even if more experimental data are needed to give statistical evidence to this fascinating hypothesis.

6. References

Abalovich, M.; Gutierrez, S.; Alcaraz, G.; Maccallini, G.; Garcia, A. & Levalle, O. (2002). Overt and subclinical hypothyroidism complicating pregnancy. *Thyroid*, 12, pp. 63-68.

Ademoglu, E., Gokkusu, C., Yarman, S. & Azizlerli, H. (1998). The effect of methimazole on oxidant and antioxidant system in patients with hyperthyroidism. *Pharmacological Research*, 3, pp. 93-96.

Agarwal, A. & Saleh, R.A. (2002). Role of antioxidants in male infertility: rationale, significance and treatment. *Urology Clinics of North America*, 29, pp. 817-827.

Aitken, R.J. & Krausz, C. (2001). Oxidative stress, DNA damage and the Y chromosome. *Reproduction*, 122, pp. 497-506.

Ansell, J.E. (1996). The blood in the hypothyroidism. In: Braverman, L.E. & Utiger, R.D. (eds), *Werner and Ingbar's The thyroid – a fundamental and clinical text*, 7th ed. Lippincott-Raven, Philadelphia, pp. 821-825.

Asayama, K., Dobashi, K., Hayashibe, H., Megata, Y. & Kato, K. (1987). Lipid peroxidation and free radical scavengers in thyroid dysfunction in the rat: a possible mechanism of injury to heart and skeletal muscle in hypothyroidism. *Endocrinology*, 121, pp. 2112-2118.

Asayama, K. & Kato, K. (1990). Oxidative muscular injury and its relevance to hyperthyroidism. *Free Radical Biology & Medicine*, 8, pp. 293-303.

Azizi, F.; Raiszadeh, F. & Solati, M. (2003). Serum paraoxonase 1 activity is decreased in thyroid dysfunction. *Journal of Endocrinological Investigation*, 26, pp. 703-109.

Bals-Pratsch, M.; De Geyter, C.; Muller, T.; Frieling, U.; Lerchl, A.; Pirke, K.M.; Hanker, J.P.; Becker-Carus, C. & Nieschlag, E. (1997). Episodic variations of prolactin, thyroid-stimulating hormone, luteinizing hormone, melatonin and cortisol in infertile women with sublinical hypothyroidism. *Human Reproduction*, 12, pp. 896-904.

Baskol, G.; Atmaca, H.; Tanriverdi, F.; Baskol, M.; Kocer, D. & Bayram, F. (2007). Oxidative stress and enzymatic antioxidant status in patients with hypothyroidism before and after treatment. *Experimental and Clinical Endocrinology & Diabetes*, 115 (8), pp. 522-526.

Bianchi, G., Solaroli, E., Zaccheroni, V., Grossi, G., Bargossi, A.M. & Melchionda, N. (1990). Oxidative stress and anti-oxidant metabolites in patients with hyperthyroidism: effect of treatment. *Hormone and Metabolic Research*, 31, pp. 620-624.

Bigazzi, M. & Nardi, E. (1981). Prolactin and relaxin: antagonism on the spontaneous motility of the uterus. *Journal of Clinical Endocrinology & Metabolism*, 53 (6), pp. 665-667.

Billings, J.J. (1972). Ovulation method of family planning. *Lancet*, 2 (7788), pp. 1193-1194.

Billings, J.J. (1981). The validation of the Billings ovulation method by laboratory research and field trials. *Acta Europaea Fertilitatis*, 22 (1), pp. 9-15.

Bohnet, H.G.; Fielder, K. & Leidenberger, F.A. (1981). Subclinical hypothyroidism and infertility. *Lancet*, 2, pp. 1278-1279.

Brown, J.B.; Blackwell, L.F.; Billings, J.J.; Conway, B.; Cox R.I.; Garrett, G.; Holmes, J. & Smithe, M.A. (1987). Natural family planning. *American Journal of Obstetrics and Gynecology*, 157 (4 Pt 2), pp. 1062-1069.

Carani, C., Isidori, A.M., Granata, A., Carosa, E., Maggi M., Lenzi, A. & Tannini, E.A. (2005). Multicenter study on the prevalence of sexual symptoms in male hypo- and hyperthyroid patients. *Journal of Clinical Endocrinology & Metabolism*, 90, 6472-6479.

Choudhury, S., Chainy, G.B.N. & Mishro, M.M. (2003). Experimentally induced hypo- and hyper-thyroidism influence on the antioxidant defense system in adult rat testis. *Andrologia*, 35, pp. 131-140.

Clifford, K., Rai, R., Watson, H. & Regan, L. (1994). An informative protocol for the investigation of recurrent miscarriage: preliminary experience of 5000 consecutive cases. *Human Reproduction*, 9 (7), pp. 1328-1332.

Coria, M.J., Pastràn, A.I., Gimenez, M.S. (2009). Serum oxidative stress parameters of women with hypothyroidism. *Acta Biomedica*, 80, pp. 135-139.

Corrales Hernandez, J.J.; Miralles Garcia, J.M. & Garcia Diez, L.C. (1990). Primary hypothyroidism and human spermatogenesis. *Archives of Andrology*, 25, pp. 21-27.

Csapo, A.I., Pulkkinen, M.O. & Wiest, W.G. (1973). Effects of luteectomy and progesterone replacement therapy in early pregnant patients. *American Journal of Obstetrics & Gynecology*, 115 (6), pp. 759-765.

Davis, L.E., Leveno, K.J. & Cunningham, F.G. (1988). Hypothyroidism complicating pregnancy. *Obstetrics & Gyencology*, 72 (1), pp. 108-112.

Daya, S., Ward, S. & Burrows, E. (1988). Progesterone profiles in luteal phase defect cycles and outcome of progesterone treatment in patients with recurrent spontaneous abortion. *American Journal of Obstetrics & Gynecology*, 158 (2), pp. 225-232.

De Groot, L. (2006). Non-thyroidal illness syndrome is a manifestation of hypothalamic-pituitary dysfunction, and in view of current evidence, shoud be treated with appropriate replacement therapy. *Critical Care Clinic*, 22, pp. 57-86

De la Balze, F.A.; Arrillaga, F.; Mancini, R.E.; Janches, M.; Davidson, O.W. & Gurtman, A.I. (1962). Male hypogonadism in hypothyroidism:a study of six cases. *Journal of Clinical Endocrinology & Metabolism*, 22, pp. 212-222.

De Souza, M.J., Miller, B.E., Loucks, A.B., Luciano, A.A., Pescatello, L.S., Campbell, C.G., & Lasley, B.L. (1998). High frequency of luteal phase deficiency and anovulation in recreational women runners; blunted elevation in follicle-stimulating hormone observed during luteal-follicular transition. *Journal of Clinical Endocrinology & Metabolism*, 83 (12), pp. 4220-4232.

Dittrich, R.; Beckmann, M.W.; Oppelt, P.G.; Hoffmann, I.; Lotz, L.; Kuwert, T. & Mueller, A. (2011). Thyroid hormone receptors and reproduction. *Journal of Reproductive Immunology*, 90 (1), pp. 58-66.

Dobrzynska, M.M., Baumgartner, A. & Anderson, D. (2004). Antioxidants modulate thyroid hormone- and noradrenaline-induced DNA damage in human sperm. *Mutagenesis*, 19(49), pp. 325-330.

Donnelly, P. & White C. (2000). Testicular dysfunction in men with primary hypothyroidism; reversal of hypogonadotrophic hypogonadism with replacement thyroxine. *Clinical Endocrinology (Oxford)*, 52, 197-201.

Doufas, A.G. & Mastorakos, G. (2000). The hypothalamic-pituitary-thyroid axis and the female reproductive system. *Annals of the New York Academy of Science*, 900, pp. 65-76.

Erdamar, H.; Demirici, H.; Yaman, H., et al (2008). The effect of hypothyroidism, hyperthyroidism, and their treatment on parameters of oxidative stress and antioxidant status. *Clinical Chemistry and Laboratory Medicine*, 46, pp. 1004-1010.

Fernandez, V., Barrientos, X., Kipreos, K., Valanzuela, A. & Videla, L.A. (1985). Superoxide radical generation, NADPH oxidase activity and cytochrome P-450 content of rat liver microsomal fractions in a experimental hyperthyroid state: relation to lipid peroxidation. *Endocrinology*, 117, pp. 496-501.

Gallagher, T.F.; Fukushima, D.K.; Noguchi, S.; Fishman, J.; Bradlow, H.L.; Cassouto, J.; Zumoff, B. & Hellman, L. (1966). Recent studies in steroid hormone metabolism in man. *Recent Progress in Hormone Research*, 22, pp. 283-302.

Gerhard, I.; Becker, T.; Eggert-Kruse, W.; Klinga, K. & Runnebaum, B. (1991). Thyroid and ovarian function in infertile women. *Human Reproduction*, 6, pp. 338-345.

Giacchi, E.; Saporosi, A.; Milardi, D.; Merola, A.M.; Pellicanò, P.; Squintani, M.C.; De Marinis, L.; Jensen, L. & Mancini A. (2001). Infertility in luteal defect due to hypothyroidism. In: *IFFS 2001 Selected Free Communication*, Monduzzi Editore, pp. 87-91.

Giacchi, E., Saporosi, A.; Leone, E.; De Marinis, L.; Pontecorvi, A.; Bompiani, A. & Mancini, A. (2007). Subclinical hypothyroidism and ovarian function: diagnostic value of the Billing's ovulation method. Abstracts of the *XIX World Congress on Fertility & Sterility*, IFFS (International Federation of Fertility Societies), Durban, South Africa, april 29-may 3, 2007, p. 125.

Ginsburg, K.A. (1992). Luteal phase defect. Etiology, diagnosis and management. *Endocrinology and Metabolism Clinics of North America*, 21 (1), pp. 85-104.

Glinoer, D., Fernandez Soto, M.L.; Bourdoux, P.; Lejeune, B.; Delange, F. ; Lemone, M. ; Klitheart, J.; Robijn, C.; Grun, J.P. & De Nayer, P. (1991). Pregnancy in patients with mild thyroid abnormalities: maternal and neonatal repercussions. *Journal of Clinical Endocrinology & Metabolism*, 73, pp. 421-427.

Gordon, G.G. & Southren, A.L. (1977). Thyroid hormone effects on steroid-hormone metabolism. *Bullettin of the New York Academy of Medicine*, 53, pp. 241-259.

Huh, K., Kwon, T.H., Kim, J.S. & Park, J.M. (1998). Role of the hepatic xanthine oxidase in thyroid dysfunction: effect of thyroid hormones in oxidative stress in rat liver. *Archives of Pharmacology Research*, 21, pp. 236-249.

Halliwell, B. & Gutteridge, J.M.C. (1994). *Free radical in biology and medicine.* Clarendon Press. 2nd ed., Oxford, 1979.

Honbo, K.S., van Herle, A.J. & Kellett, K.A. (1978). Serum prolactin levels in untreated primary hypothyroidism. *American Journal of Medicine*, 64, pp. 782-787.

Huh, K., Kwon, T.H., Kim, J.S., Park, J.M. (1998) Role of the hepatic xanthine oxidase in thyroid dysfunction: effect of thyroid hormones in oxidative stress in rat liver. *Archives of Pharmacology Research*, 21, pp- 236-249.

Huh, K., Kwon, T.H., Kim, J.S. & Park, J.M. (1998) Role of the hepatic xanthine oxidase in thyroid dysfunction: effect of thyroid hormones in oxidative stress in rat liver. *Archives of Pharmacology Research*, 21, pp. 236-249.

Insler, V. (1992). Corpus luteum defects. *Current Opinions in Obstetrics and Gynecology*, 4 (2),, pp. 203-211.

Iwasaki, A. & Gagnon, C. (1992). Formation of reactive oxygen species in spermatozoa of infertile men. *Fertility & Sterility*, 47, pp. 409-411.

Kang, D. & Hamasaki, N. (2003). Mitochondrial oxidative stress and mitochondrial DNA. *Clinical Chemistry and Laboratory Medicine* , 41, pp. 1281-1288.

Kebapcilar, L.; Akinci, B.; Bayraktar, F. et al. (2007). Plasma thiobarbituric acid-reactive substance levels in subclinical hypothyroidism. *Medical Principles and Practice*, 16, pp. 432-436.

Krassas, G.E.; Pontikides, N.; Kaltsas, Th.; Papadopoulou, Ph.; Paunkovic, J.; Paunkovic, N. & Duntas, L.H. (1999). Disturbances of menstruation in hypothyroidism. *Clinical Endocrinology (Oxford)*, 50, pp. 655-659.

Krassas, G.E. (2000). Thyroid disease, menstrual function and fertility. *Thyroid International*, 1, pp. 1-15.

Krassas, G.E., Papadopoulou, F.; Tziomalos, K.; Zeginiadou, T. & Pontikides, N. (2008). Hypothyroidism has an adverse effect on human spermatogenesis: a prospective, controlled study. *Thyroid*, 18, pp. 1255-1259.

Krassas, G.E., Tziomalos, K.; Papadopoulou, F.; Pontikides, N. & Perros, P. (2008). Erectile dysfunction in patients with hyperthyroidism: how common and should we treat? *Journal of Clinical Endocrinology & Metabolism*, 93, pp. 1815-1819.

Krassas, G.E., Poppe, K. & Glinoer, D. (2010). Thyroid function and human reproductive health. *Endocrine Review*, 31, pp. 702-705.

Lancaster, J.R. (1992). Nitric oxide in cells. *American Scientist*, 80, pp. 249-59.

Larsen, P.R.; Davies, T.F. & Hay, I.D. (1998). The thyroid gland. In: Wilson, J.D., Foster, D.W.; Kronenberg, H.M. & Larsen P.R. (eds), *Williams' textbook of Endocrinology*, 9th ed., W.B.Saunders, Philadelphia, pp. 1995-2028.

Littarru, G.P. (1994). *Energy and defence*. CESI, Roma.

Longcope, C.; Abend, S.; Braverman, L.E. & Emerson, C.H. (1990). Androstendione and estrone dynamics in hypothyroid women. *Journal of Clinical Endocrinology & Metabolism*, 70, pp. 903-907.

Mancini, A., De Marinis, L., Calabrò, F., Sciuto, R., Oradei, A., Lippa, S., Sandric, S., Littaru, G.P. & Barbarino, A. (1989). Evaluation of metabolic status in amiodarone-induced thyroid disorders: plasma coenzyme Q10 determination. *Journal of Endocrinological Investigation*, 12, pp. 511-516.

Mancini, A., De Marinis, L., Calabrò, F., Fiumara, C., Goglia, A. & Littarru, G.P. (1991). Physiopathological relevance of coenzyme Q10 in thyroid disorders: CoQ10 concentrations in normal and diseased human thyroid tissue. In: Folkers, K., Littarru, G.P., Yamagami, T. *Eds. Biomedical and Clinical Aspects of Coenzyme Q*. Amsterdam: Elsevier, pp. 441-448.

Mancini, A.; De Marinis, L.; Oradei, A.; Hallgass, M.E.; Conte, G.; Pozza, D. & Littarru, G.P. (2004). Coenzyme Q10 levels in human seminal fluid. *Journal of Andrology*, 15, pp. 591-594.

Mancini, A., Corbo, G.M., Gaballo, A., Valente, S., Gigliotti, P., Cimino, V., De Marinis, L., Principi, F. & Littarru, G.P. (2005). Relationships between plasma CoQ10 levels and thyroid hormones in chronic obstructive pulmonary disease. *Biofactors*, 25 (1-4), pp. 201-204.

Mancini, A.; Festa, R.; Silvestrini, A.; Nicolotti, N.; Di Donna V.; La Torre, G.; Pontecorvi, A. & Meucci, E. (2009). Hormonal regulation of total antioxidant capacity in seminal plasma. *Journal of Andrology*, 30 (5), 534-540.

Mancini, A., Festa, R., di Donna, V., Leone E., Littarru, G.P., Silvestrini, A., Meucci, E. & Pontecorvi, A. (2010a). Hormones and antioxidant systems: role of pituitary and pituitary-dependent axes. *Journal of Endocrinological Investigation*, 33 (6), pp. 422-433.

Mancini, A., Leone, E., Silvestrini, A., Festa, R., Di Donna, V., De Marinis, L., Pontecorvi, A., Littarru, G.P. & Meucci, E. (2010b). Evaluation of antioxidant systems in pituitary-adrenal axis diseases. *Pituitary*, 13 (2), pp. 138-145.

Marino, M.; Chiovato, L. & Pinchera, A. (2006). Graves' disease. In: De Groot, L.J. & Jameson J.L. (eds), *Endocrinology*, 5th ed. Elsevier Saunders, Philadelphia, pp. 1995-2028.

Meucci, E., Milardi, D., Mordente, A., Martorana, G.E., Giacchi, E., De Marinis, L. & Mancini A. (2003). Total antioxidant capacity in patients with varicoceles. *Fertility & Sterility*, 79, Suppl. 3, pp. 1577-1583.

Muller, A.F. & Berghout, A. (2003). Consequences of autoimmune thyroiditis before, during and after pregnancy. *Minerva Endocrinologica*, 28 (3), pp. 247-254.

Nanda, N.; Bobby, Z.; Hamide, A. et al (2007). Association between oxidative stress and coronary lipid risk factors in hypothyroid women is independent of body mass index. *Metabolism*, 56, pp. 1350-1355.

Negro, R.; Formoso, G., Mangieri, T.; Pezzarossa, A.; Dazzi, D. & Hassan, H. (2006). Levothyroxine treatment in euthyroid pregnant women with autoimmune thyroid disease: effect on obstetrical complications. *Journal of Clinical Endocrinology & Metabolism*, 91, pp. 2587-2591.

Ohye H. & Sugawara, M. (2010). Dual oxidase, hydrogen peroxide and thyroid diseases. *Experimental Biology and Medicine*, 235, pp. 424-433.

Paschke, R.; Bertelsbeck, D.S.; Tsalimalma, K. & Nieschlag, E. (1994). Association of sperm antibodies with other autoantibodies in infertile men. *American Journal of Reproductive Immunology*, 32, pp. 88-94.

Poppe, K.; Glinoer, D.; Van Steirteghem, A.; Tournaye, H.; Devroey, P.; Schiettecatte, J. & Velkeniers, B. (2002). Thyroid dysfunction and autoimmunity in infertile women. *Thyroid*, 12, pp. 997-1001.

Poppe, K. & Glinoer, D. (2003). Thyroid autoimmunity and hypothyroidism before and during pregnancy. *Human Reproduction Update*, 9, 149-161.

Poppe, K.; Glinoer, D.; Tournaye, H.; Devroey, P. ; van Steirteghem, A. ; Kaufman, L. & Velkeniers, B. (2003). Assisted reproduction and thyroid autoimmunity: an unfortunate combination? *Journal of Clinical Endocrinology & Metabolism*, 88 (9), pp. 4149-4152.

Raber, W.; Nowotny, P.; Vytiska-Binstorfer, E. & Vierhapper, H. (2003). Thyroxine treatment modified in infertile women according to thyroxine-relasing hormone testing: 5 year follow-up of 283 women referred after exclusion of absolute causes of infertility. *Human Reproduction*, 18, pp. 707-714.

Redmond, G.P. (2004). Thyroid dysfunction and women's reproductive health. *Thyroid*, 14 (Suppl. 1), pp. S5-S15.

Resch, U., Helsel, G., Tatzber, F. & Sinzinger, H. (2002). Antioxidant status in thyroid dysfunction. *Clinical Chemistry and Laboratory Medicine*, 40, pp. 1132-1134.

Rice-Evans, C. & Miller, N.J. (1994). Total antioxidant status in plasma and body fluids. *Methods in Enzymology*, 234, pp. 279-293.

Ruder, E.H.; Hartman, T.J.; Blumberg, J. & Goldman, M.B. (2008). Oxidative stress and antioxidants: exposure and impact on female fertility. *Human Reproduction Update*, 14 (4), pp. 345-357.

Ruder, E.H. Hartman, T.J. & Goldman, M.B. (2009). Impact of oxidative stress on female fertility. *Current Opinions in Obstetrics & Gynecology*, 21 (3), pp. 219-22.

Said, T.M.; Kattal, N.; Sharma, R.K.; Sikka, S.C.; Thomas A.J.; Mascha, E. & Agarwal, A. (2003) . Enhanced chemiluminescence assay vs colorimetric assay for measurement of the total antioxidant capacity of human seminal plasma. *Journal of Andrology*, 24, pp. 676-680.

Santi, A.; Duarte, M.M.; Moresco, R.N.; Menezes, C.; Bagatini,M.D.; Schetinger, M.R. & Loro, V.L. (2010). Association between thyroid hormones, lipids and oxidative stress biomarkers in overt hypothyroidism. *Clinical Chemistry and Laboratory Medicine*, 48 (11), pp. 1635-1639.

Sharma, R.; Traore, K.; Trush, M.A.; Rose, N.R.; Burek & C.L. (2008). Intracellular adhesion molecule-1 up-regulation on thyrocytes by iodine of non-obese diabetic H2(h4) mice is reactive oxygen species-dependent. *Clinical & Experimental Immunology*, 152, pp. 13-20.

Sieiro Netto, L.; Medina Coeli, C.; Micmacher, E.; Ma mede Da Costa, S.; Nazar, L.; Galvao, D.; Buescu, A. & Vaisman, M. (2004). Influence of thyroid autoimmunity and maternal age on the risk of miscarriage. *American Journal of Reproductive Immunology*, 52 (5), pp. 312-316.

Stagnaro-Green, A.; Roman, S.H.; Cobin, R.H.; El-Hazary, E.; Alvarez-Marfany, M. & Davies, T.F. (1990). Detection of at-risk pregnancy by means of highly sensitive assays for thyroid antibodies. *The Journal of the American Medical Association*, 264, pp. 1422-1425.

Stagnaro-Green, A. & Glinoer, D. (2004). Thyroid autoimmunity and hypothyroidism before and during pregnancy. *Human Reproduction Update*, 9, 149-161.

Stray-Pedersen, B. & Tray-Pedersen, S. (1984). Etiologic factors and subsequent reproductive performances in 195 couples with a prior history of habitual abortion. *American Journal of Obstetrics & Gynecology*, 148 (2), pp. 140-146.

Szlachter, N.; O'Byrne, E.; Goldsmith, L.; Steinetz, B.G. & Weiss G. (1980). Myometrial inhibiting activity of relaxin-containg extracts of human corpora lutea of pregnancy. *American Journal of Obtetrics & Gynecology*, 136 (5), pp. 584-586.

Tagawa, N.; Takano, T.; Fukata, S.; Kuma, K.; Tada, H.; Izumi, Y.; Kobayashi, Y. & Amino, N. (2001). Serum concentration of androstendiol and androstendiol sulphate in patients with hyperthyroidism and hypothyroidism. *Endocrine Journal*, 48, 345-354.

Torun, A.N.; Kulaksizoglu, S.; Kulaksizoglu, M.; Pamuk, B.O.; Isbilen, E. & Tutuncu, N.B. (2009). Serum total antioxidant status and lipid peroxidation marker malondialdehyde levels in overt and subclinical hypothyroidism. *Clinical Endocrinology (Oxford)*, 70 (3), pp. 469-474.

Trummer, H.; Ramschak-Schwarzer, S.; Haas, J.; Haberman, H.; Pummer, K. & Leb, G. (2001). Thyroid hormones and thyroid antibodies in infertile males. *Fertility & Sterility*, 76, 254-257.

Turrens, J.F. & Boveris, A. (1980). Generation of superoxyde anion by the NADH dehydrogenase of bovine mitochondria. *Biochemical Journal*, 191 (2), pp. 421-427.

Valenti, G.; Ceda, G.P.; Denti, L.; Tarditi, E. & Speroni, G. (1984). Gonadotropin secretion in hyperthyroidism and hypothyroidism. *La Ricerca in Clinica e in Laboratorio*, 14, pp. 53-63.

Vaquero, E.; Lazzarin, N.; De Carolis, C.; Valensise, H.; Moretti, C. & Romanini, C. (2000). Mild thyroid abnormalities and recurrent spontaneous abortion: diagnostic and therapeutic approach. *American Journal of Reproductive Immunology*, 43 (4), pp. 204-208.

Varela, V.; Rivolta, C.M., Esperante, S.A., Gruneiro-Papendieck, L., Chiesa, A. & Targovnik, H.M. (2006). Three mutations (p.Q36H, p.G418fsX482, and g.IVS19-2°>C) in the dual oxidase 2 gene responsible for congenital goiter and iodide organification defect. *Clinical Chemistry*, 52, pp. 182-191.

Velasquez, E.M. & Bellabarba Arata, G. (1997). Effect of thyroid status on pituitary gonadotropin and testicular reserve in men. *Archives of Andrology*, 38, pp. 85-92.

Venditti, P., Balestrieri, M., Di Meo, S. & De Leo, T. (1997). Effect of thyroid state on lipid peroxidation, antioxidant defenses and susceptibility to oxidative stress in rat tissues. *Journal of Endocrinology*, 155, pp. 151-157.

Venditti, P., Daniele, M.C., Masullo, P., Di Meo, S. (1999) Antioxidant-sensitive triiodothyronine effects on characteristics of rat liver mitochondrial population. *Cellular Physiology & Biochemistry*, 9, pp. 38-52.

Venditti, P. & Di Meo, S. (2006). Thyroid hormone-induced oxidative stress. *Cellular and Molecular Life Science*, 63(4), pp. 414-434.

Weyemi, U.; Caillou, B.; Talbot, M.; Ameziane-El-Hassani, R. ; Lacroix, L.; Lagent-Chevallier, O.; Al Ghuzlan, A. ; Roos, D. ; Bidart, J.M.; Virion, A.; Schlumberger, M. & Dupuy, C. (2010). Intracellular expression of ROS generating NADPH oxidase NOX4 in normal and cancer thyroid tissues. *Endocrine Related Cancer, 17 (1), pp. 27-37.*

World Health Organization (WHO). (1999). *Laboratory manual for the examination of human semen and semen-cervical mucus interaction*, 4th Ed. Cambridge University Press, Cambridge.

World Health Organization (2010). *WHO laboratory manual for the examination and processing of human semen*, 5th Ed. WHO Press, Geneve, Switzerland.

Wolff, S.P.; Jiang, Z.Y. & Hunt, J.V. (1991). Protein glycation and oxidative stress in diabetes mellitus and ageing. *Free Radical Biology & Medicine* , 10, pp. 339-352.

Wortsman, J.; Rosner, W. & Dufau, M.L. (1987). Abnormal testicular function in men with primary hypothyroidism. *American Journal of Medicine*, 82, pp. 207-212.

Wurfel, W. (1992). Thyroid regulation pathways and its effect on human luteal function. *Gynakologisch-Geburtshilfliche Rundschau*, 3, pp. 145-150.

7

Neurological Complications of Hypothyroidism

Hande Turker[1], Cuneyt Turker[2] and Nilgun Cengiz[1]
[1]*Ondokuzmayis University, School Of Medicine, Department of Neurology, Samsun,*
[2]*Gazi State Hospital, Clinic of Internal Medicine, Samsun*
Turkey

1. Introduction

Hypothyroidism is the most common pathological hormone deficiency (Roberts et al, 2004). The variety of end-organ effects and wide range of disease severity—from entirely asymptomatic individuals to patients in coma with multisystem failure—can make hypothyroidism an elusive clinical entity (Roberts et al, 2004). Hypothyroidism was first described in the 19 th century.

Impaired memory, slowed mental processing, depression, nerve entrapment syndromes, ataxia, muscle weakness and muscle cramps are the most common neurological symptoms which may be caused by hypothyroidism (Roberts et al, 2004). Disorders of the thyroid gland are among the most common endocrine maladies. Hypothyroidism is the most prevalent form of thyroid disease and symptoms may include memory and learning impairment, depression, psychotic behaviour, retarded locomotor ability, somnolence, progressive intellectual deterioration and, in extreme cases, coma (Anderson, 2001; Smith et al., 2002). Since the thyroid hormones dramatically affect the maturation of specific neuronal populations, the absence of these hormones during the period of active neurogenesis leads to irreversible mental retardation and is accompanied by multiple morphological alterations in the brain (Smith et al., 2002).

2. Central nervous system ınvolvement due to hypothyroıdısm

Disruption of thyroid hormone production during fetal and early neonatal development leads to a suite of permanent deficits in intelligence and sensorimotor function in humans (Dong et al, 2005).

Clinical hypothyroidism indicates a pervasive deficit in thyroid hormone actions, including modulation of calorigenesis and oxygen consumption in most tissues and additional organ-specific effects (Roberts et al, Lancet).

Brain-derived neurotrophic factor (BDNF) is a neurotrophin critical for many developmental and physiological aspects of CNS function. Severe hypothyroidism in the early neonatal period results in developmental and cognitive impairments and reductions in mRNA and protein expression of BDNF in a number of brain regions (Lasley et al., 2011).

The action of thyroid hormones (THs) in the brain is strictly regulated, since these hormones play a crucial role in the development and physiological functioning of the central nervous system (CNS) (Ahmed et al., 2008).

Transient reductions in thyroid hormone during critical periods of brain development can have devastating and irreversible effects on neurological function (Gilbert et al, 2004). The hippocampus is a brain region sensitive to thyroid hormones and is a necessary substrate for some forms of learning and memory. Subregions within the hippocampus display distinct ontogenetic profiles and have shown differential vulnerability to some indices of thyrotoxic insult. Synaptic function can be readily assessed in the hippocampus, yet little information exists on the consequences of early thyroid hormone insufficiency on the neurophysiological integrity of this structure (Gilbert et al, 2004).

Thyroid hormone deficiency during the critical period of neural differentiation produces permanent and severe alterations in the morphology and function of the nervous system leading to cretinism. Perinatal hypothyroidism results in permanent alterations of hippocampal synaptic functions in adult rats consequently causing learning and memory impairment (Calloni et al., 2005).

It has been established that both L-thyroxine (T4) and L-3,5,39-triiodothyronine (T3) are present in the adult brain. Moreover, the enzyme deiodinase type II, which is mainly responsible for converting inactive T4 to active form T3, is also present in glial and neural cells (Calza et al., 1997).

Finally, receptors for thyroid hormone T3 are localized in nuclei of glial cells and neurons in different brain areas (Calza et al., 1997).

Thyroid hormone is essential for proper development of the mammalian CNS. Previous studies have documented a decrease in the ability of neonatal hypothyroid animals to learn and to habituate to maze tests and an increase in spontaneous activity (Darbra et al, 2003). On the other hand some observers stated that children with hypothyroidism had no apparent specific impediments to learning unrelated to intelligence (England Congenital Hypothyroidism Collaborative New, 1990).

Cognitive neurological symptoms are common in myxoedema, in particular a general slowing of cognitive functions with memory impairment and apathy. This may progress insidiously to a global cognitive impairment of dementia. Appropriate treatment with replacement therapy will sometimes improve mental changes,though they are frequently only partially reversible (Osterweil et al., 1992). The longer the condition remains undiagnosed, the worse the outcome (Dennis et al., 2005).

The in vitro studies demonstrate that adult hippocampal progenitors exhibit enhanced proliferation, survival and glial differentiation in response to thyroid hormone. These results support a role for thyroid hormone in the regulation of adult hippocampal neurogenesis and raise the possibility that altered neurogenesis may contribute to the cognitive and behavioral deficits associated with adult-onset hypothyroidism (Desouzo et al., 2005).

According to a study by Bhanja et al., the results suggest that the antioxidant defence system of the developing cerebellum is sensitive to thyroid hormone deficiency and consequent alterations in oxidative stress status may play a role in regulation of cell proliferation of the cerebellum during neonatal brain development (Bhanja et al.,2010).

In vitro, THs (thyroid hormones) have been reported to modulate astrocyte morphology, differentiation, and proliferation and to regulate extracellular matrix (ECM) organization and synthesis (Dezonne et al, 2009). In vivo, THs regulate radial gliaastrocyte transition and the vimentin-GFAP (glial fibrillary acidic protein) switch, a hallmark of astrocyte differentiation, in the basal forebrain and hippocampus (Dezonne et al., 2009).

Prompt treatment of maternal hypothyroidism, identified by increased TSH, is being advocated to mitigate a negative effect on the woman and her child. However, even a moderate transient period of maternal hypothyroxinemia at the beginning of rat neurogenesis disrupts neuronal migration into cortical layers. These findings reinforce the epidemiological evidence that early maternal hypothyroxinemia—when neuronal migratory waves are starting—is potentially damaging for the child. Detection of an inappropiate first trimester FT4 surge that may not result in increased TSH, may be crucial for the prevention of learning disabilities in a significant number of unborn children (Escobar et al., 2004)

The positive effects of thyroid hormones on cognition has led to some new therapeutic approaches regarding the usage of these hormones in dementia therapy. The results of a study by Fu et al, indicate that the use of TH has some therapeutic potential in AD (Fu et al.,2009).

The congenital absence of thyroid hormone alters neuronal firing behavior during early stages of the development in rat. These changes in neuronal discharge are related to their spike ADP, which is clearly involved in the burst-firing behavior in developing CA1 pyramidal neurons (Sanchez Alonso et al., 2010; Chen et al., 2005).

The relationship between the thyroid axis and psychiatric symptoms and disease is well established. In particular, clinical hypothyroidism leads to depressive symptoms which resolve with replacement therapy. The relationship between alterations of thyroid function and primary major depression is more complex. While various abnormalities of the thyroid axis have been identified, none is specific for depression and there is no clear evidence that thyroid hypofunction is a significant etiological factor in major depression. The literature on thyroid hormone treatment of depression, particularly treatment-resistant major depression, is highly promising and warrants further investigation. Greater understanding about thyroid-brain relationships may yield important information about the etiology of major mood disorders (Joffe et al., 2009).

It is already known that hypothyroidism may alter the evoked potentials. Since 1990s some studies were performed to show this.

In order to detect the dysfunction of central and peripheral nervous systems among rats with varied duration of hypothyroidism and to elucidate the pattern of recovery after thyroxine replacement, a series of BAEP (Brainstem auditory evoked potentials) and PNCS (Peripheral Nerve Conduction Study) were conducted and compared with age-matched controls. BAEP and PNCS were performed in three groups of hypothyroid animals 1, 3 and 5 months after thyroidectomy, respectively. Following initial electrophysiological assessment, thyroxine replacement was administered to each group of hypothyroid rats, and BAEP and PNCS were performed at two month intervals, up to two successive normal studies, or six months after the initiation of therapy, whichever came first. For BAEP, prolonged I–V interpeak latency was the most consistent abnormal finding in all groups of hypothyroid rats, and longer hypothyroid states correlated well with more severe central conduction disorder (Lai et al., 1997).

Nevertheless, these abnormalities usually returned to normal after thyroxine replacement if the duration of hypothyroidism was less than 5 months. Regarding PNCS, all groups of thyroidectomized rats showed normal conduction before and after thyroxine therapy. This study indicated that, in rats: (1) the peripheral nervous system seemed to be more resistant to hypothyroidism than the central nervous system, or (2) the pathogenesis of central and peripheral nerve dysfunction in hypothyroid rats might occur through different mechanisms (Lai et al., 1997).

After thyroxine replacement, the central conduction dysfunction usually returned to normal if the hypothyroid state was not more than 5 months in duration. However, when hypothyroid state persisted over 7 months or more, there would be an incomplete recovery for central conduction disorder. This study brought out the concept of 'therapeutic window' in reversing the central nervous dysfunction caused by hypothyroidism in adult rats (Lai et al, 2000).

According to a study by MacNabb et al., the results suggested that congenital hypothyroidism impaired learning when a discrimination between correct and incorrect operations is made available (Mac Nabb et al., 1999).

Hypothyroidism was also linked to some degenerative diseases of the brain. According to a study performed by Munhoz et al., thyroid function should be assessed in parkinson patients showing worsening of symptoms that cannot be explained by disease progression or resistance to therapy adjustment (Munhoz et al., 2004).

Hypothyroidism during Iodine-therapy is associated with clinically relevant cognitive dysfunctions, especially with effortful attention demanding tasks (Munte et al.,2004).

Processes under the control of TH (thyroid hormones) range from learning and anxiety-like behaviour to sensory function. At the cellular level,TH controls events as diverse as axonal outgrowth, hippocampal synaptic activity and the patterning of opsin photopigments necessary for colour vision. Overall, TH coordinates this variety of events in both central and sensory systems to promote the function of the nervous system as a complete entity (Nunez et al., 2008).

Age at onset of hypothyroidism is suggested to be an important factor for the memory impairment induced by hypothyroidism. In a study performed by Tong et al.,the 2-month-old hypothyroid mice had significantly impaired abilities in both the olfactory discrimination and the spatial cognitive tasks relative to the 2-month-old controls. The 8-month-old hypothyroid mice had only impaired ability in the spatial cognitive task relative to the same age controls. The 15-month-old hypothyroid mice retained these cognitive abilities relative to the same age controls. These results suggested that adult-onset hypothyroidism could induce an age- and task-dependent impairment of memory in female KM mice (Tong et al.,2007).

Thyroid hormone deficiency has profound effects on the brain during development and less marked effects on the adult brain. These effects are considered to be the result of the direct regulation of specific target genes by thyroid hormone. Previous studies have shown that the expression of the neuronal gene RC3, encoding a 78-amino acid calmodulin-binding protein kinase C substrate, is under the influence of thyroid hormone in vivo (Piosik et al, 1997). In their study Piosik et al., investigated the role of thyroid hormone in RC3 mRNA expression at earlier stages of fetal development and in mature goats using in situ hybridization. Their data indicated that in both fetal and adult goats thyroid hormone, at least partly, affected the expression of RC3 mRNA in the striatum and not the cerebral cortex (Piosik et al, 1997).

It was shown that in the rat cerebellar cortex, the expression of mabN210-immunoreactivity in basket cell axons was severely suppressed in hypothyroidism while neurofilament antigen expression in other cerebellar axons seemed not to require thyroid hormones (Plioplys et al., 1986). In hypothyroid rats there is a marked supression of mabN210-immunoreactivity in the cerebral cortex and corpus callosum and, to a lesser extent, there is a reduction in staining in the internal capsule. By contrast, hypothyroidism did not reduce mabN210-immunoreactivity in the lateral olfactory tract or the stria medullaris. In rats, serum thyroid hormone starts to rise to adult levels on postnatal day 4. It appears that axons that have attained their mature distribution prior to the onset of thyroid hormone expression are not affected by hypothyroidism whereas mabN210-immunoreactivity is suppressed in those axonal tracts that reach a mature distribution after P4(Plioplys et al., 1986).

Cerebellar development on the postnatal period is mainly characterized by cellular proliferation in the external granular layer (EGL) followed by migration of granular cells in the molecular layer through the Bergmann glia (BG) fibers in order to form the granular layer in the adult. All these events are drastically affected by thyroid hormones (TH), actions of which are mainly mediated by alpha (TRα) and beta (TRβ) nuclear receptor isoforms (Portello et al., 2010).

Portello et al., analyzed the effects of a natural human mutation (337T) in the TRβ locus, which impaired T3 binding to its receptor, on the mouse cerebellum ontogenesis. They reported that target inactivation of TRβ-TH binding led to a smaller cerebellum area characterized by impaired lamination and foliation. Further, TRβ mutant mice presented severe deficits in proliferation of granular precursors, arborization of Purkinje cells and organization of BG fibers. They reported that their data suggested that the action of TH via TRβ regulated important events of cerebellar ontogenesis contributing to a better understanding of some neuroendocrine disorders. Further, their data correlated TRβ with cerebellar foliation, and provided, for the first time, evidence of a receptor-mediated mechanism underlying TH actions on this event (Portello et al., 2010).

Hypothyroidism has numerous effects on brain. It produces a hypometabolic state. Hypometabolic state following hypothermia is known to protect tissues from ischemic injury. A study by Rastogi et al., provided evidence that hypothyroidism made neuronal tissue less vulnerable to severe ischemic insult (Rastogi et al., 2006).

In a study by Rovet et al.,sixty-nine children with congenital hypothyroidism detected through thyroid screening were compared with 39 unaffected siblings for cognitive and temperamental characteristics. Intelligence test results revealed: (1) IQs of hypothyroid children were normal but lower than siblings; (2) hypothyroid children were lower than siblings in gross motor and perceptual performance abilities; (3) athyrotic children had lower IQs than those with ectopic thyroids, goiter, or hypoplastic disease; (4) athyrotic, hypoplastic, and ectopic thyroid children had lower performance than verbal IQs, but there was no scale difference for those with goiter; (5) deficits differed according to test age; and (6) age of onset of treatment was not related to IQ or pattern of deficit. Temperament test findings revealed: (1) no increase in difficult or slow-to-warm-up children, (2) lower ratings were found for hypothyroid children than siblings on approach/withdrawal and persistence scales, and (3) higher rating was given for athyrotic children than those with goiter (Rovet et al, 1984).

In a study performed by the same authors, hearing loss and its functional consequences were evaluated retrospectively in children with congenital hypothyroidism. Hearing impaired children differed from children with normal hearing in age of treatment onset (22 vs 14 days) but not disease severity or duration. A comparison of language and auditory processing skills at ages 3, 5, and 7 years revealed that early speech was delayed in hearing impaired children, whereas deficits persisted in later receptive language and auditory discrimination skills. Comparing hearing impaired children and children with normal hearing with matched control subjects at grade 3 showed that hearing impaired children were poorer readers because of less adequate phonologic processing skills (Rovet et al, 1996).

In another study that evaluated the influence of thyroid function on the activity and exploratory behaviour of rats, chronic hyperthyroidism produced a significant increase in activity, but did not affect exploration. On the other hand, hypothyroidism did not affect activity, but did increase exploration. This increase in exploration was observed in activity independent behavioural parameters, such as head dipping and glancing (Sala-Roca et al., 2002).

In a study by Sawin et al., the effects of hypothyroidism on development of cholinergic system in brain regions (prefrontal cortex and hippocampus) were evaluated by measuring choline acetyltransferase (ChAT) activity and hemicholinium-3 binding to the high-affinity choline transporter (Sawin et al., 1998). The results suggested that alterations of cholinergic system caused by perinatal hypothyroidism were associated with neurobehavioral deficits at weaning, and these developmental deviations might cause permanent impairment of cognitive function despite recovery from the hormonal imbalance at adult ages (Sawin et al., 1998).

The association of ocular abnormalities with thyroid disorders is well-known, wherein iodine plays an important role. Iodine deficiency and excess can both lead to abnormalities of thyroid function.

Neuromuscular ocular dysfunction in hypothyroidism includes ptosis, ophthalmoplegia, myokymia, cranial nerve dysfunction and cosmetic changes (Seah et al., 2009).

In addition to their role in cellular metabolic activity, thyroid hormones also regulate neural development. Central nervous system is dependent on thyroid hormones for normal maturation and function. Specifically there appears to be extensive inter-reliance between thyroid hormones and acetylcholine, nerve growth factor and hippocampal function (Smith JW et al, 2002).

Thyroid abnormalities have been associated with attention deficit/hyperactivity disorder (ADHD) and with other childhood psychiatric disorders. In a study designed to determine the relationships between thyroid hormone concentrations, neurocognitive functioning, and psychiatric diagnosis in children; thyroxine concentrations were associated with mood symptoms and unusual behaviors, and were less strongly related to attentional functioning. Thyroxine concentrations were not related to hyperactivity (Stein MA et al., 2002).

Insufficiency of thyroid hormones in the adulthood causes a wide range of cognitive dysfunctions, including deficits in learning and memory. In a study that investigated whether adult-onset hypothyroidism would alter synaptic functions in the dorsal hippocampo-medial prefrontal cortex (mPFC) pathway, a neural pathway important for learning and memory, the results suggested that alterations in synaptic plasticity of the dorsal hippocampo-mPFC pathway might contribute to understanding basic mechanisms underlying learning and memory deficits associated with adult-onset hypothyroidism (Sui et al., 2006).

Adult-onset hypothyroidism is associated with neurological changes such as cognitive dysfunction and impaired learning, which may be related to alterations of synaptic plasticity. In a study designed to investigate the consequence of adult-onset hypothyroidism on thyroid-mediated transcription events in striatal synaptic plasticity, and the effect of triiodothyronine (T3) replacement; the authors suggested that thyroid hormone modulation had a major impact on striatal synaptic plasticity of adult mice which produced in turn motor behavior modifications (Vallortigara et al.,2007).

Thyroid hormone action on brain development is essentially exerted through regulation of the expression rate of a number of genes some of which have been identified in the past 10 years (Vargiu et al., 2001).

Attention-deficit hyperactivity disorder (ADHD) is thought to have a biologic basis, but the precise cause is unknown. It is one of the neurodevelopmental abnormalities frequently observed in children with generalized resistance to thyroid hormone (GRTH), suggesting that thyroid abnormalities may be related to ADHD. According to a study by Weiss et al., the prevalence of thyroid abnormalities is higher (5.4%) in children with ADHD than in the normal population (<1%) (Weiss et al., 1993).

According to a study to assess the impact on neonatal neurobehavioral development of methimazole (MMI)-induced in-utero hypothyroxinemia and of correction by maternal-fetal thyroxine (T_4) transfer in the rat by Weller et al., prenatal T_4 treatment resulted in correction of MMI-induced delayed appearance of three different reflexes. Body-weight gain of treated pups was similar to that of controls and more rapid than development of rats treated with MMI-alone. T_4 treatment did not prevent, however, MMI-induced delay in maturation of physiological landmarks (e.g. ear opening). The authors suggested that at least a portion of the developmental delay resulting from prenatal (maternal) MMI administration might be reversed by maternal-fetal transfer of T_4 administered to the gravid dam (Weller et al, 1996).

Thyroid hormone insufficiency leads to impaired neurogenesis, behavioral alterations and cognitive deficits. Thyroid hormone receptors, expressed in brain regions involved in these behaviors, mediate the effects of thyroid hormone deficiency or excess. Thyroid hormone-regulated genes potentially responsible for the learning deficit found in TR_o/o mice include GR, RC3 and GAP-43 (Wilcoxon et al., 2007).

Developmental thyroid hormone (TH) deficiency leads to mental retardation and neurological deficits in humans. According to a study by Zamoner et al., the thyroid status could modulate the integrity of neuronal cytoskeleton acting on the endogenous NF-associated phosphorylating system and that such effect could be related to glutamate-induced excitotoxicity (Zamoner et al., 2008).

Myxoedema coma is a complication of long-standing untreated hypothyroidism. The term is largely a misnomer since most patients are not comatose. This condition is characterised by marked impairment of the central nervous system and of cardiovascular function (Jansen et al.,2006).

Hashimoto encephalopathy, also known as steroid-responsive encephalopathy associated with autoimmune thyroiditis, is a potentially fatal condition associated with a presentation of myoclonus, altered conscious state, strokelike episodes, rapid cognitive decline, and neuropsychiatric symptoms, including psychosis, hallucinations, and abulia.It is an important differential diagnosis of rapidly progressive dementia. It is also an important cause of potentially reversible dementia because with prompt and appropriate treatment its symptoms can be completely reversed. Controversially, Hashimoto encephalopathy can present in the absence of associated thyroid function abnormalities, even though it is associated with high titers of antithyroid peroxidase and antithyroglobulin antibodies. (Brodtmann et al.,, 2009)

3. Effects of hypothyroidism on the peripheral nervous system

The connection between hypothyroidism and polyneuropathy was known thouroughly even in the 70s. In a case study by Shirabe et al., it was suggested that myxoedematous polyneuropathy might be intrinsic neuropathy due to metabolic disorder of Schwann cells related to hypothyroidism, resulting in segmental demyelination, not merely compressive neuropathy due to mucinous deposits in the peripheral nerves (Shirabe et al.,1975). More case studies followed in 80s also (Martin et al., 1983).

Muscle involvement in a variety of forms is a common complication of adult-onset hypothyroidism. Hypothyroid myopathy spans a clinical spectrum that includes a number of different manifestations. The reported prevalence of hypothyroid myopathy symptoms and signs is variable. In a prospective cohort study, 79% of adult patients with hypothyroidism had muscle complaints (myalgias, cramps or weakness) . Asymptomatic CK elevation has been reported to occur in 37% to 60% of hypothyroid patients . Other significant manifestations associated with hypothyroidism include: myalgias, severe muscle weakness, polymyositis-like syndrome, rhabdomyolysis, and acute compartment syndrome (ACS). Rhabdomyolysis after withdrawal of thyroid hormone in a patient with papillary thyroid cancer has been described previously (Ramadhan et al., 2009).

The frequency of myopathy in hypothyroidism ranges from 30 to 80%. The major symptoms related are weakness, muscular cramps and myalgia. The pseudohyperthrophic form is called Hoffman's syndrome. The electrophysiological study reveals myopathy, neuropathy or mixed pattern. Laboratorial investigation generally shows increased levels of muscle enzymes and low serum thyroid hormones, with thyrotrophic-stimulating hormone (TSH) elevated. The treatment consists in hormone replacement and the prognosis is good in most of the cases (Vasconcellos LFR et al.,2003).

In a study performed by Magri et al., intraepidermal nerve fiber density reduction was evaluated as a marker of preclinical asymptomatic small-fiber sensory neuropathy in hypothyroid patients. Their findings suggested that a considerable number of untreated hypothyroid patients may have preclinical asymptomatic small-fiber sensory neuropathy (Magri et al., 2010).

According to a study by Salvi et al., visual evoked potentials in patients with thyroid-associated ophthalmopathy (TAO) identify asymptomatic optic nerve involvement. The authors observed a prolongation of the latency of the evoked cortical response in patients with TAO without subjective visual complaints and without optic nerve compression. They reported that the study of visual evoked potentials in TAO is complementary to the study of the visual field in identifying early optic nerve dysfunction in the absence of decreased visual acuity (Salvi et al, 1997).

4. Hypothyroidism and muscle disease

The relationship between hypothyroidism and muscle disease is known since 19 th century but it is precisely documented ever since 60s (Wilson et al., 1959; Fessel et al, 1968; Golding et al.,1970). In 70s hypothyroid-rheumatic diseases were also described which were defined having symptoms as muscle pain. Muscle pain and stiffness, arthralgia, synovial thickening with effusion, osteolytic lesions, hypothyroid myopathy, acroparaesthesiae, pain, cramps, and stiffness of muscles are common symptoms in hypothyroidism, and mild proximal muscle weakness occurs in over a third of patients (Golding et al., 1971). Pseudomyotonia with delayed relaxation of muscle may occur and a prolonged tendon reflex relaxation time is typical. Myoedema, the "mounding phenomenon," may be elicited in some hypothyroid patients on direct percussion of the muscle. A rare association is Hoffman's syndrome, which is characterised by muscle hypertrophy, weakness, and slowness of movement. The differential diagnosis is from other causes of painful, stiff muscles such as polymyalgia rheumatica and polymyositis. The reflex relaxation time is a useful diagnostic test, and the serum thyroid stimulating hormone concentration should be measured when the doctor is in any doubt. Increased serum activities of enzymes of muscle origin, particularly the creatine kinase isoenzyme, are found in hypothyroidism whether or not muscle symptoms are present. Serum myoglobin concentrations are also raised. Electromyographic studies show a reduction in the mean action potential duration and an increase in the number of polyphasic units in over a third of hypothyroid patients with either normal or hypertrophied muscles. Routine histopathological studies show non-specific findings, but histochemical studies have shown atrophy and reduced frequency of type 2 fibres (Taylor et al., 1983).

Muscle fibre type changes in hypothyroid myopathy were studied by serial percutaneous needle biopsy of vastus lateralis before and during treatment with L-thyroxine by Mc Karen et al. A type II fibre atrophy and loss was found, which correlated with the clinical and biochemical evidence of a myopathy. The type II fibre atrophy was corrected by L-thyroxine but type II fibre loss was still apparent in severely myopathic patients up to two years after starting treatment (Mc Karen et al.,1975). Hypothyroid myopathy has not only been reported in long standing cases of hypothyroidism.

Adult patients with myopathy associated with acute transient hypothyroidism were also described. Patients presented with severe muscle aches and cramps, stiffness and spasms. Muscle enzymes were markedly elevated and electromyography in one patient showed myopathic features. Histological changes were absent in muscle biopsy, probably because of the short duration of metabolic disturbance. The myopathy subsided promptly when the hypothyroid state was reversed (Kung et al, 1987).

Muscle weakness, aches and cramps, stiffness and delayed tendon jerk relaxation are usual features of hypothyroid myopathy (30–80%), while muscle hypertrophy, myoedema and wasting are occasionally seen. They evolve gradually over a long period of time (Bhansali et al.,1999). Hypothyroidism should be differentiated from polymyositis (Mace et al., 1980, Cabili et al.,1982).

Hypothyroidism is also a risk factor for statin-induced myopathy (SIM) and even spontaneous myopathy. Muscle aches, cramps, and weakness are the typical clinical features, irrespective of the precipitant (Bar et al., 2007).

Rhabdomyolysis, the most feared and potentially fatal complication of SIM, is also rarely caused by isolated hypothyroidism. When this is seen, it is usually characterized by a moderate rise in creatine phosphokinase (Khaleli et al., 1983). Data from clinical trials show the rate of SIM in the general population to be 0.1% to 0.2%; the rate of hypothyroid-induced myopathy is unknown. Because of these associations, patients' thyroid status should always be considered before initiating lipid-lowering medications and, for patients receiving statin therapy, thyroid function should be assessed whenever myopathic symptoms or resistance to therapy is noted (Bar et al., 2007).

5. References

Ahmed OM, El-Gareib AW, El-bakry AM, et al. Thyroid hormones states and brain development interactions. Int. J. Devl Neuroscience 2008; 147–209.

Anderson GW, Mariash CN. Molecular Aspects of Thyroid Hormone-Regulated Behavior. Hormones, Brain and Behavior 2002; 539-566.

Bar SL, Holmes DT, Frohlich J. Asymptomatic hypothyroidism and statin-induced myopathy. Canadian Family Physician • Le Médecin de famille canadien, 2007; 428-431.

Bhanja S, Chainy GBN. PTU-induced hypothyroidism modulates antioxidant defence status in the developing cerebellum. Int. J. Devl Neuroscience 2010; 251–262.

Bhansali A, Chandran V, Ramesh J, Acute myoedema: an unusual presenting manifestation of hypothyroid myopathy.

Brodtmann A. Hashimoto Encephalopathy and Down Syndrome. Arch Neurol. 2009; 663-666.

Cabili S, Pines A, Kaplinsky N, et al. Hypothyroidism masquerading as polymyositis. Postgraduate Medical Journal,1982; 545-547.

Calloni GW, Penno CA, Cordova FM et al. Congenital hypothyroidism alters the phosphorylation of ERK1/2 and p38MAPK in the hippocampus of neonatal rats. Developmental Brain Research 2005; 141- 145.

Calza L, Aloe L, Giardinos L. Thyroid Hormone-Induced Plasticity in the adult rat brain. Brain Research Bulletin 1997; 549-557.

Chen S, Yue C, Yaari Y (2005) A transitional period of Ca2_-dependent spike after depolarization and bursting in developing rat CA1 pyramidal cells. J Physiol 567:79-93.

Darbra S, Garau A, Balada F. Perinatal hypothyroidism effects on neuromotor competence, novelty-directed exploratory and anxiety-related behaviour and learning in rats. Behavioural Brain Research 2003; 209.

Dennis MS. Non-Alzheimer Dementias. Review. 2005.

Dezonne RS, Stipursky J, Gomes FCA. Effect of thyroid hormone depletion on cultured murine cerebral cortex astrocytes. Neuroscience Letters 2009; 58-62.

Dong H, Wade M, Williams A et al. Molecular insight into the effects of hypothyroidism on the developing cerebellum. Biochemical and Biophysical Research Communications 2005; 1182-1193.

Desouzo LA, Ladiwala U, Daniel SM et al. Thyroid hormone regulates hippocampal neurogenesis in the adult rat brain. Mol. Cell. Neurosci. 2005; 414 - 426.

England Congenital Hypothyroidism Collaborative New. Elementary school performance of children with congenital hypothyroidism. The Journal of Pediatrics 1990; 27-32.

Escobar GM, Obregon MJ, Escobar del Rey F. Maternal thyroid hormones early in pregnancy and fetal brain development. Best Practice & Research Clinical Endocrinology & Metabolism 2004; 225-248.

Fessel, W. J. Myopathy of hypothyroidism Ann. rheum. Dig., 1968; 590.

Gilbert ME. Alterations in synaptic transmission and plasticity in area CA1 of adult hippocampus following developmental hypothyroidism. Developmental Brain Research 2004; 11 - 18.

Golding DN. Hypothyroidism presenting with musculoskeletal symptoms. Ann. rheum. Dis., 1970:10-14.

Jansen HJ, Doebe O, Louwerse ES, et al. Status epilepticus caused by a myxoedema Coma. The Netherlands Journal of Medicine 2006; 202-205.

Joffe RT. Hypothalamic-Pituitary-Thyroid Axis . Hormones, Brain and Behavior. Elsevier (second Edition) Volume 5, Pages 2341-2355.

Khaleeli AA, Griffith Dg, Edwards RHT. The clinical presentation of hypothyroid myopathy and its relation to abnormalities in structure and function of skeletal muscle. Clin Endocrinol, 1983; 365.

Kung AWC, Ma JTC, Yu YL, et al.Myopathy in acute hypothyroidism. Postgraduate Medical Journal, 1987; 661-663.

Lai JL, Tai JT, Liu CK et al. A longitudinal study of central and peripheral nerve conduction in hypothyroid rats. Journal of Neurological Sciences 1997; 139-145.

Lai JL, Lin RT, Tai CT et al. The recovery potential of central conduction disorder in hypothyroid rats. Journal of the Neurological Sciences 2000; 113-119.

Lasley SM, Gilbert ME. Developmental thyroid hormone insufficiency reduces expression of brain-derived neurotrophic factor (BDNF) in adults but not in neonates. Neurotoxicology and Teratology. 2011; 464–472.

Mac Nabb C, O'hare E, Cleary J et al. Congenital hypothyroidism impairs response alternation discrimination behavior. Brain Research 1999; 231–239.

Mace BEW, Mallya RK, Staffhurt JS. Severe myxoedema presenting with chondrocalcinosis and polymyositis. Journal of the Royal Society of Medicine, 1980;887-888.

Magri F, Buonocore M, Oliviero A, et al. Intraepidermal nerve fiber density reduction as a marker of preclinical asymptomatic small-fiber sensory neuropathy in hypothyroid patients. Eur J Endocrinol 2010; 279-284.

Martin J, Tomkin GH, Hutchinson M. Peripheral neuropathy in hypothyroidism - an association with spurious polycythaemia (Gaisbock's syndrome). Journal of the Royal Society of Medicine 1983;187-189.

Mc Keran RO, Slavin G, Andrews M, et al.Muscle fibre type changes in hypothyroid myopathy. J. clin. Path., 1975; 659-663.

Munhoz RP, Teive HA, Troiano AR et al. Parkinson's disease and thyroid dysfunction. Parkinsonism and Related Disorders 2004; 381–383.

Munte TF, Christian L, Otting G. Cognitive changes in short-term hypothyroidism assessed with event-related brain potentials. Psychoneuroendocrinology 2004; 1109–1118.

Nunez C, Celi F, Ng L et al. Multigenic control of thyroid hormone functions in the nervous system. Molecular and Cellular Endocrinology 287 (2008) 1–12

Osterweil D, Syndulko K, Cohen SN, et al. Cognitive function in non-demented older adults with hypothyroidism. J Am Geriatr Soc. 1992; 325-35.

Piosik PA, Van Groenigen M, Baas F. Effect of thyroid hormone deficiency on RC3/neurogranin mRNA expression in the prenatal and adult caprine brain. Molecular Brain Research 1996; 227-235.

Plioplys A, Gravel C, Hawkes R. Selective suppression of neurofilament antigen expression in the hypothyroid rat cerebral cortex. Journal of the Neurological Sciences 1986; 53-68.

Portella AJ, Carvalho F, Faustino L et al. Thyroid hormone receptor β mutation causes severe impairment of cerebellar development. Molecular and Cellular Neuroscience 2010; 68–77.

Ramadhan A, Schondorf R, Tamilia M. Rhabdomyolysis and peroneal nerve compression associated with thyroid hormone withdrawal in the setting of remnant ablation: a review of the literature. Canadian Society of Endocrinology and Metabolism annual meeting on October 19, 2009 in Montreal,Canada.

Rastogi L, Godbole M, Ray M et al. Reduction in oxidative stress and cell death explains hypothyroidism induced neuroprotection subsequent to ischemia/reperfusion insult. Experimental Neurology 2006; 290–300.

Roberts CG, Ladenson PW. Hypothyroidism (Seminar). Lancet 2004; 363: 793–803.

Rovet JF, Westbrook DL, Ehrlich RM. Neonatal Thyroid Deficiency: Early Temperamental and Cognitive Characteristics. Journal of the American Academy of Child Psychiatry 1984; 10-22.

Rovet J, Walker W, Bliss B et al. Long-term sequelae of hearing impairment in congenital hypothyroidism. The Journal of Pediatrics 1996; 776-783.

Sala-Roca J, Carbonel M.A.M., Garau A et al. Effects of chronic dysthyroidism on activity and exploration. Physiology & Behavior 2002; 125- 133.

Salvi M, Spaggiari E, Neri F, et al. The Study of Visual Evoked Potentials in Patients with Thyroid-Associated Ophthalmopathy Identifies Asymptomatic Optic Nerve Involvement. The Journal of Clinical Endocrinology & Metabolism, 1997 vol. 82; 1027-1030.

Sawin S, Brodish P, Carter C, et al. Development of Cholinergic Neurons in Rat

Brain Regions: Dose-Dependent Effects of Propylthiouracil-Induced Hypothyroidism. Neurotoxicology and Teratology 1998; 627–635.

Sanchez Alonso JL, Jueavas JM, Torres MAV et al. Role of low-voltage-activated calcium current on the firing pattern alterations induced by hypothyroidism in the rat hippocampus. Neuroscience 2010; 993–1005.

Seah A., Lo YL. Ocular Aspects of Hypothyroidism: Neuro-Ophthalmological Dysfunction in Relation to Thyroid Disease and Iodine. Comprehensive Handbook of Iodine. Elsevier. Nutritional, Biochemical, Pathological and Therapeutic Aspects 2009; Ch 112: Pages 1103-1111.

Shirabe T, Tawara S, Terao A, et al. Myxoedematous polyneuropathy: a light and electron microscopic study of the peripheral nerve and muscle. Journal of Neurology, Neurosurgery, and Psychiatry, 1975; 241-247.

Smith JW, Evans AT, Costal B, Smythe JW. Thyroid hormones, brain function and cognition: a brief review. Neuroscience and Biobehavioral Reviews 2002; 45-60.

Stein MA, Weiss RE. Thyroid function tests and neurocognitive functioning in children referred for attention deficit/hyperactivity disorder. Psychoneuroendocrinology 2003; 304–316.

Sui L, Wang F, Li BM. Adult-onset hypothyroidism impairs paired-pulse facilitation and long-term potentiation of the rat dorsal hippocampomedial prefrontal cortex pathway in vivo. Brain Research 2006; 53-60.

Taylor PK, Turnbull DM. Endocrine myopathies. British Medical Journal 1983; 705-708.

Tong H, Chen GH, Liu RY et al. Age-related learning and memory impairments in adult-onset hypothyroidism in Kunming mice. Physiology & Behavior 2007; 290–298.

Vallortigara J, Alfos S, Micheau J et al. T3 administration in adult hypothyroid mice modulates expression of proteins involved in striatal synaptic plasticity and improves motor behavior. Neurobiology of Disease 2008; 378–385.

Vargiu P, Morte B, Manzano J, et al. Thyroid hormone regulation of rhes, a novel Ras homolog gene expressed in the striatum. Molecular Brain Research 2001; 1–8.

Vasconcellos RFR, Pexisoto MC, Oliveira T, et al. Hoffman's syndrome: pseudohypertrophic myopathy as initial manifestation of hypothyroidism: Case report. Arq. Neuro Psiquiatr. 2003.

Weiss RE, Stein MA, Trommer B, et al. Attention-deficit hyperactivity disorder and thyroid function. The Journal of Pediatrics 1993;539-545.

Weller A, Rozin A, Rigler O, et al. Neurobehavioral development of neonatal rats after in-utero hypothyroxinemia: efficacy of prenatal thyroxine treatment. Early Human Development 1996;63-76.

Wilcoxon JS, Nadolsky GJ, Samarut J et al. Behavioral inhibition and impaired spatial learning and memory in hypothyroid mice lacking thyroid hormone receptor. Behavioural Brain Research 2007; 109–116.

Wilson J, Walton J. Some muscular manifestations of hypothyroidism. J. Neurol. Neurosurg. Psychiat., 1959; 320-324.

Zamoner A., Heimfarth L, Pessoa-Pureur R. Congenital hypothyroidism is associated with intermediate filament misregulation, glutamate transporters down-regulation and MAPK activation in developing rat brain.

8

Thyroid Disorders and Brain Natriuretic Peptide

Hamiyet Yılmaz[1*], Barış Pamuk[2],
Derun Taner Ertugrul[3] and Erdem Yaşar[4]
[1]*Aydin State Hospital, Department of Endocrinology and Metabolism*
[2]*Bozyaka Training and Research Hospital, Department of Internal Medicine*
[3]*Kecioren Training and Research Hospital, Department of Internal Medicine*
[4]*Acıpayam State Hospital, Department of Anaesthesia*
Turkey

1. Introduction

The structure of atrial natriuretic peptide (ANP) was first discovered in 1984 (1). In following years, a molecule, which resembled ANP, was isolated from a pig brain (2). This B-type or brain natriuretic peptide (BNP) is a member of the natriuretic peptide family that has physiological effects similar to atrial natriuretic peptide (ANP), including diuretic, natriuretic, and vasorelaxant actions (3,4). Although this peptide is referred to as the brain natriuretic peptide (BNP), it is actually produced in the ventricular myocardium (5). BNP is not a prestored molecule, but if proper stimuli exist it can be produced rapidly through mRNA synthesis. The stimulus triggering the secretion of BNP by the ventricles of the heart is mainly excessive stretching of myocytes rather than the transmural pressure load (6-8). BNP is synthesized both in an inactive N-terminal fragment with 76 amino acids (NTpro-BNP) and an active hormone with 32 amino acids (BNP). ANP and related precursor peptides comprise 98% of all natriuretic peptides in healthy subjects (9).

Like ANP, BNP is induced by pathophysiological conditions of the heart, including hypertrophy, myocardial infarction, and heart failure. BNP levels have been shown to be a good predictor of left ventricular dysfunction and decompensated heart failure, and recently BNP infusion has been approved as an effective treatment for acute heart failure (10,11). Distinct physiological roles of BNP have been elucidated by generation of knockout (KO) mice. While BNP KO mice are no different from control mice with regard to blood pressure, urine volume, and urinary Na+ and K+ excretion, they have more extensive ventricular fibrosis, accompanied by increased transforming growth factor-3 (TGF-3) and collagen mRNA [81]. Studies of cultured cells indicate that BNP inhibits growth of vascular cells, as well as fibroblast proliferation and collagen production by fibroblasts (3,12). Thus, BNP may function more as an autocrine/paracrine inhibitor of cell growth in the heart, while ANP

* Corresponding Author

functions more as a traditional circulating hormone with pronounced diuretic, natriuretic, and anti-hypertensive effects. (3)

In addition to ventricular myocardium, extracardiac sources of BNP have been detected in tissues at autopsy, including the lungs, kidneys, and adrenal glands, although at much lower levels than ventricular BNP (13). BNP is produced , to a small degree, by the renal glomerular epithelial and mesangial cells (14,15) is a counter-regulatory hormone that physiologically opposes and suppresses the renin-angiotensin aldosterone system (RAAS), endothelin-1 and the sympathetic nervous system (SNS). Endogenous BNP and ANP production maintain renal function and sodium balance when cardiac function acutely deteriorates (16).

Routine BNP testing has recently been introduced as a noninvasive, low-risk test that measures circulating levels of BNP, which are elevated in individuals with both symptomatic and asymptomatic heart failure. The BNP test is used to detect preclinical heart disease or to confirm the cardiac etiology in symptomatic patients. It not only enables the early identification of patients with incipient heart failure but also provides prognostic information based on the magnitude of the increase. Also administration of exogenous intravenous (IV) BNP shown to rapidly improve hemodynamic, volume, neurohormonal, and symptomatic abnormalities in patients with acute decompensated heart failure and to decrease rates of rehospitalization (17,18). Nesiritide IV (human recombinant BNP) is approved for the treatment of acute decompensated CHF. The physiologic effects of nesiritide include veno- and arterial dilatation (without reflex tachycardia), diuresis, and natriuresis (without reduction in renal perfusion or function). Thus, nesiritide increases cardiac index and reduces pulmonary capillary wedge pressure (PCWP) (18). In addition, nesiritide is lusitropic, anti-fibrotic, and inhibits RAAS; thus, nesiritide should stabilize renal function acutely and chronically while improving cardiac function and hemodynamics in CHF patients.

The cardiovascular system is very sensitive to thyroid hormones. Hyperthyroidism and hypothyroidism induce significant changes in cardiac functions. The effects of hyperthyroidism on the heart include hemodynamic changes such as decreased systemic vascular resistance as well as increased cardiac output, heart rate, blood volume, blood pressure and impaired cardiac contractility. It may also lead to atrial arrhythmias (19). These changes result in ventricular stretch and pressure overload, which might cause concomitant rise in BNP concentrations (20). Recent attention has been drawn to the relation of BNP and hyperthyroidism. Studies suggest that plasma BNP and NT-pro-BNP concentrations are frequently increased in hyperthyroidism. This increase is partly due to hyperthyroidism-induced left ventricular dysfunction. Also in vitro animal studies have suggested that T4 and T3 stimulate BNP release from both cultured atrial and ventricular myocytes (21).

There are only a limited number of studies with contradictory results investigating the effect of thyroid function abnormalities on the measurement of BNP. Wei et al. have measured the BNP levels and left ventricular functions of 67 hyperthyroid patients and 32 healthy subjects. The average BNP level was found to be higher in the patients especially the ones with left ventricular dysfunction than the healthy individuals. Nonsignificant correlations between thyroid hormones and BNP levels were identified (19). Biondi et al. demonstrated an increase of left ventricular mass more specifically, an increase of septal and posterior wall thickness, enhanced resting systolic function and significantly impaired Doppler parameters of diastolic function (22). Smit et al. demonstrated that diastolic dysfunction was impaired in exogenous subclinical hyperthyroidism induced by levothyroxine treatment in 25 differentiated thyroid carcinoma patients (23). Two small studies suggest a beneficial effect of treatment of subclinical hyperthyroidism on cardiac function (24,25). Schultz et al. studied NT-pro-BNP levels in different thyroid function states and found that serum levels of NT-pro-BNP were strongly affected by thyroid function; the higher the thyroid function, the higher the serum levels of NT-pro-BNP. Likewise the treatment of the dysthyroid state resulted in a significant increase in NT-pro-BNP in both overt and subclinical hypothyroid patients and a decrease in both overt and subclinical hyperthyroid patients. In order to evaluate whether those findings were the direct effect of thyroid hormones or were the results of changes in heart function and structure, they compared NT-pro-BNP, thyroid function and cardiac output (CO) or resting pulse rate in a subgroup of patients under study. CO or resting pulse rate did not have any independent effect on NT-pro-BNP levels, whereas , thyroid function had a significant effect on NT-pro-BNP levels (26). Ertugrul et al evaluated the serum BNP levels in 18 overt and 47 subclinical hyperthyroid patients together with 39 subclinical and 13 overt hypothyroid patients. BNP levels were more than five times higher in hyperthyroid than euthyroid control subjects. BNP levels were also higher in subclinical hyperthyroidism than euthyroid control subjects. Free T4 and free T3 concentrations were found to be associated with high serum BNP levels. The BNP level in patients with subclinical or overt hypothyroidism was similar to that of the controls (27). On the other hand, Christ-Crain et al. found that there was no significant difference in NT-proBNP levels of euthyroid and overt hypothyroid, subclinical hypothyroid and subclinical hyperthyroid subjects, and NT-pro-BNP levels were higher in overt hyperthyroidism compared to other groups (9). Kohno et al. have found higher BNP levels in untreated hyperthyroid patients and rats with hyperthyroidism induced by thyroxine than their normal counterparts. Hypothyroid rats had lower plasma BNP concentration than the euthyroid ones. In-vitro effects of T3 and T4 on the release of BNP were investigated in newborn rat atrial and ventricular myocytes in primary culture. T3 and T4 stimulated release of BNP from both cultured atrial and ventricular myocytes in a dose-dependent manner (21). Triiodothyronine also increases BNP gene transcription and amplifies endothelin-dependent BNP gene transcription in rat ventricular myocytes (28). The effect of hyperthyroidism and subclinical hyperthyroidism on the heart may also cause an increase in BNP. At the moment, we do not know which one of these mechanisms is actually responsible for alterations in BNP levels in thyroid dysfunction. There is little known about the effects of endogenous subclinical hyperthyroidism on the heart. Faber et al. demonstrated an increase in cardiac output and a reduction in total peripheral resistance when treating subclinical hypothyroid subjects with L-T4, whereas the opposite is seen on treating subclinical hyperthyroidism with radioiodine (24).

Ertugrul et al studied BNP levels in patients with hyperthyroidism before specific treatment for hyperthyroidism and after euthyroidism was achieved. This study showed that BNP levels were significantly higher in hyperthyroid than euthyroid status of the same patients. It was found that the decrease in BNP levels was positively correlated with the decrease in fT3 and fT4 (29). Kato et al measured serum ANP and BNP levels in 130 patients with thyrotoxicosis and correlated them with serum thyroid hormone levels and with the degree of severity of the heart failure. They reported a significant elevation of BNP and atrial natriuretic peptide levels which returned to normal values after euthyroididsm was established in patients with thyrotoxicosis. It was concluded that both serum thyroid hormones and cardiovascular dysfunction contribute to the increase of serum BNP levels and atrial fibrillation is an independent contributing factor for the increase of BNP (30).

In conclusion, natriuretic peptide levels are altered in different thyroid states with a more pronounced effect in hyperthyroidism compared to hypothyroidism. This seems to reflect distinct atrial and ventricular cardiac dysfunction in thyroid hormone excess or, alternatively, mirrors a direct effect of thyroid hormones on gene expression of natriuretic peptides. As hyperthyroidism results in increased serum levels of pro-ANP, NT-proBNP and BNP levels as typically seen in mild heart failure, hyperthyroidism should be considered in patients presenting with unclear symptoms and mildly elevated natriuretic peptide levels (9). Since the treatment of hyperthyroidism is quite different than the treatment of heart failure, thyroid hormones should be checked in patients with high levels of BNP. Mild elevations in NT-pro-BNP levels should therefore always be accompanied by a thyroid function screening test (26,29).

2. References

[1] Kangawa K, Fukuda A, Minamino N, et al. Purification and complete amino acid sequence of beta-rat atrial natriuretic polypeptide (betarANP) of 5000 daltons. *Biochem Biophys Res Commun*. 1984;119:933-940.

[2] Sudoh T, Kangawa K, Minamino N, et al. A new natriuretic peptide in porcine brain. *Nature*. 1988;332:78-81.

[3] LaPointe MC. Molecular regulation of the brain natriuretic peptide gene. *Peptides* 2005; 26: 944–956.

[4] Levin ER, Gardner DG, Samson WK. Natriuretic peptides. *N Engl J Med* 1998;339:321–8.

[5] Hosoda K, Nakao K, Mukoyama M, et al. Expression of brain natriuretic peptide gene in human heart: production in the ventricle. *Hypertension*. 1991;17:1152-1155.

[6] Bruneau BG, Piazza LA, de Bold AJ. BNP gene expression is specifically modulated by stretch and ET-1 in a new model of isolated rat atria. *Am J Physiol*. 1997;273:2678-686.

[7] Wiese S, Breyer T, Dragu A, et al. Gene expression of brain natriuretic peptide in isolated atrial and ventricular human myocardium: influence of angiotensin II and diastolic fiber length. *Circulation*. 2000;102:3074-3079.

[8] Mizuno Y, Yoshimura M, Harada E, et al. Plasma levels of A- and B-type natriuretic peptides in patients with hypertrophic cardiomyopathy or idiopathic dilated cardiomyopathy. *Am J Cardiol*. 2000; 86:1036-1040.

[9] Christ-Crain M, Morgenthaler NG, Meier C, et al. Pro-A-type and N-terminal pro-B-type natriuretic peptides in different thyroid function states. *Swiss Medical Weekly*. 2005;135:549-554.

[10] Richards AM, Lainchbury JG, Nicholls MG, Troughton RW, Yandle TG. BNP in hormone-guided treatment of heart failure. *Trends Endocrinol Metab* 2002;13:151–5.

[11] Latini R, Masson S, de Angelis N, Anand I. Role of brain natriuretic peptide in the diagnosis and management of heart failure: current concepts. *J Card Fail* 2002;8:288–99.

[12] Tsuruda T, Boerrigter G, Huntley BK, Noser JA, Cataliotti A, Costello-Boerrigter LC, et al. Brain natriuretic peptide is produced in cardiac fibroblasts and induces matrix metalloproteinases. *Circ Res* 2002;91:1127–34.

[13] Gerbes AL, Dagnino L, Nguyen T, Nemer M. Transcription of brain natriuretic peptide and atrial natriuretic peptide genes in human tissues. *J Clin Endocrinol Metab* 1994;78:1307–11.

[14] McCullough PA, Joseph K, Mathur VS. Diagnostic and therapeutic utility of B-type natriuretic peptide in patients with renal insufficiency and decompansated heart failure. *Rev Cardiovasc Med* 2004;5(1):16-25.

[15] Lai KN, Leung JC, Yandle TG, et al. Gene expression and synthesis of natriuretic peptides by cultured human glomerular cells. *J Hypertension.* 1999;17:575-583.

[16] Silver M, Horton D, Ghali J, Elkayam U. Effect of nesiritide versus dobutamine on short-term outcomes in the treatment of patients with acutely decompensated heart failure. *J Am Coll Cardiol.* 2002;39:798-803.

[17] Abraham WT, Lowes BD, Ferguson DA, et al. Systemic hemodynamic, neurohormonal, and renal effects of a steady-state infusion of human brain natriuretic peptide in patients with hemodynamically decompensated heart failure. *J Card Fail.* 1998;4:37-44.

[18] Colucci WS, Elkayam U, Horton DP, et al. Intravenous nesiritide, a natriuretic peptide, in the treatment of decompensated congestive heart failure. Nesiritide Study roup. *N Engl J Med.* 2000;343:246-253.

[19] Wei T, Zeng C, Tian Y, et al. B-type natriuretic peptide in patients with clinical hyperthyroidism. *J Endocrinol Invest.* 2005;28:8-11.

[20] Tsutamoto T, Wada A, Maeda K, et al. Attenuation of compensation of endogenous cardiac natriuretic peptide system in chronic heart failure: prognostic role of plasma brain natriuretic peptide concentration in patients with chronic symptomatic left ventricular dysfunction. *Circulation.*1997;96:509-516.

[21] Kohno M, Horio T, Yasunari K, et al. Stimulation of brain natriuretic peptide release from the heart by thyroid hormone. Metabolism 1993, 42:1059-64.

[22] Biondi B, Palmieri EA, Fazio S, et al. Endogenous subclinical hyperthyroidism affects quality of life and cardiac morphology and function in young and middle-aged patients. *J Clin Endocrinol Metab.* 2000;85:4701-4705.

[23] Smit JW, Eustatia-Rutten CF, Corssmit EP, et al. Reversible diastolic dysfunction after long-term exogenous subclinical hyperthyroidism: a randomized, placebo-controlled study. *J Clin Endocrinol Metab.* 2005;90:6041-6047.

[24] Faber J, Wiinberg N, Schifter S, et al. Haemodynamic changes following treatment of subclinical and overt hyperthyroidism. *Eur J Endocrinol.* 2001;145:391-396.

[25] Sgarbi JA, Villaca FG, Garbeline B, et al. The effects of early antithyroid therapy for endogenous subclinical hyperthyroidism in clinical and heart abnormalities. *J Clin Endocrinol Metab.* 2003;88:1672-1677.

[26] Schultz M, Faber J, Kistorp C, et al. N-terminal-pro-B-type natriuretic peptide (NT-pro-BNP) in different thyroid function states. *Clin Endocrinol (Oxf).* 2004;60:54-59.

[27] Ertugrul DT, Gursoy A, Sahin M, Unal AD, Pamuk B, Berberoglu Z, Ayturk S, Tutuncu NB, Demirag NG. (2008) Evaluation of brain natriuretic peptide levels in hyperthyroidism and hypothyroidism. *J Natl Med Assoc* 100(4): 401-5.

[28] Liang F, Webb P, Marimuthu A, et al. Triiodothyronine increases brain natriuretic peptide (BNP) gene transcription and amplifies endothelindependent BNP gene transcription and hypertrophy in neonatal rat ventricular myocytes. *J Biol Chem.* 2003;278:15073-15083.

[29] Ertugrul DT, Yavuz B, Ata N, Yalçın AA, Küçükazman M, Algül B, Dal K, Akın KO, Deveci OS et al. Decreasing Brain Natriuretic Peptide Levels after Treatment for Hyperthyroidism. *Endocrine Journal* 2009, 56 (9), 1043-1048.

[30] Kato K, Murakami H, Isozaki O, Tsushima T, Takano K. Serum concentrations of ANP and BNP in patients with thyrotoxicosis. *Endocrine Journal* 2009, 56 (1), 17-27.

Part 2

Diagnose and Therapy

9

Causes of Hypothyroidism

Irena Kostic[1,2] and Francesco Curcio[2,3]
[1]*University of Kragujevac*
[2]*University of Udine Medical School, Dip. di Scienze Mediche e Biologiche*
[3]*University of Udine Teaching Hospital Santa Maria della Misericordia, Dip. di Medicina di Laboratorio*
[1]*Serbia*
[2,3]*Italy*

1. Introduction

Hypothyroidism is a common endocrine disorder resulting from deficiency of thyroid hormone or its effects on peripheral tissues. It usually is caused by an insufficient production of thyroid hormone by thyroid gland (primary hypothyroidism), but it could be also caused by inadequate secretion of either thyrotropin (ie. thyroid-stimulating hormone-TSH) from the pituitary gland (secondary hypothyroidism) or thyrotropin-releasing hormone (TRH) from the hypothalamus (tertiary hypothyroidism) (Bharaktiya, 2011).

Mixedema (previously a sinonim for hypothyroidism) is reffered to a skin and subcutaneous tissue changes in severe hypothyroid patients.

Hypothyroidism is a very common condition. It is estimated that about 2% of adult women and about 0,1-0,2% of men have clinical hypothyroidism, while the prevalence of subclinical disease is more frequent, up to 9% of adult population (Canaris et al., 2000; Danese et al., 1996 ; Vanderpump et al., 1995). The incidence however increases with age (Bharaktiya, 20111). The prevalence of hypothyroidism in newborns (congenital hypothyroidism) is about 1:3500 (LaFranchi, 1999).

2. Causes of hypothyroidism

The most common cause of hypothyroidism in adults may be summarised as follows (McPhee & Bauer, 1997):

1. Congenital:
   a. aplasia, hypoplasia, thyroid ectopy
   b. defect of hormones' synthesis and effects
2. Acquired:
   a. autoimmune thyroiditis
   b. iodide deficient diet
   c. thyroid ablation (as a consequence of radiation, surgical interventions etc)
3. Pharmacological: iodide, propylthiouracil, methimazole, lithium, thiocyanate etc

The most common cause of hypothyroidism in adults is autoimmune thyroid disease (AITD) where autoimmune thyroiditis (AT) is one of the entities. AT can begin suddenly or it can develop slowly over the years. The most frequent forms are Hashimoto's thyroiditis and atrophic thyroiditis (American Thyroid Association, 2008).

The second frequent cause is a thyroid ablation as a consequence of surgical removal of part or all of the gland in case of thyroid nodules, thyroid cancer, or Graves' disease. If part of the gland is left, it may be able to make enough thyroid hormone to keep blood levels normal. It is necessary that at least 90% of the gland be destroyed in order to develop hypothyroidism (American Thyroid Association, 2008).

Another cause of thyroid ablation is the radiation treatment during radiotherapy of neck for patients with Hodgkin's lymphoma, or cancers of the head or neck, or the use of radioactive iodine (I-131) in some patients with Graves' disease, nodular goiter, or thyroid cancer (American Thyroid Association, 2008).

Third most common are all causes of congenital hypothyroidism (in newborns), where one could find newborns without a thyroid (aplasia) or with only a partly formed one (hypoplasia). There are also babies with partial or all thyroid tissue in the wrong place (ectopic thyroid) or in some cases the thyroid is in place, but biosynthetic enzymes are defective (American Thyroid Association, 2008).

Although autoimmune thyroiditis is the most frequent cause of hypothyroidism, there are also a few forms of infective processes in thyroid. According to the duration, infective thyroiditis could be acute (generally caused by bacteria) or subacute (generally caused by viral agents). During the course of infective thyroiditis there could be a transient episode of thyroid hormones liberation in circulation from destroyed or damaged thyroid cells, called thyrotoxicosis. Subsequently if more than 90% of thyroid tissue is destroyed, hypothyroidism develops (McPhee & Bauer, 2007).

In some cases, medicines could be the cause of hypothyroidism, usually by interfering with normal thyroid hormone synthesis. Very often it is found in patients taking amiodarone, lithium, interferon alpha, and interleukin-2. These drugs are most likely to trigger hypothyroidism in patients who have a genetic tendency to develop AITD (American Thyroid Association, 2008). Potassium perchlorate could be used to treat thyrotoxicosis and hypothyroidism induced by amiodarone (Wolff, 1998). Perchlorate is a competitive inhibitor of the sodium-iodide symporter (NIS) that can suppress T3 and T4 production. Also, the drugs used for the hyperthyroidism treatment such as methimazole and propylthiouracil, could cause hypothyroidism.

In 1998 it is estimated that about one third of world's population lived in iodine-deficient areas, primarily in Africa, Southeast and Central Asia, but also in some European countries (like Germany, Belgium, France and Italy) (Dunn, 1996). Since iodine is the essential factor for thyroid hormone synthesis and it is concentrated in thyroid, any disequilibrium (too much or too little) in circulating iodine levels could cause or worsen hypothyroidism. Since more than 90% of dietary iodine is excreted in the urine, the World Health Organization (WHO) has determined 100mcg/L of urinary iodine as cut-off level for iodine deficiency (WHO, UNICEF & ICCID, 2001). In areas of the world with very low iodine intake in the diet (like India, Chile, Ecuador, Himalayas), severe hypothyroidism can be seen in 5% to 15% of the population (Mathur, 2011).

If the pituitary or hypothalamus are damaged by a tumor, radiation, or surgery, hypothyroidism could be developed (secondary or tertiary hypothyroidism, respectively), characterized by diminished both, TSH and thyroid hormone levels.

Finally, in some cases the deposit of abnormal substances in the thyroid, could be the cause of hypothyroidism. For example, in the course of amyloidosis there can be deposit of amyloid protein, in the course of sarcoidosis there can form granulomas, and in the course of hemochromatosis there can be deposit iron (American Thyroid Association, 2008)

3. Pathogenesis of autoimmune thyroid disease (AITD)

3.1 The role of genetic factors in the development of AITD

It is generally believed that AITD is a complex of several entities that could overlap: Hashimoto's thyroiditis (HT), Graves' disease (GD) and orbitopathy. The majority of autoimmune endocrinopathies are inherited as complex genetic traits, with multiple genetic and environmental factors interactions which confer susceptibility to such disorders. The genetic factors remain largely unknown, with the exception of the human leukocyte antigen (HLA). It is known that AITD are more frequent in families with HLA DR3 and DR5 HLA alleles. Predominantly involved are women. Indeed, HT is 5 to 10 times more common in women than in men. Since the basis for autoimmune diseases may have a common origin, it is possible that patients with HT or their first degree relatives, have one or more other autoimmune diseases such as type 1 diabetes mellitus or pernicious anemia (with antibodies against gastric parietal cells or B12) (Mathur, 2011).

In recent years however, considerable efforts have been made to discover other genetic factors responsible for autoimmune endocrinopathies (Vaidya & Pearce, 2004). There are several studies confirming that genetic polymorphism of the cytotoxic T lymphocyte antigen (CTLA)-4 alleles on 2q33 chromosome have been associated with HT (Awata et al., 1998; Donner et al., 1997; Nithiyananthan et al., 2002; Tomoyose et al., 2002). CTLA-4 is a co-stimulatory molecule expressed on the surface of activated T cells (Brunet et al., 1987). CTLA-4 (49) A/G allele was significantly more frequent in the group of HT patients compared to the healthy controls. Additionally, linkage and association of CTLA-4 with the presence of thyroid antibodies have also been reported (Tomer et al., 2001; Zaletel et al., 2002).

3.2 Autoimmune mechanisms

The thyroid is a major target for autoimmune disease, as exemplified by autoimmune thyroiditis (which include HT type 1 and 2, and atrophic thyroiditis), and GD with opposite clinical outcomes. Both diseases, but particularly HT, are characterized by lymphocytic infiltration of the gland which can result in tissue destruction, fibrosis and hypothyroidism. The follicular spaces shrink and colloid is absent or sparse. Fibrosis may be completely absent or present in degrees ranging from slight to moderate. Heuer and coll. (Bernet et al., 1996; Heuer et al., 1996) found increased expression of IFN-gamma, IL-2 and CD25 positive T cells in the thyroid specimens of patients with HT.

Although the two disorders, HT and GD, have striking differences in clinical symptoms, they share the same histopathological features: lymphocytic infiltration and aberrant expression of HLA class II molecules on thyrocytes (Bernet et al., 1996). It is possible that HT and GD are caused by a similar immunologic dysfunction because similar autoantibodies (Abs) have been found in these patients.

The cause of the autoimmune process is probably a combination of an inherited tendency and an as yet unknown trigger (American Thyroid Association, 2008). Previous studies have shown that HLA class II–expressing thyrocytes could stimulate the proliferation of autologous T cells grown from thyroid glands during autoimmune diseases (Dayan et al., 1991; Londei et al., 1984; Weetman et al., 1986). Local up-regulation of the antigen-presenting function on thyrocytes may be an early event in the development of AITD (Dayan et al., 1991). Autoantigen presentation by thyrocytes is more efficient than by professional antigen-presenting cells (APC), because the thyroid autoantigens thyroid peroxidase and thyrotropin (TSH) receptor are membrane proteins. These proteins can be recycled and presented by class II molecules, and the effective concentration of these antigens on thyroid epithelial cells may be higher than when picked up by other antigen-presenting cells (Feldmann et al., 1992). However, lack of expression of costimulators such as B7.1 (CD80) or B7.2 (CD86) by thyrocytes undermines their ability to present antigens. Instead, class II–expressing thyrocytes may induce tolerance in autoreactive CD4+T cells (Matsuoka et al., 1996).

On the other hand, increased expression of intercellular adhesion molecule-1 (ICAM-1) has been shown present in specimens from patients with HT, while expression was less or absent in GD (Bagnasco et al., 1991; Ciampolillo et al., 1993; Pesce et al., 2002; Weetman et al., 1990). ICAM-1 is a member of the Ig gene superfamily and present on the surface of various cell types, serves as a ligand for lymphocyte function associated antigen-1 (LFA-1), and can be induced by various stimuli, such as cytokines (IL-1, tumor necrosis factor [TNF]-alpha, interferon [IFN]-gamma), hormones, cellular stresses (H2O2), and other environmental factors (Roebuck & Finnegan, 1999). Upon up-regulation it promotes cell–cell interactions, providing intense signals to the immune system that cause the T cells to home in on the inflamed site (Bonita et al., 2002).

An earlier investigation had found that elevated (rather than reduced) plasma levels of soluble CTLA-4 (sCTLA-4) protein were more frequent in patients with AITD than in healthy controls (Oaks & Hallett, 2000). CTLA-4 molecule, together with CD28 co-stimulatory molecule (both expressed on the T cell surface), plays a critical role in the T cell response to antigen presentation. For T cell activation two signals are needed: TCR engages antigen (the first signal), which is bound to a HLA class II molecule on the surface of an APC, and a co-stimulatory signal, that could be stimulatory or inhibitory. This stimulatory second signal is provided mainly by the interaction of CD28 with its ligands, B7.1 (CD80) and B7.2 (CD86) on APC. CTLA-4 also binds to the same B7 ligands (CD80 and CD86) but it delivers inhibitory signals to T-cell activation (Walunas et al., 1994). In the absence of a stimulatory second signal, the antigen–TCR engagement is ineffective, and causes functional inactivation of the T cell (anergy) or induces apoptosis of the cell (Alegre et al., 2001).

Soluble CTLA4 molecules (sCTLA4), more frequently found in AITD patients, could compete with membrane-bound CTLA-4 for CD80 / CD86-binding sites and cause a reduction of inhibitory signaling (Vaida & Pearce, 2004). Thus, autoreactive T cells will become activated leading to autoimmune process. The altered levels of sCTLA-4 could lead to either blockade of available B7 ligands, leading to a decreased stimulatory signal (if sCTLA-4 is increased), or to an inability of membranous CTLA-4 to bind the B7 ligand, leading to subsequently less inhibitory signal (if sCTLA-4 is decreased).

3.3 The possible role of iodide excess on thyroid mild inflammation and the development of hypothyroidism

Many epidemiological studies have demonstrated the toxic effects of iodide excess on thyroid function. In one study, about 10% of European patients receiving 0.5 mg of iodide per day for 6 months developed lymphocytic infiltration of the thyroid gland, accompanied by hypothyroidism or less often hyperthyroidism. Both the infiltration and the hypofunction were reversible upon discontinuation of iodide (Kahaly et al., 1998). The thyroid response to excess iodide is known as thyroid autoregulation. Most commonly, studies that examined the effects of toxic doses of iodide were usually performed in Fisher's rat thyroid low-serum-5 (FRTL-5) cells, which can synthesize and secrete thyroglobulin (Tg), absorb and transport iodide, and produce thyroid peroxidase (Ambesi-Impiombato et al., 1980). Although iodide doses over 10 mM caused toxic effects on the thyroid gland in vivo (Li & Boyages, 1994), higher concentrations of iodide were needed in order to influence cell proliferation (Becks et al., 1987; Eng et al., 2001; Smerdely et al., 1993) or even to induce apoptosis (Smerdely et al., 1993; Vitale et al., 2000) in cell culture.

Possible sources of excess iodide for humans are: amiodarone, povidone-iodine, iodinated radiographic contrast media, Lugol's 5% solution (used as 0,1-0,3ml for the treatment of simple goiter, equivalent of 12,5-37,5 mg of iodine) (Gennaro, 1995), dry or powdered algae (in many vitamin-mineral supplements and preparations for weight-loosing programs and herbal products).

The U.S. recommended daily intake (RDI) for dietary iodine is 150 mcg for adults, 220 mcg for pregnant women, and 270 mcg during lactation (Surks et al., 2004). The safe upper limit has been set at 1,000 mcg (1 mg) as a result of studies assessing TSH levels with supplementation. Iodine intake over 1 mg daily could potentially contribute to an underlying thyroid pathology-AITD, or even could exacerbate nodularities in euthyroid individuals in those taking over 20 mg of iodide (Burgi et al., 2001; Dunn et al., 1998; Robison et al., 1998). Population studies have shown that an excess of iodine intake may increase the prevalence of autoimmune thyroiditis (HT and atrophic thyroiditis) in animals and humans, increasing the risk of clinically evident hypothyroidism (Teng et al., 2006).

Iodide excess could influence thyroid cell growth and immunological profile. It is known that Lugol's solution given a couple of days before surgery in GD patients reduced HLA class I and II mRNA expression in thyroid cells in vivo and in vitro (Schuppert et al., 1996). It has also been reported that ICAM-1 mRNA was doubled in suspensions of isolated human thyroid follicles incubated with 10 mM sodium iodide (NaI) (Yamazaki et al., 2003). Furthermore, iodide excess did not change Tg level in FRTL-5 cells (Pregliasco et al., 1996), but it inhibited iodine organification (Davies et al., 1989), thyroid hormone secretion (Sato et al., 1990), and cAMP production and secretion (Miyazaki et al., 1999) in isolated human thyroid follicles. Recently, it was reported (Kostic et al., 2009) that iodide excess inhibited human primary thyroid cell proliferation and gradually increased ICAM-1 on cell surface. In the presence of low-dose IFN-gamma, KI additionally augmented ICAM-1 expression, and such effect could induce lymphocytic infiltration in the thyroid gland and secretion of proinflammatory cytokines. Decreased Tg production in the presence of KI excess and IFN-gamma could explain the development of hypothyroidism after iodide dietary addition in patients that already have lymphocytic infiltration and/or mild inflammation in the thyroid gland.

Among the subjects exposed to iodine supplementation for the prevention of iodine deficiency or fed diet with high iodine intake, besides a few cases of focal and reversible lymphocyte infiltration of the thyroid, severe cases of hypothyroidism, not reversed by the suspension of iodine administration, with severe lymphocyte infiltration and parenchymal destruction have been described.

Various animal strains genetically susceptible to autoimmune thyroiditis have been described, such as Cornell and obese strain (OS) chickens, BB/Worcester and Buffalo rats, and diabetic non-obese mice NOD.H-2h4.

NOD mice expressing the H-2Jg7 allele of MHC class II, are genetically predisposed to develop type I diabetes and other autoimmune diseases, such as spontaneous autoimmune thyroiditis, which appears with low incidence. On the contrary, transgenic mice NOD.H-2h4, expressing the H-2Ak allele on the NOD background, do not develop diabetes but develop, with higher frequency, a spontaneous autoimmune thyroiditis (SAT). Moreover, as in BB/Worcester rats, SAT is increased by the addition of iodide in the drinking water. In these animals, deletion of IFN-gamma is associated with a strong reduction of anti-TG antibodies and of thyroid infiltration with B, T and plasma cells.

High iodide doses transiently inhibit Tg iodination by thyroperoxidase (TPO) (Wolff-Chaikoff effect). This is because, at high iodide to Tg ratios (mM to microM), iodide peroxidation to molecular iodine (I2) by TPO prevails over iodination of tyrosyl residues of Tg (Km 6 x 10-3M and 8 x 10-5, respectively). The iodination of tyrosyl residues leads to the production of one mole of OH- ions per mole of tyrosyl residue formed, whereas the peroxidation of iodide to I2 leads to the formation of two moles of OH- ions per mole of I2 produced. Hydrogen peroxide (H2O2), produced by the NADPH-oxidase of the apical membrane of thyroid epithelial cells (TECs), is the limiting electron acceptor in the TPO-catalized reactions. Its production leads to the production of superoxide anion (O2-) as an intermediate. Excess I- ions inhibit both the enzymatic degradation of H2O2 by TPO and non enzymatic oxidation of H2O2 by I2.

However, in dog thyroid slices, iodide excess seems to inhibit H2O2 generation, through the formation of oxidized iodine compounds. Thus, excess iodide inhibits thyroid functions by multiple mechanisms, which include, besides true anion effects, the oxidative modification and/or iodination of important enzymes, the inhibitory effect of the products of the iodination or peroxidation of polyunsaturated fatty acid, which, in turn, can act as free radicals. An imbalanced production of free radicals and/or dysfunctions of enzymes involved in their detoxication, such as glutathione peroxidase, catalase and superoxide dismutase, have been associated with aging, neurodegenerative diseases, cancer and autoimmune diseases.

At persistingly high doses, iodide can determine thyroid involution. Preliminary studies showed the accumulation of lipid peroxidation products, with necrosis and inflammation of murine and human thyroid exposed to toxic iodide doses (23, 24). More recently, it has been demonstrated that thyroid cell apoptosis is the prevalent cause of TEC death in thyroid iodide-dependent involution in goitrogen-treated rats. However, TEC necrosis induced by iodide excess has been indicated as a preliminary step in a model of the development of autoimmune thyroiditis.

Iodide excess induces apoptosis in thyroid cultured cells, through a p53-independent oxidative mechanism. Diminished levels of bcl-2 gene expression and increased levels of bax gene expression have been found in the brain and the thyroid of guinea-pigs exposed to excess iodide. In OS chickens, the TEC damage, preceding the development of autoimmune thyroiditis, is mediated by the production of ROS. H2O2 induces apoptosis in cultured pig thyroid cells.

Cellular products of thyroid iodinated lipids include arachidonic acid derivatives, such as 6-iodo-5-hydroxy-8,11,14-eicosatrienoic acid and 14-iodo-15-hydroxy-5,8,11 eicosatrienoic acid (I-OH-A), and their respective delta and omega iodolactones (IL-d and IL-ω). IL-ω inhibits iodide organification in dog thyroid slices, by inhibiting H2O2 production (31). IL-ω and IL-d inhibit the proliferation of rat FRTL-5 cultured thyroid cells and cause the involution of thyroid in goitrogen-treated rats. IL-d inhibits inositol-3-phosphate production and EGF and beta FGF signal transduction in human and pig thyroid cells. 2-iodoesadecanal (2-IHDA), produced from the rat thyroid exposed to iodide, inhibits adenylate cyclase activity and cAMP-stimulated activities of NADPH oxidase and TPO. The non-iodinated products derived from arachidonic acid oxidation induce apoptosis in smooth muscle vessel cells. 4-Hydroxynonenal, the most important product of arachidonic acid oxidation, induces apoptosis in a number of cell types, including endotelial cells. As with iodide in the thyroid, it can do so through a p53-idependent mechanism

The current vision of the pathogenesis of autoimmunity favors the triggering role of the exposure of cryptic self epitopes. It has been demonstrated that a hormonogenic carboxy-terminal fragment of Tg , beginning at residue 2384, was released during enzymatic iodination or metal-catalyzed oxidation of Tg in vitro, as well as during oxidative stress in vivo. Because it was recognized by autoantibodies of patients affected with autoimmune thyroid disease (AITD), it was suggested that oxidative proteolysis can expose immunopathogenetic cryptic epitopes.

In vitro iodination of murine Tg , used to immunize susceptible rats, determined the transformation of a T-cell epitope (residues 2495-2511) from cryptic to immunodominant in vivo. It is well known that the iodination of Tg with TPO in vitro is accompanied by the formation of proteolytic peptides, whose amount is related to their iodine and hormone content.

Thyroid autoantigens could be also transferred to thyroidal dendritic cells (DC) and cross-presented to T lymphocytes. Apoptosis of TECs, induced by iodide excess, could play a pivotal role in this process. Apoptotic cells are a preferred source of antigens for cross-presentation, being captured by DCs via alpha(v)-beta5 or alpha(v)-beta 5 integrins and CD36. Although DC can cross-present both apoptotic and necrotic cells, MHC class II-restricted presentation can occur with both of them, while MHC class I-restricted presentation can only occur with apoptotic cells. Moreover, even if immature DCs phagocytose efficiently both apoptotic and necrotic cells, the exposition to the latter is necessary in order to induce their maturation to APC, with optimal abilities of antigen processing and presentation and elevate levels of CD38, DC-LAMP, and CD40 and CD86 co-stimulatory molecules. Moreover, DC can cross-activate CTL by the internalization of heat shock proteins gp96 and Hsp70 loaded with antigenic peptides. Finally, the processing and the class II-restricted presentation are increased by receptor-mediated internalization of mannosylated antigens, such as Tg.

3.4 Other cell stressors that could induce hypothyroidism

It has been shown that human primary thyroid cells increase HLA-DR surface expression in response to a variety of cell stressors, such as IFN-gamma (Montani et al., 1998; Otten et al., 1998; Wu et al., 1999) and ionizing radiations (Czirjak et al., 1990) or transiently modify HLA-DR expression in vitro in the presence of iodide excess (Kostic et al., 2009). Recently, Kostic et al. (Kostic et al., 2010) showed that HLA-DR expression was also transiently increased 24 hours after UVC treatment of human primary thyroid cells in vitro, and subsequently returned to normal level 48 h after irradiation. This local up-regulation of antigen presenting function on thyrocytes in vivo could be sustained by a local inflammatory network (formed by cytokines and other cells of the immune system) and it may be an early event in the development of AITD (Botazzo et al., 1983; Liu et al., 2008).

Another consequence of UVC as physical mutagen is a cell cycle arrest or apoptosis induction in human primary thyroid cells. As already mentioned, the local up-regulation of HLA-DR by thyrocytes together with the expression of proteins from apoptotic cells may represent an early event in the development of AITD (Botazzo et al., 1983).

The model for the cellular response of human thyroid cells after UVC irradiation (Kostic et al., 2010) suggested that UV induced dimers lead to activation of p53 that is in turn able to induce G0 / G1 cell cycle arrest in order to repair DNA damage. Cells that are able to repair damaged DNA or that do not have a large DNA damage enter S phase of the cell cycle, but secondary lesions generated during replication, induce apoptosis. The cells that are severely damaged after UVC irradiation, diminish Bcl-2 expression in the mitochondria and start apoptosis.

It has also been shown that in microgravity conditions the thyroid cells FRTL5 in culture do not respond to TSH treatment and present an irregular shape with condensed chromatin, a modification of the cell membrane with shedding of the TSH-receptor in the culture medium, and an increase of sphingomyelin-synthase and bax proteins. It is possible that microgravity induces a rearrangement of specific sections of the cell membrane, which act as platforms for molecular receptors, thus influencing thyroid cell function in astronauts during space missions.

It has been recently reported that FTRL-5 cells cultured in the presence or absence of TSH in the International Space Mission during the Eneide and Experia missions presented a similar cell growth pattern, which indicates an absence of response to TSH in space (Albi et al., 2010). It is difficult to establish whether this modification that occurs in space is due to cosmic radiation or microgravity.

It was previously reported that simulated weightlessness changed the cytoskeleton of normal thyroid cells (Infanger et al., 2004), increased the extracellular matrix proteins (Infanger et al., 2006), reduced thyroglobulin, FT3 and FT4 secretion, (Grimm et al., 2002), and induced apoptosis (Kossmehl et al., 2002, Grimm et al., 2002) of thyroid carcinoma cells. These data were supported by exposing mitochondria-rich thyroid carcinoma cells and normal thyroid cells to simulated microgravity conditions and obtaining apoptotic cells (Kossmehl et al., 2003). We reported for the first time the modifications of thyroid cells under real microgravity conditions.

We have shown that, in microgravity, the FRTL5 cells appeared aggregated and presented chromatin condensation, the TSH-induced cAMP production was significantly attenuated, and the TSHR was increased about 4.4 fold in the culture medium. At Earth's gravity, the TSHR was unaltered, and the cells responded to TSH treatment with normally high levels of cAMP production (Albi et al., 2011).

It is possible that the loss of TSHR from the cells in microgravity was due to the disorganization of microdomains within the cell membrane, depending on Sphingomyelin and Cholesterol incorporation from the culture medium that yielded a more rigid membrane structure. These data were consistent with the observation that a medium lacking TSH caused cessation of FRTL-5 cell proliferation due to the decrease in membrane lipid fluidity, which in turn was caused by an absolute increase of membrane cholesterol.

It has been shown that microgravity induced the FRTL5 cells treated with TSH to release Cholesterol and Sphingomyelin to the culture medium probably by modifying the microdomain structure (Albi et al., 2011). The lower amount of TSHR in the culture medium after TSH stimulation with respect to the TSH- samples may have been due to the fact that raft-TSHR complexes are regulated by TSH, which stimulates the formation of monomers and allows their rapid exit from the rafts (Latif et al., 2003). Therefore, the modification of lipid rafts consequent to the removal of Cholesterol and Sphingomyelin may have been preceded by a transfer of the receptor, which would explain the reduction but not the absence of the cAMP response. The disorganization of microdomains in microgravity was confirmed by the presence of caveolin 1 in the pellet obtained after fixation, which was absent in the samples maintained in Earth's gravity.

4. Types of AITD

The types of AITD may be summarised as follows:

- Type 1 (Thyroiditis chronica Hashimoto type 1):
    - euthyroidism with anti-TPO Abs and
        - 1A: with goiter;
        - 1B: without goiter
- Type 2 (Thyroiditis chronica Hashimoto type 2):
    - hypothyroidism with anti-TPO Abs and
        - 2A with goiter; 2B without goiter;
        - 2C transitory forms (postpartal hypothyroidism, Hashitoxicosis)
- Type 3 (Morbus Graves):
    - 3A hyperthyroidism with

  - stimulating anti-TSH R Abs;
  - anti-TPO Abs and anti-Tg Abs +/-
- 3B Euthyroidism with supressed TSH and anti-TSH R Abs
- 3C Hypothyroidism. Orbitopathy and anti-TPO Abs +/-

The Abs present in the sera of patients with AITD are only the witnesses of autoimmune destruction or activation of thyroid gland.

The most frequent in HT are Abs against thyroperoxidase (anti-TPO), Abs associated with euthyroidism (HT type 1) or hypothyroidism (HT type 2) and accompanied or not by goiter. On the other hand, in GD (AITD type 3) Abs against Tg (anti-Tg Abs) in AITD type 3A, and stimulating or inhibiting Abs against TSH receptor (anti-TSHR Abs) may also be found.

According to the prevalence of stimulating or blocking anti-TSHR Abs, GD patients could develop hyperthyroidism (stimulating anti-TSHR Abs), hypothyroidism (inhibiting anti-TSHR Abs) or be euthyroid (GD type 3B).

Of great interest is the relationship between Interferon and Autoimmune Thyroid Disease. Three different types of thyroid dysfunction associated with IFN treatment have been reported: (1) autoimmune (often subclinical) hypothyroidism; (2) destructive thyroiditis; and (3) Graves' hyperthyroidism.

These abnormalities can occur at any time during IFN therapy, from as early as 4 weeks until as late as 23 months after initiation, and there is no clear difference between the three types, with a median date of onset of 17 weeks after start of IFN treatment. Pooling of several studies shows that hypothyroidism seems to be more frequent than thyrotoxicosis.

The majority of patients with hypothyroidism also have TPO antibodies (87%), indicating the autoimmune nature of this event. According to most studies hypothyroidism can be transient, subsiding after discontinuation of IFN. In a large Italian survey, hypothyroidism was, however, permanent in 59% of the patients. A similar result was found in the review of the literature (Koh et al.), which showed that 56% of the patients had permanent hypothyroidism. In a recent long-term follow-up study, it was found (Carella et al.) that 10 of 36 (28%) TPO antibody-positive patients lost their antibodies at 6 years after discontinuation. On the other hand, 26 patients remained antibody-positive at that time, and subclinical hypothyroidism was detected in seven of them

5. Conclusion

Hypothyroidism is a common endocrine disorder resulting from deficiency of thyroid hormone. It usually is a primary process in which the thyroid gland produces insufficient amounts of thyroid hormone. It can also be secondary—that is, lack of thyroid hormone secretion due to inadequate secretion of either thyrotropin (ie, thyroid-stimulating hormone [TSH]) from the pituitary gland or thyrotropin-releasing hormone (TRH) from the hypothalamus (secondary or tertiary hypothyroidism). The patient's presentation may vary from asymptomatic to, rarely, coma with multisystem organ failure (myxedema coma).

Localized disease of the thyroid gland that results in decreased thyroid hormone production is the most common cause of hypothyroidism.

The most common cause of hypothyroidism in adults is autoimmune thyroid disease (AITD. The second frequent cause is a thyroid ablation as a consequence of surgical removal of part or all of the gland. Third most common are all causes of congenital hypothyroidism (in newborns). There are also a few forms of infective processes in thyroid.

In some cases, medicines could be the cause of hypothyroidism, usually by interfering with normal thyroid hormone synthesis.

Because all metabolically active cells require thyroid hormone, deficiency of the hormone has a wide range of effects. Systemic effects are due to either derangements in metabolic processes or direct effects by myxedematous infiltration (ie, accumulation of glucosaminoglycans in the tissues).

The myxedematous changes in the heart result in decreased contractility, cardiac enlargement, pericardial effusion, decreased pulse, and decreased cardiac output. In the GI tract, achlorhydria and decreased intestinal transit with gastric stasis can occur. Delayed puberty, anovulation, menstrual irregularities, and infertility are common. Decreased thyroid hormone effect can cause increased levels of total cholesterol and low-density lipoprotein (LDL) cholesterol and a possible change in high-density lipoprotein (HDL) cholesterol due to a change in metabolic clearance. In addition, hypothyroidism may result in an increase in insulin resistance.

6. Acknowledgment

We are very grateful to Drs. Massimo Moretti Ph.D., Federico Ferro Ph.D., and Renza Spelat MS. This work was partially supported by a grant from the Agenzia Spaziale Italiana MoMa project

7. References

Albi E., Ambesi-Impiombato F.S., Villani M., De Pol I., Spelat R., Lazzarini R. & Perrella, G. (2010) Thyroid cell growth: sphingomyelin metabolism as non-invasive biomarker for cell damage acquired during space flight. *Astrobiol.* Vol.10, N.8, pp. 811-20.

Albi E., Ambesi-Impiombato F.S., Peverini M., Damaskopoulou E., Fontsanini E., Lazzarini R., Curcio F. & Perrella G. (2011) Thyrotropin receptor/membrane interactions in FRTL-5 thyroid cell strain in microgravity. *Astrobiol.* Vol. 11, N.1, pp. 57-64

Alegre M.L., Frauwirth K.A. & Thompson C.B. (2001). T-cell regulation by CD28 and CTLA-4. *Nature Reviews Immunology.* Vol.1, pp. 220-228.

Ambesi-Impiombato F.S., Parks L.A.M. & Coon H.G. (1980) Culture of hormone-dependent functional epithelial cells from rat thyroids. *Proc Natl Acad Sci U S A.* Vol.77, pp. 3455–3459.

American Thyroid Association: Hypothyroidism brochure. (2008) Available from http://www.thyroid.org/patients/patient_brochures/hypothyroidism.html#causes.

Awata T., Kurihara S., Iitaka M., Takei S., Inoue I., Ishii C. et al. (1998). Association of CTLA-4 gene A-G polymorphism (IDDM12 locus) with acute-onset and insulin-depleted IDDM as well as autoimmune thyroid disease (Graves' disease and Hashimoto's thyroiditis) in the Japanese population. *Diabetes.* Vol.47, pp. 128–129.

Bagnasco M., Caretto A., Olive D., Pedini B., Canonica G.W. & Betterle C. (1991). Expression of ICAM-1 on thyroid epithelial cells in Hashimoto's thyroiditis but not in Graves' disease or papillary thyroid cancer. *Clin Exp Immuno*. Vol.l, N.83, pp. 309–313.

Becks G.P., Eggo M.C. & Burrow G.N. (1987). Regulation of differentiated thyroid function by iodide: preferential inhibitory effect of excess iodide on thyroid hormone secretion in sheep thyroid cell cultures. *Endocrinology*. Vol.120, pp. 2569–2575.

Bernet V. & Burman K. Autoimmune thyroid disease. (1996) In: Rich R.R., Fleisher T.A., Schwartz B.D., Shearer W.T. & Strober W, eds. Clinical immunology: principles and practice. St Louis, MO: Mosby. pp. 1482-6

Bharaktiya S. (2011). In: Griffing GT, ed. Hypothyroidism. Available form http://emedicine.medscape.com/article/122393-overview

Bonita R.E., Rose N.R., Rasooly L., Caturegli P. & Burek C.L. (2002) Adhesion molecules as susceptibility factors in spontaneous autoimmune thyroiditis in the NOD-H2h4 mouse. *Exp Mol Pathol*. Vol.73, pp. 155–163.

Botazzo G.F. , Pujol-Borrell R. , Hanafusa T. & Feldmann M. (1983) Role of aberrant HLA-DR expression and antigen presentation in induction of endocrine autoimmunity. *Lancet*. Vol.2, N.8359, pp. 1115–1119.

Brunet J.F., Denizot F., Luciani M.F., Roux-Dosseto M., Suzan M., Mattei M.G. et al. (1987) A new member of the immunoglobulin superfamily - CTLA-4. *Nature*. Vol.328, pp. 267–270.

Burgi H., Schaffner T.H. & Seiler J.P. (2001) The toxicology of iodate: a review of the literature. *Thyroid*. Vol.11, pp. 449-456.

Canaris G.J., Manowitz N.R., Mayor G. & Ridgway E.C. (2000) The Colorado thyroid disease prevalence study. *Arch Intern Med*. Vol.160, N.4, pp. 526-534.

Carella C., Mazziotti G., Morisco F., Manganella G., Rotondi M., Tuccillo C., Sorvillo F., Caporaso N. & Amato G. (2001) Longterm outcome of interferon-induced thyroid autoimmunity and prognostic influence of thyroid autoantibody pattern at the end of treatment. *J Clin Endocrinol Metab*. Vol.86, pp. 1925-1929.

Ciampolillo A., Napolitano G., Mirakian R., Miyasaki A., Giorgino R. & Botazzo G.F. (1993) ICAM-1 in Graves' disease: contrast between in vivo and in vitro results. *Clin Exp Immunol*. Vol.94, pp. 478–485

Czirjak L., Danko K., Gaulton G.N. & Stadecker M.J. (1990) Thyroid-derived epithelial cells acquire alloantigen-presenting capabilities following X-irradiation and class II antigen induction . *Eur J Immunol*. Vol.20, pp. 2597–2601.

Danese M.D., Powe N.R., Sawin C.T. & Ladenson P.W. (1996) Screening for mild thyroid failure at the periodic health examination: a decision and cost-effectiveness analysis. *JAMA*. Vol.276, N.4, pp. 285-292.

Davies T.F., Yang C. & Platzer M. (1989) The influence of antithyroid drugs and iodine on thyroid cell MHC class II antigen expression. *Clin Endocrinol*. Vol.31, pp. 125–135.

Dayan C.M., Londei M., Corcoran A.E., Grubeck-Loebenstein B., James R.F., Rapoport B. & Feldman M. (1991) Autoantigen recognition by thyroid-infiltrating T cells in Graves' disease. *Proc Natl Acad Sci USA*. Vol.88, pp. 7415–7419.

Donner H., Braun J., Seidl C., Rau H., Finke R., Ventz M. et al. (1997) Codon 17 polymorphism of the cytotoxic T lymphocyte antigen 4 gene in Hashimoto's thyroiditis and Addison's disease. *Journal of Clinical Endocrinology and Metabolism*. Vol.82, pp. 4130–4132.

Dunn J.T. (1996) Seven deadly sins in confronting endemic iodine deficiency, and how to avoid them. *J Clin Endocrinol Metab.* Vol.81, pp. 1332-1335.

Dunn J.T., Semigran M.J. & Delange F. (1998) The prevention and management of iodine-induced hyperthyroidism and its cardiac features. Thyroid. Vol.8, pp. 101-106.

Eng P.H., Cardona G.R., Previti M.C., Chin W.W. & Braverman L.E. (2001) Regulation of the NIS by iodide in FRTL-5 cells. *Eur J Endocrinol.* Vol.144, pp. 139–144.

Feldmann M., Dayan C., Rapoport B. & Londei M. (1992) T cell activation and antigen presentation in human thyroid autoimmunity. J Autoimmun. Vol.5, pp. 115–121.

Gennaro A.S. Remington: The Science and Practice of Pharmacy. (1995) 19th ed. Easton, PA: Mack Pub Co.

Grimm D., Bauer J., Kossmehl P., Shakibaei M., Schöberger J., Pickenhahn H., Schulze-Tanzil G., Vetter R., Eilles C., Paul M. & Cogoli, A. (2002) Simulated microgravity alters differentiation and increases apoptosis in human follicular thyroid carcinoma cells. *FASEB J.* Vol.16, pp. 604-606.

Heuer M, Aust G, Ode-Hakim S, Scherbaum WA. (1996) Different cytokine mRNA profiles in Graves' disease, Hashimoto's thyroiditis, and nonautoimmune thyroid disorders determined by quantitative reverse transcriptase polymerase chain reaction (RT-PCR). *Thyroid.* Vol.6, pp. 97-106

Infanger M., Kossmehl P., Shakibaei M., Schulze-Tanzil G., Cogoli A., Faramarzi S., Bauer J., Curcio F., Paul, M. & Grimm D. (2004) Long term conditions of mimicked weightlessness influences the cytoskeleton in thyroid cells. *J. Gravit. Physiol.* Vol.11, pp. 169-172.

Infanger M., Kossmehl P., Shakibaei M., Bauer J., Kossmehl-Zorn S., Cogoli A., Curcio F., Oksche A., Wehland M., Kreutz R., Paul M. & Grimm D. (2006) Simulated weightlessness changes the cytoskeleton and extracellular matrix proteins in papillary thyroid carcinoma cells. *Cell Tissue Res.* Vol.324, pp. 267-277.

Kahaly G.J., Dienes H.P., Beyer J. & Hommel G. (1998) Iodide induces thyroid autoimmunity in patients with endemic goitre: a randomised, double-blind, placebo-controlled trial. *Eur J Endocrinol.* Vol.139, pp. 290–297.

Koh L.K.H., Greenspan F.S. & Yeo P.P.B. (1997) Interferon-induced thyroid dysfunction: three clinical presentations and a review of the literature. *Thyroid.* Vol.7, pp. 891-896.

Kossmehl P., Shakibaei M., Cogoli A., Pickenhahn H., Paul M. & Grimm, D. (2002) Simulated microgravity induces programmed cell death in human thyroid carcinoma cells. *J. Gravit. Physiol.* Vol.9, pp. 295-296.

Kossmehl P., Shakibaei M., Cogoli A., Infanger M., Curcio F., Schönberger J., Eilles C., Bauer J., Pickenhahn H., Schulze-Tanzil G., Paul M. & Grimm, D. (2003) Weightlessness induced apoptosis in normal thyroid cells and papillary thyroid carcinoma cells via extrinsic and intrinsic pathways. *Endocrinology.* Vol.144, pp. 4172-4179.

Kostic I., Toffoletto B., Fontanini E., Moretti M., Cesselli D., Beltrami C.A., Ambesi Impiombato F.S. & Curcio F. (2009) Influence of iodide excess and interferon-gamma on human primary thyroid cell proliferation, thyroglobulin secretion, and intracellular adhesion molecule-1 and human leukocyte antigen-DR expression. Thyroid. Vol.19, N.3, pp. 283-291

Kostic I., Toffoletto B., Toller M., Beltrami C.A., Ambesi-Impiombato F.S. & Curcio F. (2010)UVC radiation-induced effect on human primary thyroid cell proliferation and HLA-DR expression. *Horm Metab Res.* Vol.42, N.12, pp. 846-53.

LaFranchi S. (1999) Congenital hypothyroidism: etiologies, diagnosis, and management. *Thyroid.* Vol.9., N.7, pp. 735-40.

Li M. & Boyages S.C. (1994) Iodide induced lymphocytic thyroiditis in the BB/W rat: evidence of direct toxic effects of iodide on thyroid subcellular structure. *Autoimmunity.* Vol.18, pp. 31–40.

Liu C., Papewalis C., Domberg J., Scherbaum W.A. & Schott M. (2008) Chemokines and autoimmune thyroid diseases. *Horm Metab Res.* Vol.40, pp. 361–368.

Londei M., Lamb J.R., Bottazzo G.F. & Feldmann M. (1984) Epithelial cells expressing aberrant MHC class II determinants can present antigen to cloned human T cells. *Nature.* Vol.312, pp. 639–641.

Mathur R. In: Shiel WC, ed. What causes hypothyroidism. (2011). Available from http://www.medicinenet.com/hypothyroidism/article.htm

Matsuoka N., Eguchi K., Kawakami A., Tsuboi M., Nakamura H., Kimura H., Ishikawa N., Ito K. & Nagataki S. (1996) Lack of B7.1/B80 and B7.2/B86 expression on thyrocytes of patients with Graves' disease. Delivery of costimulatory signals from bystander professional antigen-presenting cells. *J Clin Endocrinol Metab.* Vol.81, pp. 4137–4143.

McPhee S. & Bauer D.C. (1997) Pathology of disease. New York, Lange Medical Books/McGraw-Hill,

Miyazaki A., Shimura H., Endo T., Haraguchi K. & Onaya T. (1999) Tumor necrosis factor-a and interferon-g suppress both gene expression and deoxyribonucleic acid-binding of TTF-2 in FRTL-5 cells. *Endocrinology.* Vol.140, pp. 4214–4220.

Montani V., Taniguchi S.I., Shong M., Suzuki K., Ohmori M., Giuliani C., Napolitano G., Saji M., Fiorentino B., Reimold A.M., Ting J.P., Kohn L.D. & Singer D.S. (1998) Major histocompatibility class II HLA DR gene expression in thyrocytes: counter regulation by the class II transactivator and the thyroid Y box protein. *Endocrinology.* Vol.139, pp. 280 – 289

Nithiyananthan R., Heward J.M., Allahabadia A., Franklyn J.A. & Gough S.C. (2002) Polymorphism of the CTLA-4 gene is associated with autoimmune hypothyroidism in the United Kingdom. *Thyroid.* Vol.12, pp. 3–6.

Oaks M.K. & Hallett K.M. (2000) A soluble form of CTLA-4 in patients with autoimmune thyroid disease. *Journal of Immunology.* Vol.164, pp. 5015–5018

Otten L.A., Steimle V., Bontron S. & Mach B. (1998) Quantitative control of MHC class II expression by the transactivator CIITA . Eur J Immunol;28: 473 – 478

Pesce G., Fiorino N., Riccio A.M., Montagna P., Torre G., Salmaso C., Altrinetti V. & Bagnasco M. (2002) Different intrathyroid expression of intercellular adhesion molecule-1 in Hashimoto's thyroiditis and Graves' disease: analysis at mRNA level and association with B7.1 costimulatory molecule. *J Endocrinol Invest.* Vol.25, pp. 289–295.

Pregliasco L., Bocanera L., Krawiec L., Silberscmidt D., Pisarev M. & Juvenal G. (1996) Effects of iodide on thyroglobulin biosynthesis in FRTL-5 cells. *Thyroid.* Vol.6, pp. 319–323.

Robison L.M., Sylvester P.W., Birkenfeld P., et al. (1998) Comparison of the effects of iodine and iodide on thyroid function in humans. *J Toxicol Environ Health A*. Vol.55, pp. 93-106.

Roebuck K.A. & Finnegan A. (1999) Regulation of ICAM 1 gene expression. J Leukoc Biol. Vol.66, pp. 876–888.

Sato K., Satoh T., Shizume K., Ozawa M., Han D.C., Imamura H., Tsushima T., Demura H., Kanaji Y. & Ito Y. (1990) Inhibition of 125I organification and thyroid hormone release by interleukin- 1, tumor necrosis factor-alpha, and interferon-gamma in human thyrocytes in suspension culture. *J Clin Endocrinol Metab*. Vol.70, pp. 1735–1743.

Schuppert F., Taniguchi S., Schroder S., Dralle H., von zur Muhlen A. & Kohn L.D. (1996) In vivo and in vitro evidence for iodide regulation of major histocompatibility complex class I and class II expression in Graves' disease. *J Clin Endocrinol Metab*. Vol.81, pp. 3622–3628.

Smerdely P., Pitsiavas V. & Boyages S.C. (1993) Evidence that the inhibitory effects of iodide on thyroid cell proliferation are due to arrest of the cell cycle at G0/G1 and G2/M phases. Endocrinology. Vol.133, pp. 2881–2888.

Surks M.I., Ortiz E., Daniels G.H., et al. (2004) Subclinical thyroid disease: scientific review and guidelines for diagnosis and management. *JAMA*. Vol.291, pp. 228-238.

Teng W., Shan Z., Teng X., et al. (2006) Effect of iodine intake on thyroid diseases in China. *N Engl J Med*. Vol.354, pp. 2783-2793.

Tomer Y., Greenberg D.A., Barbesino G., Concepcion E. & Davies T.F. (2001) CTLA-4 and not CD28 is a susceptibility gene for thyroid autoantibody production. *Journal of Clinical Endocrinology and Metabolism*. Vol.86, pp. 1687–1693.

Tomoyose T., Komiya I., Takara M., Yabiku K., Kinjo Y., Shimajiri Y. et al. (2002) Cytotoxic T-lymphocyte antigen-4 gene polymorphisms and human T-cell lymphotrophic virus-1 infection: their associations with Hashimoto's thyroiditis in Japanese patients. *Thyroid*. Vol.12:, pp. 673–677.

Vaidya B. & Pearce S. (2004) The emerging role of the CTLA-4 gene in autoimmune endocrinopathies. *Eur J Endocrinol*. Vol.150, pp. 619-626

Vanderpump M.P., Tunbridge W.M., French J.M., Appleton D., Bates D., Clark F., et al. (1995) The incidence of thyroid disorders in the community : a twenty-year follow-up of the Whickham survey. *Clin Endocrinol (Oxf)*. Vol.43, N.1, pp. 55-68

Vitale M., di Matola T., D'Ascoli F., Salzano S., Bogazzi F., Fenzi G., Martino E. & Rossi G. (2000) Iodide excess induces apoptosis in thyroid cells through a p53-independent mechanism involving oxidative stress. *Endocrinology*. Vol.141, pp. 598–605.

Walunas T.L., Lenschow D.J., Bakker C.Y., Linsley P.S., Freeman G.J., Green J.M. et al. (1994) CTLA-4 can function as a negative regulator of T cell activation. *Immunity*. Vol.1, pp. 405–413.

Weetman A.P., Volkman D.J., Burman K.D., Margolick J.B., Petrick P., Weintraub B.D. & Fauci A.S. (1986) The production and characterization of thyroid-derived T-cell lines in Graves' disease and Hashimoto's thyroiditis. *Clin Immunol Immunopathol*. Vol.39, pp. 139–150.

Weetman A.P., Freeman M., Borysiewicz L. & Makgoba M.W. (1990) Functional analysis of intercellular adhesion molecule-1 expressing human thyroid cells. *Eur J Immunol.* Vol.20, pp. 271–275.

WHO, UNICEF & ICCIDD. (2001) Assessment of the Iodine Deficiency Disorders and Monitoring their Elimination. WHO/NHD/01.1. Geneva, Switzerland: World Health Organization; pp. 1-107

Wolff J. (1998) Perchlorate and the thyroid gland. *Pharmacol Rev.* Vol.50, pp. 89-10

Wu Z., Biro P.A., Mirakian R., Hammond L., Curcio F. & Ambesi-Impiombato F.S. (1999) HLA-DMB expression by thyrocytes: indication of the antigen processing and possible presenting capability of thyroid cells. *Clin Exp Immunol.* Vol.116, p. 62–69

Yamazaki K., Yamada E., Kanaji Y., Yanagisawa T., Kato Y., Takano K., Obara T. & Sato K. (2003) Genes regulated by thyrotropin and iodide in cultured human thyroid follicles: analysis by cDNA microarray. *Thyroid.* Vol.13, pp. 149–158.

Zaletel K., Krhin B., Gaberscek S., Pirnat E. & Hojker S. (2002) The influence of the exon 1 polymorphism of the cytotoxic T lymphocyte antigen 4 gene on thyroid antibody production in patients with newly diagnosed Graves' disease. *Thyroid.* Vol.12, pp. 373–386

10

The Role of Real-Time Thyroid Ultrasonography in the Assessment and Management of Patients with Hashimoto's Thyroiditis

Jack R. Wall* and Bernard Champion
Department of Medicine, the University of Sydney, Nepean Hospital, Penrith, New South Wales, Australia

1. Introduction

The most common cause of hypothyroidism is the autoimmune disorder Hashimoto's thyroiditis, the stages of which can be accurately and objectively assessed by serial, real-time thyroid ultrasonography. Early stages of chronic thyroiditis include; increased vascularity and a patchy heterogeneous texture reflecting the inflammatory infiltrations, enlargement of the thyroid gland and sometimes associated lymphadenopathy. As the autoimmune destruction of the thyroid gland continues the normal thyroid texture progressively changes until the tissue is replaced by empty spaces, so called end-stage. We can follow the course of the thyroiditis, which typically proceeds over several years, correlating with clinical features, thyroid [thyroid peroxidase (TPO), thyroglobulin (Tg)] antibody titres and serum levels of thyroid stimulating hormone (TSH) and free thyroxin (T4). We can confirm change in thyroid status from Hashimoto's thyroiditis to Graves' disease when TSH-receptor antibodies are additionally produced, document remission in young patients with Hashimoto's thyroiditis and we can obtain diagnostic information in patients with the rare but serious Riedel's thyroiditis. In the hands of an experienced operator real-time thyroid ultrasonography can provide information about the underlying autoimmune process. For example, ultrasound abnormalities can be correlated with; the eye changes that are found in about 25% of patients (1), serum levels of calsequestrin and collagen XIII antibodies (2-5), serum levels of thyroid antibodies and other parameters of the autoimmune process including phenotypes and numbers of infiltrating T lymphocytes in the thyroid.

In this chapter, we will highlight the use of real-time ultrasound in the assessment of patients with Hashimoto's thyroiditis, not only for clinical purposes but also to provide information about the pathogenesis of Hashimoto's thyroiditis and its variants such as silent and post partum thyroiditis and Riedel's thyroiditis.

---

* Corresponding Author

2. Serial studies in Hashimoto's thyroiditis

In the hands of a single operator using standard criteria for assessing the ultrasound changes of Hashimoto's thyroiditis, real-time thyroid ultrasonography is a valuable new tool for diagnostic and management purposes. Images can be stored and changes compared serially in individual patients and correlated with immune parameters in cohorts of patients in research studies. Fine needle aspiration (FNA) biopsy can characterise any nodules and features of the Hashimoto's thyroiditis process itself, such as numbers of lymphocytes and other mononuclear cells and overall architectural changes. Typically, the most classical appearance in early thyroiditis is the formation of small cystic areas throughout the gland which reflect the lymphoid infiltrations (fig 1) which progresses to a stage of multi-cystic disease (fig. 2). Later, there is increased destruction of the thyroid follicles, scarring and pseudo nodule formation (fig. 3) and the gland becomes shrunken and avascular (fig 4). Finally, in long standing cases, there may be tissue calcification (fig. 4). The full process takes from many months to 2-3 yr although this needs to be shown in a long term prospective study of patients who were diagnosed early, i.e. with no symptoms, normal TSH and positive serum thyroid antibodies, correlating ultrasound changes with parameters of thyroid function and the autoimmune reactions. We have followed a few such patients

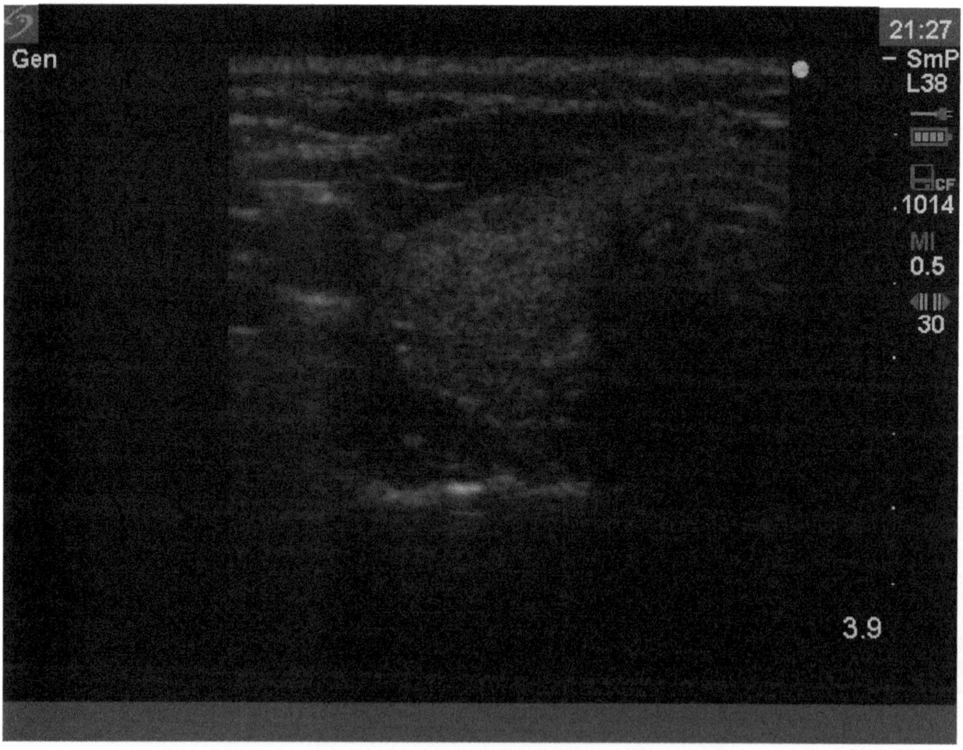

Fig. 1. Thyroid ultrasound changes in a 23 yr old female with early Hashimoto's thyroiditis and subclinical hypothyroidism (normal fT4, TSH 4.5) showing minimal cystic changes and a patchy texture, reflecting the autoimmune reactions.

with Hashimoto's thyroiditis over a course of the natural history of the disease before and after treatment with thyroxin, observing that the correlation between findings on real time ultrasound, thyroid function and thyroid antibody levels are indeed close (Wall, Champion *et al* unpublished observations). Moreover, ultrasonographic changes correlate closely with serum TSH and T4 values and clinical features of both the thyroiditis (tender painful gland, goitre) and hypothyroidism and can indicate accurately the stage of the disease and whether or not a patient needs to be treated with thyroxin.

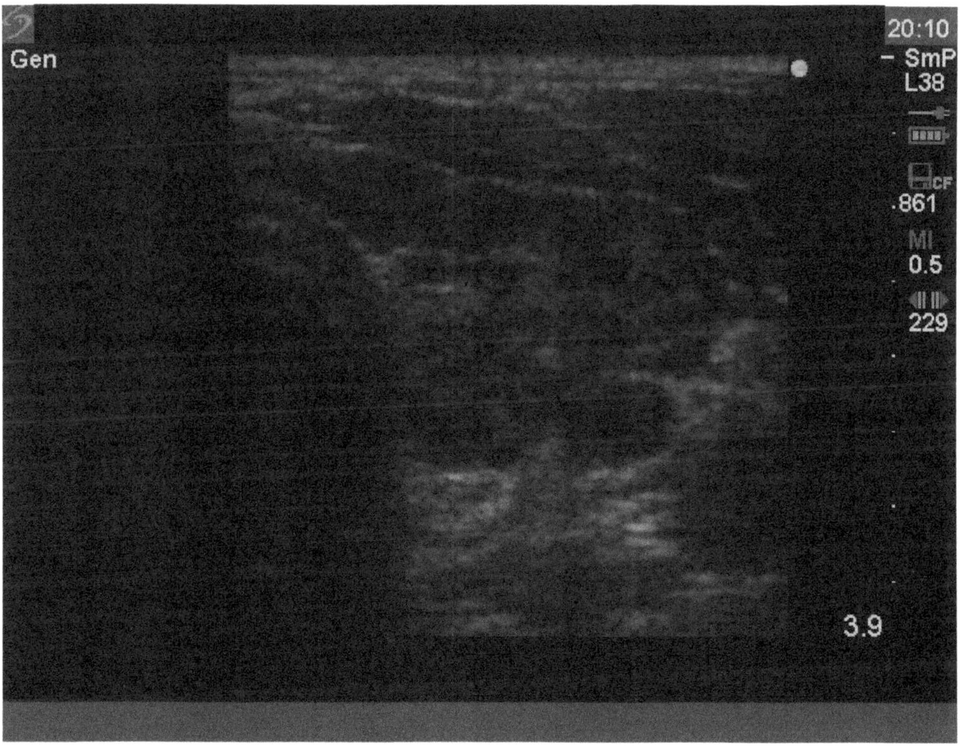

Fig. 2. Ultrasound changes in a 30 yr old male with more severe Hashimoto's thyroiditis and overt hypothyroidism showing extensive cystic changes throughout the lobe, especially in the upper parts, scarring and pseudo nodule formation.

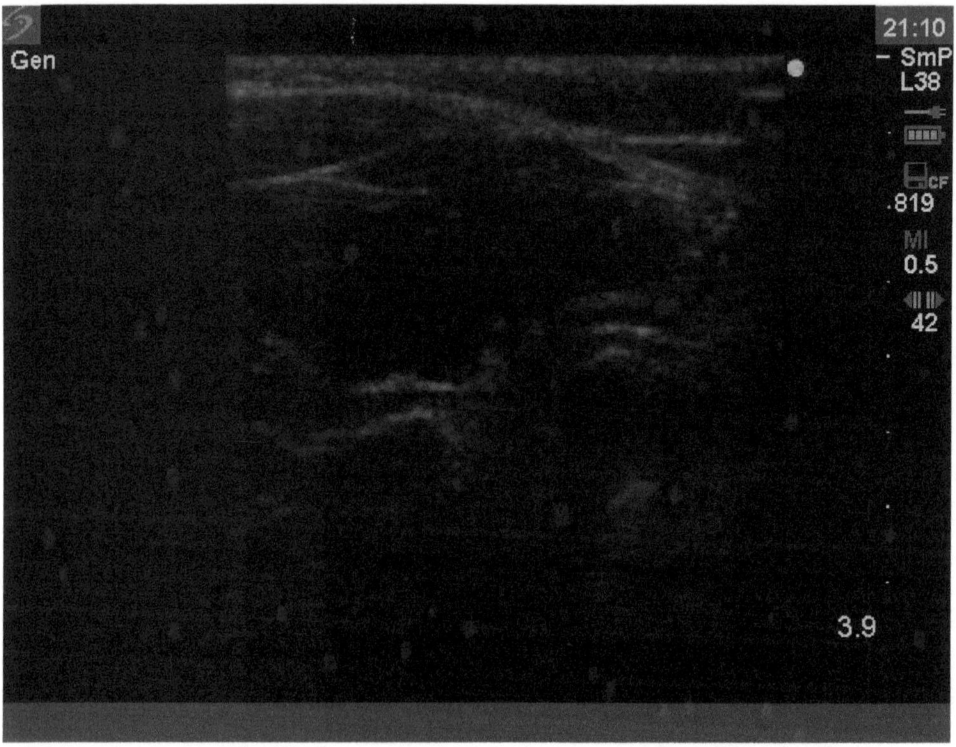

Fig. 3. Typical ultrasound changes in a 50 yr old female with long standing hypothyroidism due to Hashimoto's thyroiditis. The thyroid tissue has been destroyed and replaced by empty spaces (seen as black areas) and linear scarring, giving the appearance of pseudo nodules. This can be called "end stage" disease. In this patient, the gland is slightly enlarged although with time it becomes shrunken and small.

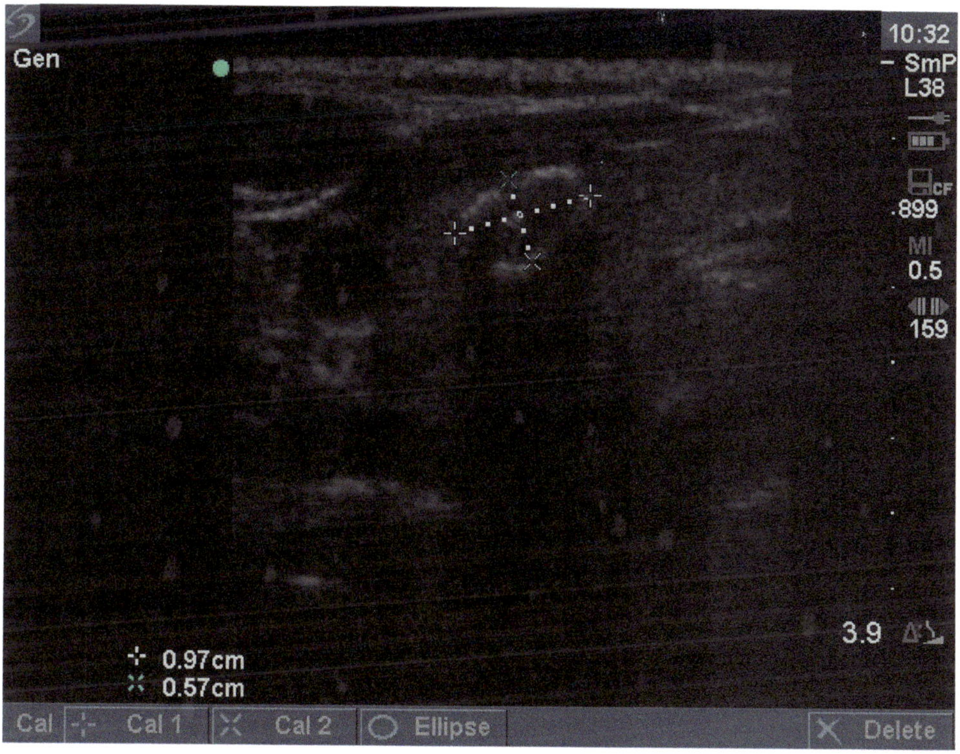

Fig. 4. Late stage Hashimoto's thyroiditis in a 45 yr old female showing chronic, egg shell, calcification seen as a 1 cm calcified ball with shadowing (due to inability of the ultrasound waves to penetrate the calcified material).

3. Thyroid nodules in Hashimoto's thyroiditis

There is an increased prevalence of thyroid cancer in patients with Hashimoto's thyroiditis (6) so any nodules (fig. 5) should be carefully documented, assessed for signs of malignancy and ultrasound-guided fine needle aspiration biopsy (FNA) performed where appropriate. The possibility that the number and/or size of any nodules might reflect the severity and extent of the autoimmune process or represent a surrogate for the development of ophthalmopathy, could be studied.

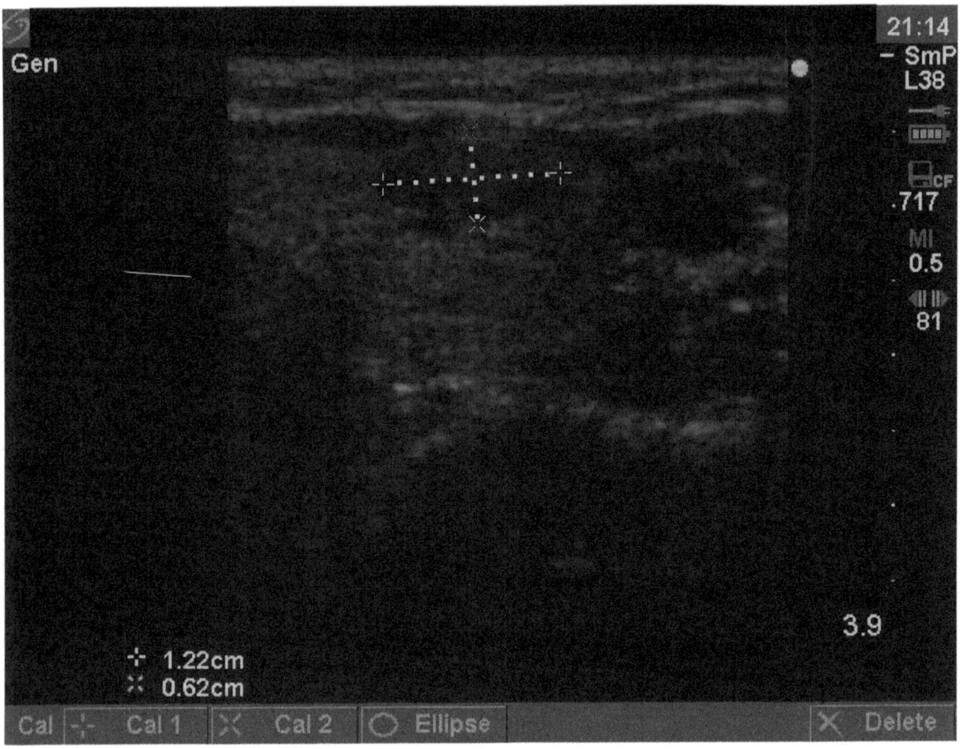

Fig. 5. A suspicious hypo echoic nodule in the thyroid of a 35 yr old female patient with early Hashimoto's thyroiditis. Apart from a few small cystic areas around the nodule and mild patchiness throughout, the texture of the gland itself is relatively normal

4. Conversion of Hashimoto's thyroiditis to Graves' hyperthyroidism

Changes in the status of the autoimmune reactions of Hashimoto's thyroiditis can be quantified by measurement of serial TPO, Tg and TSH-receptor antibodies and some patients show dramatic changes from one disorder to the other, particularly development of Graves' disease even after the apparent destruction of the thyroid gland by the Hashimoto's thyroiditis process. We have studied a 14 yr old female patient who presented with profound hypothyroidism due to Hashimoto's thyroiditis with high levels of TSH and unmeasurable T4 and ultrasound appearances typical of end stage Hashimoto's thyroiditis who later converted to Graves' hyperthyroidism with the development of TSH-r antibodies (7). We were able to show by serial real time thyroid US, destruction of the thyroid gland initially then re filling with newly formed follicular cells through the action of the TSH receptor antibodies, followed by overall thyroid enlargement and finally, the typical heterogeneous appearance of Graves' hyperthyroidism that reflect the lymphoid infiltration, including increased vascularity (fig. 6a, 6b). This is the first documented observation of change from hypothyroidism to hyperthyroidism recorded by real time thyroid ultrasonography (7).

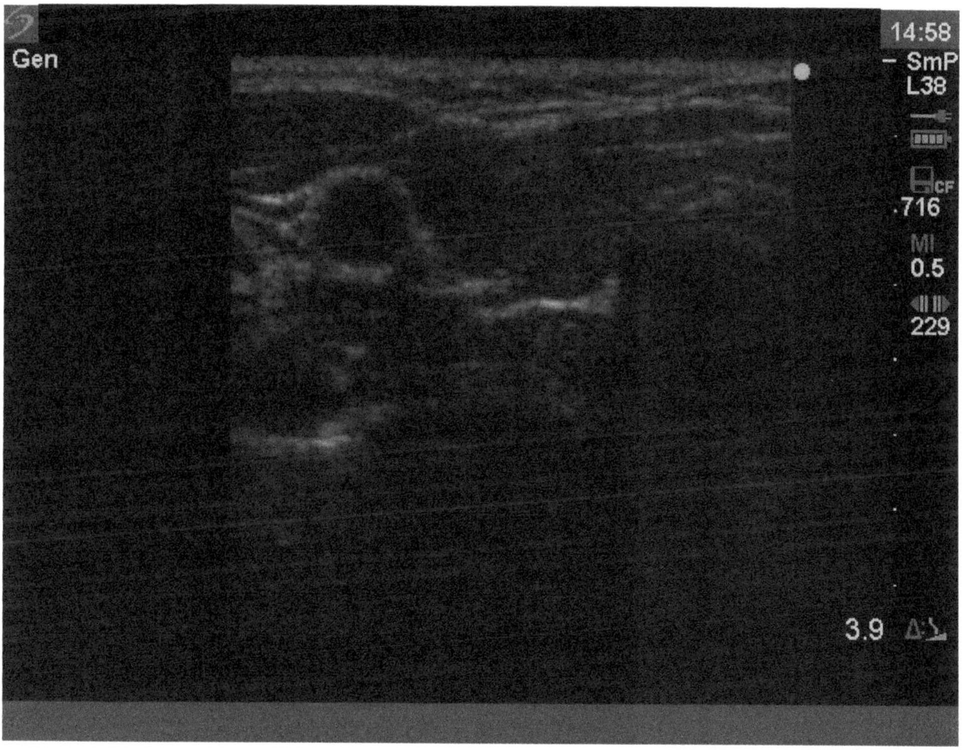

Fig. 6a. Ultrasound appearance of the thyroid gland in a 14 year old female patient 10 months after presenting with Hashimoto's thyroiditis and profound hypothyroidism and 9 months after biochemical and clinical conversion to Graves' hyperthyroidism. The typical appearances of Hashimoto's thyroiditis namely, a small, shrunken lobe and isthmus and generalized hypo echoicity due to inflammation of the thyroid tissue, are still present.

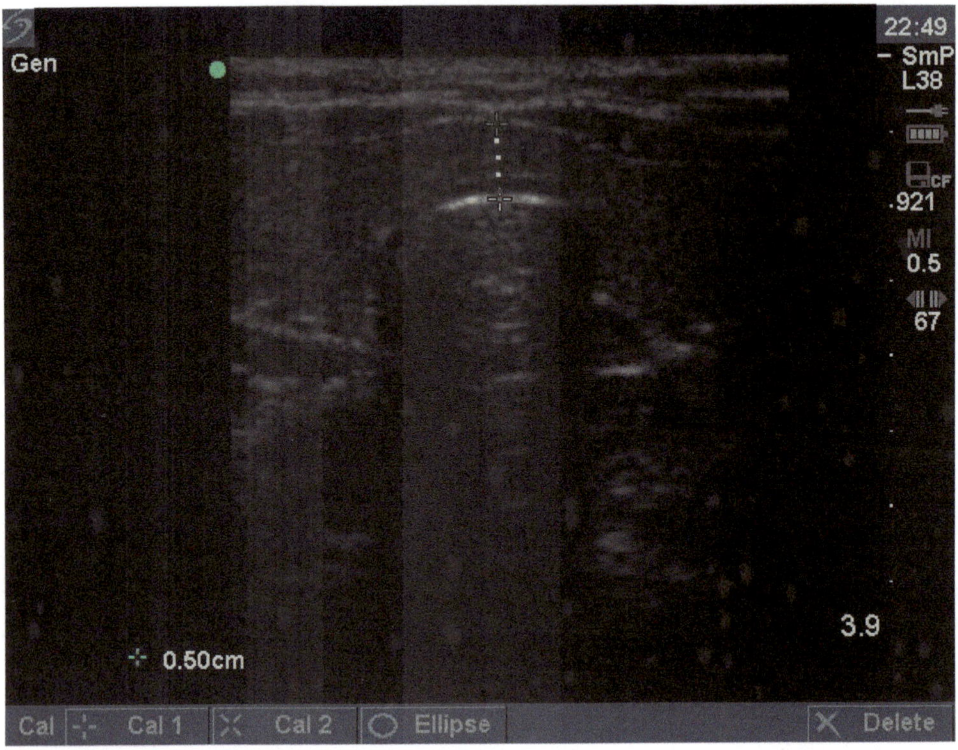

Fig. 6b. Thyroid ultrasonography 16 months later (30 months after biochemical and clinical conversion from Hashimoto's hypothyroidism to Graves' hyperthyroidism). The thyroid is larger, particularly the isthmus, more hyper echoic throughout and typical of fully established Graves' hyperthyroidism

5. Remission in young patients with Hashimoto's thyroiditis

We have studied a 12 yr old girl with Hashimoto's thyroiditis was initially euthyroid and later treated with 50 µg l-thyroxin (L-T4) when her fT4 had declined from 17 to 7 pmol/L (normal range, 8-22 pmol/L). At this time her TSH was 4.1 mIU/L (normal range, 0.30-4.0 mIU/L) and thyroid ultrasonography demonstrated features of early inflammation. Two years later, while on the same dose of T4, ultrasound examination revealed severe end-stage Hashimoto's thyroiditis (fig 7a) and thyroid function tests showed a T4 of 14.0 pmol/L and TSH of 0.81 mIU/L. Twelve months later, however, the thyroid ultrasound had returned to almost normal with only minimal features of inflammation (fig 7b). Thyroid function tests showed an fT4 of 12.8 pmol/L and TSH of 0.75 mIU/L. Her T4 treatment was then stopped. Eight, 17, and 30 weeks after this, her fT4 levels were 16.8, 9.7, and 13.9 pmol/L, respectively. Twelve months later her goitre suddenly enlarged and became tender; ultrasound revealed that she now had features of end stage disease with a huge empty thyroid gland (fig 7c) and fT4 level was low (8 pmol/L) and TSH elevated (11 mU/L) and she was again treated with thyroxin, this time permanently. This is the first recording of serial thyroid ultrasound changes in a patient with Hashimoto's thyroiditis that paralleled changes in thyroid function. This case (8) indicates that thyroiditis can have a fluctuating course, including go into remission in some children. Thyroid ultrasound may be useful to make presumptive therapeutic decisions in children and adolescents with Hashimoto's thyroiditis whose dose of thyroid hormone seems to be less than is full replacement. Thyroid function tests, however, should ultimately guide T4 dosage. It is well recognised that Hashimoto's thyroiditis can be transient in about a third of young patients whereas it is presumed that in adults in all cases it is progressive into end stage destruction and hypothyroidism which is permanent. Use of real time thyroid ultrasonography provides an additional aid to studies of cohorts of children and teenagers to objectively characterise the natural history of the disease.

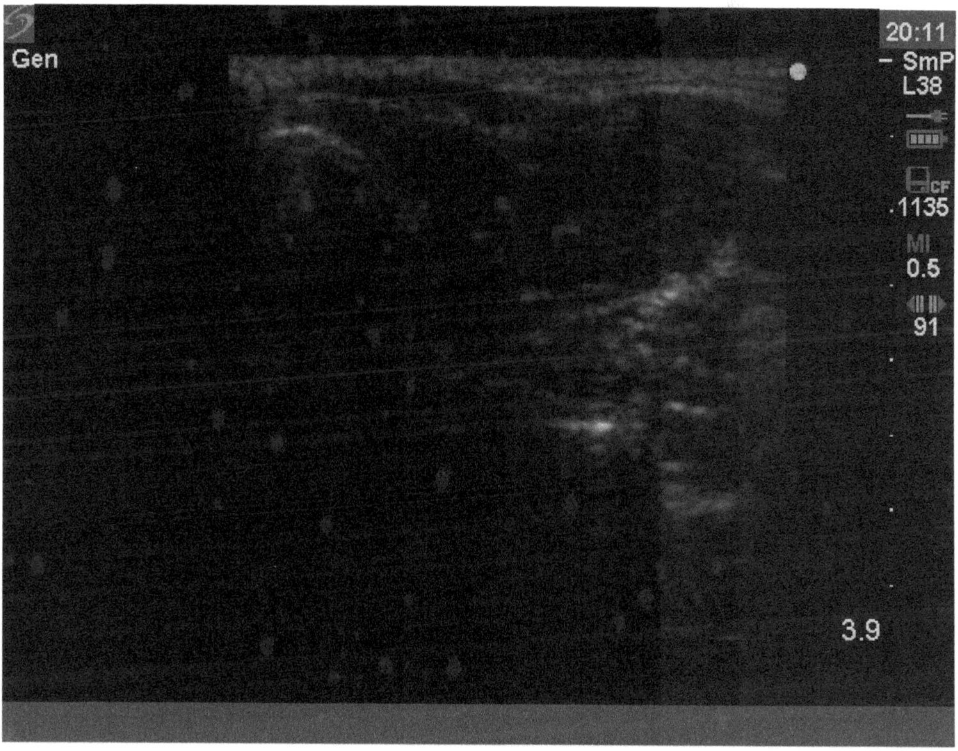

Fig. 7a. Thyroid ultrasonography in a 12-year-old girl with Hashimoto's thyroiditis who was initially euthyroid and later treated with 50 µg l-thyroxin (L-T4) when her fT4 had declined from 17 to 7 pmol/L (normal range, 8-22 pmol/L). At this time her TSH was 4.1 mIU/L (normal range, 0.30-4.0 mIU/L) and thyroid ultrasonography demonstrated features of severe thyroiditis similar to those seen in fig. 3.

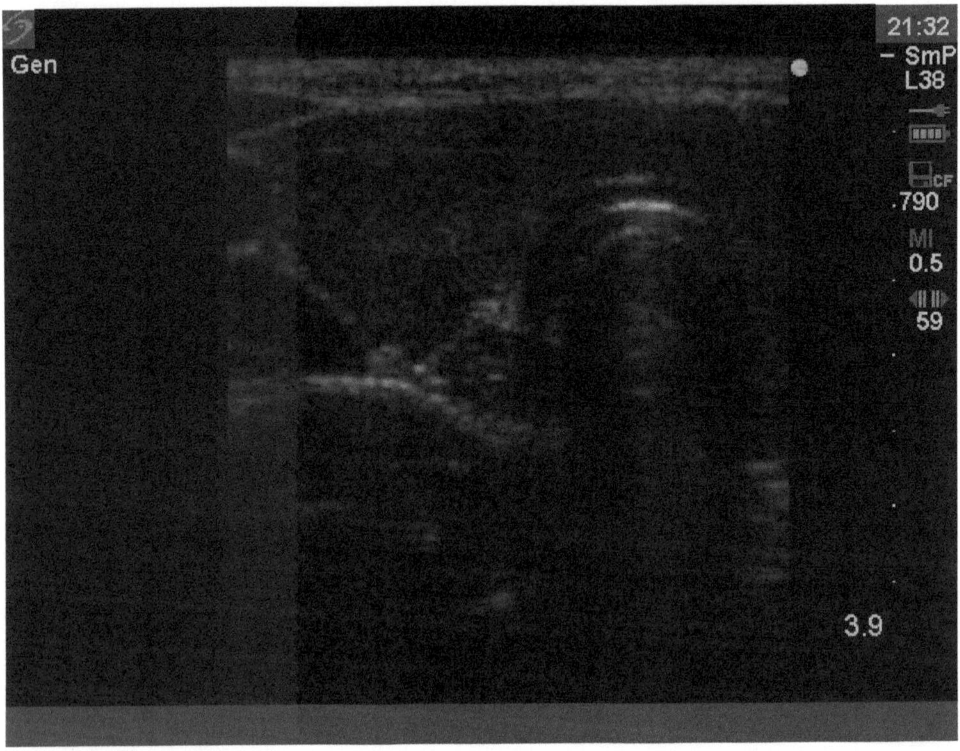

Fig. 7b. Eighteen months later, the thyroid ultrasound in this patient has returned to almost normal with only minimal features of inflammation. Thyroid function tests showed an fT4 of 12.8 pmol/L and TSH of 0.75 mIU/L and she was clinically euthyroid and well.

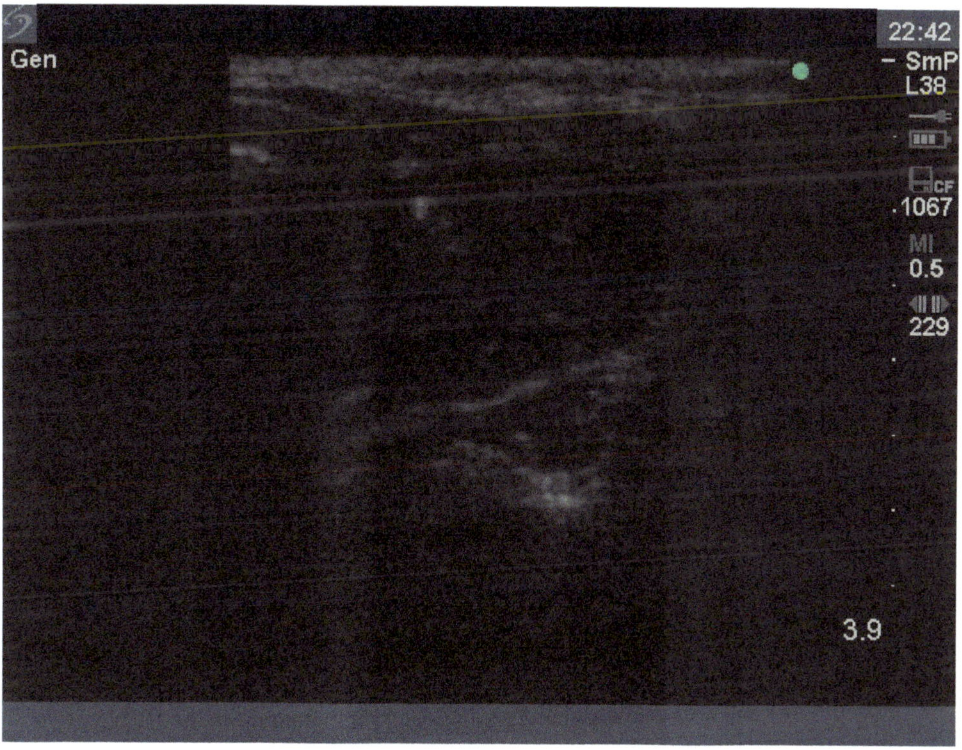

Fig. 7c. Twelve months later this patient's goitre suddenly enlarged greatly and was tender; ultrasound revealed that she now had features of end stage disease with a huge empty thyroid gland and fT4 level was low (8 pmol/L) and TSH elevated (11 mU/L) and she was again treated with thyroxin, this time permanently.

6. Riedel's thyroiditis

A female aged 25 with a very large, firm goitre, strongly positive thyroid antibodies and marked and resistant hypothyroidism was studied by ultrasound. Her gland was non-tender, stony hard to palpation, diffusely enlarged with no associated adenopathy. (fig. 8). On ultrasound (fig. 8), the texture was quite different to that found in classical Hashimoto's thyroiditis (see above) and consistent with massive fibrosis. Indeed, this patient also had evidence for generalised fibrotic process with radiologically and biopsy proven retroperitoneal fibrosis causing bilateral ureteric obstruction. She was treated with thyroxin as well as glucocorticoids and azathiaprine to control her systemic fibrotic process. Tamoxifen, with anti-transforming growth factor (TGF) beta properties, is also another potential therapeutic strategy.

Riedel thyroiditis, or Riedel's thyroiditis, is a rare, chronic inflammatory disease of the thyroid gland characterized by a dense fibrosis that replaces normal thyroid parenchyma (9). At the Mayo clinic, 37 cases were diagnosed in a series of 57,000 thyroidectomies that were performed between 1920 and 1984. The operative incidence was 0.06% and the overall incidence in outpatients was 1.06 per 100,000 (10). The fibrotic process invades adjacent structures of the neck and extends beyond the thyroid capsule. This feature differentiates Riedel's thyroiditis from other inflammatory or fibrotic disorders of the thyroid. Because of the encroachment beyond the thyroid capsule, other problems can be associated with Riedel's thyroiditis, including hypoparathyroidism, hoarseness (due to recurrent laryngeal involvement), and stridor (due to tracheal compression). Approximately one third of Riedel's thyroiditis cases are associated with clinical findings of multifocal fibrosclerosis at the time of diagnosis. Riedel's thyroiditis is also associated with other fibrous inflammatory processes, including retroperitoneal fibrosis, orbital pseudotumor, mediastinal fibrosis, sclerosing cholangitis and fibrosis in other organ systems.

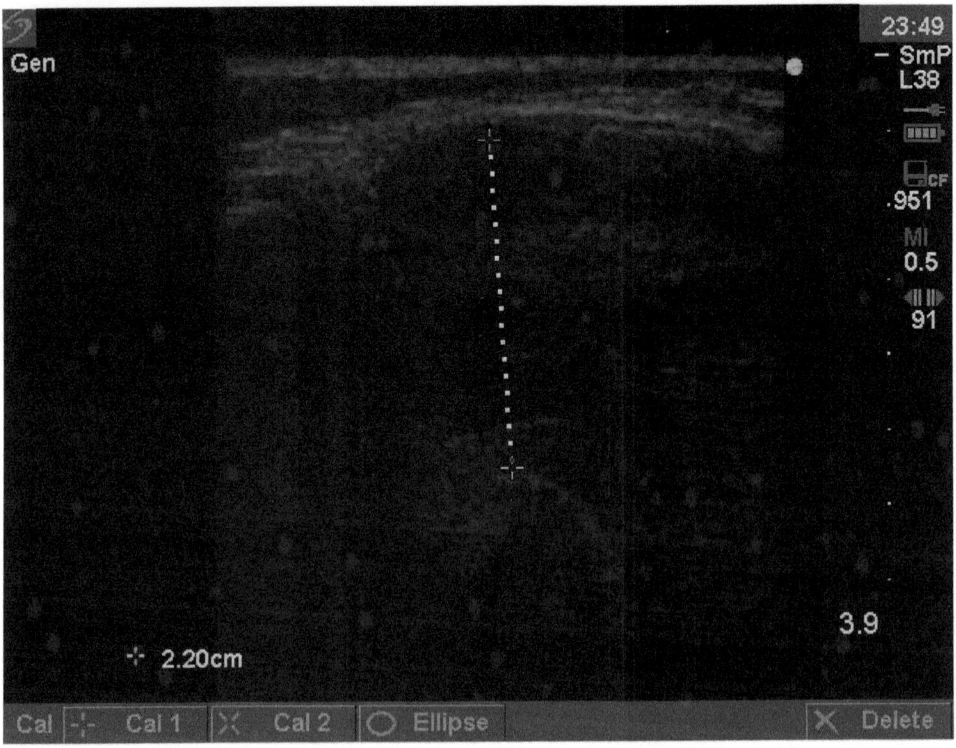

Fig. 8. Thyroid ultrasound in a 32 yr old woman with Riedel's thyroiditis, a very large goiter, a systemic fibrotic reaction, strongly positive thyroid antibodies and marked and resistant hypothyroidism. The isthmus is 2.20 cm thick, approximately 3 times normal, and the texture of the thyroid contents is quite different from that found in classical end-stage Hashimoto's thyroiditis (see above), with large oblong hypo echoic spaces scattered among more iso echoic areas, consistent with a combination of thyroiditis and diffues fibrosis, respectively.

7. Eye changes in patients with Hashimoto's thyroiditis

Mild eye signs (ophthalmopathy) are common in patients with Hashimoto's thyroiditis (1) if looked for (since the main and sometimes only sign is upper eyelid lag) and correlate fairly closely with a variety of eye muscle antibodies which are probably secondary to the putative inflammation of the levator palpebrae superioris muscle. We have studied patients with Graves' hyperthyroidism, addressing whether the thyroid size - as a surrogate for the severity of the "thyroiditis" - is a marker for associated ophthalmopathy (Oliffe, Wall submitted). While we did not demonstrate a significant correlation between bigger thyroid size and ophthalmopathy we have not yet studied patients with Hashimoto's thyroiditis in whom goitre size varies a lot and could - in the early stages before destruction - provide a better marker for subsequent eye signs. Ultrasound changes can also be correlated with serum titres of calsequestrin and collagen XIII antibodies and eye signs in patients with Hashimoto's thyroiditis.

8. Relationship between thyroid and orbital immune reactions in pregnant patients with Hashimoto's thyroiditis

Changes in the thyroid and orbital inflammatory processes may run in parallel or diverge in pregnancy and real-time ultrasound has been used to study patients with Graves' disease and Hashimoto's thyroiditis from pre-pregnancy through pregnancy and in the post-partum period. Changes in the status of Hashimoto's thyroiditis is common during pregnancy and afterwards. We are studying whether these abnormalities are reflected in ultrasound changes, goitre size and thyroid antibody titres and whether they run parallel to changes in eye signs and serum titres of calsequestrin and collagen XIII antibodies or run divergent courses. Preliminary results suggest that thyroid and eye muscle antibody levels fall in parallel during pregnancy and rebound together in the post partum period and correlate with changes in eye signs in patients with Graves' disease and Hashimoto's thyroiditis (Wall, Champion et al., unpublished observations). This suggests that the ophthalmopathy of both Graves' disease and Hashimoto's thyroiditis is closely linked with the thyroid autoimmune process in both disorders, although this study is ongoing. In Hashimoto's thyroiditis the eye changes are usually mild and confined to the upper eyelids with mild proptosis, but the underlying process seems to be the same. While most workers (11-13) believe that the reason for the association is due to cross reactive antibodies targeting the TSHr in the thyroid follicular cell and orbital fibroblast and pre adipocyte TSHr antibodies are not always detected in patients with eye signs (1). For this reason we propose that there may be a primary eye muscle reaction against calsequestrin. and possibly collagen XIII (2-5, 14).

9. Conclusions

Real-time thyroid ultrasonography is an under utilised tool for the assessment of Hashimoto's thyroiditis and hypothyroidism in individual patients and in research studies. Use of real-time thyroid ultrasonography gives us a unique opportunity to directly observe the consequences of the thyroid autoimmune process in the thyroid gland. We have shown how the ultrasonographic changes closely reflect the nature of the immune reactions, their effects on thyroid follicles and tissue architecture in general and on the ability of the thyroid gland to produce thyroid hormones.

There are limitations to ultrasonography, in particular that we have not proven that the observed visual changes can be directly extrapolated to the immune reactions in the thyroid. However, as technology improves, for example when we can characterise and quantify the lymphoid patches, we can expect to be able to better correlate what is seen on ultrasound with the underlying autoimmune reactions.

10. References

[1] Tjiang H, Lahooti H, McCorquodale T, Parmar KR, Wall JR 2010 Eye and eyelid abnormalities are common in patients with Hashimoto's thyroiditis Thyroid 20:287-290

[2] Gopinath B, Tani J, Bao N, Wall JR 2007 Eye signs and serum eye muscle and collagen XIII antibodies in patients with transient and progressive thyroiditis Thyroid 17: 1-7.

[3] Tani J, Gopinath B, Nuygen B, Wall JR 2007 Immunological mechanisms for the eye muscle and orbital connective tissue reactions of thyroid-associated ophthalmopathy. Expert Reviews in Clin Immunol 3:299-311.

[4] Gopinath B, Musselman R, Beard N, Tani J, Adams C, Wall JR 2006 Antibodies targeting the calcium binding skeletal muscle protein calsequestrin are sensitive and specific markers of ocular myopathy in patients with Graves' disease. Clin Exp Immunol 145:56-62.

[5] Gopinath B, Musselman R, Adams C, Tani J, Beard N, Wall JR 2006 Study of serum antibodies against three eye muscle antigens and the connective tissue antigen collagen XIII in patients with Graves' disease with and without ophthalmopathy - correlation with clinical features. Thyroid 16: 967-974.

[6] Büyükaşık O, Hasdemir AO, Yalçın E, Celep B, Sengül S, Yandakçı K, Tunç G, Küçükpınar T, Alkoy S, Cöl C The association between thyroid malignancy and chronic lymphocytic thyroiditis: should it alter the surgical approach? Endokrynol Pol. 2011;62(4):303-8.

[7] Champion B, Gopinath B, Ma G, El-Kaissi S, Wall JR 2008 Conversion of Hashimoto's thyroiditis to Graves' hyperthyroidism observed by real-time thyroid ultrasonography. Thyroid (Letter to Editor) 18:1135-37.

[8] Nanan R, Lahooti H, Wall JR 2010 Remission of Hashimoto's thyroiditis at puberty in a 12 year old girl documented by changes in thyroid ultrasonography. Thyroid 20:1187-1190.

[9] Schwaegerle SM, Bauer TW, Esselstyn CB: Riedel's thyroiditis. Am J Clin Pathol 1988, 90:715-722.

[10] De Boer WA (May 1993). Riedel's thyroiditis, retroperitoneal fibrosis, and sclerosing cholangitis: diseases with one pathogenesis? Gut 34 (5): 714

[11] Eckstein AK, Plicht M, Lax H, Neuhäuser M, Mann K, Lederbogen S, Heckmann C, Esser J, Morgenthaler NG 2006 Thyrotropin receptor autoantibodies are independent risk factors for Graves' ophthalmopathy and help to predict severity and outcome of the disease. J Clin Endocrinol Metab 91:3464-3470.

[12] Paschke R, Vassart G, Ludgate M 1995 Current evidence for and against the TSH receptor being the common antigen in Graves' disease and thyroid associated ophthalmopathy. Clin Endocrinol (Oxf) 42:565-569.

[13] Weetman AP 2000 Graves' disease. N Engl J Med 343:1236-1248.

[14] Lahooti H, Parmar K R, Wall JR 2010 Pathogenesis of Thyroid Eye Disease: important role of autoimmunity against calsequestrin and collagen XIII. Pathogenesis of Thyroid Eye Disease: important role of autoimmunity against calsequestrin and collagen XIII. A review. Clin Ophthalmol. 14:417-25.

11

Options of Replacement Therapy in Hypothyroidism

Valentine V. Fadeyev[1,2], Galina A. Melnichenko[1,2] and Tatyana Morgunova[1]
[1]*I.M. Sechenov First Moscow State Medical University, Department of Endocrinology;*
[2]*Federal Endocrinological Research Centre*
Russia

1. Introduction

1.1 History of replacement therapy of hypothyroidism

Before the middle of XX century treatment of hypothyroidism implied prescription to the patients animals' thyroid extracts, containing both, thyroxine and triiodothyronine [*Oppenheimer JH, 1995*]. Those drugs, in which it was almost impossible to measure the dose of thyroid hormones precisely, could not adequately provide euthyroidism. Moreover, it was rather difficult to prescribe proper doses. Furthermore there weren't any objective control parameter for dose adjustment like modern TSH-assays. Synthetic preparations of levothyroxine (L-T4) have been used since about 1958, and levotriiodothyronine (L-T3) - since 1956 (**figure 1**).

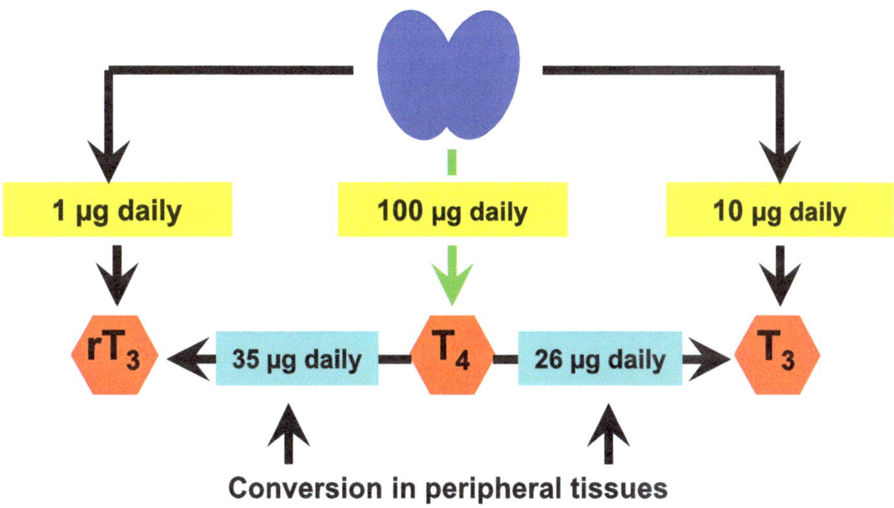

Fig. 1. Production of thyroid hormones

Based on the concept that the thyroid gland produces two hormones - thyroxine (T4) and triiodothyronine (T3), there was a long-term understanding that in the treatment of hypothyroidism it is preferable to use a combination of L-T3 and L-T4, rather than monotherapy with one of those drugs [*Oppenheimer JH, 1995*]. In the 70s, it was shown that the majority of circulating in blood T3 (80%) is produced not by the thyroid gland, but is formed by deiodination of T4 in peripheral tissues [*Braverman LE, 1970; Surks MI, 1973*]. These data allowed to consider T4 as prohormone to T3, which shows a stronger affinity to the receptors of thyroid hormones than T4. In addition, it was demonstrated, that L-T3 has unfavorable pharmacokinetics: it is rapidly and almost completely gets absorbed, the serum level of T3 reaches a peak after 2 - 4 hours, but after 6 - 8 hours it considerably declines. Thus, after taking the L-T3, the serum level of T3 reaches a non-physiological level for a short time and then rapidly gets metabolized [*Toft, 1994*]. These data led to the concept of the predominant use of replacement monotherapy with L-T4 (**figure 2**).

Year	Event
1891	Treatment with animals' thyroid extracts
1926	Description of the structure and synthesis of T4
1952	Description of the structure and synthesis of T3
1956	Start of treatment with synthetic L-T3
1958	Start of treatment with synthetic L-T4 (200-400 μg daily)
1973-74	Recommended dose of L-T4 100-150 μg daily
	The widespread use of combination with L-T4 + T3
1980-85	Appearance of highly sensitive methods for determination of TSH
	Concept of preferable use of replacement monotherapy with L-T4

Fig. 2. History of replacement therapy of hypothyroidism

Together with fundamental studies, which investigated the thyroid hormones metabolism intensive development of laboratory diagnostics led to the development of modern concepts of replacement therapy with thyroid hormones. Thus, while determining the TSH level with methods of poor sensitivity in the lower range of values (unable to distinguish the suppressed level of TSH from the low-normal value) in the 1960s a replacement dose of L-T4 was recommended, ranged between 200 and 400 micrograms daily, which was accompanied by a significant increase in T4 level in serum [*Toft, 1999*].

The situation changed in the 1980s with appearance of highly sensitive methods for the determination of TSH levels. It became obvious that the doses of L-T4, leading to suppression of TSH, even in normal levels of T4 and T3 in blood, were accompanied by similar, but less evident changes in the liver, heart, kidneys and bones, like in thyrotoxicosis [*Gow,1987*]. Thus, by the early 1980s the concept of preferable use of replacement monotherapy with L-T4 was formulated. TSH level, determined by methods of high sensitivity, has become the main indicator for assessment the adequacy of hypothyroidism replacement therapy.

1.2 The principles of generally recommended replacement therapy

Overt hypothyroidism is an absolute indication for replacement therapy with thyroid hormones. According to current recommendations, monotherapy with L-T4 is the "gold standard" of replacement therapy, because a single daily dose of the drug can maintain euthyroid state.

To date, L-T4 is the most commonly prescribed hormonal drug. The replacement dose of L-T4 is initially calculated as 1.6 μg per kilogram of body mass. In most cases, full replacement dose for women is about 100-150 μg of L-T4 daily and about 125-200 μg for men. How long it takes to reach full replacement doses of thyroid hormones, depends on several factors, first of all on the patient's age, history and severity of hypothyroidism, and presence of comorbidity and above all, cardiac diseases. In most cases, a full replacement dose of L-T4 can be prescribed to young patients immediately. Herewith, to date there is insufficient number of studies that could investigate the advantages and disadvantages of immediate prescribing of the full replacement dose of L-T4 as compared with slow titration. The results of recently published prospective randomized double-blind study compared the safety of the prescribing immediately the full replacement dose of L-T4 (1.6 μg per kg body mass) vs. the beginning with low-dose (25 μg daily) and gradual increase every four weeks in patients with newly diagnosed overt hypothyroidism without cardiac disease history [*Roos A, 2005*]. Safety was assessed by frequency of cardiac symptoms or acute cardiovascular events, and effectiveness – by the levels of TSH, freeT4, symptoms of hypothyroidism dynamics and quality of life. Fifty patients were randomized into two groups; the groups were comparable in terms of baseline TSH levels (61 vs. 48 mU/l), fT4 (7.2 vs. 8.2 pmol/l) and age (47 vs. 47 years). During the study at baseline and after 12 and 24 weeks, there were no cardiac symptoms or acute cardiovascular events. Hypothyroidism compensation was achieved more quickly in the group of treatment with full replacement dose initition, as compared with initial low-dose treatment: in 13 and 1 patients compensation was achieved after 4 weeks, in 19 and 3 patients after 8 weeks, in 19 and 9 patients after 12 weeks, in 20 and 14 patients over 16 weeks, in 20 and 18 patients after 20 weeks and in 21 and 20 patients in 24 weeks respectively ($p = 0.005$). Nevertheless, the dynamics of hypothyroidism symptoms and quality of life parameters in both groups were rather similar. Based on these results, the authors concluded that the prescribing of a full replacement dose of L-T4 immediately in patients with overt hypothyroidism without cardiac disease anamnesis is safe and may be more convenient and cost-effective as compared with the beginning with low doses of L-T4. However, in clinical practice traditionally the most widely used is the beginning of replacement therapy with relatively low doses of L-T4, with a subsequent increase to a full replacement ("start slow and go low"). Exceptions are only pregnant women with hypothyroidism.

As a rule, L-T4 preparations are recommended to take in the morning upon starving, 30-40 minutes before breakfast and taking other drugs. When taken per os, about 70-80% of the dose gets absorbed: 20% of the drug is absorbed in the duodenum and 40% - in the upper part of the ileum, the remaining 40% - in the lower ileum. The peak absorption of the drug is reached between 30 and 60 minutes after the administration, the drug is absorbed completely in 90 minutes [*Centanni M., 2006*].

The adequacy of replacement therapy of hypothyroidism is estimated over 6-8 weeks after the beginning of a full replacement dose of L-T4 or dose adjustment. The normal TSH level is the main criterion of hypothyroidism compensation. If necessary to adjust (decrease or increase) the dose, the "step" of L-T4 is 12.5-25 μg. After reaching euthyroidism, it is necessary to monitor the adequacy of therapy annually. In some cases, adjustment of the dose may be required and, therefore, further assessment of the therapy adequacy. Thus, the necessity to increase doses of L-T4 may occur in the following situations: use of the drugs that increase L-T4 clearance (phenobarbital, carbamazepine, rifampicin, phenytoin, sertraline, chloroquine); use of the drugs that hinder the absorption of L-T4 in the gut (calcium carbonat, cholestyramine, sucralfate, aluminum hydroxide, sulphate of iron, fiber supplements); in conditions of increased concentrations of thyroxine-binding globulin due to pregnancy or estrogen administration; in malabsorption or celiac disease [*Arafah B., 2000; Havrankova J., 1992; Singh N., 2000*]. Besides, thyroxine dose adjustment may be required in such diseases as lactose deficiency, hypoacidic gastritis, atrophic gastritis, chronic gastritis, associated with Helicobacter pylori, intestinal parasitic diseases [*Centanni M., 2006*].

1.3 Factors, that influence on the quality of compensation of replacement therapy

In general, replacement therapy with thyroid hormones is rather simple, but despite this fact, according to different authors, the part of patients receiving L-T4 replacement therapy and remains in decompensation varies from 32.5 to 62% [Diez J.J., 2002; Canaris G.J., 2000; Parle J., 1991].

Thus, in the study by Diez J.J., patients over 55 years with hypothyroidism, receiving replacement therapy with L-T4 were screened for TSH level. Among 385 patients, hypothyroidism was compensated only in 67.5%, and decompensated in 32.5%. The degree of compensation depended on the hypothyroidism duration, but was independent on age, sex, history and severity of hypothyroidism [Diez, 2002].

In a large-population Colorado study, which included 25 862 people, it was shown that among 1525 patients treated with L-T4, only 916 patients (60.1%) were compensated. Among 609 patients with decompensated hypothyroidism overt hypothyroidism was detected in 11 patients (0.7%) and subclinical hypothyroidism in 269 patients (17.6%) , in 13 (0.9%) - overt hyperthyroidism, and in 316 patients (20.7%) subclinical hyperthyroidism were found [*Canaris GJ, 2000*]. It is remarkable, that 92% of patients visited a physician less than one year prior to enrollment in the study.

In a small study, performed by Parle J. et al., among 97 patients with primary hypothyroidism, who received monotherapy with L-T4, 46.8% of patients were decompensated, of whom 26.8% (26 patients) had elevated TSH (and in 13 (50 %) - above 10 mU/l), while in 21% (20 patients) the TSH was decreased [*J. Parle, 1991*].

So, what are the reasons for decompensation in so many patients with hypothyroidism? It is well known, that control of any chronic disease, including hypothyroidism, is at least partly dependents on patient compliance. **Compliance** is a patient's adherence to the recommended course of treatment. According to a number of studies the main reason for decompensation of hypothroidism is poor compliance of patients [*Hueston W., 2001; Hanna F., 1999*].

The study conducted by Leese G.P. et al. has shown that among 1180 patients, receiving replacement therapy with L-T4, *58.5%* had a decreased level of TSH, 3.5% - increased TSH, and only in 38% of patients the TSH level was within the normal range. In patients with suppressed TSH recommended dose of L-T4 was usually higher than in the group with normal TSH (114.2 ± 56.9 µg as compared with 100.4 ± 45.9 µg, $p < 0.01$). In the group with elevated TSH, the situation was different: in patients treated with lower doses of L-T4 the reason for decompensation was insufficient dose of the drug, while in patients receiving high dose of L-T4 (137.1 ± 58.8 µg) the decompensation was due to poor compliance [*Leese G., 1993*].

In clinical practice, there are some methods to improve the quality of compensation: patient's education, using of registers (patients with compensated hypothyroidism are included in the database, and their status is evaluated annually). However, the registers' formation, despite their potential economic benefits, remains difficult to be updated [*Hanna F., 1999*].

In the study by Cuthbertson D.J. et al. authors evaluated the compensation of hypothyroidism in 6205 patients, entered in the electronic register. The following parameters were entered into the database: etiology of hypothyroidism, levels of TSH and free T4 at baseline, type of the replacement therapy. The levels of TSH for patients entered in the register were measured every 18 months. In step of the of L-T4 dose adjustment, the patients were invited for a follow-up visit every 6 months. The L-T4 dose adjustment was made in accordance with the level of TSH: if TSH was above 4 mU/l, the daily dose was increased by 25 µg; if the TSH level was normal or reduced (in the range 0.03 - 0.4 mU/l), the dose remained unchanged, but if the TSH level was below 0.03 mU/l, the dose was reduced by 50 µg (with the dose of L-T4 within 225-300 µg), or 25 µg (with the dose of L-T4 175 - 200 µg). With the dose less than 150 µg a reduction was recommended only in case of increased level of free T4 above 24 pmol/l. The study demonstrated, that there were 58.5% of patients with suppressed TSH (<0.03 mU/l) before 1991. Later the rate of patient with decompensation of hypothyroidism decreased markedly to 15,7 ± 3,6% in the period from 1993 to 2001 [*Cuthbertson DJ, 2006*].

One of the reasons for decompensation of hypothyroidism could be the changing of **L-T4 preparation even in the same dose**. To date, several L-T4 preparations produced by different manufacturers are available in the pharmaceutical market. Preparations of L-T4 produced by different companies may be insufficiently bioequivalent. In addition, even drugs produced by one company but with different technologies may be not bioequivalent. That is why the problem of bioequivalence and interchangeability of L-T4 is recently under discussion.

In addition to the above-mentioned reasons, it has been suggested, that the **psychological state of patients** can affect the quality of compensation. In particular, patients with depression rarely take medicines regularly and correctly [*Sevinc A., 2004*]. It is well known, that depression is diagnosed more frequently in patients with hypothyroidism than in general population; herewith, it is irrespective of the quality of the disease compensation. Sometimes hypothyroidism can be manifested with the symptoms of depression [*Lindsay RS, 1997, Weetman AP, 1997, Demet, 2003; Joffe RT, 1992; Rack SK, 2000*]. For the first time the relationship between hypothyroidism and depression was mentioned more than 100 years ago, in 1888 [*Oppenheimer J.H., 1995*]. According to some studies, the prevalence of depression in patients with hypothyroidism may be as high as 40% [*Haggerty JJ, 1995*], which is often accompanied by psychomotor retardation and a moderate decrease in cognitive function [*Pies RW, 1997*]. Thus, Munoz-Cruzado Poce et al. while examining 108 patients with depression, has found previously undiagnosed thyroid abnormalities in 24.1% of them, hypothyroidism was diagnosed in 7.4% of cases [*Munoz-Crusado Poce, 2000*]. In a similar study made by Gold MS et al., hypothyroidism was diagnosed in 20 out of 250 patients with depression [*Gold MS, 1981*]. In addition, depression may often be the first sign of subclinical hypothyroidism.

We have organized a study with the aim of investigating medical and social factors, affecting the quality of compensation in hypothyroid patients on L-T4 replacement therapy [*Fadeyev, 2006*]. The study included 200 patients with overt hypothyroidism taking L-T4 for a year or more. Patients were examined at the baseline and after 6 months. The symptoms of hypothyroidism, thyroid hormone levels and lipid profiles were analyzed. In case of decompensation, we were trying to clarify the main reasons thereof: accuracy and regularity of taking the medication and its dose; and in case of incorrect admission or taking inadequate doses of L-T4 we identified the main reasons for that (the doctor did not explain, the patient supposed the regular use of medication as unnecessary, the patient noted subjective changes in well-being, while taking the full replacement dose of L-T4). As a result only 58% (84/200) of patients were euthyroid in the beginning of the study while 26% of them had increased TSH level and 16% had low TSH.

In nearly in one third of patients (24/84; 28.6%) the main reason of decompensation was medication incompliance (the drug was taken after a meal or less than 30 minutes before breakfast; dividing the dose - one part before breakfast, another one before dinner; taking L-T4 together with calcium or iron supplements). Six months later, after the education, the hypothyroidism was decompensated only in 8 patients from this group (8/19, 42.1%). The reason for decompensation in the other 11 patients was also the incompliance in taking of medication or self-changing (increase or decrease) of the L-T4 dose. Only in 13 of 84 patients with decompensated hypothyroidism the main reason for that was the inadequate recommendations of a doctor. In this group, in 6 months after the dose adjustment, out of 9 re-examined patients the hypothyroidism was compensated in 8 cases (88.9%).

2. Challenges of the replacement therapy

2.1 Dissatisfaction with monotherapy of hypothyroidism

It is well known that in clinical practice there is a significant number of patients, who still complains about unspecific symptoms similar to hypothyroid despite the compensation of hypothyroidism and normal TSH level. The most common of them are: fatigue, muscle pain, impaired mood and poor memory [*Wekking E., 2005*]. The presence of these complaints affects the overall well-being and quality of life. The most interesting are results of the study performed in the UK by Saravanan P. et al. [*Saravanan P., 2002*]. The study included 961 patients with hypothyroidism at the age of 18 - 75 years, taking L-T4 for at least four months. The control group included healthy people of the same age. Patients completed two questionnaires: General Health Questionnaire - GHQ-12 and Thyroid symptom questionnaire - TSQ. All the participants were divided into three groups: general group of patients (n = 597), a subgroup of patients with normal TSH (n = 397) and control group (n = 551). The study showed that the mean score under 36-point GHQ scale in patients receiving L-T4 was 12.1, in patients with compensated hypothyroidism - also 12.1, whereas in control group it was 11.4 (p = 0,03 and 0.01 as compared to control, respectively), indicating greater dissatisfaction with their well-being in patients receiving L-T4. Similarly, according to the TSQ, in patients receiving L-T4 results were even worse than in other patients (12.6, 12.8 and 11.5 points respectively; p <0.001). These differences remained after the assessment with regard to other chronic illnesses, including depression. The authors concluded that patients, receiving replacement therapy with L-T4, even normal TSH have lower indicators of overall health than in the people without hypothyroidism.

It is still not quite clear, whether the results of these studies are specific to hypothyroidism, or they reflect the reducing of the overall well-being in patients with any chronic disease, sometimes regardless of its compensation, often from a patient's awareness of their illness [*Ladenson P., 2002*].

2.2 Quality of life and cognitive functioning in patients with compensated hypothyroidism

The assessment of quality of life associated with health, allows us to study the effect of the disease and its treatment on the indictors of the patient's quality of life. A questionnaire is the standard research tool in the quality of life assessment.

In general, according to various authors, the development of hypothyroidism leads to a decline of the patients' quality of life. In most cases, achieving the compensation of disease is accompanied by improvement of well-being of patients and, consequently, improves the quality of life. However, according to some authors, despite the adequate replacement therapy and stable achieving of normal TSH level, the number of parameters of quality of life of those patients (in general groupe) remains decreased compared with healhy control [*Wekking E.M., 2005; Bianchi P., 2004*].

This can be confirmed by the results of the study carried out by Wekking EM et al. [*Wekking EM, 2005*], where the authors assessed the neurocognitive function and quality of life in the patients with hypothyroidism. The study included 141 patients with compensated hypothyroidism aged from 18 to 70 years. The quality of life was assessed by the questionnaire RAND-36 (Dutch version of the questionnaire MOS SF-36). The results of the quality of life assessment were compared with the quality of life of a representative sample of the population of Denmark (n = 1063). It was shown that the levels of vitality and mental health by questionnaire RAND-36 were significantly lower in patients receiving L-T4, as compared with those in representative sample.

We also assessed the quality of life of patients with hypothyroidism and compared it with the quality of life of patients with nodular euthyroid goiter and people without thyroid disease. Thirty patients with compensated primary hypothyroidism (aged from 25 to 55 years), 28 patients with nodular (multinodular) euthyroid goiter of the same age not receiving L-T4, and 30 healthy people were assessed (**figure 3, 4**). The scores for the Short-Form 36 (SF-36) and Beck Depression Inventory Scale were analyzed. Almost all scales of the questionnaire SF-36 (except for general health and role emotional functioning) in patients with compensated hypothyroidism were significantly lower (p 0.05), than in healthy people. While comparing quality of life in patients with hypothyroidism with quality of life in patients with nodular goiter the rates of role physical functioning (p = 0.042), vitality (p = 0.015), social functioning (p = 0.0) and psychological health (p = 0.021) of patients with hypothyroidism were significantly lower compared with patients with euthyroid goiter. In assessing the severity of depression we have shown that the value on a scale of depression in patients with compensated hypothyroidism was significantly higher compared with the results of patients with nodular goiter and healthy individuals (p = 0.014). So, in patients with compensated hypothyroidism in almost all parameters the quality of life is worse than in people without thyroid disease, and on many scales (role physical functioning, vitality, social functioning and psychological health) is worse than in patients with euthyroid goiter. Severity of depression in patients with compensated hypothyroidism is higher compared to patients with nodular goiter and healthy people, which may be one of the reasons for the decrease of quality of life of these patients [*Morgunova T., Manuilova Yu.,2010*].

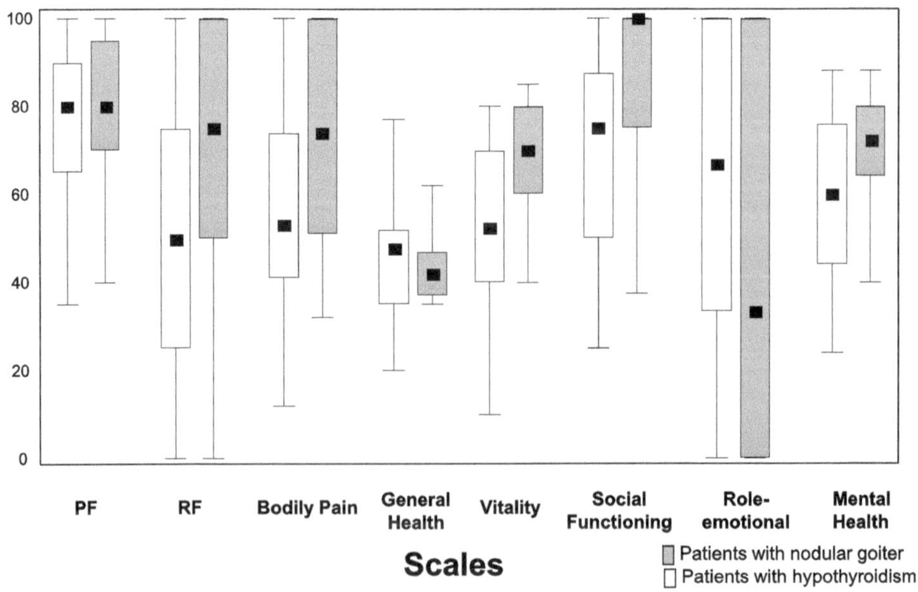

Fig. 3. Quality of life for patients with compensated hypothyroidism and with nodular goiter

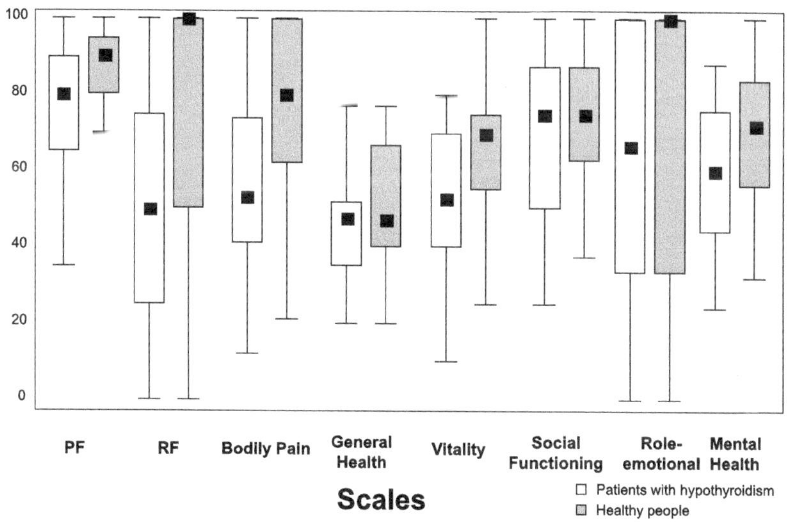

Fig. 4. Quality of life for patients with compensated hypothyroidism and healthy people

2.3 Modification of L-T4 intake (evening vs. morning)

General recommendation that L-T4 should be taken upon starving, 30-40 minutes before breakfast can lead to the poor compliance of the patients. On the other hand, failure to comply with this recommendation could result in significant worsening of the L-T4 absorption. However, as an alternative, patients can take drugs L-T4 in the evening or at night, finding the optimal time for an intake. Currently, in literature there is a discussion on a possibility of clinically significant change in TSH levels when changing the time of taking of L-T4. However, to date there are insufficient data on the feasibility and effectiveness of changing the time of taking the L-T4 drugs.

Elliott D.P. et al. have shown that the TSH level did not significantly change when shifting the time of L-T4 intake from morning (1-2 hours before breakfast) to evening hours (midnight) [*Elliott DP., 2001*].

2.4 Circadian rhythms of TSH and thyroid hormones

One of the factors which should be considered while adjusting the replacement dose of thyroid hormones is the physiological fluctuation of TSH and thyroid hormones, which is based on circadian rhythm secretion thereof. Normally, the TSH secretion occurs in a pulsating mode, whereas frequency and amplitude of pulsation increases at night, resulting in the circadian changes in TSH levels. TSH level is rising after midday, reaching a maximum of 2 - 4 hours in the morning, followed by a "plateau" for several hours and then decreasing to minimum values at midday [*Darzy KH, 2005, Persani L, 1995*]. Thus, fluctuations in TSH during the day can range from 1 to 3 mU/l. Thyroid hormone levels during the day also varies, but far less than the TSH. Thus, the study of Lucke C. et al. has shown that the level of T4 reached a maximum from 8 to 12 a.m., and reached the minimum values from 11 p.m. to 3 a.m. T3 level was highest from 7 a.m. to 1 p.m. and the lowest - from 11 p.m. to 3 a.m. Herewith, those changes in hormone levels were insignificant and did not exceed the normal indicators [*Lucke C., 1977*].

The clinical significance of TSH circadian variability is defined, first of all, by the diagnostics of thyroid dysfunction. If in a number of patients, whose level of TSH is identified in the early morning hours, allows to diagnose subclinical hypothyroidism, but when the test is made later, the TSH level in some patients falls within the reference range. Thus, in a prospective study, performed by Scobbo R.R. et al., in 97 out of 100 of outpatients, the level of TSH, identified early in the morning was approximately by 26.4% higher as compared with the repeated tests made later in the afternoon. Based on the second (later) TSH tests, in 6% of patients the diagnosis of subclinical hypothyroidism was renounced [*Darzy KH, 2005*].

Similar results were obtained by in our study of 27 healthy persons at the age of 18–60 years. Measurements of serum TSH, fT4, fT3 were performed at 8.00–9.00 and 14.00–16.00 during the day and at 8.00–9.00 in 4–6 weeks. The median of TSH concentrations in the morning was 2.28 mU/l, at the daytime - 1.6 mU/l (p 0.05). The amplitude of TSH circadian variability reached 58% (Me = 21.45%). According to the current TSH reference ranges (0.4–4.0 mU/l) all participants had an euthyroidism in the morning and at the daytime (**figure 5**). According to the proposed TSH reference ranges (0.4–2.5 mU/l) 12 participants (44.4%) in the morning and 4 participants (14.8%) at the daytime have been classified as having a hypothyroidism. TSH levels in 4–6 weeks differed from initial on 42.8–7.71% [*Sviridonova M., 2010*].

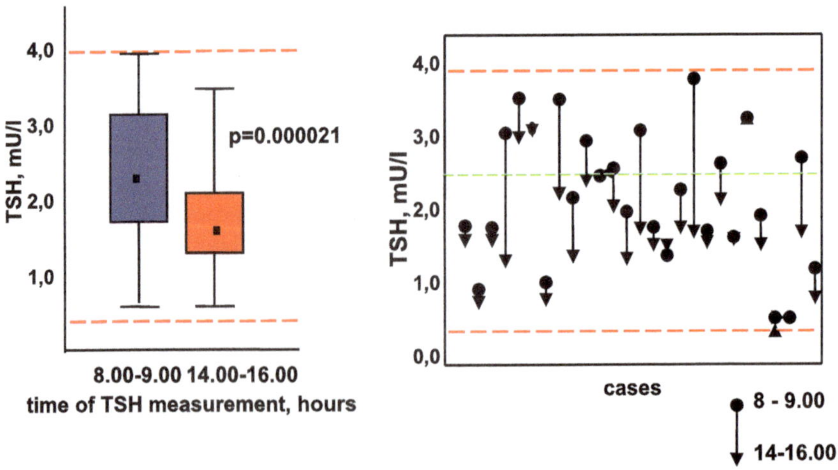

Fig. 5. Circadian variability of TSH in subjects with euthyroidism

In addition, of course, the data on circadian rhythms of TSH secretion plays an important role in assessing the adequacy of replacement therapy with thyroid hormones. Herewith, if the patients with overt hypothyroidism lose typical to healthy people increase in amplitude and frequency of TSH secretion during the night [*Adriaanse R, 1992*], the prescribing of adequate replacement therapy with thyroid hormones leads to restore of circadian rhythm of TSH secretion [*Persani L, 1995*].

2.5 Combined therapy with T3 and T4

2.5.1 Controlled trials comparing L-T4 and L-T4 + L-T3

In the last decade the problem of combined therapy with L-T4+LT3 was in the centre of attention for many publications and some controlled randomized studies were performed. There are some publications where the authors, referring to their own clinical experience in treating of patients with hypothyroidism, are in favor of combined therapy of L-T3 + L-T4. For example, according to Mazzaferri E.L., some patients taking the preparations of thyroid gland extracts of animals (containing T3 and T4) over decades, noted the deterioration of well-being during switching to monotherapy with L-T4 [*Mazzaferri EL, 1999*].

First studies about comparison of two types of treatments, mono- and combined therapy with thyroid hormones were made in the 1970s. Thus, in 1970, Smith R.N. et al. published results of a double-blind crossover study. The study included 99 patients with primary hypothyroidism (postsurgical or after treatment with radioactive iodine), previously treated with L-T4 in the doses of 200-300 µg/day. All patients were randomized into 2 groups and within 2 months received L-T4 (200 or 300 µg) or L-T3 + L-T4 (2 or 3 tablets, respectively, 20 µg of L-T3 and 80 µg of L-T4 in each tablet). After 2 months, the treatment mode has been changed: patients from group 1 received L-T3 + L-T4, and those from group 2 received L-T4. Among 87 patients who completed the study, 42 patients (48%) did not prefer any type of therapy, 29 (33%) preferred monotherapy with L-T4 and 16 (18%) - a combination of L-T3+L-T4. During the study, a higher frequency of side effects was observed (palpitations, nervousness, feeling short of breath, etc.) on the combination of L-T3 + L-T4, as compared to monotherapy with L-T4. Authors concluded that tolerability of monotherapy with L-T4 is better as compared with the combination of L-T3 + L-T4, as well as the fact that L-T4 is effective as monotherapy and is preferable because of a longer half-life [*Smith RN, 1970*]. However, it should be noted that in this study rather large doses of thyroid hormones were prescribed, especially L-T3 (40-60 µg/day), which could lead to a high frequency of side effects.

In a relatively small study by Bunevičius R. et al., which however, attracted a high interest, the authors also compared the efficacy of monotherapy and combination therapy with L-T4 and L-T3 in patients with primary hypothyroidism. The study involved 33 patients with primary hypothyroidism, developed as a result of chronic autoimmune thyroiditis (16 patients) or after thyroidectomy due to a cancer (17 patients). All the patients at the moment of enrollment received a replacement or suppressive therapy with L-T4. Patients were randomized into 2 groups: patients from group 1 received L-T4 for 5 weeks, and then a combination of L-T4 + L-T3 for 5 weeks (when changing the type of therapy, the L-T4 dose was reduced by 50 µg and supplemented with 12,5 µg of L-T3); in group 2 patients initially received L-T3 + L-T4, followed by L-T4. The results showed that the levels of cholesterol and triglycerides in both groups were similar, whereas the level of SHBG (sex hormone-binding globulin) was significantly higher on combined therapy. The authors noted that on the combined therapy, the pulse rate at rest was slightly higher, but blood pressure and results of neurophysiologic tests were similar on both regimens of treatment. To assess cognitive function and mood 17 tests were performed. Among 17 tests the results in 16 patients of both groups were normal. However, in six of 16 tests they were better or patients reported a better mood on the combined therapy with L-T4 and L-T3, rather than with L-T4 monotherapy. These results were confirmed by visual analogue scales. None of the performed tests demonstrated better results with L-T4 monotherapy versus combination therapy with L-T4 and L-T3. According to the results of the study, the authors concluded that: in patients with hypothyroidism, the use of combined therapy L-T3 and L-T4 leads to improved psychological and neurophysiological parameters, and the prescription of a combined therapy of L-T3 and L-T4 leads to a better quality of life than monotherapy with L-T4 [*Bunevičius R., 1999*]. Among disadvantages of this study that coud be mentioned, firstly - short treatment period (5 weeks), which is sufficient only for reaching the stable thyroid status after changing of the therapy [*Walsh JP, 2001*], but insufficient for assessment of the dynamics of the lipids, and secondly, the lack of adequate assessment of the cardiovascular system, which could help to identify possible changes in heart rate. Finally small number of patients was included in the study [*Walsh JP, 2001*].

Later, the results of some other similar studies were published. It should be noted, that these studies differed in the number of patients, monitoring duration and the ratio of L-T4 to L-T3 in the combined regimens. The majority of studies found no benefits of combined therapy L-T4 + L-T3, as compared with monotherapy L-T4 [*Levitt A., 2002; Sawka AM, 2003; Clyde PW, 2003; Siegmund, 2004; Rodriquez, 2005*].

One of the most interesting studies, comparing mono- and combination therapy of hypothyroidism was conducted by Walsh JP et al. [*Walsh J.P., 2003*]. The double-blind controlled study with crossover design included 110 patients with compensated hypothyroidism receiving L-T4. The patients enrolled in the study were satisfied or dissatisfied with their well-being on the replacement therapy. Patients were randomized into 2 groups: one group continued to receive monotherapy with L-T4, and the patients of the second group were switched to a combined therapy with L-T4 + L-T3, while the dose of L-T4 was reduced by 50 μg and L-T3 dose of 10 μg was added. After 10 weeks of therapy and a follow-up washout period (4 weeks of monotherapy with L-T4) replacement therapy was adjusted: the patients from group 1 were switched to a combination of L-T4 + L-T3, while the patients from the second group - to L-T4 monotherapy. All patients at each stage of treatment have undergone psychological tests (General Health Questionnaire 28 - GHQ-28, a visual analog scale), quality of life assessment (Short Form 36 - SF-36) and tests for hypothyroidism symptoms (Zulewski et al. scale, Thyroid Symptom Questionnaire - TSQ), which determined the level of TSH, freeT4, freeT3, SHBG, deoxypyridinoline, osteocalcin, alkaline phosphatase and cholesterol. The study included only women, whose average age was 47.7 ± 11.7 years. According to the results, during the combined therapy with L-T4 + L-T3, the TSH level was significantly higher than that demonstrated on monotherapy with L-T4. Increased TSH was due to inadequate replacement of L-T4 50 μg by L-T3 10 μg, and there was no L-T4 dose adjustment during the study. Thus, according to the authors, the tentative positive changes in the transition to a combination of L-T4 + L-T3 were balanced by high TSH [*Walsh J.P., 2003*]. No dynamics in the body mass and blood pressure was noted during the study. It was shown that on the combined therapy L-T4 + L-T3, the score as per Zulewski scale and total cholesterol were significantly higher than on the L-T4 monotherapy. However, given the significant increase in TSH during the combination therapy, the authors also identified a group of patients, whose TSH levels did not change. The analysis in this subgroup showed that on the L-T4 + L-T3 combined therapy, the level of freeT4 was lower than on the L-T4 monotherapy, while the total cholesterol, the sum of Zulewski scale scores and pulse rate were the same. Quality of life and psychological state of patients did not differ on those types of therapy. At the same time, indictors of anxiety were significantly higher in the combination therapy.

We also conducted a study to compare two types of replacement therapy in hypothyroidism. We conducted a randomized controlled trial with a crossover design in 36 premenopausal women with hypothyroidism. All patients were divided into two groups: Group A (n=20) was randomized to L-T4; Group B received the combined therapy first, followed by the monotherapy. The treatment periods lasted for 6 months. No significant difference between monotherapy and combined therapy was demonstrated on TSH level, ECG monitoring, densitometry, thyroid symptoms score. The lipid profiles were better during combined treatment than L-T4 alone. In the Group B during combined treatment the levels of cholesterol and LDL decreased, in the Group A during treatment with L-T4 alone the levels of cholesterol and LDL were unchanged. The levels of osteocalcin were unchanged, but the level of deoxypyridinoline decreased during combined treatment. According to other authors, there were no significant differences in total cholesterol and lipoproteins during monotherapy with L-T4 and the combination of L-T4+L-T3 [*Clyde P.W., 2003, Bunevicius R., 1999, Saravanan P., 2005*]. Apparently, the registered changes in lipoprotein profiles can be explained by the homogeneity of the groups, i.e., in this study 36 premenopausal women without any concomitant diseases were enrolled. Other studies, on the contrary, were conducted on both men and women, and the women group consisted both from women of reproductive age and women in peri- and postmenopause. According to our results, compared with L-T4 alone, replacement treatment with combination of L-T4+L-T3 shows beneficial changes in serum lipids, but higher activation of bone resorbtion [*Fadeyev, 2010*].

However, despite the lack of obvious advantages in influencing the psycho-emotional status, patients often prefer the combination compared with monotherapy L-T4 [*Saravanan P., 2005, Escobar-Morreale H.F., 2005, Appelhof B., 2005*]. According to *Escobar-Morreale H.F. et al*, of the 26 patients, 18 preferred the combination of L-T4+L-T3 [*Escobar-Morreale H.F., 2005*]. A similar result was confirmed in a large study, conducted by Appelhof B. et al [*Appelhof B., 2005*]. In this study 141 patients were randomized to receive monotherapy with L-T4, the combination of L-T4+L-T3, ratio 10:1 and L-T4+L-T3, ratio 5:1. Studied therapy was preferred to usual treatment by 29,2%, 41,3% and 52,2% in the L-T4, 10:1 ratio and 5:1 ratio groups respectively. Although patients preferred combined L-T4+L-T3 therapy to usual L-T4 therapy, but changes in mood, fatigue, well-being and neurocognitive functions could not satisfactorily explain why the primary outcome (i.e. preference of the treatment) was in favor of L-T4+L-T3 combination therapy. According to our results from 36 patients completing the study 10 preferred L-T4+L-T3 treatment (27,8 %) and 8 preferred L-T4 treatment (22,2%). It is an interesting that 50% of the patients (18 from 36) had no preference.

Among the reasons why the patients chose monotherapy with L-T4 the main ones were the following: absence of anxiety and irritability, quiet sleep. Besides, a strong reason for the patients taking 100 μg of L-T4 (i.e. 1 pill of «L-thyroxin-100») was convenient administration. Patients who preferred combination of L-T4+L-T3 noticed, improvement of mood, higher working capacity, body weight reduction (in those patients who were initially overweight; but this difference was not significant) *[Fadeyev, 2010]*.

2.5.2 Levels of thyroid hormones on the replacement monotherapy with L-T4 and combination of LT4+L-T3

Several studies have shown that in patients on replacement monotherapy with L-T4 with normal serum levels of TSH and T3, an increased level of T4 is observed [*Fish LH, 1987, Ross DS, 2001, Salmon D., 1982*]. On the contrary the normal serum levels of T4 and TSH are often accompanied by lower values of T3 than in healthy people [*Woeber KA, 2002*]. Thus, the ratio of T4 to T3 is significantly higher in patients with hypothyroidism on the replacement monotherapy with L-T4 than in healthy controls. According to Woeber K.A., a higher ratio of T4 to T3 is due to the suppression of the residual T3 secretion by the thyroid gland and low conversion of T4 to T3 in the peripheral tissues on the exogenous L-T4 therapy. It has been demonstrated in earlier studies, that replacement therapy of hypothyroidism with L-T4 is accompanied by increased ratio of T4 to T3 in the blood [*Pearce CJ, 1984, Rendell M., 1985, Stock JM, 1974*], and this ratio grows up with increasing doses of L-T4.

According to Woeber K.A., higher level of T4 and lower level of T3 during the replacement therapy with L-T4, as compared with healthy people is because TSH secretion is regulated mainly by T4. Therefore, the normal level of TSH on the monotherapy with L-T4 may be accompanied by the decreased level of T3. According to Woeber K.A., among 35 patients treated with L-T4, four patients had a reduced T3 level, and three of them had it in the lower limit of normal range [*Woeber KA, 2002*]. In addition, according to Bunevicius R. et al., in patients who received monotherapy with L-T4, total serum T3 was close to the lower limit of normal range [*Bunevičius R., 1999*]. Similar results were obtained by Alevizaki M. et al. in a large group of patients (114 healthy people and 130 patients with hypothyroidism on L-T4 monotherapy) the serum level of T3 and T3/T4 ratio in patients on the L-T4 therapy were significantly lower than in the healthy group [*Alevizaki M., 2002*].

A number of studies have shown that switching of patients with hypothyroidism from L-T4 to the combination of L-T4+L-T3 results in a reduction of FT4 levels [*Bunevičius R.,1999, Clyde P.W., 2003*], while FT3 levels increase [*Clyde P.W., 2003, Levitt A., 2002*] or remain unchanged [*Bunevičius R.,1999, Walsh J.P., 2003*]. This is most likely caused by the use of different L-T4 and L-T3 doses since there are no comprehensive recommendations for L-T4 and L-T3 dose calculation for combined therapy. Moreover, it is not clear how the L-T4 dose should be reduced after the addition of L-T3. According to available publications, the additional prescription of 10 μg [*Walsh J.P., 2003*] or 12.5 μg [*Bunevičius R.,1999*] L-T3 is associated with a reduction of L-T4 by 50 μg. However, in the study of Walsh et al, it was reported that after replacement of 50 μg of L-T4 with 10 μg of L-T3, TSH concentrations increased considerably [*Walsh J.P., 2003*]. According to Walsh et al, the increase of TSH level may be caused either by a decrease of T4 level in serum, which is considered to play the main role in the regulation of TSH production, or by the incorrect concept about the required T3:T4-ratio, which is in fact about 4:1 or even 3:1, but not 5:1 [*Walsh J.P., 2003*].

We also conducted a study to assess the level of thyroid hormones in patients with hypothyroidism receiving L-T4 monotherapy or combination therapy with L-T4 + L-T3.Fifty-eight women with primary hypothyroidism receiving L-T4 were enrolled in the study. The patients were randomised into two groups: Group 1 (n=42) patients continued monotherapy with L-T4, and Group 2 (n=16) patients were switched to combined therapy with L-T4+L-T3 (25 µg L-T4 was replaced with 12.5 µg L-T3). The final examination was carried out 6 months thereafter. There was also a third group of 20 healthy women (control group). Under monotherapy with L-T4, serum FT4 levels were higher ($p < 0.05$) and FT3 lower ($p < 0.05$) than in the control group.

Serum FT4 under combined therapy was significantly lower than in both control and monotherapy groups. FT3 levels did not differ between the two groups of combined and monotherapy subjects; the highest FT3 levels were in the control group (**figure 6**). So, monotherapy with L-T4 in hypothyroidism is associated with non-physiologically high FT4 and low FT3 levels; but therapy with L-T3 once a day does not simulate the normal production of T3 by the thyroid [*Fadeyev V., 2005*].

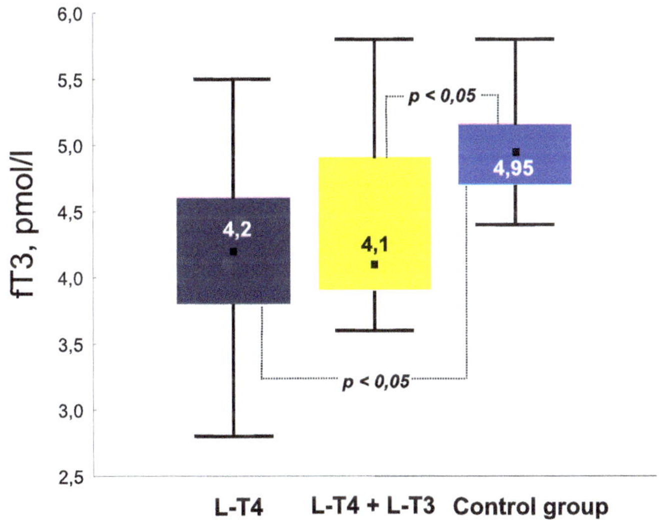

Fig. 6. Free T3 levels in patients with hypothyroidism on different replacement regimens and in controls (Me [25; 75])

2.6 Peripheral markers of thyroid hormones effects on tissues

The level of TSH is the main indicator which helps to assess the adequacy of replacement therapy of hypothyroidism. However, it reflects thyroid hormones action only on hypothalamic-pituitary axis.

Herewith, the issue of peripheral markers of replacement therapy adequacy in hypothyroidism is discussed in literature. At the same time, in clinical practice the identification of essential markers of the thyroid hormones peripheral action is difficult. In general, according to various authors, the markers of peripheral thyroid hormone effects may include: the level of total cholesterol, sex hormone-binding protein (SHBG), angiotensin-converting enzyme and markers of bone metabolism (bone formation and bone resorption) [*Ferretti E., 1999; Meier C., 2003*]. The soluble receptors of interleukin-2 may serve as a marker of the action of thyroid hormones on the lymphocytes [*Toft A.D., 2003*].

3. Target TSH level in L-T4 replacement therapy

The adequacy of the replacement therapy of hypothyroidism is estimated by the TSH level. To date, the reference range for TSH is generally accepted as 0.4 - 4.0 mU/l. However, in general population in 97% of people the TSH level is less than 5 mU/l, and upon exclusion from the sample persons with anti-thyroid-antibodies and those with goiter or close relatives with thyroid pathology, only in 8% of people the TSH level is higher than 2.5-3 mU/l [*Hollowell J., 2002*]. In 2003, the U.S. National Academy of Clinical Biochemistry has published the data that the TSH level more than 2.5 mU/l can be a predictor of hypothyroidism in the future. In addition, recommendations were given on a closer monitoring of persons with "high-normal" TSH level [*Baloch Z, 2003*].

However, to date there is insufficient evident data about advantages and disadvantages of maintaining "low-" or "high-normal" TSH levels on L-T4 replacement therapy. In 2006 were published results of a double-blind study examining the psycho-emotional state, cognitive function and some biochemical parameters in patients with hypothyroidism taking different doses of L-T4 [*Walsh J.P., 2006*]. The study included 56 women with hypothyroidism taking L-T4 and having normal TSH level at the time of enrollment. Patients took L-T4 in small, medium and high doses (dose was changed to 25 μg) for 8 weeks at each stage. According to the results, statistically significant changes were observed in the level of biochemical markers of thyroid hormones effects: the level of sex hormone binding globulin (SHBG), total cholesterol, alkaline phosphatase and deoxypyridinoline. The levels of SHBG, alkaline phosphatase and deoxypyridinoline with high L-T4 dose were significantly higher, and total cholesterol level was lower than the parameters with low-dose of L-T4. However, there was no statistically significant dynamics in quality of life parameters, symptoms of hypothyroidism and cognitive function when the dose of L-T4 was changed. The authors concluded that there are no clear advantages to maintain "low-normal" TSH levels in patients receiving L-T4 in terms of impact on psycho-emotional status and quality of life [*Walsh J.P., 2006*].

Thus, by now according to clinical studies there is not enough evidance to recommend maintenance of TSH levels in the lower range of normal values for patients with hypothyroidism on L-T4 replacement therapy.

Interesting results were obtained in the study of McDermott M.T. et al. According to a survey conducted among members of the American Thyroid Association (ATA) and general practitioners, it was found that more than 40% of the ATA-members considered the target TSH levels on L-T4 replacement therapy should be within the range of 0.5-2.0 mU/l and for elderly patients - 1.0-4.0 mU/l. GPs more often designated the target TSH levels within 0.5 - 5.0 mU/l [*McDermott M.T., 2001*].

4. Replacement therapy of hypothyroidism in specific conditions

4.1 Elderly patients with concomitant disorders

The question of the beginning of replacement therapy in elderly patients especially in the presence of concomitant cardiac pathology should be discussed separately. It is generally recommended and agreed to start replacement therapy in these situations with small doses of L-T4 (12.5 - 25 μg) with a gradual increase to full replacement during 4 – 6 months or sometimes even longer. Although treatment of hypothyroidism with L-T4 could improve myocardial function and reduce peripheral vascular resistance, it could increase the need for oxygen in the myocardium. In patients with an already compromised myocardial blood supply due to coronary atherosclerosis, L-T4 treatment may provoke anginal symptoms. Patients with preexisting angina should be evaluated for obstructive coronary lesions before the beginning of L-T4 therapy.

4.2 Secondary hypothyroidism

Replacement therapy with thyroid hormones in the secondary hypothyroidism (SH) has some special features. First of all, as secondary hypothyroidism in adults is often associated with deficit of other pituitary hormones, the symptoms of thyroid hormone deficiency are "disguised" by deficiency of other hormones. In addition the level of TSH in SH is often normal at the time of diagnosis [*Ferretti E.,1999, Alexopoulou, 2004*], and decreases after the beginning of replacement therapy (in 2/3 of patients) [*Carrozza V, 1999*]. Corticosteroids taking for secondary hypocorticism also lead to reducing the TSH level. Thus, the TSH level cannot be a criterion for the compensation of SH. That is why generally recommended marker for its compensation is free T4 level which suggested to be in the upper third of the reference range in combination with normal level of free T3. Although the T3 level in spite of L-T4 substitution is often reduced. Thus, according to Alexopoulou et al, the level of free T3 is reduced in more than half of patients, despite normal levels of freeT4 [*Alexopoulou, 2004*].

Monotherapy with L-T4 is a preferred method of treatment in secondary hypothyroidism. Estimated dose, as in the situation with primary hypothyroidism, is about 1.6 μg per kilogram of body weight on average. However, the dose of L-T4 may differ significantly between patients often due to the effect of some medications. Most frequently, the L-T4 dose adjustment is required when patients are taking injections of growth hormone leading to increase of T4 to T3 deiodination in peripheral tissues finally leading to increase of L-T4 dose. The same situation could be due to estrogens replacement therapy in women. The adequacy of replacement therapy with L-T4 should be assessed in 4 - 6 weeks after the appointment of full replacement dose. After the adjustment of adequate L-T4 dose, the level of thyroid hormones is also advisable to control at least once per year.

4.3 Pregnancy

The recommended treatment of hypothyroidism during pregnancy is with oral L-T4. According to Guidelines of the American thyroid association the goal of L-T4 treatment is to normalize maternal serum TSH values within the trimester-specific pregnancy reference range (first trimester, 0,1-2,5 mIU/L; second trimester, 0,2-3,0 mIU/L; third trimester, 0,3-3,0 mIU/L).

Clinical studies have confirmed that the increased requirement for L-T4 occurs beginning from 4-6 weeks of gestation. About 50-85% of women with compensated hypothyroidism (receiving L-T4) need to increase the dose of L-T4 during pregnancy [*Abalovich M., 2002, Mandel S.J., 1990, Alexander E.K., 2004*]. The greater dose increase will required to the patients with hypothyroidism after radioablation, surgery in comparison with women with autoimmune thyroiditis [*Kaplan M.M., 1996, Loh J.A., 2009*].

4.4 Subclinical hypothyroidism

Whether or not subclinical hypothyroidism in adults should be treated was and still is hotly debated; there are strong defenders as well as strong opponents to levothyroxine treatment. Pregnancy or the desire to become pregnant in case of infertility are the indications for replacement therapy.

5. References

[1] Abalovich M, Gutierrez S, Alcaraz G, Maccallini G, Garcia A, Levalle O. //Overt and subclinical hypothyroidism complicating pregnancy.// Thyroid-2002-12:63-68.

[2] Adriaanse R., Romijn J.A., Endert E., Wiersinga W.M. //The nocturnal TSH surge is absent in overt but present in mild primary hypothyroidism and equivocal in central hypothyroidism //Acta Endocrinol. (Copenh). -1992.- P. 126 206–126212.

[3] Alevizaki M., Mantzou E., Cimponeriu A.T., et al. //Evidence for tissue hypothyroidism in treated hypothyroid patients with "euthyroid" TSH levels. // J. Endocrinol. Invest. – 2002 – Vol. 25 – Suppl. to no.7 – P.083.

[4] Alexander EK, Marqusee E, Lawrence J, Jarolim P, Fischer GA, Larsen PR. //Timing and magnitude of increases in levothyroxine requirements during pregnancy in women with hypothyroidism//N Engl J Med. Jul -2004-15;351(3):241-9.

[5] Alexopoulou O, Beguin C, De Nayer P, Maiter D.// Clinical and hormonal characteristics of central hypothyroidism at diagnosis and during follow-up in adult patients// Eur J Endocrinol. 2004 Jan;150(1):1-8.

[6] Appelhof B, Fliers E, Wekking EM et al. //Combined therapy with levothyroxine and liothyronine in two ratios, compared with levothyroxine monotherapy in primary hypothyroidism: a double-blind, randomized, controlled clinical trial. J Clin Endocrinol Metab 90: 2666-2674.

[7] Arafah B. "Increased need for thyroxine in women with hypothyroidism during estrogen therapy"// The New England journal of medicine. – 2000 – vol. 344, №23. - p.1743-1749.

[8] Baloch Z., Carayon P., ConteDevolx B. et al. Guidelines Committee, National Academy of Clinical Biochemistry. Laboratory medicine practice guidelines. Laboratory support for the diagnosis and monitoring of thyroid disease // Thyroid. 2003. V. 13. P. 3–126

[9] Bianchi P., Zaccheroni V., Solaroli E., Vescini F., Cerutti R., Zoli M., Marchesini G. "Health-related quality of life in patients with thyroid disorders"// Quality of Life Research. – 2004. – vol.13, №1. – p.45-54.

[10] Braverman L.E., Ingbar S.H., Sterling K. // Conversion of thyroxine (T4) to triiodothyronine (T3) in athyreotic human subjects. // The Journal of clinical investigation. – 1970. – Vol. 49, N 5. – P. 855-864.

[11] Bunevičius R., Kažanavičius G., Žalinkevičius R., Prangc A.J. // Effects of thyroxine as compared with thyroxine plus triiodothyronine in patients with hypothyroidism. // The New England Journal of Medicine. – 1999. – Vol. 340, N 6. – P. 424-429.

[12] Canaris G., Manowitz N., Mayor G., Ridgway E. "The Colorado thyroid disease prevalence study"// Arch. Internal medicine. – 2000. - vol.160. -p.526-534

[13] Carrozza V, Csako G, Yanovski JA, Skarulis MC, Nieman L, Wesley R, Pucino F. //Levothyroxine replacement therapy in central hypothyroidism: a practice report.//Pharmacotherapy. 1999 Mar;19(3):349-55.

[14] Centanni M, Gargano L, Canettieri G et al "Thyroxine in goiter, helicobacter pylori infection, and chronic gastritis"//N Engl J Med – 2006; №354, p.1787-1795

[15] Clyde P.W.; Harari A. E.; Getka E. J.; Shakir K. M. // Combined Levothyroxine Plus Liothyronine Compared With Levothyroxine Alone in Primary Hypothyroidism. // JAMA - 2003 – Vol. 290, N. 22 – P. 2952-2958.

[16] Cuthbertson D., Flynn R., Jung R., Leese G. "Optimisation of thyroid hormone replacement using an automated thyroid register."// Int J Clin Pract. – 2006. – vol. 60, №6 - p. 660-664.

[17] Darzy K.H., Shalet S.M. Circadian and stimulated thyrotropin secretion in cranially irradiated adult cancer survivors // J. Clin. Endocrinol. Metab. 2005. V. 90. P. 6490–6497.

[18] Demet M., Ozmen B., Deveci A. et al. "Depression and anxiety in hypothyroidism"// West Indian Med.J. – 2003.– vol. 52, № 3. – p.233-237

[19] Diez J.J. "Hypothyroidism in patients older than 55 years: an analysis of the etiology and assessment of the effectiveness of therapy"// J.gerontol a boil sci med sci. - 2002. – vol.57, № 5. - p.315-320.

[20] Elliott DP. Effect of levothyroxine administration time on serum TSH in elderly patients// Ann Pharmacother. 2001 May;35(5):529-32.

[21] Escobar-Morreale HF, Botella-Carretero JI, Gomez-Bueno M, Galán JM, Barrios V, Sancho J, 2005 Thyroid Hormone Replacement Therapy in Primary Hypothyroidism: A Randomized Trial Comparing L-Thyroxine plus Liothyronine with L-Thyroxine Alone. Ann Intern Med 142: 412–424

[22] Fadeyev V., Morgunova T., Manuylova Y. "L-thyroxine replacement therapy: factors of compensation quality"// 33th Annual Meeting of the ETA-Sep, 2008.

[23] Fadeyev V., Morgunova T., Melnichenko G. "TSH and thyroid hormones concentrations in patients with hypothyroidism receiving replacement therapy with L-thyroxine alone or in combination with L-triiodothyronine"// Hormones 2005, 4(2):101-107

[24] Fadeyev V., Morgunova T., Melnichenko G., Dedov I. "Combined Therapy With L-Thyroxine and L-Triiodothyronine Compared to L-Thyroxine Alone in the Treatment of Primary Hypothyroidism"// Hormones 2010, 9(3):245-252

[25] Ferretti E., Persani L., Jaffrain-Rea M.L., et al. // Evaluation of the adequacy of levothyroxine replacement therapy in patients with central hypothyroidism. // J Clin Endocrinol Metab – 1999 – Vol. 84 – N.3 – P. 924-932

[26] Fish L.H., Schwartz H.L., Cavanaugh J. et al. // Replacement dose, metabolism, and bioavailability of levothyroxine in the treatment of hypothyroidism. Role of

triiodothyronine in pituitary feedback in humans. // N. Engl. J. Med. - 1987. - Vol. 316. - P. 764.

[27] Gold M., Pottash A., Extein I. "Hypothyroidism and depression. Evidence from complete thyroid function evaluation".//JAMA. - 1981. - 15; 245(19).-p. 1919-1922.

[28] Gow S.M., Caldwell G., Toft A.D. et al. // Relationship between pituitary and other target organ responsiveness in hypothyroid patients receiving thyroxine replacement. // The Journal of clinical endocrinology and metabolism. - 1987. - Vol. 64, N 2. - P. 364-370.

[29] Haggerty J., Prange A.// "Borderline hypothyroidism an depression"// Annual review of medicine. - 1995. - vol.46. - p.37-46.

[30] Hanna F., Lazarus H., Scanlon M. "Controversial aspects of thyroid disease"// British medical journal. - 1999. - vol.319.-p.894-898

[31] Havrankova J., Lahaie R. "Levothyroxine binding by sucralfate"// Annals of internal medicine - 1992-117-p.445-446.

[32] Hollowell J., Staehling N., Flanders W. et al. "Serum TSH, T4 and thyroid antibodies in the United States population (1988 to 1994): National Health and Nutrition Examination Survey (NHANES-III)"//J.clinical endocrinology and metabolism. - 2002. - vol.87, №2. - p.489-499.

[33] Hueston W. "Treatment of hypothyroidism"// American family physician. - 2001- vol. 64. -p. 1717-1724.

[34] Joffe R., Levitt A. "Major depression and subclinical (grade 2) hypothyroidism".// Psychoneuroendocrinology. - 1992.- vol. 17, №2-3. - p.215-221.

[35] Kaplan MM. 1996 Management of thyroxine therapy during pregnancy// Endocr Pract. 1996 Jul-Aug;2(4):281-6.

[36] Ladenson P. "Psychological wellbeing in patients".//Clinical endocrinology. - 2002. - vol.57-p.575-576.

[37] Leese G., Jung R., Scott A., Waugh N., Brouning M. "Long-term follow-up of treated hyperthyroid and hypothyroid patients."// Health bull (Edinburg). - 1993. - vol.51, №3. - p.177-183.

[38] Levitt A., Silverberg J. // T4 plus T3 treatment for hypothyroidism: a double-blind comparison with usual T4.// 74th Annual Meeting of the American Thyroid Association. Los Angeles, California, October 10-13, 2002.

[39] Lindsay R., Toft A., "Hypothyroidism".// Lancet. - 1997. - vol.349, № 9049. - p.413-417.

[40] Loh JA, Wartofsky L, Jonklaas J, Burman KD. 2009 The magnitude of increased levothyroxine requirements in hypothyroid pregnant women depends upon the etiology of the hypothyroidism// Thyroid. 2009 Mar;19(3):269-75.

[41] Lucke C, Hehrmann R, von Mayersbach K, von zur Mühlen A. // Studies on circadian variations of plasma TSH, thyroxine and triiodothyronine in man // Acta Endocrinol (Copenh) - 1977- Sep;86(1):81-8.

[42] Mandel SJ, Larsen PR, Seely EW, Brent GA. 1990 Increased need for thyroxine during pregnancy in women with primary hypothyroidism// N Engl J Med. Jul 12;323(2):91-6.

[43] Mazzaferri E.L. // The New England Journal of Medicine. - 1999. - Vol. 340, N 6. - P. 430.

[44] McDermott M., Haugen B., Lezotte D., Seggelke S., Ridgway E. "Management practices among primary care physicians and thyroid specialists in the care of hypothyroid patients."// Thyroid. - 2001. - vol.11, №8. - p. 757 - 764.

[45] Meier C., Trittibach P., Guglielmetti M., Staub JJ., et al. // Serum thyroid stimulating hormone in assessment of severity of tissue hypothyroidism in patients with overt

primary thyroid failure: cross sectional survey // BMJ - 2003 - Vol. 326 - P. 311-312
[46] Morgunova T., Manuilova Yu., Madyarova M.,Lichodei N., Fadeyev V. Quality of life in patients with hypothyroidism // Клиническая и экспериментальная тиреоидология 2010 N2 стр.62
[47] Munoz-Cruzado Poce M., Carcia Navas A., Moreno Gomez M. et al. "Prevalence of thyroid disorders in patients diagnosed with depression."// Attention primaria. - 2000. - vol.26, №3. - p.176-179.
[48] Oppenheimer J.H., Braverman L.E., Toft A. et al. // A therapeutic controversy. Thyroid hormone treatment: when and what? // J. Clin. Endocrinol. Metab. - 1995. - Vol. 80, N 10. - P. 2873-2876.
[49] Parle J., Franklyn J., Cross K., Jones S., Sheppard M. "Prevalence and follow-up of abnormal thyrotrophin (TSH) concentration in the elderly in the United Kingdom."// Clin. Endocrinology (Oxford). - 1991. - vol.34, №1. -p.77-83.
[50] Pearce C.J., Himsworth R.L. // Total and free thyroid hormone concentrations in patients receiving maintenance replacement treatment with thyroxine. // British medical journal. - 1984. - Vol. 288, N 6418. - P. 693-695.
[51] Persani L., Terzolo M., Asteria C. et al. Circadian variations of thyrotropin bioactivity in normal subjects and patients with primary hypothyroidism//J. Clin. Endocrinol. Metab. 1995. V. 80. P. 2722–2728.
[52] Pies R.W. "The diagnosis and treatment of subclinical hypothyroidism states in depression patients".// Gen.Hosp.Psychiatry. - 1997. - vol.19, №5. - p.344-354.
[53] Rack S., Makela E. "Hypothyroidism and depression: a therapeutic challenge".// The annals of pharmacotherapy. - 2000. - vol.34, №1. - p.1142-1145.
[54] Rendell M., Salmon. // 'Chemical hyperthyroidism': the significance of elevated serum thyroxine levels in L-thyroxine treated individuals. // Clinical endocrinology. - 1985. - Vol. 22, N 6. - P. 693-700.
[55] Roos A, Linn-Rasker SP, van Domburg RT, Tijssen JP, Berghout A. The starting dose of levothyroxine in primary hypothyroidism treatment. A prospective, randomized, double-blind trial. Arch Int Med 2005; 165: 1714-1720.
[56] Ross D.S. // Endocrinology and metabolism clinics of North America. - 2001. - Vol. 30, N 2. - P. 245-264.
[57] Salmon D., Rendell M., Williams J. et al. // Chemical hyperthyroidism: serum triiodothyronine levels in clinically euthyroid individuals treated with levothyroxine. // Archives of internal medicine. - 1982. - Vol. 142, N 3. - P. 571-573.
[58] Stagnaro-Green A, Abalovich M, Alexander E, Azizi F, Mestman J, Negro R, Nixon A, Pearce EN, Soldin OP, Sullivan S, Wiersinga W. 2001 Guidelines of the american thyroid association for the diagnosis and management of thyroid disease during pregnancy and postpartum// Thyroid. Oct; 21(10):1081-125.
[59] Saravanan P., Chau F., Roberts N., Vedhara K., Greenwood R., Dayan C.M. "Psychological well-being in patients on 'adequate' doses of L-thyroxine".// Clinical endocrinology.- 2002. - vol.57, №5 - p.577-585.
[60] Saravanan P, Siddique H, Simmons DJ, Greenwood R, Dayan CM. Twenty-four hour hormone profiles of TSH, Free T3 and free T4 in hypothyroid patients on combined T3/T4 therapy. Exp Clin Endocrinol Diabetes. 2007 Apr;115(4):261-7.
[61] Saravanan P, Simmons DJ, Greenwood R, Peters TJ, Dayan CM, 2005 Partial Substitution of Thyroxine (T4) with Tri-Iodothyronine in Patients on T4

Replacement Therapy: Results of a Large Community-Based Randomized Controlled Trial. J Clin Endocrinol Metab 90: 805-812.
[62] Sawka A. M., Gerstein H. C., Marriott M. J., et al // Does a Combination Regimen of Thyroxine (T4) and 3,5,3'-Triiodothyronine Improve Depressive Symptoms Better Than T4 Alone in Patients with Hypothyroidism? Results of a Double-Blind, Randomized, Controlled Trial. // J. Clin. Endocrinol. And Metab. – 2003 – Vol. 88 – N. 10 – P. 4551-4555.
[63] Sevinc A., Savli H. "Hypothyroidism masquerading as depression: the role of noncompliance".// J.Natl.Med.Assoc. – 2004. – vol.96, №3. - p.379-382.
[64] Singh N., Singh P., Hershman J. "Effect of calcium carbonate on the absorption of levothyroxine."//JAMA. – 2000. – vol.283, №21. - p.2822-2825.
[65] Smith R.N., Taylor S.A., Massey J.C. // Controlled clinical trial of combined triiodothyronine and thyroxine in the treatment of hypothyroidism. // British Medical Journal. – 1970. – Vol. 4. - P. 145-148.
[66] Stock J.M., Surks M.I., Oppenheimer J.H. // Replacement dosage of L-thyroxine in hypothyroidism. A re-evaluation. // N. Engl. J. Med. – 1974. – Vol. 290. – P. 529-533.
[67] Surks M.I., Schadlow A.R., Stock J.M., Oppenheimer J.H. // Determination of iodothyronine absorption and conversion of L-thyroxine (T 4) to L-triiodothyronine (T 3) using turnover rate techniques. // The Journal of clinical investigation. – 1973. – Vol. 52, N 4. – P. 805-811.
[68] Sviridonova M.A., Fadeyev V.V., Ilyin A.V. Circadian and individual variability of TSH and thyroid hormones in subjects with euthyroidism// Клиническая и экспериментальная тиреоидология 2010 N1, стр.39
[69] Toft AD // Thyroxine therapy. // The New England journal of medicine. – 1994. – Vol. 331, N 3. – P. 174-180.
[70] Toft A.D. // Thyroid hormone replacement--one hormone or two? // N. Engl. J. Med. - 1999. – Vol. 340. – P. 469-470.
[71] Toft A.D., Beckett G.J. // Thyroid function tests and hypothyroidism // BMJ - 2003 - Vol. 326- P. 295-296
[72] Walsh JP, Shiels L, Lim EE, et al, 2003 Combined thyroxine/liothyronine treatment does not improve well-being, quality of life, or cognitive function compared to thyroxine alone: a randomized controlled trial in patients with primary hypothyroidism. J Clin Endocrinol Metab 88: 4543-4550.
[73] Walsh J.P., Stuckey B.G.A. // Med. J. Aust. – 2001. – Vol. 174. – P. 141-143.
[74] Walsh J., Ward L., Burke V., Bhagat C. et al. "Small changes in thyroxine dosage do not produce measurable changes in hypothyroid symptoms, well-being or quality of life: results of a double blind, randomized clinical trial."// J Clin Endocrinol Metab. – 2006. – vol.91. - p. 2624 – 2630.
[75] Weetman A. //Hypothyroidism: screening and subclinical disease.// British medical journal. – 1997. – vol. 314. – p. 1175-1178.
[76] Wekking E., Appelhof B., Fliers E., Schene A. et al. "Cognitive functioning and well-being in euthyroid patients on thyroxine replacement therapy for primary hypothyroidism."// European journal of endocrinology. – 2005. -vol.153 - issue 6. – p.747-753.
[77] Woeber K.A. // Levothyroxine therapy and serum free thyroxine and free triiodothyronine concentrations.// J Endocrinol. Invest. – 2002. – Vol. 25. – P. 106-109.

12

Hypothyroidism and Radioiodine Therapy

Otakar Kraft
Clinic of Nuclear Medicine, University Hospital Ostrava, Ostrava and Faculty of Medicine, University of Ostrava, Ostrava, Czech Republic

1. Introduction

Thyroid diseases are the most common endocrinopathies. In the Czech Republic they make up 80 to 90% workload of the endocrine centers. Thyroid diseases requiring treatment or at least follow up affect at least 5% of our population, for women middle-aged and older 10 to 15%.

In some thyroid diseases radioiodine ^{131}I has been used for treatment.

Hypothyroidism arises most often in the Czech Republic on the basis of chronic autoimmune thyroiditis, hypothyroidism is relatively common as artificial - after surgical or radioiodine therapy (RAIT) of various diseases of the thyroid gland.

2. Hyperthyroidism

In hyperthyroidism three major treatment modalities are currently available: antithyroid drugs, radioiodine and surgery, each of which presents advantages and restrictions (Surk et al.,1990). RAIT is considered as the most comfortable and economical approach of hyperthyroidism treatment caused by Graves´ disease or toxic nodular goiter. Such treatment is indicated in patients with/or without functional autonomy to normalize thyroid function, and to reduce thyroid volume (Meier et al., 2002).

The therapeutic use of radioiodine to treat hyperthyroidism from Grave's disease was first reported by Saul Hertz in 1941. Hertz administered produced a I-130 - I-131 mixture as a therapeutic dose to the first human patient with Graves' disease at Massachusetts General Hospital. This was the first successful treatment of humans with an artificially produced radioactive material. Gradually a series of 29 patients were treated and documented (http://en.wikipedia.org/wiki/Saul_Hertz#cite_note-10). The Journal of the American Medical Association published in May 1946 the paper with results of a five year follow up study of the 29 patients and documented the successful treatment and safety of radioactive iodine for the treatment of hyperthyroidism. The follow-up study firmly launched the use of RAIT as a standard treatment for Graves´ disease (Hertz & Roberts, 1946).

RAIT is applied mostly in hyperthyroid adults. However, it has recently gained appreciation also in children (Brown, 2009). In children radioiodine treatment should be considered in recurrent toxic goiter and in cases of ineffective thyrostatic drugs (Cooper, 2003). RAIT of

Graves' disease was introduced 70 years ago, and it is estimated that more than one million individuals have been treated with ^{131}I for hyperthyroidism (Chapman, 1983). The use of radioactive iodine has been detailed for more than 1200 children (Rivkees et al., 1998). Patients as young as 1 yr of age have been treated with ^{131}I with excellent outcomes (Rivkees et al.1998). Some studies have reported remission rates that exceed 95%, with very rare complications (Levy et al., 1988, Read et al., 2004, Rivkees et al.1998). Properly administered radioactive iodine remains an ideal form of treatment for Graves' disease in the pediatric population and it is an effective cure for Graves' disease which is associated with few acute side effects (Rivkees & Dinauer 2007). When radioiodine is used at appropriate doses, there is a very high cure rate without increased risks of thyroid cancer or genetic damage (Rivkees, 2001). Also data of Moll & Patel (Moll & Patel, 1997) from nearly 8 years experience with ^{131}I therapy support consideration of RAIT within 3 to 6 months of diagnosis of pediatric Graves´ disease as an effective, efficient, and probably safe alternative approach to the traditional antithyroid therapy of Graves´ disease in children.

For 70 years radioidine has been used to treat most cases of Graves´ disease and thyroid autonomies. The thyroid gland utilizes iodine for the synthesis of thyroid hormones. The cells do not differentiate between stable and radioactive iodine. If radioactive iodine is administered, it is trapped and then organified by thyroid follicular cells like nonradioactive iodine. The therapeutic effects of ^{131}I sodium iodide are due to the emission of ionizing radiation from the decaying radionuclide. The therapy is based on short-range beta radiation from radioactive ^{131}I. The beta particles, due to their high mean energy (190 keV, with typical beta-decay spectra present) have a tissue penetration of 0.6 to 2 mm (Skugor, 2006). Radioiodine administration should be preceded by pharmacological normalization of fT4 and fT3 levels, beacause post-radiation thyrocyte destruction and thyroid hormone release can lead to hyperthyroidism exacerbation (Gurgul & Sowinski, 2011). In some cases it is possible to withdraw antithyroid drugs 10-14 days before radioiodine administration to restore appropiate iodine uptake. It is known that one of the cause of reduced ^{131}I uptake and shortened effective half life is pre-treatment with antithyroid drugs (ATD), which may have an additional radio-protective effect. It can influence the outcome of ^{131}I therapy (Sabri et al., 2001, Walter et al., 2002) with possibility a risk of treatment failure for lower delivered radioiodine doses to the target tissue (Dunkelmann et al., 2005). Tuttle et al. describe that antithyroid drug therapy has been associated with relative radioresistance and with a decrease in radioiodine therapy effectiveness (Tuttle et al., 1995). A similar effect as longer discontinuation of ATD (10-14 days) can be obtained when ATD is discontinued 24 hours before ^{131}I administration („bounce effect") (Gurgul & Sowinski, 2011). But in severe hyperthyreoidism it is not possible to withdraw ATD for a long time, that is why discontinuation of ATD starting two or three days before ^{131}I is now widely accepted (Walter et al., 2002). 2-day ATD withdrawal prior to radioiodine administration sufficiently increases the radioiodine uptake and does not exacerbate hyperthyroidism compared to 7-day withdrawal in Graves´ disease patients. There is not significant diference in RAIT outcomes between 2-day and 7-day groups. In order to prevent serum thyroid hormone increase after ATD withdrawal and RAIT, a 2-day ATD withdrawal period before RAIT may be useful for high-risk patients such as the elderly and patients with cardiac complications (Kubota et al., 2006). Pretreatment with propylthiouracil but not methimazole, discontinued even 15 days before radioiodine administration, reduces the rate of success of ^{131}I therapy. Propylthiouracil pretreatment and large goiters are related to failure of radioiodine therapy.

Propylthiouracil should be avoided if radioiodine is considered in the management of hyperthyroid patients with Graves´ disease (Santos et al., 2004). Bonnema et al. (Bonnema et al., 2004) have shown, in a randomized set-up, that propylthiouracil treatment before ^{131}I therapy for hyperthyroid diseases approximately halves the cure rate at 1 year and that after classification the outcome into two categories, cured (euthyroidism or hypothyroidism) or not cured (recurrence), the treatment failure rate in patients with toxic nodular goiter was approximately 4 times as high in the propylthiouracil pretreatment group as in the group without propylthiouracil pretreatment, whereas the diference among patients with Graves' disease was less obvious. Andrade et al. have demonstrated that thyroid hormone levels stabilize or decrease after RAIT in patients with Graves' hyperthyroidism who are not pretreated with ATD (Andrade et al., 1999). Andrade et al. proved that short term increase in thyroid hormone levels in patients with Graves' hyperthyroidism receiving RAIT occurs mainly as a result of discontinuing antithyroid drug therapy. Among patients who received RAIT without pretreatment, serum thyroid hormone levels did not change or decreased in the 30-day interval after radioiodine administration. They postulated that RAIT without pretreatment with ATD can be safely prescribed (Andrade et al., 1999). Burch et al. (Burch et al., 2001) concluded that pretreatment with ATD does not protect against worsening thyrotoxicosis after radioiodine, but this pretreatment provides a measure of protection by establishing lower baseline values should an exacerbation of thyrotoxicosis occur. The findings support the recommendation that most patients with Graves' disease do not require antithyroid drug pretreatment before receiving radioiodine.

In benign conditions such as Graves´ disease, division of some metabolically active cells is prevented by the effect of the ionizing radiation of radioiodine. Cell death is another mechanism activated when the cells are exposed to high levels of radiation, for example in autonomous adenoma, where the suppressed normal thyroid tissue is essentially spared with delivery of a very high concentration to the cells of the autonomous adenoma (toxic nodule). Cell death is followed by replacement with connective tissue, which may lead to hypothyroidism, depending on the number of cells destroyed and replaced by fibrous nonfunctioning tissue. Since 90% of the radiation effects of ^{131}I are due to beta radiation, which has a short range in tissue, the extrathyroid radiation, and consequently the side effects, are minimal.

The potential risk after radioiodine therapy of hyperthyroidism that is most extensively discussed in the literature is cancer induction (Lacko et al., 2001, Reiners, 1997, Vlček & Neumann, 2002). Since the 1980s, large-scale, long-term (15–17 years) follow-up studies of cancer risk in patients treated with radioiodine for hyperthyroidism have been reported (Franklyn et al., 1999, Goldman et al., 1988, Hoffman et al., 1982, Holm et al., 1991) with conflicting results. The first 2 longterm studies were continuations of the Cooperative Thyrotoxicosis Therapy Follow-up Study (Hoffman et al., 1982, Goldman et al., 1988). Hoffman et al. (Hoffman et al., 1982) reported no difference between 1005 women treated with radioactive iodine and 2141 women treated with surgery for hyperthyroidism in total cancer incidence, breast cancer, or leukemia. Although based on a small number of cases, an elevated risk of cancer was observed in the thyroid gland and other organs that concentrate radioiodine (salivary glands, digestive tract, kidney, and bladder) (Hoffman et al., 1982). In a study of Goldman et al. (Goldman et al., 1988) the cancer incidence of 1762 hyperthyroid women (80% treated with radioactive iodine) did not differ from that of US white women. In a large population-based study of 10552 Swedish patients who received RAIT for hyperthyroidism, significantly elevated overall cancer incidence was observed compared with the Swedish population (Holm et al., 1991). Among 10-year survivors, significantly elevated risks were seen for cancers of the stomach, brain, and kidney (Holm et al., 1991). In a population-based study of 7417 patients treated with radioiodine for hyperthyroidism in Birmingham (UK), the overall cancer incidence and mortality decreased, but the incidence and mortality of cancers of the small bowel and the thyroid gland were increased compared with expected rates (Franklyn et al., 1999). According to the American Cooperative Thyrotoxicosis Therapy Follow-up Study (Ron et al., 1998) RAIT of hyperthyroidism was linked to a slightly increased risk for thyroid cancer. Metso proved that cancer incidence, especially cancer of the stomach, kidney, and breast, was higher in patients treated with radioiodine for hyperthyroidism (Metso et al., 2007). On the other hand, a Swedish follow-up study did not reveal any increased risk of thyroid cancer (Holm et al., 1991). Although radioactive iodine is being used in progressively younger ages, it is not known if there is an age below which high-dose ^{131}I therapy should be avoided. Risks of thyroid cancer after external irradiation are highest in children younger than 5 yr of age and progressively decline with advancing age (Boice, 1998, 2006, Dolphin, 1968, Read et al., 2004). If there is residual thyroid tissue in young children after RAIT, there is a theoretical risk of thyroid cancer. It may therefore be prudent to avoid RAIT in children younger than 5 years (Rivkees & Dinauer, 2007). In addition to thyroid cancer, potential influences of ^{131}I therapy on other cancers need to be considered. Follow-up from the large cohort of the Cooperative Thyrotoxicosis Therapy Follow-Up Study did not find increased risks of leukemia in the ^{131}I -treated group, as compared with the drug- and surgery-treated groups (Saenger et al., 1968). No increase in overall cancer mortality was seen in the ^{131}I-treated patients either (Ron et al., 1998). In one other study, excess thyroid cancer mortality after ^{131}I therapy for Graves' disease was observed during early, but not late, follow-up (Hall et al., 1992a). Yet this was related to increased cancer surveillance and detection, not ^{131}I effects (Hall et al., 1992a). Edmonds and Smith (Edmonds & Smith, 1986) reported a small but significant excess of incidence and mortality of leukemia in 258 patients treated with high-activity radioiodine for thyroid cancer (2960 MBq to 5550 MBq). However, no increased risk for malignancies of the hematopoietic system was found in the study of Metso et al. (Metso et al., 2007), which is in the agreement with earlier studies on patients treated with radioactive iodine (370 MBq to 555 MBq) for hyperthyroidism (Franklyn et al., 1999, Hall et al., 1992b, Hoffman et al., 1982, Holm et al., 1991). No increase in the risk of thyroid malignancies has been observed in patients treated with radioiodine for hyperthyroidism in most of the published long-term follow-up studies (Augusti et al., 2000, Goldman et al., 1988, Holm et al., 1991).

Several factors affect the therapeutic activity to be administered to patients suffering from hyperthyroidism including factors related to gland itself, particularly its size, the level of radioiodine uptake, the rate of iodine turnover in the gland (measured by the effective half-life), scintigraphic findings of uniform or nonuniform uptake, and whether nodules are present. The dose (in Gray) is dependent on how the nuclear medicine physician defines the goals of therapy. If the control of hyperthyroidism is the most important consideration, the total activity (in megabecquerels - MBq) or the dose per gram of estimated thyroid tissue weight will be higher than when the physician is trying to avoid or delay hypothyroidism. In our department we use individually calculated therapeutic radioiodine activity (in MBq) using Marinelli´s formula (Marinelli et al., 1948):

$$\text{Activity} = K * \frac{\text{Absorbed Dose} * \text{Volume}}{\text{Max. Uptake}\ (\%) * \text{eff. Half - life}}$$

K = 24,94; absorbed dose in Gray-Gy; volume of target thyroid tissue in ml or weight in g; effective half time in days

We calculate it from a formula referring to thyroid volume, radioiodine uptake and its half-life time. But it is difficult to determine the radioiodine sensitivity of thyroid tissue which depends on the structure of normal sized thyroid or goiter and is individually variable. This parameter cannot be estimated and that is why it is difficult to predict the effectiveness of RAIT. While waiting for the effects of the RAIT, thyroid function should be controlled regularly. If hyperthyreoidism is still present 4-6 months after ^{131}I administration, the therapy can be repeated. However, in some patients the therapeutic effects can be observed up to 12 months later (Cooper, 2003, Gurgul & Sowinski, 2011, Nygaard et al., 1999b). In our opinion calculated radioiodine activity is advantageous and we prefer it in RAIT, but some authors prefer fixed activities (Leslie et al., 2003).

2.1 Graves´ disease

Thyroid scintigraphy shows uniform uptake throughout thyroid gland (Fig. 1) or varying degrees of nonuniform uptake.

This nonuniformity is related predominantly to different stages of involution of the disease with variable amounts of fibrosis based on the duration of the disease. Infiltration of extraocular muscles by an inflammatory reaction consisting predominantly of lymphocytes is the main pathological feature of ophtalmopathy. These lymphocytes are sensitized to antigens common to the orbital muscles and thyroid gland.

Indications for RAIT include recurrent hyperthyroidism after thyrostatic treatment or thyroidectomy. It is also recommended in patients with concomitant severe diseases (Gurgul & Sowinski, 2011). The first activity of ^{131}I is sufficient in 70% of patients with Graves´ disease (Cooper, 2003). The rest requires repeated RAIT.

Absolute contraindications to ^{131}I therapy is pregnancy and breastfeeding (Sisson et al., 2011).

Although there is general consensus that radioiodine is a safe and effective treatment for Graves' hyperthyroidism, debate remains in terms of the optimal method for calculating the activity (in MBq) and even what the criteria should be for defining optimal. Sustained euthyroidism would clearly be the most desirable outcome, but this appears to be a futile objective, because high rates of cumulative hypothyroidism are reported in most series.

Findings of Leslie et al. (Leslie et al., 2003) confirm this result, with the vast majority developing permanent hypothyroidism and very few with euthyroidism. Therefore, the objective of eradicating hyperthyroidism at the lowest effective radioiodine dose may well be the preferred strategy. This has led some groups to suggest a larger initial radioiodine dose (in Gy) and activity (in MBq) to minimize the need for retreatment and the morbidity and medical costs associated with ineffective primary treatment. Alternatively, others favor a low activity approach (185 MBq), at least for those with mild disease and without complications (Nordyke & Gilbert, 1991). Allahabadia et al. (Allahabadia et al., 2001), who use fixed therapetic activity reported these results: patients given a single activity of 370 MBq had a higher cure rate than those given 185 MBq, but an increase in hypothyroidism incidence at 1 year. There was no difference in cure rate between the groups with Graves' disease and those with toxic nodular goiter, but Graves' patients had a higher incidence of hypothyroidism. Males had a lower cure rate than females, whereas younger patients (<40 years) had a lower cure rate than patients over 40 years old (Allahabadia et al., 2001).

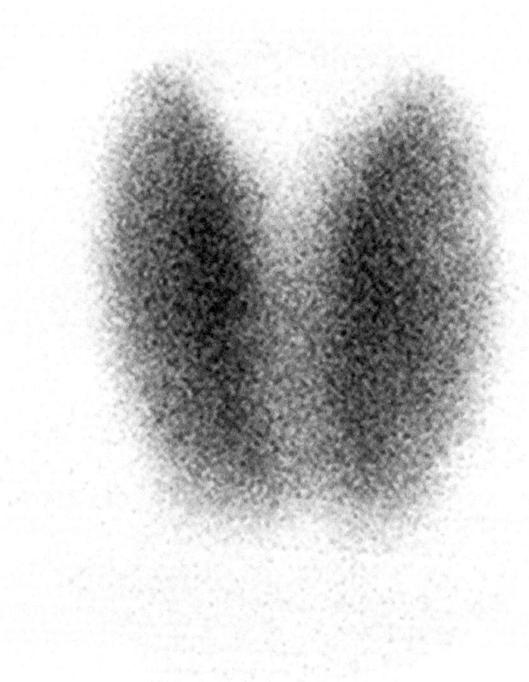

Fig. 1. Thyroid scintigraphy – diffuse goiter in Graves´ disease

2.2 Toxic nodular goiter (Plummer´s disease)

It means hyperthyroidism in glands with both single and multiple toxic nodules. The toxic nodular goiter contains nodules that are not hyperactive.

Therapy of Graves´ disease and toxic nodular goiter can be conservative with drugs, surgical and by radioiodine. Surgery is connected with higher risk, RAIT is indicated most often. RAIT in the world today is the most common and the least expensive therapy. It is indicated mainly for failure of conservative treatment, also in the organ complications, especially circulation (atrial fibrillation, circulatory failure), or where the operation is contraindicated for other reasons. In toxic nodular goiter radioiodine is used mostly in recurrent goiter. This therapy reduces thyroid volume by approximately 40%. The efficiency of RAIT is estimated at 70% (Nygaard et al., 1999b).

Late complication after radioiodine therapy is the development of transient or permanent hypothyroidism. The early transient hypothyroidism is that which arose within six months of treatment with radioiodine. It is a block of hormonogenesis after radioiodine. It is caused by an immunological mechanism.

As the early permanent hypothyroidism we consider a steady increase of TSH levels within 1 year after therapeutic application of radioiodine. In the permanent hypothyroidism the failure of hormonogenesis is involved in addition to immunological processes, damage of the follicular cell nuclei, which leads to accelerated aging and cell death. Hypothyroidism develops after radioiodine therapy like postoperatively in patients with hyperthyroidism. Hypothyroidism after RAIT gradually increases with time, several years after this therapy. It is detected at several tens of percent of such treated patients. Hypothyroidism develops in 10-30% of patients treated with radioiodine, especially due to Graves´ disease (Cooper, 2003). However, it cannot be considered as a side-effect of such therapy. Hypothyroidism ocurrence is estimated at 1-2% per year (Cooper, 2003). Despite the numerous attempts to design dosage schedules aiming at euthyroidism, hypothyroidism occurs in the majority of patients throughout life (Pauwels et al., 2000).

Hypothyroidism occurs at a linear rate on a permanent basis (Staffurth, 1987, Taylor et al., 1984). Besides permanent hypothyroidism, transient hypothyroidism may be seen in patients 2-5 months (or in the first year) after RAIT with spontaneous recovery in the following months (Connell et al., 1983, Dorfman et al., 1977).

^{131}I activities are typically calculated to deliver the desired amount of radiation based on gland size and radioactive iodine uptake (Quimby et al., 1970). Some centers administer to all patients the same fixed activity of ^{131}I with excellent outcome (Nebesio et al., 2002). When children are treated with the dose more than 200–250 Gy/g, hypothyroidism is achieved in nearly 95% of patients (Rivkees & Cornelius, 2003). But in our opinion these doses per gram are too high. Gland size also influences treatment outcome, as higher doses of ^{131}I are needed to induce hypothyroidism when large glands are present (up to 60 g) (Rivkees & Cornelius, 2003). When thyroid size exceeds 80 g, remission rates after ^{131}I therapy are poor (Peters et al., 1996). Thus, surgery is preferred when thyroid gland size is large (>60–80 g). Hamburger reported the largest series of pediatric patients with Graves´ disease in which ^{131}I therapy resulted in relatively uncomplicated clinical courses, except for hypothyroidism requiring lifelong thyroid hormone replacement in 89% (Hamburger, 1985).

Several studies have attempted to determine the optimal activity of radioiodine for curing hyperthyroidism, while avoiding the development of permanent hypothyroidism. Regimens used have included low activity 80 MBq (Franklyn et al., 1991, Lowdell et al., 1985, Nordyke & Gilbert 1991), various fixed activity (185, 370, and 555 MBq) (Franklyn et al., 1991, Jarlov et al., 1995, Nordyke & Gilbert, 1991, Watson et al., 1988), and activities calculated on the basis of thyroid size, the uptake of radioiodine, or the turnover of radioiodine (Franklyn et al., 1991, Jarlov et al., 1995, Sridama et al., 1984). Most dosimetric methods have the benefit of including a measure of thyroid size in their formulas, thereby administering a dose of radioiodine proportional to size of the gland and theoretically increasing the probability of cure, because this has been considered to be an important prognostic factor for success after RAIT. In addition, the use of isotope uptake measurements, as part of the activity calculation protocol, can confirm the absence of thyroiditis and identify patients with values at the extreme ends of the reference range of isotope uptake or turnover, which may predict failure of RAIT (Kaplan et al., 1998). Despite these potential benefits of calculated acitivities, several studies have failed to demonstrate improvements in cure rate over fixed activities (Catargi et al., 1999, Jarlov et al., 1995, Peters et al., 1995). Furthermore, there is little evidence that using a calculated activity has any advantage over a fixed-activity regimen, in terms of preventing hypothyroidism (Turner et al., 1985, Sridama et al., 1984), so many centers and clinicians prefer the use of a fixed-activity regimen (Hedley et al., 1992, Franklyn, 1994).

Although low fixed activities (185 MBq) are associated with a reduced early incidence of hypothyroidism, they often result in unacceptably low cure rates. Moreover, the development of long-term hypothyroidism seems to be inevitable, irrespective of the amount of radioiodine administered, with an annual incidence of 2–3% many years after therapy (Franklyn et al., 1991, Hennemann et al., 1986). Some clinicians now prefer to give a large ablative activity (555 MBq and upwards), which results in early hypothyroidism, so that the need for long-term follow-up of thyroid function in euthyroid patients is obviated.

2.3 Endocrine orbitopathy

Very advanced endocrine orbitopathy has a significant symptomatology. Therapy of endocrine orbitopathy complicated thyreotoxicosis is done with the cooperation with ocularist. RAIT may increase the inflammatory process and exacerbate the ophtalmological symptoms. This is due to radiation thyroiditis, which releases thyroid antigens and stimulates antithyroid antibody production. Therefore, in these patients, high doses of ^{131}I are recommended to assure complete thyroid tissue destruction, especially when high thyroid stimulating hormone receptor antibody (TRAb) levels are observed. The elimination of thyroid antigens and lymphocytes infiltration may reduce the autoimmunological process that is responsible for hyperthyroidism and endocrine orbitopathy (Gurgul & Sowinski, 2011). After calming of thyrotoxicosis we must think of definitive therapy - thyroidectomy followed by ablative radioiodine therapy. Of course then the patient is without the thyroid gland, with rapid development of hypothyroidism. The hormonal replacement therapy is necessary.

2.4 Thyroid autonomies

Autonomously functioning thyroid tissue is characterized by the ability to function without TSH. Neither the antibodies nor TSH is involved. The group of follicular cells just continues autonomously to produce excess amount of thyroid hormones. For clinical diagnosis, radioiodine or ^{99m}Tc-pertechnetate imaging of the thyroid gland is performed. Normally the scan would show increased radionuclide uptake by the autonomous thyroid area (with or without nodule) compared with surrounding normal thyroid tissue. Histological examinations of tissue corresponding to scintigraphically autonomous areas show different architectural patterns and histological features of follicular cells compared with normal quiescent tissue (Kraft, 2006).

The main cause of functional autonomies of the thyroid is iodine deficiency. A higher prevalence of functional autonomies in thyroid tissue have been described in areas with an endemic iodine deficiency (Belfore et al., 1983, Guglmann et al., 1995), the prevalence in countries replete with iodine is below (Hamburger, 1980).

The main pathologic attribute of thyroid functional autonomies is the loss of regulation in the axis of hypothalamus-hypophysis-thyroid.

The histopathology of goiter varies with etiology and age of the goiter. Initially, uniform follicular epithelial hyperplasia (diffuse goiter) is present with an increase in thyroid mass. As the disorder persists, the thyroid architecture loses uniformity, with the development of areas of involution and fibrosis interspersed with areas of focal hyperplasia. This process results in multiple nodules. On scintigraphy, some nodules are "hot," with a high radionuclide uptake (in the end autonomous), or "cold," with a low radionuclide uptake, compared with the normal thyroid tissue. The development of nodules correlates with the progression of functional autonomy and a reduction in TSH levels. Clinically, the natural history of a nontoxic goiter is growth, nodule production, and functional autonomy, resulting in thyrotoxicosis in a minority of patients (Lee & Ananthakrishnan http://www.emedicine.com/med/TOPIC919).

Functional autonomous tissue can present as an autonomous adenoma with nodule (Fig. 2), multifocal functional autonomy in multinodular goiter (MFA) (Fig. 3), or unifocal functional autonomy in thyroid glands without nodules (UFA) or diffuse functional autonomy (DFA).

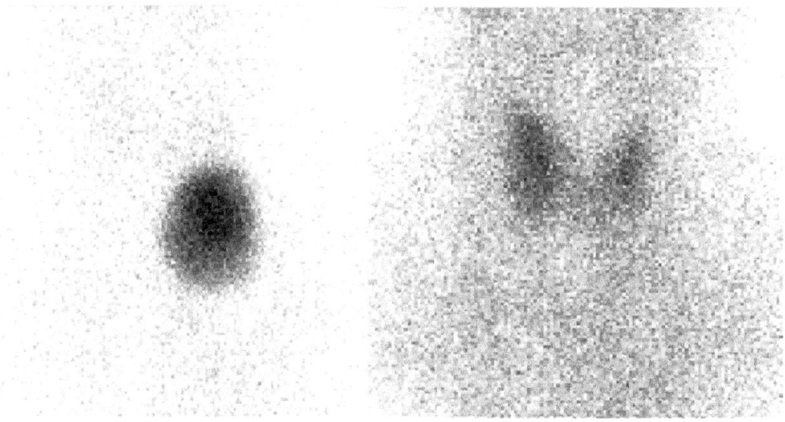

Fig. 2. Thyroid scintigraphy - autonomous adenoma before (on the left) and after (on the right) successful RAIT

Thyroid adenomas (and most nodules in goiters), even if morphologically heterogenous, are true benign tumors (Studer & Derwahl, 1995).

For the diagnostics of thyroid fuctional autonomy and the evaluation of the radioiodine therapeutic effect of functional autonomies, a thyroid scintigraphy is the basic and necessary procedure. Decisions concerning the definitive treatment of thyroid autonomy should take into account previous episodes of hyperthyroidism, objective parameters of risk stratification in euthyroid patients, concomitant diseases, and the probability of future iodine exposure.

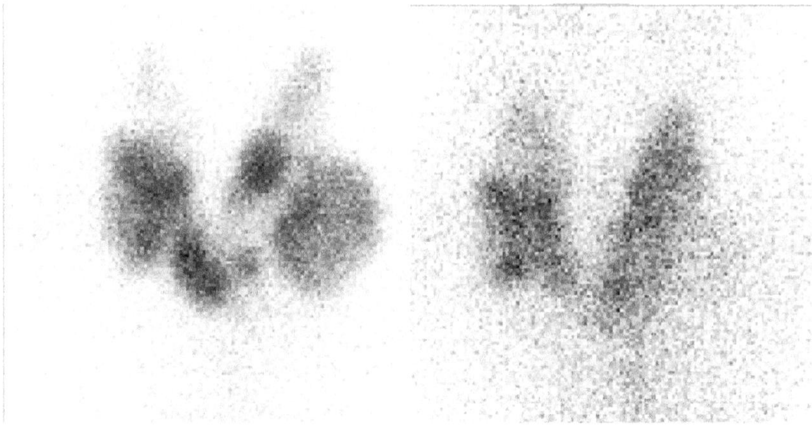

Fig. 3. Thyroid scintigraphy - multifocal functional autonomy in multinodular goiter before (on the left) and after (on the right) successful RAIT

Autonomous adenoma in single thyroid nodule or unifocal or multifocal thyroid autonomies can secrete sufficient thyroid hormones to cause hyperthyroidism. In autonomous adenoma palpable nodule can suppress paranodular tissue (decompensated adenoma) with suppressed TSH with normal or higher fT3 and/or fT4 or the function of the surrounding tissue is preserved (compensated adenoma). Initial thyreosuppressive conservative therapy cannot have permanent effect and we cannot expect remission and it should be treated with radioiodine or operate.

Patients with autonomy who develop hyperthyroidism spontaneously or after iodine excess carry a high risk of recurrence, ranging from 55% up to 81% (Voth et al., 1990). There is general agreement that if hyperthyroidism occurs or has occurred in autonomy, definitive treatment is indicated. RAIT is indicated in patients with functionally relevant autonomy to normalize thyroid function, to remove functional autonomy, and to reduce thyroid volume (Meier et al., 2002).

Radioiodine treatment should be preferred over surgery in patients with smaller goiters (volume <100 ml), the absence of cold nodules or cysts, or the lack of suspicion for malignancy, as well as in those who have undergone previous surgery or would be at increased risk from a surgical intervention. On the other hand, surgery should be preferred in all patients who do not meet these criteria, as well as in the presence of compression symptoms and when there is a need for an immediate therapeutic effect. The risk of relapse on medical treatment with ATD alone is very high, exceeding 80% and long-term antithyroid treatment is not safe in elderly patients, mainly because of poor compliance or a dose reduction by inexperienced physicians. Ablative treatment should be preferred in patients with overt hyperthyroidism owing to functional autonomy. RAIT represents the most comfortable and economic approach (cost of radioiodine and short hospitalization is lower than surgery or long-term conservative therapy). The aim of RAIT in autonomy is the destruction of autonomous tissue with restoration of euthyroidism. Some groups have successfully used standard activities without any activity calculation. We advocate individual pretherapeutic dosimetry to determine the activity necessary to achieve a targeted radiation dose in autonomously functioning tissue. If the elimination of hyperthyroidism in patients with autonomy is achieved, RAIT can be considered successful. The normalization of serum TSH has been proposed as a criterion in the evaluation of a post-therapeutic outcome. Serum TSH >0,5 mU/l excludes autonomous thyroid function with a probability of 88% in an iodine deficiency area (Becker et al., 1992). Therefore, the normalization of this parameter following radionuclide treatment usually indicates a favorable result. Long-term suppressed serum TSH after ^{131}I, on the other hand, has a low predictive potential, as it is often decreased for a prolonged period, despite therapeutic success (Seeger et al., 1995).

In our great group of 868 patients with unifocal and multifocal functional autonomy, and disseminated functional autonomy who received at least one treatment of radioiodine side-effects were minimal. Postradiation hypothyroidism was diagnosed in 38 patients (4,4%). Such a low incidence of hypothyroidism can be influenced by these factors: 1. A very low number of patients had previous treatment with methimazole, which is associated with a faster progression toward hypothyroidism (Ceccarelli et al., 2005); 2. Before ^{131}I therapy in patients with functional autonomy, the degree of nonautonomous thyroid tissue suppression was high, and this tissue was not influenced by radioiodine beta rays (radioiodine is absorbed only in autonomous nodule or tissue, therefore it destroys only this area and does not damage the remaining thyroid tissue); 3. follow-up of our patients was 2 years long, and certainly later, the number of hypothyroid patients can (but maybe not) increase (Ceccarelli et al., 2005). In the literature, the incidence of hypothyrodism after RAIT for functional autonomy of the thyroid is described in 10%–20% cases (Reiners & Schneider, 2002) and even in 60% (Ceccarelli et al., 2005). 4. pretherapeutic dosimetry with a treatment by means of individually calculated ^{131}I activity (Kraft & Stepien, 2007). Generally, in thyroid autonomies, focused radioiodine absorption only or almost only in autonomous areas results in selective destruction of these areas. Low TSH levels decreases radioiodine uptake in surrounding tissue, which additionally protects healthy thyroidal tissue. Therefore, the effectiveness of RAIT in thyroid autonomies is very high and the risk of hypothyroidism is low (Gurgul & Sowinski, 2011). This is in contrast to the situation for example in RAIT of Graves´ disease and toxic nodular goiter. Non-suppressed serum TSH before ^{131}I therapy has been mentioned as a risk factor for development of hypothyroidism (Farrari et al., 1996). Nygaard (Nygaard et al., 1999a) had a cure-rate of 75% within 3 months when treating autonomous solitary thyroid nodules with ^{131}I in 62 patients. The thyroid volume was reduced by 35% within 3 months and 45% after 2 years. Side effects were few and consist of hypothyroidism in 8% with a median follow-up of 5 years (Nygaard et al., 1999a).

3. Euthyroid goiter

Small eufunctional goiter usually does not carry any trouble. The growth of goiter gradually creates local problems and in advanced stages we can objectively find the compression of the trachea and esophagus, abnormal innervation of the larynx, possibly obturation of the upper aperture. On scintigraphy the diffuse goiter accumulates homogeneously, in nodular goiter some areas accumulate with reduced and often with increased activity (Fig.4).

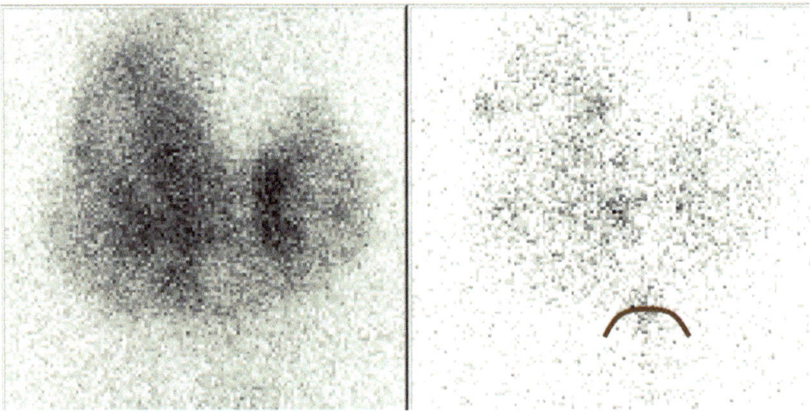

Fig. 4. Thyroid scintigraphy – nodular goiter with normal function and mechanical syndrome

Goiter with mechanical syndrome is a disease that has to be solved urgently and radically (Fig.5). In the first place surgery comes. If thyroidectomy is contraindicated, the use of RAIT is appropriate.

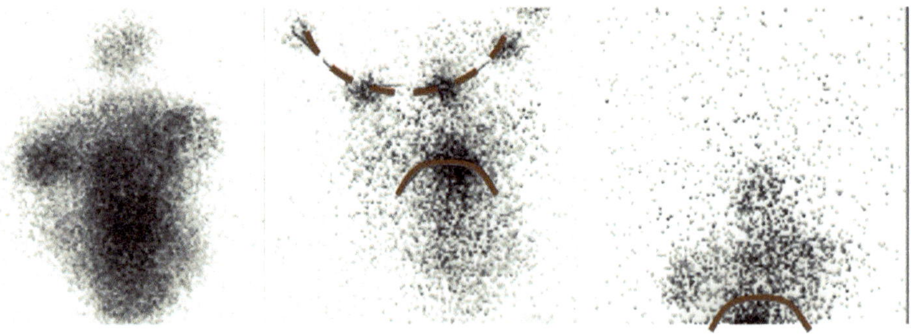

Fig. 5. Thyroid scintigraphy – retrostrernal goiter after thyroidectomy with mechanical syndrome

After this treatment, postradiation hypothyroidism is a common finding with need to use replacement therapy of thyroid hormones.

4. Differentiated Thyroid Cancers (DTC)

Radioiodine is the mainstay of therapy for residual, recurrent, and metastatic thyroid cancer that takes up iodine and cannot be resected. About 90% or more of thyroid carcinomas are well differentiated (papillary or follicular types), which take up iodine and accordingly can be successfully treated with ^{131}I. The therapeutic effects on differentiated thyroid cancer is based on destruction of cells by high dose of administered radioiodine. RAIT is defined as the systemic administration of ^{131}I - sodium or potassium iodide for selective irradiation of thyroid remnants, microscopic DTC or other nonresectable or incompletely resectable DTC, or both purposes. Based on the primary goal of the RAIT, there are two main forms of the procedure (Luster et al., 2008). The first form, radioiodine ablation, is a post-surgical adjuvant modality. It seeks to eliminate thyroid remnants to increase the sensitivity and specificity of follow-up testing for DTC persistence or recurrence, namely, of assays of serum thyroglobulin (Tg) as a tumour marker and of diagnostic whole-body scintigraphy (dxWBS) (Fig. 6). Ablation also allows sensitive "post-therapy" whole-body scintigraphy (rxWBS) (Fig. 7) that may detect previously occult metastases (Dietlein et al., 2007) and serves to treat any microscopic tumour deposits.

Ablation, therefore, may reduce long-term morbidity and possibly, mortality (Dietlein et al., 2007, Sawka et al., 2004, Pacini et al., 2005). Ablation success is evaluated 6–12 months after the ablation procedure. The second form of RAIT, radioiodine treatment of nonresectable or incompletely resectable lesions, e.g. microscopic disease, macroscopic local tumour or lymph node or distant metastases, is performed as curative or paliative therapy either as a component of primary treatment of DTC or to address persistent or recurrent disease (Luster et al., 2008). Radioiodine ablation after total or near-total thyroidectomy is a standard procedure in patients with DTC. When radioiodine uptake is scintigraphically proven before or after RAIT, then RAIT of nonresectable or incompletely resectable tumour, e.g. local recurrences, lymph node metastases or disseminated iodineavid lung metastases or other distant lesions, has shown to be effective in eradicating disease, slowing disease progression or providing symptomatic relief (Durante et al., 2006). Decision on whether or not to give RAIT with the intention of cure or palliation should be individualised to the patient and should consider several factors, among others also the patient health status – inability to tolerate surgery or other potential therapeutic interventions, e.g. chemotherapy.

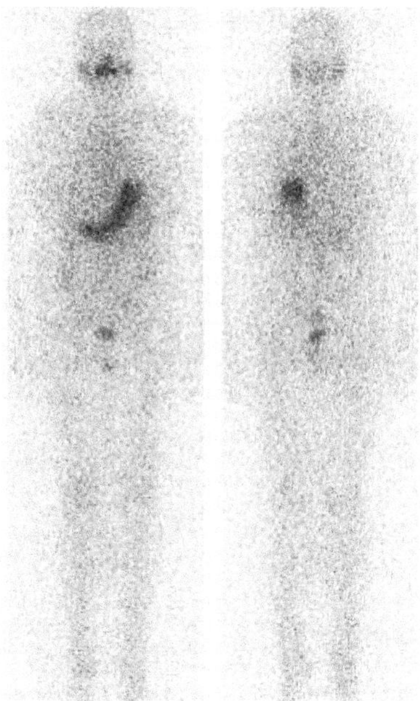

Fig. 6. Diagnostic whole-body scintigraphy - normal finding

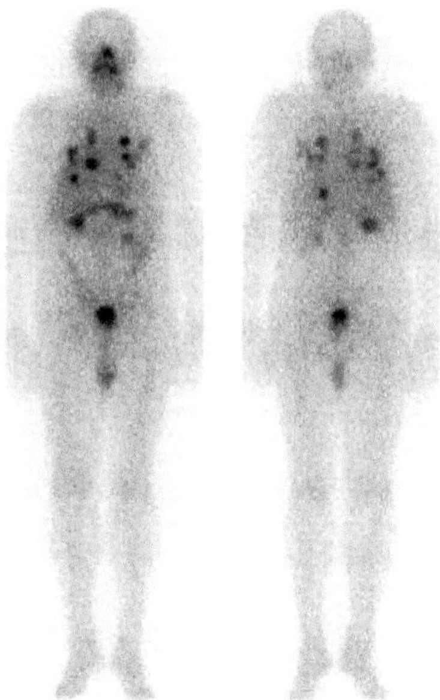

Fig. 7. Post-therapy whole-body scintigraphy. Multiple lung metastases which accumulate radioiodine

It can make RAIT the preferred or the only therapeutic option; conversely, where use of recombinant human thyroid-stimulating hormone (rhTSH) is not economically feasible, inability to tolerate hypothyroidism could rule out RAIT.

Absolute contraindications of RAIT is pregnancy and breastfeeding (as in RAIT in hyperthyroidism).

The effectiveness of RAIT depends on the patient's serum TSH level being sufficiently elevated. A TSH level of ≥30 mU/l is believed to increase sodium iodine symporter (NIS) expression and thereby to optimise radioiodine uptake (Cooper et al., 2006). Such TSH elevation can be reached by waiting at least 3 weeks after thyroidectomy or 4–5 weeks after discontinuing treatment with levothyroxine (T4). Triiodothyronine (T3) may be substituted for T4 until 2 weeks before RAIT in an attempt to decrease the duration of hypothyroidism. When thyroid hormone is withheld, it should be initiated or resumed 2 days after radioiodine administration. Traditional thyroid hormone withdrawal has the major drawback of causing weeks to months of hypothyroid symptoms in most patients (Duntas & Biondi, 2007, Luster et al., 2005, Dow et al., 1997, Schroeder et al., 2006). Such physical and psychological morbidity may include fatigue, depression, impaired ability to concentrate, sleep disturbance, weight gain, constipation, dry skin, hoarseness, puffy face or hands, cardiovascular abnormalities, impaired renal function and exacerbation of dyslipidemia (Billewicz et al., 1969, Botella-Carretero et al., 2003, 2004, 2005, 2006, Luster et al., 2005, Tagay et al., 2005). These manifestations in turn frequently significantly decrease patient quality of life, cause absenteeism from or impaired performance in work or study or lead to debilitating or even life-threatening worsening in psychological, cardiovascular, renal or other concomitant conditions (Borget et al., 2007, Dow et al., 1997, Duntas & Biondi, 2007,

Haugen et al., 1999, Ladenson et al., 1997, Leclere et al., 2000, Luster et al., 2005, Nijhuis et al., 1999, Schroeder et al., 2006).

An alternative to thyroid hormones withdrawal for attaining TSH elevation is rhTSH administration. In Europe and elsewhere, this drug has been approved for use in adults as preparation for serum Tg testing, dxWBS or both or for radioiodine ablation (Luster, 2006).

Radiosensitivity of thyroid gland is relatively high. For destruction and ablation of normal thyroid gland is needed higher activity than for destruction of tumor tissue.

Because of the larger dose of radioiodine and the lower uptake by the tissue in thyroid cancer, more side effects can be seen, particularly transient sialoadenitis, than in the therapy of hyperthyroidism. The mortality of patients treated with less than total thyroidectomy and limited ^{131}I treatment was found to be three to four times higher than that of patients treated with total thyroidectomy and RAIT to ablate known foci of radioiodine uptake. Thyroglobulin is the major tumour marker for thyroid cancer of the follicular epithelium. It is not only specific for tumour tissue but is also specific component of normal thyroid tissue. Since thyroglobulin is produced exclusively by thyroid tissue, only very small amounts can be found in the blood after thyroidectomy and ablative radioiodine therapy. Any post-therapeutic elevation of its levels indicates either remnant of thyroid tissue, requiring further ablative therapy, or the presence of metastases or local recurrence. Following total or near-total thyroidectomy, TSH elevation reaches a maximum in 4-6 weeks. In the follow-up care, patients are maintained on suppressive doses of thyroid hormone. The goals of follow-up after initial therapy are to maintain adequate levothyroxine (T4) therapy and to detect persistent or recurrent thyroid carcinoma. All patients with thyroid cancer must be treated with thyroid hormone after thyroidectomy for correction of surgically induced hypothyroidism and to suppress stimulated growth of persistent or recurrent thyroid cancer by reducing TSH levels. Thus thyroid hormone therapy ensures „replacement" therapy, which corrects hypothyroidism, and „suppressive" therapy, which inhibits TSH secretion. Thyroid cell proliferation and differentiation is mainly TSH dependent. Therefore TSH secretion must be inhibited by thyroid hormone therapy in all patients with differentiated thyroid cancers. Thyroid hormone is a basic principle that is included in the guidelines of thyroid cancer therapy. Before administration of radioiodine, thyroid homone therapy has to be interrupted for diagnosis or treatment. Radioiodine uptake, thyroglobulin synthesis and its secretion by thyroid cancer cells will be stimulated by increased TSH. Neoplastic as wel as normal thyroid cell differentiation depends on TSH. Accordingly, metastases take up radioiodine only if the patient is hypothyroid with high serum TSH levels, while no uptake is seen when the patient is on hormone suppressive therapy with low or undetectable serum TSH concentrations. Serum TSH level should be taken into account when interpreting the serum thyroglobulin value as the presence or absence neoplastic disease. In most patients with persistent or recurrent neoplastic disease, thyroglobulin concentration will increase dramatically during hypothyroidism following withdrawal of thyroid hormone treatment. If there is histologically confirmed thyroid cancer, then 6-8 weeks after thyroidectomy the patient is admitted for radioiodine thyroablation. The patient comes in a fully developed deep clinical hypothyroidism (TSH level usually above 100 mU/l). To achieve sufficient accumulation of radioiodine in the thyroid remnants it is needed to be TSH higher than 30 mU/l. Then we perform ablation of thyroid remnant by radioiodine, which in addition to destruction of the remaining thyroid tissue removed also possible intrathyroidal metastases.

After radioiodine therapy the suppressive therapy is started. 6 to 12 months after ablation the control whole-body scintigraphy is performed in hypothyroidism after 4 weeks withdrawal of thyroid hormones.

In the postoperative monitoring of patients with differentiated thyroid cancer should be solved a serious problem that is disturbing the patient life. This is hypothyroidism, which is a prerequisite for the implementation of thyroablation, whole body radioiodine scintigraphy and any further RAIT. It must be deep enough, which can be in actively working patients after withdrawal of suppressive therapy considerable difficult. Fortunately the rapid tumor growth is rarely stimulated by a brief rise in TSH concentration. The usual scheme is to carry out the treatment or control of patients during hospitalization after discontinuation of levothyroxine replacement for approximately 4-5 weeks. This has lead to profound hypothyroidism. In a small number of patients on long-term suppressive therapy we have observed only a moderate response to TSH after withdrawal of T4. Another option is to combine T4 and triiodothyronine (T3). Short-term administration of T3 alleviates some of the symptoms of prolonged hypothyroidism and must be stopped 2 weeks before radioiodine administration. This procedure also achieves a corresponding increase in TSH levels and hypothyroid patients subjectively perceived better. The third option is administration of recombinant human thyrotropin (rhTSH - Thyrogen) which stimulates thyroid tissue without requiring the discontinuation of thyroid hormone therapy. rhTSH can be used for diagnostic purposes (determination of thyroglobulin, scintigraphy) and before RAIT. Thyrogen should be used in patients who are either unable to mount an adequate endogenous TSH response to thyroid hormone withdrawal or in whom withdrawal is medically contraindicated. The use of Thyrogen allows for radioiodine imaging while the patient are euthyroid on levothyroxine. The clearance of radioiodine is approximately 50% greater in euthyroid patients than in hypothyroid patients, who have decreased renal function. Thus, radioiodine retention is less in euthyroid patients at the time of imaging and this factor should be considered when selecting the activity of radioiodine for imaging. Thyrotropin also stimulates the production of thyroglobulin and increases the usefulness of this tumour marker in patients treated with thyroid hormone who have had thyroid tissue ablated. For its high price Thyrogen unfortunately cannot be used in all patients with thyroid cancer.

Suppression of endogenous secretion of TSH should be always maintained in patients with differentiated thyroid cancer. In low risk patients considered as cured, the levothyroxine dose is modified to maintain a low but detectable serum TSH concentration (0,1 to 0,5 mU/l). In high risk patients with persistent/recurrent disease and even those considered as cured, higher doses of levothyroxine are continued, with the objective of attaining a serum TSH level of 0,1 mU/l or less, the free triiodothyronine concentration should be maintained within the normal range to avoid any significant overdosage. Reduction of serum thyroglobulin concentration is achieved with doses of thyroid hormone that reduce serum TSH to very low levels.

5. Conclusion

This chapter describes treatment options for some kinds of benign thyroid disease and differentiated thyroid cancers with radioactive iodine and context of this therapy with the development of post-radiation hypothyroidism. Moreover, deliberately induced hypothyroidism by thyroablation and in the further course also by the withdrawal of substitution and suppressive thyroid hormone therapy is used in the diagnosis and treatment of differentiated thyroid carcinomas.

6. References

Allahabadia, A., Daykin, J., Sheppard, M.C., Gough, S.C. & Franklyn J.A. (2001). Radioiodine treatment of hyperthyroidism-prognostic factors for outcome. J Clin Endocrinol Metab, Vol.86, No.8, (2001), pp. 3611-3617, ISSN 0021-972X

Andrade, V.A., Gross, J.L. & Maia, A.L. (1999). Effect of methimazole pretreatment on serum thyroid hormone levels after radioactive treatment in Graves' hyperthyroidism. J Clin Endocrinol Metab, Vol.84, (1999), pp. 4012–4016, ISSN 0021-972X

Angusti, T., Codegone, A., Pellerito, R. & Favero, A. (2000). Thyroid cancer prevalence after radioiodine treatment of hyperthyroidism. J Nucl Med, Vol. 41, (2000), pp. 1006–1009, ISSN 0161-5505

Becker, W., Börner, W. & Rendl, J. (1992). Ist ein TSH-Screening zur Diagnose oder zum Ausschluß der Autonomie der Schilddrüse sinnvoll? Nuklearmedizin, Vol.31, (1992), pp. 132, ISSN 0029-5566

Belfore, A., Sara, L., Runello, L. & al. (1983). Solitary autonomously functioning thyroid nodules and iodine deficiency. J Clin Endocrinol Metab, Vol. 56, (1983), pp. 283, ISSN 0021-972X

Billewicz, W.Z., Chapman, R.S., Crooks, J., Day, M.E., Gossage, J., Wayne, E. & al. (1969). Statistical methods applied to the diagnosis of hypothyroidism. Q J Med, Vol.38, No.150, (1969), pp. 255–66, ISSN 0033-5622

Boice Jr, J.D. (1998). Radiation and thyroid cancer—what more can be learned? Acta Oncol, Vol.34, (1998), 321–324, ISSN 0284-186X

Boice Jr, J.D. (2006). Thyroid disease 60 years after Hiroshima and 20 years after Chernobyl. J Am Med Assoc, Vol.3295, (2006), pp. 1060–1062, ISSN 00987484

Bonnema, S.J., Bennedbaek, F.N., Veje, A., Marving, J. & Hegedüs, L. (2004). Propylthiouracil before 131I Therapy of Hyperthyroid Diseases: Effect on Cure Rate Evaluated by a Randomized Clinical Trial. J Clin Endocrinol Metab, Vol.89, (2004), pp. 4439-4444, ISSN 0021-972X

Borget, I., Corone, C., Nocaudie, M., Allyn, M., Iacobelli, S., Schlumberger, M. & De Pouvourville, G. (2007). Sick leave for follow-up control in thyroid cancer patients: comparison between stimulation with Thyrogen and thyroid hormone withdrawal. Eur J Endocrinol, Vol.156, No.5, (2007), pp. 531–8, ISSN 0804-4643

Botella-Carretero, J.I., Galan, J.M., Caballero, C., Sancho, J. & Escobar-Morreale, H.F. (2003). Quality of life and psychometric functionality in patients with differentiated thyroid carcinoma. Endocr Relat Cancer, Vol.10, No.4, (2003), pp. 601–10, ISSN 1351-0088

Botella-Carretero, J.I., Gomez-Bueno, M., Caballero, C. & al. (2004). Chronic thyrotropin-suppressive therapy with levothyroxine and short-term overt hypothyroidism after thyroxine withdrawal are associated with undesirable cardiovascular effects in patients with differentiated thyroid carcinoma. Endocr Relat Cancer, Vol.11, No.2, (2004), pp. 345–56, ISSN 1351-0088

Botella-Carretero, J.I., Prados, A., Manzano, L., Montero, M.T., Escribano, L., Sancho, J. & Escobar-Morreale, H.F. (2005). The effects of thyroid hormones on circulatingmarkers of cell-mediated immune response, as studied in patients with differentiated thyroid carcinoma before and during thyroxine withdrawal. Eur J Endocrinol, Vol.153, No.2, (2005), pp. 223–30, ISSN 0804-4643

Botella-Carretero, J.I., Álvarez-Blasco, F., Sancho, J. & Escobar-Morreale, H.F. (2006). Effects of thyroid hormones on serum levels of adipokines as studied in patients with differentiated thyroid carcinoma during thyroxine withdrawal. Thyroid, Vol.16, No.4, (2006), pp. 397–402, ISSN 1050-7256

Brown, R.S. (2009) Autoimmune thyroid disease; unlocking a complex puzzle. Current opinion in paediatrics, Vol.21, (2009), pp. 523-528, ISSN 1040-8703

Burch, H.B., Solomon, B.L., Cooper, D.S., Ferguson, P., Walpert, N. & Howard, R. (2001). The Effect of Antithyroid Drug Pretreatment on Acute Changes in Thyroid Hormone Levels after 131I Ablation for Graves' Disease. J Clin Endocrinol Metab, Vol.86, (2001), pp. 3016–3021, ISSN 0021-972X

Catargi, B., Leprat, F., Guyot, M., Valli, N., Ducassou, D. & Tabarin, A. (1999). Optimized radioiodine therapy of Graves' disease: analysis of the delivered dose and of other possible factors affecting outcome. Eur J Endocrinol, Vol.141, (1999), pp.117–121, ISSN 0804-4643

Ceccarelli, C., Bencivelli, W., Vitti, P.& al. (2005). Outcome of radioiodine-131 therapy in hyperfunctioning thyroid nodules: a 20 year retrospective study. Clin Endocrinol, Vol. 62, (2005), pp. 331, ISSN 0300-0664

Connell, J.M., Hilditch, T.E., McCruden, D.C. & Alexander, W.D. (1983). Transient hypothyroidism following radioiodine therapy for thyrotoxicosis. Br J Radiol, Vol. 56, No.665, (1983), pp. 309-313.

Cooper, D.S. (2003). Hyperthyroidism. Lancet, Vol.362, (2003), pp. 459-468, ISSN 0140-6736

Cooper, D.S., Doherty, G.M., Haugen, B.R. & al. (2006). Management guidelines for patients with thyroid nodules and differentiated thyroid cancer. Thyroid, Vol.16, No.2, (2006), pp. 109–42, ISSN 1050-7256

Dietlein, M., Dressler, J., Eschner, W., Grünwald, F., Lassmann, M., Leisner, B., Luster, M., Moser, E., Reiners, C., Schicha, H. & Schober, O. (2007). Procedure guidelines for radioiodine therapy of differentiated thyroid cancer (version 3). Nuklearmedizin, Vol.46, No.5, (2007), pp. 213–9, ISSN 0029-5566

Dolphin, G.W. (1968). The risk of thyroid cancers following irradiation. Health Phys, Vol.15, (1968), pp. 219–228, ISSN 0017-9078

Dorfman, S., Young, R.L. & Carretta, R.F. (1977). Transient hypothyroidism. Arch Intern Med, Vol.137, No.2, (1977), pp. 256-257, ISSN 0003-9926

Dow, K.H., Ferrell, B.R. & Anello, C. (1997). Quality-of-life changes in patients with thyroid cancer after withdrawal of thyroid hormone therapy. Thyroid, Vol.7, No.4, (1997), pp. 613–9, ISSN 1050-7256

Dunkelmann, S., Neumann, V., Staub, U. & al. (2005). Results of a risk adapted and functional radioiodine therapy in Graves´ disease. Nuklearmedizin, Vol.44, (2005), pp. 238-242, ISSN 0029-5566

Duntas, L.H. & Biondi, B. (2007). Short-term hypothyroidism after levothyroxine-withdrawal in patients with differentiated thyroid cancer: clinical and quality of life consequences. Eur J Endocrinol, Vol.156, No.1, (2007), pp. 13–9, ISSN 0804-4643

Durante, C., Haddy, N., Baudin, E. & al. (2006). Long-term outcome of 444 patients with distant metastases from papillary and follicular thyroid carcinoma: benefits and limits of radioiodine therapy. J Clin Endocrinol Metab, Vol.91, No.8, (2006), pp. 2892–9, ISSN 0021-972X

Edmonds, C.J. & Smith, T. (1986). The long-term hazards of the treatment of thyroid cancer with radioiodine. Br J Radiol, Vol.59, (1986), pp. 45–51, ISSN 0007-1285

Farrari, C., Reschini, E. & Paracchi, A. (1996). Treatment of the autonomous thyroid nodule: a review. Eur J Endocrinol, Vol.135, (1996), pp. 383–390, ISSN 0804-4643

Franklyn, J.A., Daykin, J., Drolc, Z., Farmer, M., & Sheppard, M.C. (1991). Long-term follow-up of treatment of thyrotoxicosis by three different methods. Clin Endocrinol (Oxf), Vol.34, (1991), pp. 71–76, ISSN 0300-0664

Franklyn, J.A. (1994). The management of hyperthyroidism. N Engl J Med, Vol.330, (1994), pp. 1731–1738. ISSN 0028-4793

Franklyn, J.A., Maisonneuve, P., Sheppard, M., Betteridge, J. & Boyle, P. (1999). Cancer incidence and mortality after radioiodine treatment for hyperthyroidism: a population-based cohort study. Lancet, Vol.353, (Vol.1999), pp. 2111–2115, ISSN 0140-6736

Goldman, M.B., Maloof, F., Monson, R.R., Aschengrau, A., Cooper, D.S. & Ridgway, E.C. (1988). Radioactive iodine therapy and breast cancer. A follow-up study of hyperthyroid women. Am J Epidemiol, Vol.127, (1988), pp. 969–980, ISSN 0002-9262

Guglmann, C.A., Seybold, S., Rendl, J. & al. (1995). Epidemiology and diagnostic of functional thyroidal autonomy. [in German]. Nuklearmediziner, Vol.18, (1995), pp. 251, ISSN 0723-7065

Gurgul, E. & Sowinski, J. (2011). Primary hyperthyroidism - diagnosis and treatment. Indications and contraindications for radioiodine therapy. Nucl Med Rev Cent E Eur, Vol.14, No.1, (2011), pp. 29-32, ISSN 1506-9680

Hall, P., Berg, G., Bjelkengren, G., Boice Jr, J.D., Ericsson, U.B., Hallquist, A., Lidberg, M., Lundell, G., Tennvall, J. & Wiklund, K. (1992a). Cancer mortality after iodine 131I treatment of hyperthyroidism. Int J Cancer, Vol.50, (1992), pp. 886–890, ISSN 1097-0215

Hall, P., Boice Jr, J.D., Berg, G. & al. (1992b). Leukaemia incidence after iodine-131 exposure. Lancet, Vol.340, (1992), pp.1–4. ISSN 0140-6736

Hamburger, J.L. (1980). Evolution of toxicity in solitary nontoxic autonomously functioning thyroid nodules. J Clin Endrocrinol Metab, Vol.50, (1980), pp. 1089, ISSN 0021-972X

Hamburger, J.I. (1985). Management of hyperthyroidism in children and adolescents. J Clin Endocrinol Metab, Vol.60, (1985), pp. 1019-1024, ISSN 0021-972X

Haugen, B.R., Pacini, F., Reiners, C. & al. (1999). A comparison of recombinant human thyrotropin and thyroid hormone withdrawal for the detection of thyroid remnant or cancer. J Clin Endocrinol Metab, Vol.84, No.11, (1999), pp. 3877–85, ISSN 0021-972X

Hedley, A.J., Lazarus, J.H., McGhee, S.M. & al. (1992). Treatment of hyperthyroidism by radioactive iodine. Summary of aUKnational survey prepared for the Royal College of Physicians Committee on Endocrinology and Diabetes. J Roy Coll Phys Lond, Vol.26, (1992), pp. 348–351, ISSN 0035-8819

Hennemann, G., Krenning, E.P. & Sankaranarayanan, K. (1986). Place of radioactive iodine in treatment of thyrotoxicosis. Lancet, Vol.1, (1986), pp.1369–1372, ISSN 0140-6736

Hertz, S. & Roberts, A. (1946) Radioactive Iodine in the Study of Thyroid Physiology: VII. The Use of Radioactive Iodine Therapy in Hyperthyroidism. J Am Med Assoc, Vol.131, No.2, (1946), pp. 81-86, ISSN 00987484

Hoffman, D.A., McConahey, W.M., Fraumeni J.F. Jr & Kurland L.T. (1982). Cancer incidence following treatment of hyperthyroidism. Int J Epidemiol, Vol.11, (1982), pp. 218–224, ISSN 0300-5771

Holm, L.E., Hall, P., Wiklund, K. & al. (1991). Cancer risk after iodine-131 therapy for hyperthyroidism. J Natl Cancer Inst, Vol.83, (1991), pp. 1072–1077, ISSN 0027-8874

http://en.wikipedia.org/wiki/Saul_Hertz#cite_note-10

Chapman, E.M. (1983). History of the discovery and early use of radioactive iodine. J Am Med Assoc, Vol. 250, (1983), pp. 2042–2044, ISSN 00987484

Jarlov, A.E., Hegedüs, L., Kristensen, L.O., Nygaard, B. & Hansen, B.M. (1995). Is calculation of the dose in radioiodine therapy of hyperthyroidism worthwhile? Clin Endocrinol (Oxf), Vol.43, (1995), pp. 325–329, ISSN 0300-0664

Kaplan, M.M., Meier, D.A. & Dworkin, H.J. (1998). Treatment of hyperthyroidism with radioactive iodine. Endocrinol Metab Clin N Am, Vol.27, (1998), pp 205-223. ISSN 0889-8529

Kraft, O. (2006). Radioiodine therapy of thyroid functional autonomies: experience at a single University Referral Hospital Centre in Czech Republic.World J Nucl Med, Vol.5, (2006), pp. 104-108, ISSN 1450-1147

Kraft, O. & Stepien, A. (2007). Functional autonomies of thyroid and efficacy of radioiodine therapy. Cancer Biother Radiopharm, Vol.22, No.2, pp. 261-267, ISSN 1084-9785

Kubota, S., Ohye, H., Yano, G., Nishihara, E., Kudo, T., Ito, M., Fukata, S., Amino, N., Kuma, K.& Miyauchi, A. (2006). Two-day thionamide withdrawal prior to radioiodine uptake sufficiently increases uptake and does not exacerbate hyperthyroidism compared to 7-day withdrawal in Graves´ disease. Endocrine Journal, Vol.53, (2006), pp. 603-607. ISSN 1348-4540

Lacko, A., Bestvina, D. & Schóber, A. (2001). Influence of radiation on organism on cells level [in Slovak]. Military Academy, Liptovský Mikuláš, Slovak Republic.

Ladenson, P.W., Braverman, L.E., Mazzaferri, E.L. & al. (1997). Comparison of administration of recombinant human thyrotropin with withdrawal of thyroid hormone for radioactive iodine scanning in patients with thyroid carcinoma. N Engl J Med, 1997; Vol. 337, No.13, (1997), pp. 888–96, ISSN 0028-4793

Leclere, J., Nunez, S., Dejaz, C., Sohmer, V. & Schvartz, C. (2000). Quantitative and qualitative consequences of l-T4 suppressive withdrawal. Satellite symposium presentation, EANM Annual Congress, Paris, France, September 2000

Lee, S.L. & Ananthakrishnan, S. Goiter, Nontoxic. eMedicine Specialties, Endocrinology, Thyroid, online: http://www. emedicine.com/med/TOPIC919.htm

Leslie, W.D., Ward, L., Salamon, E.A., Ludwig, S., Rowe, R.C. & Cowden, E.A. (2003). A randomized comparison of radioiodine doses in Graves' hyperthyroidism. J Clin Endocrinol Metab, Vol.88, (2003), pp. 978–983, ISSN 0021-972X

Levy, W.M., Schumacher, O.P. & Gupta, M. (1988). Treatment of childhood Graves' disease. A review with emphasis on radioiodine treatment. Cleveland Clin J Med, Vol.55, (1988), pp. 373–382, ISSN 0891-1150

Lowdell, C.P., Dobbs, H.J., Spathis, G.S., McCready, V.R., Cosgrove, D.O. & Harmer, C.L. (1985). Low-dose 131I in treatment of Graves' disease. J R Soc Med, Vol.78, (1985), pp. 197-202, ISSN 0141-0768

Luster, M., Felbinger, R., Dietlein, M. & Reiners, C. et al. (2005). Thyroid hormone withdrawal in patients with differentiated thyroid carcinoma: a one hundred thirty-patient pilot survey on consequences of hypothyroidism and a pharmacoeconomic comparison to recombinant thyrotropin administration. Thyroid, Vol.15, No.10, (2005), pp. 1147–55. ISSN 1050-7256

Luster, M. (2006). Acta Oncologica Lecture. Present status of the use of recombinant human TSH in thyroid cancer management. Acta Oncol, Vol.45, No.8, (2006), pp. 1018–30, ISSN 0284-186X

Luster, M., Clarke, S.E., Dietlein, M., Lassmann, M., Lind, P., Oyen, W.J.G., Tennvall, J. & Bombardieri, E. (2008). Guidelines for radioiodine therapy of differentiated thyroid cancer. Eur J Nucl Med Mol Imaging, Vol.35, No.10, (2008), pp. 1941-1959, ISSN 1619-7070

Marinelli, L.D., Quimby, E.H. & Hine, G.J. (1948). Dosage determination with radioactive isotopes. Practical consideration in therapy and protection. Am J Roentgenol, Vol.59, (1948), pp.260-281, ISSN 0361-803X

Meier, D.A., Brill, D.R., Becker, D.V. & al. (2002). Society of Nuclear Medicine Procedure guideline for therapy of thyroid disease with 131-iodine. J Nucl Med, Vol.43, (2002), pp. 856-861, ISSN 0161-5505

Metso, S., Auvinen, A., Huhtala, H., Salmi, J., Oksala, H. & Jaatinen, P. (2007). Increased cancer incidence after radioiodine treatment for hyperthyroidism. Cancer, Vol.109, (2007), pp. 1972–9. ISSN 1097-0142

Moll, G.W. & Patel, B.R. (1997). Pediatric Gravesš disease: Therapeutic options and experience with radioiodine at the University of Mississippi Medical Center. Southern Medical Journal, Vol.90, No.10, (1997), pp. 1017-1022, ISSN 00384348

Nebesio, T.D., Siddiqui, A.R., Pescovitz, O.H. & Eugster, E.A. (2002). Time course to hypothyroidism after fixed-dose radioablation therapy of Graves' disease in children. J Pediatr. Vol.141, (2002), pp. 99–103, ISSN 0022-3476

Nijhuis, T.F., van Wepperen, W. & de Klerk, J.M.H. (1999). Costs associated with the withdrawal of thyroid hormone suppression therapy during the follow-up treatment of well-differentiated thyroid cancer. Tijd Nucl Geneeskd, Vol.21, (1999), pp. 98–100

Nordyke, R.A. & Gilbert, F.I. (1991). Optimal iodine-131 dose for eliminating hyperthyroidism in Graves' disease. J Nucl Med, Vol.32, (1991), pp. 411–416, ISSN 0161-5505

Nygaard, B., Hegedüs, L., Nielsen, K.G., Ulriksen, P. & Hansen, J.M. (1999a) Long-term effect of radioactive iodine on thyroid function and size in patients with solitary autonomously functioning toxic thyroid nodules. Clin Endocrinol, Vol.50, (1999), pp. 197–202, ISSN 0300-0664

Nygaard, B., Hegedüs, L., Ulriksen, P., Nielsen, K.G. & Hansen, J.M. (1999b). Radioiodine therapy for multinodular toxic goiter. Arch Intern Med, Vol.159, (1999), pp.1364-1368, ISSN 0003-9926

Pacini F., Schlumberger M., Harmer C. & al. (2005). Post-surgical use of radioiodine (131I) in patients with papillary and follicular thyroid cancer and the issue of remnant ablation: a consensus report. Eur J Endocrinol, Vol.153, No.5, (2005), pp. 651–9, ISSN 0804-4643

Pauwels, E.K.J., Smit, J.W.A., Slats, A., Bourguignon, M. & Overbeek, F. (2000). Health effects of therapeutic use of 131I in hyperthyroidism. Q J Nucl Med, Vol.44, No.4, (2000), pp. 333-339, ISSN 1125-0135

Peters, H., Fischer, C., Bogner, U., Reiners, C. & Schleusener, H. (1995) Radioiodine therapy of Graves' hyperthyroidism: standard vs. calculated 131iodine activity. Results from a prospective, randomized, multicentre study. Eur J Clin Invest, Vol.25, (1995), pp. 186–193, ISSN 0014-2972

Peters, H., Fischer, C., Bogner, U., Reiners, C. & Schleusener, H. (1996). Reduction in thyroid volume after radioiodine therapy of Graves' hyperthyroidism: results of a prospective, randomized, multicentre study. Eur J Clin Invest, Vol.26, (1996), pp. 59–63, ISSN 0014-2972

Quimby, E.M., Feitelberg, S. & Gross, W. (1970). Radioactive nuclides in medicine and biology. Lea and Febiger, Philadelphia, USA, 1970.

Read Jr, C.H., Tansey, M.J., & Menda, Y. (2004). A 36-year retrospective analysis of the efficacy and safety of radioactive iodine in treating young Graves' patients. J Clin Endocrinol Metab, Vol.89, (2004), pp. 4229–4233, ISSN 0021-972X

Reiners, Ch. (1997). Zum Krebs- und genetischen Risiko nach Radioiodtherapie der Hyperthyreose. Nuklearmediziner, Vol.20, (1997), pp. 331-334, ISSN 0723-7065

Reiners, C. & Schneider, P. (2002). Radioiodine therapy of thyroid autonomy. Eur J Nucl Med Mol Imaging, (Suppl.2) (2002) p. S471, ISSN 1619-7070

Rivkees, S.A., Sklar, C. &, Freemark, M. (1998). Clinical review 99: the management of Graves' disease in children, with special emphasis on radioiodine treatment. J Clin Endocrinol Metab, Vol.83, (1998), pp. 3767–3768, ISSN 0021-972X

Rivkees, S.A. (2001). The use of radioactive iodine in the management of hyperthyroidism in children. Current Drug Targets - Immune, Endocrine & Metabolic Disorders Vol.1, (2001), pp. 255-264, ISSN 1568-0088

Rivkees, S.A. & Cornelius, E.A. (2003). Influence of iodine-131 dose on the outcome of hyperthyroidism in children. Pediatrics, Vol.111, pp. 745–749, ISSN 0031 4005

Rivkees, S.A. &, Dinauer, C. (2007). Controversy in clinical endocrinology. An optimal treatment for pediatric Graves' disease is radioiodine. J Clin Endocrinol Metab, Vol.92, (2007), pp. 797–800, ISSN 0021-972X

Ron, E., Doody, M.M., Becker, D.V., Brill, A.B., Curtis, R.E., Goldman, M.B., Hartus 3rd, B.S., Hoffman, D.A., McConahey, W.M., Maxon, H.R., Preston-Martin, S., Warshauer, M.E., Wong, F.L. & Boice, Jr, J.D. (1998). Cancer mortality following treatment for adult hyperthyroidism. Cooperative Thyrotoxicosis Therapy Follow-Up Study Group. J Am Med Assoc, Vol.280, pp. 347–355, ISSN 00987484

Sabri, O,, Zimny, M.. Schreckenberger, M., Reinartz, P. & al. (2001). Characteristics of radioiodine therapy failures in Graves´ disease without simultaneous antithyroid agent. Nuklearmedizin, Vol.40, (2001), pp. 1-6, ISSN 0029-5566

Saenger, E.L., Thoma, G.E. & Tompkins, E.A. (1968). Incidence of leukemia following treatment of hyperthyroidism. Preliminary report of the Cooperative Thyrotoxicosis Therapy Follow-Up Study. J Am Med Assoc, Vol.205, (1968), pp. 855–862, ISSN 00987484

Santos, R.B., Romaldini, J.H. & Ward L.S. (2004). Propylthiouracil reduces the effectiveness of radioiodine treatment in hyperthyroid patients with Graves´ disease Clinical research report. Thyroid, Vol.14, No.7, (2004), pp. 525-530, ISSN 1050-7256

Sawka, A.M., Thephamongkhol, K., Brouwers M. & al. (2004). Clinical review 170: a systematic review and metaanalysis of the effectiveness of radioactive iodine remnant ablation for well-differentiated thyroid cancer. J Clin Endocrinol Metab, Vol.89, No.8, (2004), pp. 3668–76, ISSN 0021-972X

Seeger, T., Emrich, D. & Sandrock, D. (1995). Radiojodtherapie der funktionellen Autonomie unter Verwendung des funktionelle autonomen Volumens. Nuklearmedizin, Vol.34, (1995), pp.135, ISSN 0029-5566

Schroeder, P.R., Haugen, B.R., Pacini, F. & al. (2006). A comparison of short-term changes in health-related quality of life in thyroid carcinoma patients undergoing diagnostic evaluation with recombinant human thyrotropin compared with thyroid hormone withdrawal. J Clin Endocrinol Metab, Vol.91, No.3, (2006), pp. 878–84, ISSN 0021-972X

Sisson, J.C., Freitas, J., McDougall, I.R., Bauer, L.T., Hurley, J.R., Brierley, J.D., Edinboro, C.H., Rosenthal, D., Thomas, M.J., Wexler, J.A., Asamoah, E., Avram, A.M., Milas, M. & Greenlee, C. (2011). Radiation safety in the treatment of patiens with thyroid diseases by radioiodine 131I: Practice recommendations of the American Thyroid Association. Thyroid, Vol.21, No.4, (2011), pp. 335-346, ISSN 1050-7256

Skugor, M. (2006) Thyroid Disorders (A Cleveland Clinic Guide) in Cleveland Clinic Press. 2006, pp. 82. ISBN 9781596240216

Sridama, V., McCormick, M., Kaplan, E.L., Fauchet, R. & DeGroot, L.J. (1984). Longterm follow-up study of compensated low-dose 131I therapy for Graves' disease. N Engl J Med, Vol.311, (1984), pp. 426–432, ISSN 0028-4793

Staffurth, J.S. (1987). Hypothyroidism following radioiodine treatment of thyrotoxicosis. J Roy Coll Phys Lond, Vol.21, No.1, (1987), pp. 55-57, ISSN 0035-8819

Studer, H.. & Derwahl, M. (1995). Mechanisms of non-neoplastic endocrine hyperplasia—a changing concept: A review focussed on the thyroid gland. Endocr Rev, Vol.16, (1995), pp. 411, ISSN 0163-769X

Surks, M.I., Chopra, I.J., Mariash, C.N., Nicoloff J.T. & Solomon, D.H. (1990). American Thyroid Association guidelines for use of laboratory tests in thyroid disorders. J Am Med Assoc, Vol.263, (1990), pp. 1529-1532, ISSN 00987484

Tagay, S., Herpertz, S., Langkafel, M. & al. (2005). Health-related quality of life, anxiety and depression in thyroid cancer patients under short-term hypothyroidism and TSH-suppressive levothyroxine treatment. Eur J Endocrinol, Vol.153, No.6, (2005), pp. 755–63, ISSN 0804-4643

Taylor, K.P., Keir, M.J. & Ross, W.M. (1984). Ablative radioiodine therapy for hyperthyroidism: long term follow up study. Br Med J Clin Res Ed, Vol.289, No.6441, (1984), pp. 361-363, ISSN 0267-0623

Turner, J., Sadler, W., Brownlie, B. & Rogers, T. (1985). Radioiodine therapy for Graves' disease: multivariate analysis of pretreatment parameters and early outcome. Eur J Nucl Med, Vol.11, (1985), pp. 191–193, ISSN 1619-7070

Tuttle, R.M., Patience, T. & Budd, S. (1995). Treatment with propylthiouracil before radioactive iodine therapy is associated with a higher treatment failure rate than therapy with radioactive iodine alone in Graves' disease. Thyroid, Vol.4, (1995), pp. 243–247. ISSN 1050-7256

Vlček, P., & Neumann, J. (2002). Thyroid cancer, postsurgery follow-up of patients. [in Czech]: Maxdorf, 218 pp., ISBN 80-85912-50-3, Prague, Czech Republic.

Voth, E., Dickmann, N., Schicha, H. & Emrich, D. (1990). Rezidivrisiko nach thyreostatischer Therapie immunogener und nicht immunogener Hyperthyreosen. Nuklearmedizin, Vol.29, (1990), pp. 1–6, ISSN 0029-5566

Walter, M.A., Christ-Crain, M., Müller, B. & Müller-Brand, J. (2002). Radioiodine uptake and thyroid hormone levels on or off simultaneous carbimazole medication: A ptrospective paired comparison. Nuklearmedizin, Vol.44, (2002), pp. 33-36, ISSN 0029-5566

Watson, A.B., Brownlie, B.E., Frampton, C.M., Turner, J.G. & Rogers, T.G. (1988). Outcome following standardized 185 MBq dose 131I therapy for Graves' disease. Clin Endocrinol (Oxf), Vol.28, (1988), pp. 487–496, ISSN 0300-0664

13

Treatment Related Hypothyroidism, a Viewpoint from Cancer Therapy and Hematopoietic Stem Cell Transplantation

Chao-Jung Tsao and Yin-Hsun Feng
Chi-Mei Medical Center
Taiwan

1. Introduction

Hypothyroidism is the most common disorder of thyroid dysfunction. Sometimes, it can be caused by a variety of medical treatments that leads to a decrease in thyroidal production and secretion of thyroxine and triiodothyronine. Radiation treatment, either radioactive iodine treatment of hyperthyroidism or external radiation treatment for cancer therapy is a major cause of treatment related hypothyroidism. Others include various drugs associated with thyroid suppression, include lithium, iodine, iodine-containing drugs, radiographic contrast agents and cytotoxic chemotherapy. Thyroid dysfunction is one of the most common complications in endocrine system after hematological stem cell transplantation. This chapter will discuss certain type of primary hypothyroidism, including those encountered commonly in clinical practice, such as radioactive iodine therapy, tyrosine kinase inhibitor, hematological stem cell transplantation or other entities.

2. Causes of treatment related hypothyroidism

Thyroid ablation	Surgery
	Radioactive iodine
	External radiotherapy
Pharmacological agent	Lithium
	Interferon-alpha
	Interleukin-2
	Amiodarone
	Tyrosine kinase inhibitor
	Cytotoxic chemotherapy
	Aminoglutethimide
	Ethionamide
	Sulfonamides
Hematological stem cell transplantation	Autologous stem cell transplantation
	Allogeneic stem cell transplantation

Fig. 1. Causes of treatment-related hypothyroidism

2.1 Hypothyroidism due to thyroid ablation

Radioactive iodine therapy

Thyroid ablation using radioactive iodine for thyroid cancer is one of the most common causes of nonspontaneous hypothyroidism since the treatment modality is an important step in adjuvant or palliative setting of thyroid cancer. Radioactive iodine is an effective agent for delivering high radiation doses to the thyroid tissue with low spillover to other portions of the body. The radiation dose to the thyroid tissue is related to the tissue concentration, the ratio between the total tissue uptake and the volume of functional tissue, and the effective half-life of radioactive iodine in the tissue. Radioactive iodine therapy generally results in hypothyroidism, necessitating levothyroxine treatment. In thyroid cancer, total ablation of thyroid function can be achieved after administration of either 100 mCi or 30 mCi in more thane 80% of patients who had at least a near-total thyroidectomy. After less extensive surgery, ablation can be achieved in only two thirds of patients with 30 mCi.

External radiotherapy

Radiotherapy is a frequently applied treatment in patients with head and neck cancer, and sometimes in patients with inoperative thyroid cancer as well as lymphoma. Despite its beneficial effects on locoregional tumor control, radiation may also cause a variety of acute or late side effects, which may be progressive and hamper health-related quality of life (Langendijk et al. 2008). Hypothyroidism may develop within the first year after radiotherapy, especially in patients under 20 years of age. After external radiotherapy, hypothyroidism develops at a median interval of 1.4-1.8 (range 0.3-7.2) years, but may continue to develop many years following therapy (Mercado et al. 2001; Tell et al. 2004). Approximately 30% of patients with solid tumors of the head and neck cancer treated with external radiotherapy develop hypothyroidism (Tami et al. 1992). In stem cell transplantation, hypothyroidism occurs in approximately 9% to 16 % of adults who undergo total body irradiation (Al-Fiar et al. 1997). From a 30 years' experience at the Fred Hutchinson Cancer Research Center in treating children with stem cell transplantation, hypothyroidism is the most common type of thyroid dysfunction as 30% developed hypothyroidism at various times after stem cell transplantation. The incidence of hypothyroidism increased with total body irradiation and the use of busulfan-based regimen (Sanders et al. 2009).

2.2 Hypothyroidism due to therapeutic pharmacological agents

Several drugs can cause hypothyroidism by interfering with thyroid hormone production or provoking thyroid autoimmunity. Pharmacological iodine, such as those to which patients treated with amiodarone or other iodine-containing compounds are exposed, can inhibit thyroid hormone production, especially when combined with underlying autoimmune thyroiditis, and cause hypothyroidism.

Amiodarone

Amiodarone is a commonly prescribed anti-arrhythmic drug because of its ability to treat various types of cardiac arrhythmia including ventricular arrhythmia, paroxysmal supraventricular tachycardia, atrial fibrillation and flutter with minimal negative inotropic and proarrhythmic effects. It is benzofuran derivative containing 37.5% iodine by weight. Daily maintenance dosages of 100 to 600 mg result in a 35 to 140 fold excess in recommended daily iodine intake of 100 to 150 μg. Such a high iodine content and inherent effects of amiodarone and its active metabolite desethylamiodarone are postulated to result in thyroid dysfunction in 14 to 18 % subjects after 2 to 3 years of treatment (Martino et al. 2001). Amiodarone induced hypothyroidism is due to the inhibition of iodine oxidation because of excess intrathyroidal iodine, which is known as the Wolff-Chaikoff effect (Eng et al. 1999). In addition to iodine related effects, amiodarone can alter the activity of deiodinase enzymes. The inhibition of iodothyronine deiodinase activity in peripheral tissues results in decreased triiodothyronine concentration, increased total thyrosine concentration and increased reverse triiodothyronine concentration in serum (Martino et al. 2001). Whether to discontinue amiodarone is still controversial. Withdrawal of the drug may precipitate dysrhythmia, especially as most other alternative anti-arrhythmics are seldom as effective. The treatment of choice for amiodarone induced hypothyroidism is levothyroxine. Amiodarone can be continued at discretion of the cardiologist, keeping in mind that spontaneous remission of hypothyroidism may occur. If amiodarone treatment is discontinued, the decision to initiate thyroid hormone replacement can be delayed (Cohen-Lehman et al. 2010).

Lithium

One in 200 people receives lithium for treatment of bipolar disorder. Lithium has many actions on thyroid physiology. The most important clinical relevant action is the inhibition of thyroid hormone release. The effect of lithium on inhibition of cyclic AMP-mediated cellular events and its inhibitory effect on the phosphoinositol pathway help to explain the intracellular disturbances, but the full mechanism is still not clear. The immunological influence of lithium on thyroid antibody concentrations leads to a more rapid onset of thyroid autoimmunity characterized usually by goiter and hypothyroidism. The clinical side effects of the drug are goiter in up to 40% and hypothyroidism in about 20% (Lazarus 2009). Treatment of lithium-induced hypothyroidism with levothyroxine is no different from treatment of primary hypothyroidism. In these cases there is often a concern that even mild hypothyroidism may contribute to depressive symptoms and that increased thyroid stimulating hormone levels may favor further growth of goiter. The presence of thyroid abnormalities alone is almost never a reason for lithium discontinuation, as this medication is often crucial in maintaining these patients free of the most severe manifestations of their psychiatric illness (Barbesino 2010).

Interferon alpha

Interferon alpha is used for the treatment of hepatitis B and C, as well as various neoplasms, including malignant carcinoid, Kaposi's sarcoma and hairy cell leukemia. Dose-limited side effects of interferon alpha are common, most frequently malaise, depression and hematological side effects. Thyroid dysfunction during interferon alpha is also quite common. Hypothyroidism was initially described as a side effect of interferon alpha therapy in patients receiving long-term interferon alpha treatment for breast cancer (Fentiman et al. 1985). Thyroid effects of interferon alpha have been classified as autoimmune and nonautoimmune, mostly based on the presence or absence of markers of thyroid autoimmunity such as serum thyroid peroxidase and / or thyroglobulin antibodies (Mandac et al. 2006). The observed incidence of interferon alpha associated hypothyroidism in patients with hepatitis C has been reported from approximately 6% to 10% (Deutsch et al. 1997; Koh, Greenspan, and Yeo 1997). Transient hypothyroidism occurs more commonly with interferon alpha therapy than does persistent hypothyroidism, although pooled data from several series indicates that 30% to 44% of patients who develop hypothyroidism during interferon alpha treatment develop persistent thyroid failure (Preziati et al. 1995).

Interleukin-2

Interleukin-2 is used in the treatment of melanoma and renal cell carcinoma. In one series, 32% of 111 patients with cancer developed hypothyroidism during interleukin-2 treatment, and 14% had hypothyroidism postimmunotherapy, persisting from 44 to greater than 149 days (Schwartzentruber et al. 1991). Earlier studies showed a higher incidence of hypothyroidism up to 21% after treatment of interleukin-2 in combination with lymphokine-activated killer cells (Atkins et al. 1988). Most patients who developed hypothyroidism had positive thyroglobulin or thyroid peroxidase antibodies, suggesting autoimmune thyroiditis. Similarly to interferon alpha-induced thyroid disorders, hypothyroid patients are easily treated with thyroid hormone, while destructive thyrotoxicosis only requires symptom control with beta-blockers.

Tyrosine kinase inhibitors

Tyrosine kinase inhibitors have recently emerged as promising chemotherapeutic agents in several types of malignant neoplasms, including thyroid cancer. Several tyrosine kinase inhibitors exert distinctive effects on thyroid function. Tyrosine kinase inhibitors affect thyroid function through two major mechanisms: by increasing thyroid hormone requirements in patients on thyroid hormone replacement and by causing primary hypothyroidism in patients with previously normal thyroid function. In a small clinical report, imatinib caused a fourfold increase in thyroid stimulating hormone level in all eight patients taking levothyroxine after total thyroidectomyt for medullary thyroid cancer. The effect was reversible after discontinuation of treatment and it could be corrected by a doubling in the daily levothyroxine dosage in some patients. There was no change in total thyroxine to suggest increased serum protein binding of thyroid hormone as a possible explanation. Hence, these effects of imatinib are most likely related to increase liver metabolism of thyroid hormone (Barbesino 2010; de Groot et al. 2005). Sunitinib is an oral, multitargeted tyrosine kinase inhibitor of vascular growth receptors, stem cell factor receptor and platelet-derived growth factor receptors. It has been approved for the treatment of gastrointestinal stromal tumor and metastatic renal cell carcinoma. Hypothyroidism has been observed as an adverse event and a clinically relevant toxicity of sunitinib. In one study, 36% of patients with gastrointestinal stromal tumor treated with sunitinib, developed primary hypothyroidism (Desai et al. 2006). Rini et al reported that hypothyroidism occurred in 56 (85%) of 66 patients with metastatic renal cell carcinoma (Rini et al. 2007). Although the mechanism behind this complication remains unclear, it is considered that treatment with levothyroxine can control subclinical and overt hypothyroidism. There have been cases of thyroid atrophy following sunitinib treatment, suggesting a direct effect of sunitinib that leads to degeneration of thyroid follicular cells (Shinohara et al. 2011).

Cytotoxic chemotherapy

Cytotoxic chemotherapy can alter thyroid function in a small proportion of patients. An increased incidence of primary hypothyroidism has been documented in patients treated with multiple drug regimens (Yeung et al. 1998). There is some evidence that L-asparaginase can cause pituitary hypothyroidism, which is resulted from reducing the thyroid stimulating hormone response to thyroid releasing hormone (Heidemann, Stubbe, and Beck 1981). In patients with testicular cancer who received combinations of cisplatin, bleomycin, vinblastine, etoposide, and dactinomycin, 4 of 27 individuals (15%) developed hypothyroidism. In particular, the cumulative doses of cisplatin and vincristine seem to exacerbate these symptoms (Stuart et al. 1990). Forty-four percent of patients who received six cycles of MOPP regimen (mechlorethamine, vinblastine, procarbazine, and prednisolone) for Hodgkin's disease developed an elevated serum thyroid stimulating hormone concentration (Sutcliffe, Chapman, and Wrigley 1981).

2.3 Hypothyroidism after hematopoietic stem cell transplantation

Thyroid dysfunction is an important problem in patents receiving hematopoietic stem cell transplantation and several forms of thyroid disorders have been reported including hypothyroidism, euthyroid sick syndrome, transfer of autoimmune thyroiditis, graft-versus-host disease, and secondary thyroid tumors (Kami et al. 2001). Hypothyroidism is one of the common forms of thyroid disorder after hematopoietic stem cell transplantation. Its frequency was found to be as high as 40% (Borgstrom, and Bolme 1994; Sklar, Kim, and Ramsay 1982) and it appeared to increase with the duration of post-transplant follow-up. In less common instance, patients appeared to have hyperthyroidism after stem cell transplantation, even six months later from clinical reports (Feng et al. 2008). Development of hypothyroidism has been attributed largely to exposure to radiation (Sanders 1990), but it also does occur after chemotherapy-based preparative regimens.

Mechanism of thyroid dysfunction after hematopoietic stem cell transplantation

Hematopoietic stem cell transplantation is a potentially curative procedure for a variety of malignant and non-malignant conditions. When developed initially, hematopoietic stem cell transplantation was considered an approach to rescue patients from toxic side effects of supralethal doses of radiation and chemotherapy used to treat various underlying diseases by transplanting hematopoietic stem cells, which had the ability to reconstitute hematopoiesis. In allogeneic hematopoietic stem cell transplantation, healthy hematopoietic stem cell s are harvested from a separate, related or unrelated, ideally human leukocyte antigen-matched donor, and used to replace the patient's own abnormal hematopoietic stem cells. Conditioning regimen for allogeneic hematopoietic stem cell transplantation often combine total body irradiation and high-dose chemotherapy to eradicate the patient's malignant cell population at the cost of partial or complete bone marrow ablation. Autologous hematopoietic stem cell transplantation requires the extraction of hematopoietic stem cells from the patient. The harvested hematopoietic stem cells return to the patient's body to resume normal blood cell production after conditioning treatment. Individuals successfully treated with hematopoietic stem cell transplantation are at risk of developing post-transplant complications as a result of drug and radiation toxicity, as are those treated with allogeneic hematopoietic stem cell transplantation as a consequence of graft versus host disease. Endocrine complications are among the most prevalent late effects observed in hematopoietic stem cell transplantation recipients (Chemaitilly, and Sklar 2007; Hows et al. 2006). Several thyroid abnormalities have been described following hematopoietic stem cell transplantation. These include therapy-induced primary hypothyroidism, autoimmune thyroid disease, and thyroid neoplasms.

Autologous hematopoietic stem cell transplantation

Autologous hematopoietic stem cell transplantation is performed more frequently than any allogeneic type of organ transplantation worldwide. The endocrine system is one of the most common targets of post-transplant complications. The relative risk of developing endocrine disorders was found to be related to underlying diseases, previous treatments, use of radiation therapies and type of irradiation schedule, post-transplant treatment and age (Brennan, and Shalet 2002; Shalet et al. 1995). Carlson et al. described hypothyroidism developed in 20 of 111 (18%) individuals after autologous stem cell transplantation and the incidence of hypothyroidism was more frequent in patients treated with total body irradiation (Carlson et al. 1992). There were some reports on development of hypothyroidism after non-total body irradiation preparative regimens (Michel et al. 1997; Toubert et al. 1997). Considering the wide differences in the total doses of radiation applied, during treatment of Hodgkin's disease versus preparative conditioning for hematopoietic stem cell transplantation, the incidence of hypothyroidism after hematopoietic stem cell transplantation remains striking. These findings suggest that irradiation of the thyroid gland may not be the sole cause of hypothyroidism after hematopoietic stem cell transplantation. Early effect of thyroid dysfunction was reported by Tauchmanova in patients first year after autologous hematopoietic stem cell transplantation. Subclinical hypothyroidism was diagnosed in 10% of patients and worsened progressively in all but one patient (Tauchmanova et al. 2005).

Allogeneic hematopoietic stem cell transplantation

Hypothyroidism haven been reported to be as high as 52% of patients with allogeneic hematopoietic stem cell transplantation (Al-Hazzouri et al. 2009; Bailey et al. 2008; Berger et al. 2005; Sanders et al. 2009). The time course of developing hypothyroidism after hematopoietic stem cell transplantation varied based on the conditioning regimen. In one study, patients who received single fraction total body irradiation developed compensated hypothyroidism at a mean of 3.2 (range 1-8.2) years after hematopoietic stem cell transplantation and progressed to overt hypothyroidism about 1-2 years later (Thomas et al. 1993). Hypothyroidis was recognized between 0.9 and 7.3 (median 4.1) years after hyperfractionated radiation and at a median of 4.2 years in patients conditioned with busulfan and cyclophosphamide (Boulad et al. 1995). In a 30 year-surveillance of post-transplant, 30% of children developed hypothyroidism at various times after hematopoietic stem cell transplantation and among these 20% were treated with thyroid hormone. Thyroid dysfunction continues to occur as long as 28 years after hematopoietic stem cell transplantation conditioning with total body irradiation and as long as 10 years after busulfan-cyclophosphamide preparative regimen (Sanders et al. 2009).

The mechanism for hypothyroidism after transplant is unknown. Donor antibody transfers, immune-mediated injury, conditioning treatment effects, post-transplant medications and patient susceptibility may play a role in post-hematopoietic stem cell transplantation hypothyroidism. Case studies have shown that a donor with autoimmune thyroid disorder may transfer cell capable of injuring the recipient's thyroid gland after hematopoietic stem cell transplantation (Lee et al. 2001; Marazuela, and Steegman 2000). Immune-mediated thyroid injury arising in the host has been suggested in other studies and may be a form of graft-versus-host-disease (Kami et al. 2001; Katsanis et al. 1990; Somali et al. 2005). Patients receiving single-agent graft-versus-host-disease prophylaxis were found to have a 9.5 times greater risk of developing hypothyroidism than patients with multi-agent prophylaxis (Katsanis et al. 1990). From an immunological standpoint, stem cells from matched sibling donors are though to be less immunologically reactive than those from unrelated donors. Patients who received stem cells from an unrelated donor had over an eightfold increased risk of hypothyroidism compared to those who received matched sibling stem cells (Bailey et al. 2008). Total body irradiation is a well established risk factor for hypothyroidism after hematopoietic stem cell transplantation and used of fractionated instead of single-dose total body irradiation decreases its risk (Boulad et al. 1995). Other risk factor for developing hypothyroidism after hematopoietic stem cell transplantation includes young age at transplantation and stem cell transplantation during second complete remission (Berger et al. 2005; Ishiguro et al. 2004). A study focused on reduced-intensity conditioning regimen in hematopoietic stem cell transplantation disclosed that the incidence of post-transplant hypothyroidism was similar in myeloablative or reduced-intensity conditioning regimen (Al-Hazzouri et al. 2009).

3. Conclusions

The endocrine system is one of the most common targets of post-treatment complications in cancer survivors. The relative risk of developing endocrine disorders was found to be related to underlying diseases, previous treatments, use of radiation therapies, and post-transplant treatments. Thyroid dysfunction has been frequently reported after hematopoietic cell transplantation. Radiation has been considered the main cause for this and for thyroid malignancies, but in the context of hematopoietic cell transplantation, total body irradiation has been considered to be the major cause. The incidence of post-transplant thyroid disorder ranging from 0% to 57% was reported previously. Sick euthyroid syndrome was more frequently observed. Most patients developed a mild compensated primary hypothyroidism that may be transient and can be resolved spontaneously. Hypothyroidism can be an early complication but is usually considered as a late complication identified several years after hematopoietic cell transplantation. Approximately 15 % of patients develop overt primary hypothyroidism and 30% have compensated hypothyroidism. The incidence is lower in patients treated with autologous hematopoietic cell transplantation or conditioned with chemotherapy alone.

With the cumulative experiences in hematopoietic cell transplantation and advances in supportive care, the number of long-term survivors has increased. Knowledge about increased risk for long term complications due to cancer therapy and pre-hematopoietic cell transplantation preparative regimen should encourage each physician to improve their quality of care.

4. References

Al-Fiar, F. Z., R. Colwill, J. H. Lipton, G. Fyles, D. Spaner, and H. Messner. (1997). Abnormal thyroid stimulating hormone (TSH) levels in adults following allogeneic bone marrow transplants. *Bone Marrow Transplant,* Vol. 19, No.10, pp. 1019-22, ISSN 0268-3369.

Al-Hazzouri, A., Q. Cao, L. J. Burns, D. J. Weisdorf, and N. S. Majhail. (2009). Similar risks for hypothyroidism after allogeneic hematopoietic cell transplantation using TBI-based myeloablative and reduced-intensity conditioning regimens. *Bone Marrow Transplant,* Vol. 43, No. 12, pp. 949-51, ISSN 1476-5365.

Atkins, M. B., J. W. Mier, D. R. Parkinson, J. A. Gould, E. M. Berkman, and M. M. Kaplan. (1988). Hypothyroidism after treatment with interleukin-2 and lymphokine-activated killer cells. *N Engl J Med,* Vol. 318, No. 24, pp. 1557-63, ISSN 0028-4793.

Bailey, H. K., M. S. Kappy, R. H. Giller, and J. Gralla. (2008). Time-course and risk factors of hypothyroidism following allogeneic hematopoietic stem cell transplantation (HSCT) in children conditioned with fractionated total body irradiation. *Pediatr Blood Cancer,* Vol. 51, No. 3, pp. 405-9, ISSN 1545-5017.

Barbesino, G. (2010). Drugs affecting thyroid function. *Thyroid,* Vol. 20, No. 7, pp. 763-70, ISSN 1557-9077.

Berger, C., B. Le-Gallo, J. Donadieu, O. Richard, A. Devergie, C. Galambrun, P. Bordigoni, E. Vilmer, E. Plouvier, Y. Perel, G. Michel, and J. L. Stephan. (2005). Late thyroid toxicity in 153 long-term survivors of allogeneic bone marrow transplantation for acute lymphoblastic leukaemia. *Bone Marrow Transplant,* Vol. 35, No. 10, pp. 991-5, ISSN 0268-3369.

Borgstrom, B. and P. Bolme. (1994). Thyroid function in children after allogeneic bone marrow transplantation. *Bone Marrow Transplant,* Vol. 13, No. 1, pp. 59-64, ISSN 0268-3369.

Boulad, F., M. Bromley, P. Black, G. Heller, K. Sarafoglou, A. Gillio, E. Papadopoulos, and C. Sklar. (1995). Thyroid dysfunction following bone marrow transplantation using hyperfractionated radiation. *Bone Marrow Transplant,* Vol. 15, No. 1, pp. 71-6, ISSN 0268-3369.

Brennan, B. M. and S. M. Shalet. (2002). Endocrine late effects after bone marrow transplant. *Br J Haematol,* Vol. 118, No. 1, pp. 58-66, ISSN 0007-1048.

Carlson, K., G. Lonnerholm, B. Smedmyr, G. Oberg, and B. Simonsson. (1992). Thyroid function after autologous bone marrow transplantation. *Bone Marrow Transplant,* Vol. 10, No. 2, pp. 123-7, ISSN 0268-3369.

Chemaitilly, W. and C. A. Sklar. (2007). Endocrine complications of hematopoietic stem cell transplantation. *Endocrinol Metab Clin North Am,* Vol. 36, No. 4, pp. 983-98, ISSN 0889-8529.

Cohen-Lehman, J., P. Dahl, S. Danzi, and I. Klein. (2010). Effects of amiodarone therapy on thyroid function. *Nat Rev Endocrinol,* Vol. 6, No. 1, pp. 34-41, ISSN 1759-5037.

de Groot, J. W., B. A. Zonnenberg, J. T. Plukker, W. T. van Der Graaf, and T. P. Links. (2005). Imatinib induces hypothyroidism in patients receiving levothyroxine. *Clin Pharmacol Ther,* Vol. 78, No. 4, pp. 433-8, ISSN 0009-9236.

Desai, J., L. Yassa, E. Marqusee, S. George, M. C. Frates, M. H. Chen, J. A. Morgan, S. S. Dychter, P. R. Larsen, G. D. Demetri, and E. K. Alexander. (2006). Hypothyroidism after sunitinib treatment for patients with gastrointestinal stromal tumors. *Ann Intern Med,* Vol. 145, No. 9, pp. 660-4, ISSN 1539-3704.

Deutsch, M., S. Dourakis, E. K. Manesis, A. Gioustozi, G. Hess, A. Horsch, and S. Hadziyannis. (1997). Thyroid abnormalities in chronic viral hepatitis and their relationship to interferon alfa therapy. *Hepatology,* Vol. 26, No. 1, pp. 206-10, ISSN 0270-9139.

Eng, P. H., G. R. Cardona, S. L. Fang, M. Previti, S. Alex, N. Carrasco, W. W. Chin, and L. E. Braverman. (1999). Escape from the acute Wolff-Chaikoff effect is associated with a decrease in thyroid sodium/iodide symporter messenger ribonucleic acid and protein. *Endocrinology,* Vol. 140, No. 8, pp. 3404-10, ISSN 0013-7227.

Feng, Y. H., B. A. Su, C. Y. Lin, W. T. Huang, and C. J. Tsao. (2008). Hyperthyroidism as a latent complication of autologous hematopoietic stem cell transplantation. *Int J Hematol,* Vol. 88, No. 2, pp. 237-9, ISSN 0925-5710.

Fentiman, I. S., B. S. Thomas, F. R. Balkwill, R. D. Rubens, and J. L. Hayward. (1985). Primary hypothyroidism associated with interferon therapy of breast cancer. *Lancet,* Vol. 1, No. 8438, pp. 1166, ISSN 0140-6736.

Heidemann, P. H., P. Stubbe, and W. Beck. (1981). Transient secondary hypothyroidism and thyroxine binding globulin deficiency in leukemic children during polychemotherapy: an effect of L-asparaginase. *Eur J Pediatr,* Vol. 136, No. 3, pp. 291-5, ISSN 0340-6199.

Hows, J. M., J. R. Passweg, A. Tichelli, A. Locasciulli, R. Szydlo, A. Bacigalupo, N. Jacobson, P. Ljungman, J. Cornish, A. Nunn, B. Bradley, and G. Socie. (2006). Comparison of long-term outcomes after allogeneic hematopoietic stem cell transplantation from matched sibling and unrelated donors. *Bone Marrow Transplant,* Vol. 38, No. 12, pp. 799-805, ISSN 0268-3369.

Ishiguro, H., Y. Yasuda, Y. Tomita, T. Shinagawa, T. Shimizu, T. Morimoto, K. Hattori, M. Matsumoto, H. Inoue, H. Yabe, M. Yabe, O. Shinohara, and S. Kato. (2004). Long-term follow-up of thyroid function in patients who received bone marrow transplantation during childhood and adolescence. *J Clin Endocrinol Metab,* Vol. 89, No. 12, pp. 5981-6, ISSN 0021-972X.

Kami, M., Y. Tanaka, S. Chiba, T. Matsumura, U. Machida, Y. Kanda, K. Nakagawa, T. Mitsuhashi, and H. Hirai. (2001). Thyroid function after bone marrow transplantation: possible association between immune-mediated thyrotoxicosis and hypothyroidism. *Transplantation,* Vol. 71, No. 3, pp. 406-11, ISSN 0041-1337.

Katsanis, E., R. S. Shapiro, L. L. Robison, R. J. Haake, T. Kim, O. H. Pescovitz, and N. K. Ramsay. (1990). Thyroid dysfunction following bone marrow transplantation: long-term follow-up of 80 pediatric patients. *Bone Marrow Transplant,* Vol. 5, No. 5, pp. 335-40, ISSN 0268-3369.

Koh, L. K., F. S. Greenspan, and P. P. Yeo. (1997). Interferon-alpha induced thyroid dysfunction: three clinical presentations and a review of the literature. *Thyroid,* Vol. 7, No. 6, pp. 891-6, ISSN 1050-7256.

Langendijk, J. A., P. Doornaert, I. M. Verdonck-de Leeuw, C. R. Leemans, N. K. Aaronson, and B. J. Slotman. (2008). Impact of late treatment-related toxicity on quality of life among patients with head and neck cancer treated with radiotherapy. *J Clin Oncol,* Vol. 26, No. 22, pp. 3770-6, ISSN 1527-7755.

Lazarus, J. H. (2009). Lithium and thyroid. *Best Pract Res Clin Endocrinol Metab,* Vol. 23, No. 6, pp. 723-33, ISSN 1532-1908.

Lee, W. Y., E. S. Oh, C. K. Min, D. W. Kim, J. W. Lee, M. I. Kang, W. S. Min, B. Y. Cha, K. W. Lee, H. Y. Son, S. K. Kang, and C. C. Kim. (2001). Changes in autoimmune thyroid disease following allogeneic bone marrow transplantation. *Bone Marrow Transplant,* Vol. 28, No. 1, pp. 63-6, ISSN 0268-3369.

Mandac, J. C., S. Chaudhry, K. E. Sherman, and Y. Tomer. (2006). The clinical and physiological spectrum of interferon-alpha induced thyroiditis: toward a new classification. *Hepatology,* Vol. 43, No. 4, pp. 661-72, ISSN 0270-9139.

Marazuela, M. and J. L. Steegman. (2000). Transfer of autoimmune hypothyroidism following bone marrow transplantation from a donor with Graves' disease. *Bone Marrow Transplant,* Vol. 26, No. 11, pp. 1217-20, ISSN 0268-3369.

Martino, E., L. Bartalena, F. Bogazzi, and L. E. Braverman. (2001). The effects of amiodarone on the thyroid. *Endocr Rev,* Vol. 22, No. 2, pp. 240-54, ISSN 0163-769X.

Mercado, G., D. J. Adelstein, J. P. Saxton, M. Secic, M. A. Larto, and P. Lavertu. (2001). Hypothyroidism: a frequent event after radiotherapy and after radiotherapy with chemotherapy for patients with head and neck carcinoma. *Cancer,* Vol. 92, No. 11, pp. 2892-7, ISSN 0008-543X.

Michel, G., G. Socie, F. Gebhard, F. Bernaudin, I. Thuret, J. P. Vannier, F. Demeocq, G. Leverger, J. L. Pico, H. Rubie, F. Mechinaud, J. Reiffers, N. Gratecos, X. Troussard, J. P. Jouet, G. Simonin, E. Gluckman, and D. Maraninchi. (1997). Late effects of allogeneic bone marrow transplantation for children with acute myeloblastic leukemia in first complete remission: the impact of conditioning regimen without total-body irradiation--a report from the Societe Francaise de Greffe de Moelle. *J Clin Oncol,* Vol. 15, No. 6, pp. 2238-46, ISSN 0732-183X.

Preziati, D., L. La Rosa, G. Covini, R. Marcelli, S. Rescalli, L. Persani, E. Del Ninno, P. L. Meroni, M. Colombo, and P. Beck-Peccoz. (1995). Autoimmunity and thyroid function in patients with chronic active hepatitis treated with recombinant interferon alpha-2a. *Eur J Endocrinol,*Vol 132, No. 5, pp. 587-93, ISSN 0804-4643.

Rini, B. I., I. Tamaskar, P. Shaheen, R. Salas, J. Garcia, L. Wood, S. Reddy, R. Dreicer, and R. M. Bukowski. (2007). Hypothyroidism in patients with metastatic renal cell carcinoma treated with sunitinib. *J Natl Cancer Inst,* Vol. 99, No. 1, pp. 81-3, ISSN 1460-2105.

Sanders, J. E. (1990). Late effects in children receiving total body irradiation for bone marrow transplantation. *Radiother Oncol,* Vol. 18 Suppl 1, pp. 82-7, ISSN 0167-8140.

Sanders, J. E., P. A. Hoffmeister, A. E. Woolfrey, P. A. Carpenter, B. E. Storer, R. F. Storb, and F. R. Appelbaum. (2009). Thyroid function following hematopoietic cell transplantation in children: 30 years' experience. *Blood,* Vol. 113, No. 2, pp. 306-8, ISSN 1528-0020.

Schwartzentruber, D. J., D. E. White, M. H. Zweig, B. D. Weintraub, and S. A. Rosenberg. (1991). Thyroid dysfunction associated with immunotherapy for patients with cancer. *Cancer,* Vol. 68, No. 11, pp. 2384-90, ISSN 0008-543X.

Shalet, S. M., M. Didi, A. L. Ogilvy-Stuart, J. Schulga, and M. D. Donaldson. (1995). Growth and endocrine function after bone marrow transplantation. *Clin Endocrinol (Oxf),* Vol. 42, No. 4, pp. 333-9, ISSN 0300-0664.

Shinohara, N., M. Takahashi, T. Kamishima, H. Ikushima, N. Otsuka, A. Ishizu, C. Shimizu, H. Kanayama, and K. Nonomura. (2011). The incidence and mechanism of sunitinib-induced thyroid atrophy in patients with metastatic renal cell carcinoma. *Br J Cancer,* Vol. 104, No. 2, pp. 241-7, ISSN 1532-1827.

Sklar, C. A., T. H. Kim, and N. K. Ramsay. (1982). Thyroid dysfunction among long-term survivors of bone marrow transplantation. *Am J Med,* Vol. 73, No. 5, pp. 688-94, ISSN 0002-9343.

Somali, M., V. Mpatakoias, A. Avramides, I. Sakellari, C. Smias, A. Anagnostopoulos, A. Papachristou, and A. Antoniadou. (2005). Thyroid dysfunction in adult long-term survivors after hemapoeitic stem-cell transplantation (HSCT). *Horm Metab Res,* Vol. 37, No. 8, pp. 494-9, ISSN 0018-5043.

Stuart, N. S., C. M. Woodroffe, R. Grundy, and M. H. Cullen. (1990). Long-term toxicity of chemotherapy for testicular cancer--the cost of cure. *Br J Cancer,* Vol. 61, No. 3, pp. 479-84, ISSN 0007-0920.

Sutcliffe, S. B., R. Chapman, and P. F. Wrigley. (1981). Cyclical combination chemotherapy and thyroid function in patients with advanced Hodgkin's disease. *Med Pediatr Oncol,* Vol. 9, No. 5, pp. 439-48, ISSN 0098-1532.

Tami, T. A., P. Gomez, G. S. Parker, M. B. Gupta, and D. A. Frassica. (1992). Thyroid dysfunction after radiation therapy in head and neck cancer patients. *Am J Otolaryngol,* Vol. 13, No. 6, pp. 357-62, ISSN 0196-0709.

Tauchmanova, L., C. Selleri, G. De Rosa, M. Esposito, C. Di Somma, F. Orio, S. Palomba, G. Lombardi, B. Rotoli, and A. Colao. (2005). Endocrine disorders during the first year after autologous stem-cell transplant. *Am J Med,* Vol. 118, No. 6, pp. 664-70, ISSN 0002-9343.

Tell, R., G. Lundell, B. Nilsson, H. Sjodin, F. Lewin, and R. Lewensohn. (2004). Long-term incidence of hypothyroidism after radiotherapy in patients with head-and-neck cancer. *Int J Radiat Oncol Biol Phys,* Vol. 60, No. 2, pp. 395-400, ISSN 0360-3016.

Thomas, B. C., R. Stanhope, P. N. Plowman, and A. D. Leiper. (1993). Endocrine function following single fraction and fractionated total body irradiation for bone marrow transplantation in childhood. *Acta Endocrinol (Copenh),* Vol. 128, No. 6, pp. 508-12, ISSN 0001-5598.

Toubert, M. E., G. Socie, E. Gluckman, S. Aractingi, H. Esperou, A. Devergie, P. Ribaud, N. Parquet, M. H. Schlageter, J. P. Beressi, J. D. Rain, and P. Vexiau. (1997). Short- and long-term follow-up of thyroid dysfunction after allogeneic bone marrow transplantation without the use of preparative total body irradiation. *Br J Haematol,* Vol. 98, No. 2, pp. 453-7, ISSN 0007-1048.

Yeung, S. C., A. C. Chiu, R. Vassilopoulou-Sellin, and R. F. Gagel. (1998). The endocrine effects of nonhormonal antineoplastic therapy. *Endocr Rev,* Vol. 19, No. 2, pp. 144-72, ISSN 0163-769X.

Part 3

New View

14

Thyroid Hormones and Motoneurons Development

Farzaneh Ganji
Department of Biology, Faculty of Science,
Golestan University, Gorgan
Iran

1. Introduction

It is well known that postnatal maturation of the central nervous system is critically dependent on thyroid hormone levels (Thompson & Potter, 2000) and this might influence the neuromuscular system (Barakat-Walter et al., 2000). Previous neuroanatomical and biochemical investigations demonstrated that development of skeletal muscles including the masseter is affected by both neuronal and thyroid hormonal effects (Adams et al., 1999; d' Albis et al., 1989, 1990; Butler-Browne et al. 1984; Gambke et al., 1983; Rubinstein et al., 1988). Under normal condition the phenotypic properties of motoneurons and muscle fibers in the neuromuscular unit are matched (Copray & Kernell, 2000; Hughes & Salinas, 1999; Akihiko Ishihara, Kawano, Okiura, Morimatsu, & Ohira, 2005).

A pronounced shift in oromotor behavior occurs with the transition from sucking to chewing in humans and other mammals (Green et al., 1997; Saito, Ohnuki, Yamane, & Saeki, 2002). It has been reported that the transition from neonatal to adult fast MHC is however dependent on thyroid hormone (Soukup & Jirmanová, 2000). In the rat there is a significant rise to peak T4 serum levels at 15 days followed by a slight decline to mature values (Gambke et al., 1983). The diameter of muscle fibers enlarges progressively from slow to fast type in order to adapt to the rapid functional changes from weaning to chewing motion (Miyata et al., 1996).

During development, hyporthyroidism results in an inhibition in the expression of adult fast MHC isoforms and a persistence of the slow isoforms in the masseter muscle (Agbulut et al., 2003; Butler-Browne et al., 1987; Pette & Staron, 2000) which is also associated with a decrease in fiber diameter of the masseter muscle (Sugasawa & Mori, 1998). The increase in the circulating levels of thyroid hormone in suckling rats is involved in development of the masseter (Maeda et al., 1981a, 1981b). This effect is explained first as a result of an orthograde mechanism through the trophic factors secreted by different motoneuron types at the neuromuscular junction. The second explanation invokes a retrograde mechanism, so that, once muscle fibers are differentiated into slow or fast types they may modify properties of motoneurons via retrograde transport of substances (Barakat-Walter & Riederer, 1996; Munson et al., 1997). Based on these hypotheses, Sickles et al. (Sickles et al., 1987) and Bakels et al. (Bakels et al., 1998) reported considerable alteration in the adult rats' soleus motoneurons morphology due to hyper- and hypo-thyroidism respectively. In regard to the masseter muscle, neuroanatomical evidence related to the mechanisms of shifting from sucking to biting was first reported by Kubota et al. in mice (Kubota et al., 1988). Upon their observation the differentiation of the trigeminal motoneurons related to biting is rapidly accelerated after birth. Miyata et al. have reported morphometric alteration of superficial masseter motoneurons from sucking to chewing in normal rats in a way that the diameter of the largest motoneurons increases rapidly from 5 to 21 postnatal days (Miyata et al., 1996).

Calcitoin-gene related peptide (CGRP), a co-transmitter, along with acetylcholine in the neuromuscular system is released at motor end plates, where the muscle cells demonstrate binding sites for CGRP (Popper & P. E. Micevych, 1989; Terrado et al., 1997). In fact, CGRP is synthesized in the motoneuron cell bodies, transported down to the motor terminals, stored in dense-core vesicles and released upon nerve stimulation (Buffelli et al., 2001). This neuropeptide exerts a variety of effects on skeletal muscle such as spontaneous acetylcholine release from motor nerve terminals, enhancement of neurally evoked muscle contraction and regulation of the rate of the acetylcholine receptor (AChR) at the neuromuscular junction (Kimura, 1998; van Rossum, Hanisch, & Quirion, 1997). CGRP functions are mediated by cell membrane receptors that belong to the family of G-protein-coupled receptors (van Rossum et al., 1997). CGRP may thus serve as an anterograde trophic agent released by motoneurons that contributes to the maintenance of a high density of neuromuscular junctional AChRs (H L Fernandez, Chen, I Nadelhaft, & Durr, 2003; Roa & Changeux, 1991). Indeed, motoneuronal CGRP acts as a physiological transducer through its complex receptors in muscle motor endplates (Hugo L. Fernandez, Ross, & Irving Nadelhaft, 1999). It has been proposed that the levels of CGRP present in individual motoneurons are related to the type of muscle unit that is innervated by the respective motoneuron (Popper & P. E. Micevych, 1989). It has also been claimed that there is a relationship between the type of myosin composition of different rat muscles and the CGRP mRNA expression in conveying motoneurons (Blanco, Popper, & P. Micevych, 1997). Hypothyroid muscles show a nearly 50% reduction in AChRs density when compared to the control muscles (Kragie & Smiehorowski, 1993), therefore during weaning, when feeding behavior needs to transform from suckling to chewing (Saito et al., 2002), prenatal slow myosin persists, preventing faster muscular contraction due to severe decrease in the density of neuro- muscular junction AChRs (Miyata et al., 1996). According to the available target, motoneuronal CGRP levels alter in relation to the type of muscle fibers (Blanco et al., 1997; Popper & P. E. Micevych, 1989).

A review of literature regarding to motoneurons development shows that detailed morphometric data on the developing masseter innervation has been neglected in prenatal hypothyroid rats. Thus in this chapter the morphological features of the developing masseter motoneurons labeled by injection of HRP into the superficial masseter muscle were analyzed in normal and congenital hypothyroid rat's offspring. HRP retrograde reaction product is observed as dark blue intracellular granules varying in quantity from motoneuron to motoneuron even in the same trigeminal motor nucleus (Kawagishi et al., 1992). As hypothyroidism reduces neuronal process growth, synaptogenesis, axonal transport velocity (Biesiada et al., 1996; Stein et al., 1991) and neurotransmitter synthesis (Barakat-Walter et al., 2000; Behzadi & Ganji, 2005), it was of especial interest to investigate the alteration in the morphological characteristics of masseter motoneurons as well as HRP uptake and transport from the neuromuscular junction. In this regard the labeling quality of HRP backfilled masseteric motoneurons along with their size distribution profile under developmental hypothyroidism were evaluated. Furthermore the oro-facial motoneuronal CGRP immunoreactive responses under the congenital thyroid hypofunction were examined and also usig the Golgi staining method, the morphology of the masseteric motoneurons including their dendritic arborization pattern in normal and hypothyroid weaned rat pups was studied. These studies may lead to better understanding of the ontogenic changes in mastication.

2. Materials and methods

2.1 Animals

Timed pregnant Sprauge-Dawley rats (Pasteur's Institute, Tehran, Iran) were housed individually in plastic cages with free access to food and water. The animal room was maintained at constant 22-24° C temperature under a 12 hour light/ 12 hour dark cycle. The studies were performed according to the guidelines for laboratory animal use and care set forth by the research council at Shahid Beheshti University of Medical Sciences (Tehran-Iran). Neonatal hypothyroidism was induced by adding 50mg/liter PTU (Sigma) to the drinking water of pregnant dams beginning at gestational day 16 to postnatal day 23. It should be noted that this concentration represents the same amount of PTU which is received by the pups during suckling period (Blake & Henning, 1985). Control dams received tap water. Usually litters were culled to 8 pups on postnatal day 1 for each dam.

2.2 Intramasseter HRP injection

On the 1st, 5th, 13th and 21st days after birth several male pups in each age group were anesthetized by i.p. injection of Ketamine (100mg/Kg) and Xylazine (5mg/Kg). A small incision was made in the chick skin to expose the surface of the superficial masseter muscle. Then 1-5µlit of 40% HRP (type VI- Sigma) dissolved in sterile saline was injected slowly into the 2-5 loci above as well as under the parotid duct in the left masseter using a Hamilton syringe as demonstrated by Kawagishi et al. (Kawagishi et al., 1992). After each injection the needle was left in situ for 1 min to avoid backflow of the injected HRP, following which the needle was removed, the injection sites were cleaned with sterile saline, and the opening was sutured.

2.2.1 Histochemical procedure

After 24-48h of survival time, the pups were deeply anesthetized and perfused transcardially with 20-50 ml saline (37°C) followed by 50-100 ml of fixative (1.25% glutaraldehyde and 1% paraformaldehyde in 0.1 M phosphate buffer at pH 7.4, 4°C). Following perfusion and fixation the lower brainstems were removed and post fixed for 24h. The blocks of tissue were cut serially into 50µm thick coronal sections using a Vibratome. Then the sections were processed for HRP reaction using TMB method (Mesulam, 1982) and counterstained with 0.1% neutral red.

2.2.2 Microscopic study

In each experimental group, three pups with the most reliable labeling in their trigeminal motor nucleus (Mo5) were chosen for microscopic study. From rostral to caudal part of Mo5, eight cross sections were selected per animal for each age group of normal and hypothyroid pups. The HRP labeled motoneurons showing a nucleolus or with visible primary dendrites were counted and upon their HRP labeling profile they were semi-quantitatively divided into strong (S) and weak (W) intensities. The cell body area of 500 HRP labeled neurons with both intensities were measured through the cross sections using a computer based image analysis system (Olympus BX60, DP12, Olysia soft imaging system, Japan). To measure the soma areas images of labeled cells were displayed on a monitor and their cell bodies perimeters in continuous with soma-dendritic transitional regions were outlined. Photomicrographs were arranged using CorelDRAW12.

2.2.3 Statistics

Differences between normal and hypothyroid groups were analyzed with two tailed student's t-test. Two- way analysis of variance (ANOVA) was employed to assess the variation of soma size in relation to labeling intensity of masseteric motoneurons in different groups. The level of significance was set at $P<0.05$. Values are means ± SEM

2.3 CGRP immunohistochemistry

At the onset of weaning period (post natal day 23), 12 deeply anaesthetized (100 mg/kg ketamine and 5 mg/kg xylazine) male pups (6 hypothyroid and 6 controls) underwent transcardial perfusion with saline followed by 4% paraformaldehyde, 1.33% picric acid and 0.1% glutaraldehyde in phosphate buffer, pH 7.4. The brainstems of all 12 rats were cut serially into 50 micron thick coronal sections with a Vibratome. Tissue sections were collected in phosphate buffered saline (PBS) containing 0.3% Triton X-100 (PBST) and 0.3% hydrogen peroxide. The sections were rinsed with bovine serum albumin (0.1% in PBST, for 1 h) and then they were incubated in a rabbit polyclonal CGRP antibody solution (Sigma, USA, 1:2500 dilution) at 4 ◦C for 72 h. Thereafter, the sections were washed in PBST and incubated in biotinylated goat anti-rabbit IgG (Vector Laboratories, 1:2000 dilution) at 4 ◦C overnight with stirring. After two further rinses, the sections were placed in a 1:1000 dilution of avidin-biotin complex (Vector Laboratories) for 2 h. The immunohistochemical reaction product was revealed with 0.05% 3, 3'-diaminobenzidine (DAB, Sigma) and 0.5% nickel in Tris-HCl buffer, pH 7.6, in the presence of 0.005% hydrogen peroxide. Finally, tissue sections were washed in Tris-HCl buffer, mounted on gelatinized slides and counterstained with neutral red before coverslipping

2.3.1 Microscopic study

Eight sections containing main and accessory trigeminal (Mo5 and Mo5-AC) and facial (Mo7) motor nuclei were selected per animal. A semiquantitative CGRP-like intensity of these motoneurons was unilaterally evaluated as strong, moderate, weak and negative staining. The mean soma diameter of the motoneurons showing a nucleus were obtained by taking the average of two diameters, measured at the maximal and minimal axes of soma (Honma et al. 2002; Ishihara et al. 1988), using a computer- based image analysis system (Olympus BX60, DP12, Olysia soft imaging system, Japan). Photomicrographs were arranged using CorelDRAW12. Statistical significance was analyzed by Student's *t*-test. The level of significance was set at $P < 0.05$.

2.4 Golgi staining method

Time pregnant female Wistar rats weighing 180 g were randomly divided into control and PTU-treated groups. PTU-treated group received 50ppm propylthiouracil (PTU) in their drinking water from 16th day of pregnancy, continued to 22nd day post-partum. Control group received tap water. After transcardial perfusion, brain stems of 6 male 23 day old pups in each experimental group were processed for Golgi-Hortega staining method. Using rotary microtome brain stem paraffin embedded blocks were cut to 70 micron slices. Mo5 tissue sections were selected for photomicrography and morphological analysis. Using Image Analysis Starter software (Olympus, Japan) the cross section area of selected motoneurons in both experimental groups were measured and their primary and secondary dendrites were counted. Dendritic tree arborization pattern was analyzed with altered Sholl's concentric circles method (Ristanović,et al. 2006) . Statistical analysis including Student's t-test and ANOVA tests was done using SPSS software.

3. Results

3.1 Experimental hypothyroidism

For induction of prenatal hypothyroidism, at first, a range of 0.050 and 0.075 % of PTU was tested, but the survival of the pups dropped sharply beyond the second postnatal week and and finally the 0.005% concentration of this drug was used which induced a mild hypothyroidism and allowed us to have hypothyroid pups with a moderate rate of mortality until the time of weaning. In accordance with previous observations (Blake & Henning, 1985; Sawin, Brodish, Carter, Stanton, & Lau, 1998), PTU treated pups displayed the skeletal and morphological deformities characteristic of hypothyroidism including blunt snouts, unfolded ears and rounded bodies compared to normal pups, eye opening was delayed for 2 days. In this study, PTU-treated pups were weighed at different times from birth to 23 days after birth (Fig 1). At the time of weaning hypothyroid pups weighed 50% under normal weight.

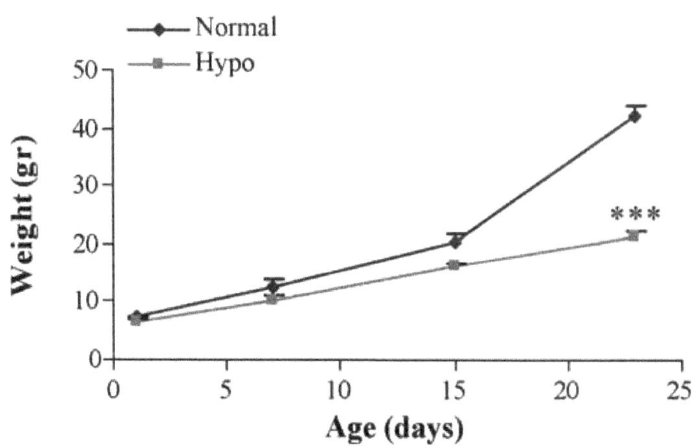

Fig. 1. Body weight profile (mean ± S.E.M.) of hypothyroid offspring was significantly reduced compared to the controls by postnatal day 15 up to 23 ($P < 0.001$).

3.2 Masseter HRP labeled motoneurons

In accordance to Mizuno et al., the masseteric labeled motoneurons were located in the dorsolateral part of the trigeminal motor nucleus (Mizuno et al. 1975). No contralateral neuronal labeling was observed. Unlabeled motoneurons were excluded from the study. The labeled motoneurons of normal and hypothyroid pups at days1, 7, 15 and 23 are shown in Fig 2. The number of labeled motoneurons in control pups was not significantly different from those found in their hypothyroid homologues (table 1). In addition, the total number of strongly labeled motoneurons (S) was higher than weakly labeled (W) ones in both normal and hypothyroid pups during postnatal development. Indeed, the most obvious morphological changes in hypothyroid masseter motoneurons could be detected from day 15 to 23, in that the hypothyroid masseteric motoneurons showed less primary dendrites with shorter processes and slightly more weakly HRP labeled soma compared to normal pups (fig. 3).

Pups	day 1	day 7	day 15	day 23
Normal	190±18.8	170±13.9	195±19.1	174±17.0
Hypothyroid	182±24.0	182±22.7	199±13.5	176± 7.8

Table 1.

The correlative results between soma size and HRP labeling intensity of 500 measured motoneurons in each group were as follows:

Day 1

At day 1 after birth, a similar number of HRP-positive neurons was found in hypothyroid and in normal pups. The soma area of the labeled motoneurons ranged between 80-400μm^2. Among them, the number of smaller motoneurons (soma area < 200μm^2) was about 2/3 of all the labeled cells (Fig 4A). In addition, about 60% of them were strongly labeled (table 2).

Day 7

One week after birth the masseter motoneurons grew rapidly and about 4/5 of total labeled cells reached a soma area of 200 up to 500μm^2 and the ratio of S /W neurons was about 2/1 in both normal and hypothyroid pups (tables 2,3).

Day 15

The medium size motoneurons appeared at the 15th postnatal day with a significantly lower value in hypothyroid pups (P<0.001, table 2). In contrast their small sized weakly labeled motoneurons (<500μm^2) were higher than normal (P<0.01, table 2,3). Regardless of the labeling intensity a higher frequency of smaller motoneurons (<300μm^2) and a lower frequency of larger motoneurons were observed in hypothyroid pups when compared to normal pups (fig. 5A). Both the intense and weakly hypothyroid labeled neurons displayed quite shorter processes in comparison to normal animals (Figs 2, 3).

Day 23

The most pronounced changes in soma area and labeling intensity were observed at the time of weaning. Small motoneurons in normal pups comprised less than 20% of all labeled

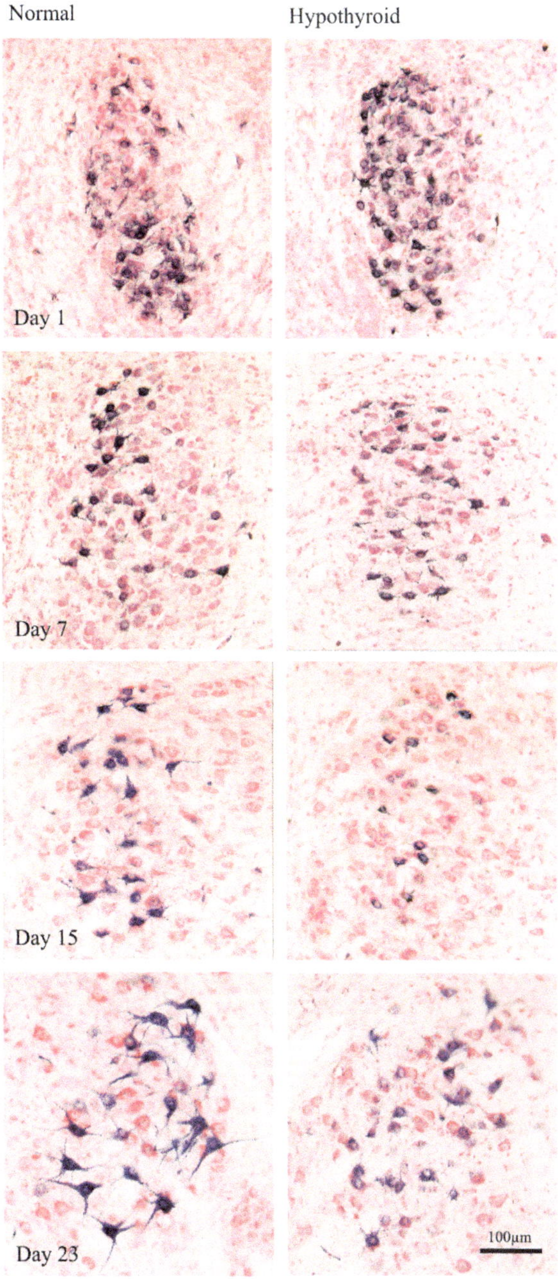

Fig. 2. Photomicrographs showing superficial masseter HRP labeled motoneurons from day 1 to day 23 in normal and hypothyroid trigeminal motor nucleus. At day 23 initial parts of dendrites of normal labeled motoneurons exhibit a Golgi-like labeling appearance with visibly longer extension than those of their hypothyroid homologues.

motoneurons, whereas hypothyroid Mo5 contained 2 fold more of small motoneurons ($P<0.001$).The medium size motoneurons had almost an equal quantitative pattern (~ 45% and 50%) in both normal and hypothyroid pups respectively. While the number of large motoneurons reached to 40% of total number of labeled motoneurons in normal pups, the hypothyroid masseteric motor pool contained 15% of large cells ($P<0.001$), (See fig. 5B in details). The pattern of labeling intensity showed larger and strongly HRP labeled motoneurons in normal pups versus smaller and strong intensity of HRP labeled motoneurons in hypothyroid pups. In normal animals, the Golgi-like labeled motoneuron pool had numerous dedritic processes that extended in both ventral and transverse directions. However in hypothyroid motoneurons the primary dendritic processes were shortened remarkably in all any directions (Fig. 3, B, b).

Peak frequency distributions of labeled motoneurons with different soma size revealed a trimodal pattern of masseter muscle innervation at the time of weaning in both groups: Small size motoneurons with soma area <500μm^2, medium size motoneurons 500-700μm^2 and large motoneurons >700μm^2 are presented in table 2.

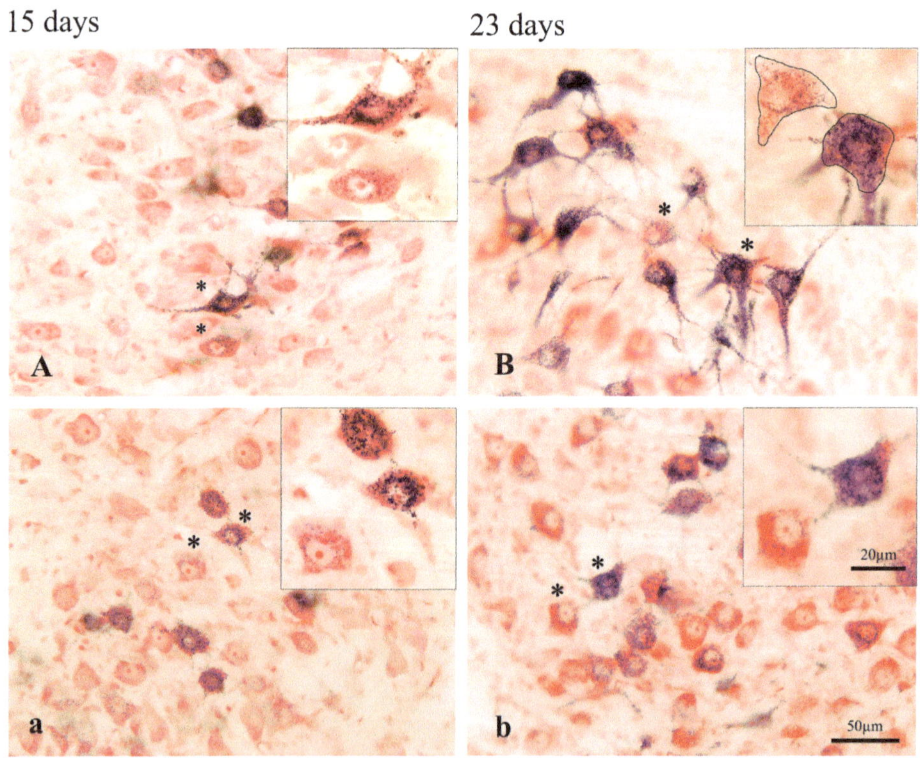

Fig. 3. Masseteric motoneurons labeled with HRP at 15 and 23 postnatal days in normal (A, B) and hypothyroid (a, b) pups. Insets illustrate high magnification of strong and weakly labeled motoneurons (asterisks). Examples of outlined motoneurons are shown in B (inset). Note that hypothyroid motoneurons possess remarkably shorter dendritic processes compared to those of normal pups.

	Strongly labeled cells						Weakly labeled cells					
	small		medium		large		small		medium		large	
	N	H	N	H	N	H	N	H	N	H	N	H
Day 1	96± 3.9	96+ 4.8	0	0	0	0	71± 8.4	70± 6.1	0	0	0	0
Day 7	117± 8.0	106± 5.7	0	0	0	0	51± 2.7	61± 7.0	0	0	0	0
Day 15	97± 3.1	92± 2.1	15± 0.3	6± 0.9***	0	0	43± 1.5	62± 3.6**	13± 0.6	4± 0.7***	0	0
Day 23	17± 0.9	40± 3.0**	44± 3.8	50± 4.2	52± 3.2	13± 1.5***	15± 1.1	31± 2.1**	24± 1.9	26± 3.3	15± 2.3	6± 0.6***

N; normal, H; hypothyroid. * P<0.05, ** P<0.01, *** P<0.001

Table 2.

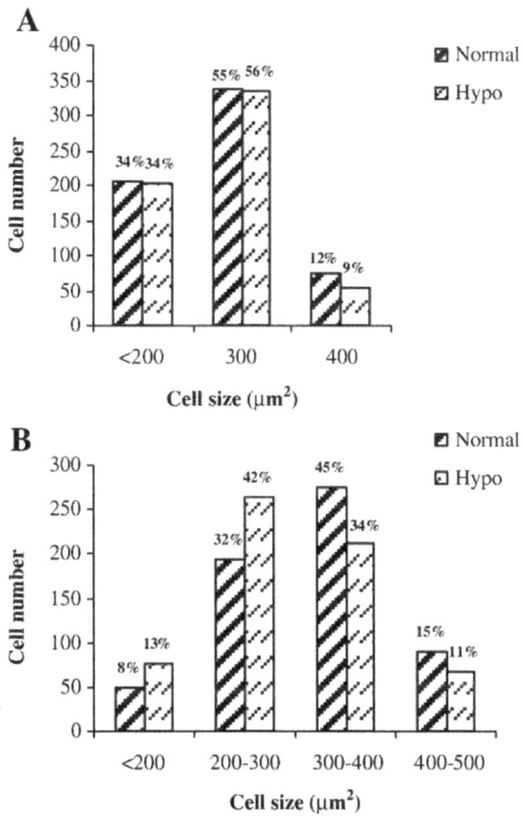

Fig. 4. Frequency distributions in soma area of labeled motoneurons innervating superficial masseter muscle in both normal and hypothyroid pups at 1 day of age (A) and 7 days of age (B).There was no significant difference between normal and hypothyroid pups in both age groups, although at 7 days of age in hypothyroid pups the number of smaller cells (up to 300 μm2) was more and that of larger cells (300–500 μm2) was less than the normal pups.

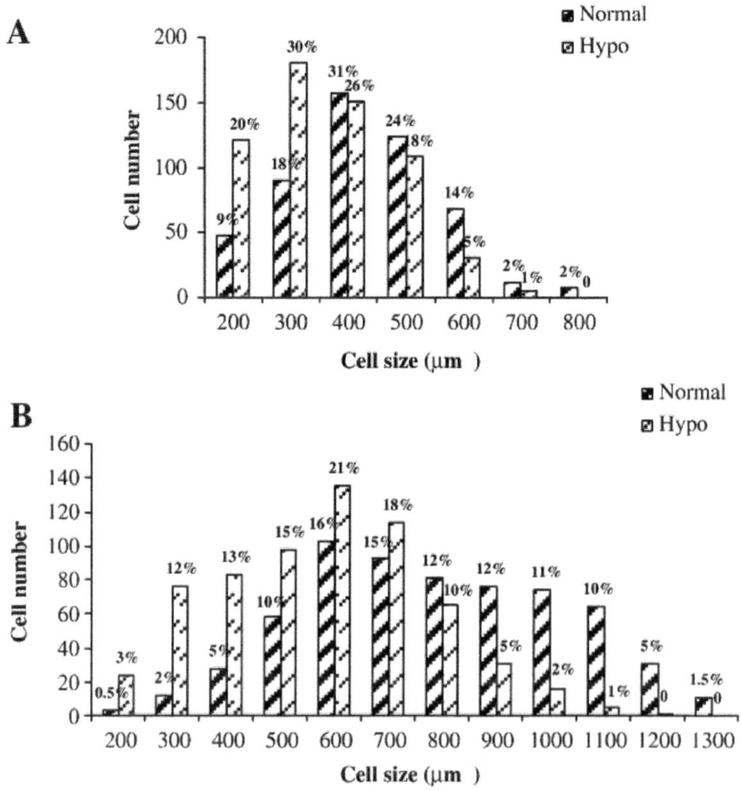

Fig. 5. Frequency distributions in soma area in both normal and hypothyroid pups at 15 days of age (A) and 23 days of age (B). At day 23, neurons in both control and hypothyroid pups were composed of three populations with lower quantity of small, large size and higher quantity of medium-sized motoneurons in peaks. Note that in normal pups there are significantly more larger and less smaller motoneurons than in hypothyroid pups.

3.3 CGRP Histochemistry

To analyze the effect of prenatal thyroid hypofunction on the CGRP immunoreactive intensity, distribution of CGRP containing motoneurons was quantified through Mo5, Mo5-AC and Mo7 nuclei (Fig. 6). CGRP immunoreactivity is extensively and differentially expressed in oro-facial motoneurons somata and primary processes.

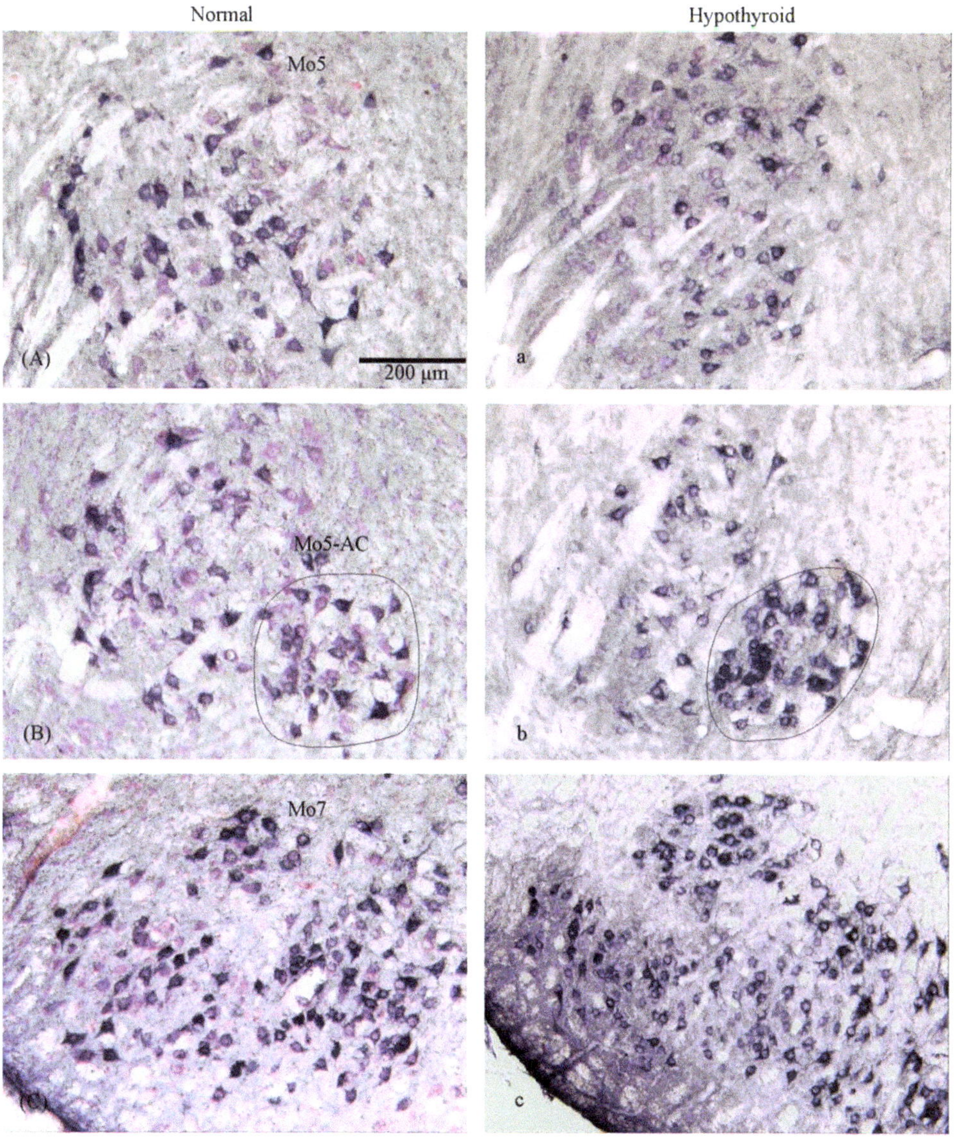

Fig. 6. Low-power photomicrographs of frontal sections through brainstem showing the distribution of CGRP immunoreactive motoneurons through the trigeminal (Mo5), trigeminal accessory (Mo5-AC, outlined area) and facial (Mo7) motor nuclei in the normal (A–C) and in the hypothyroid (a–c) weaned pups.

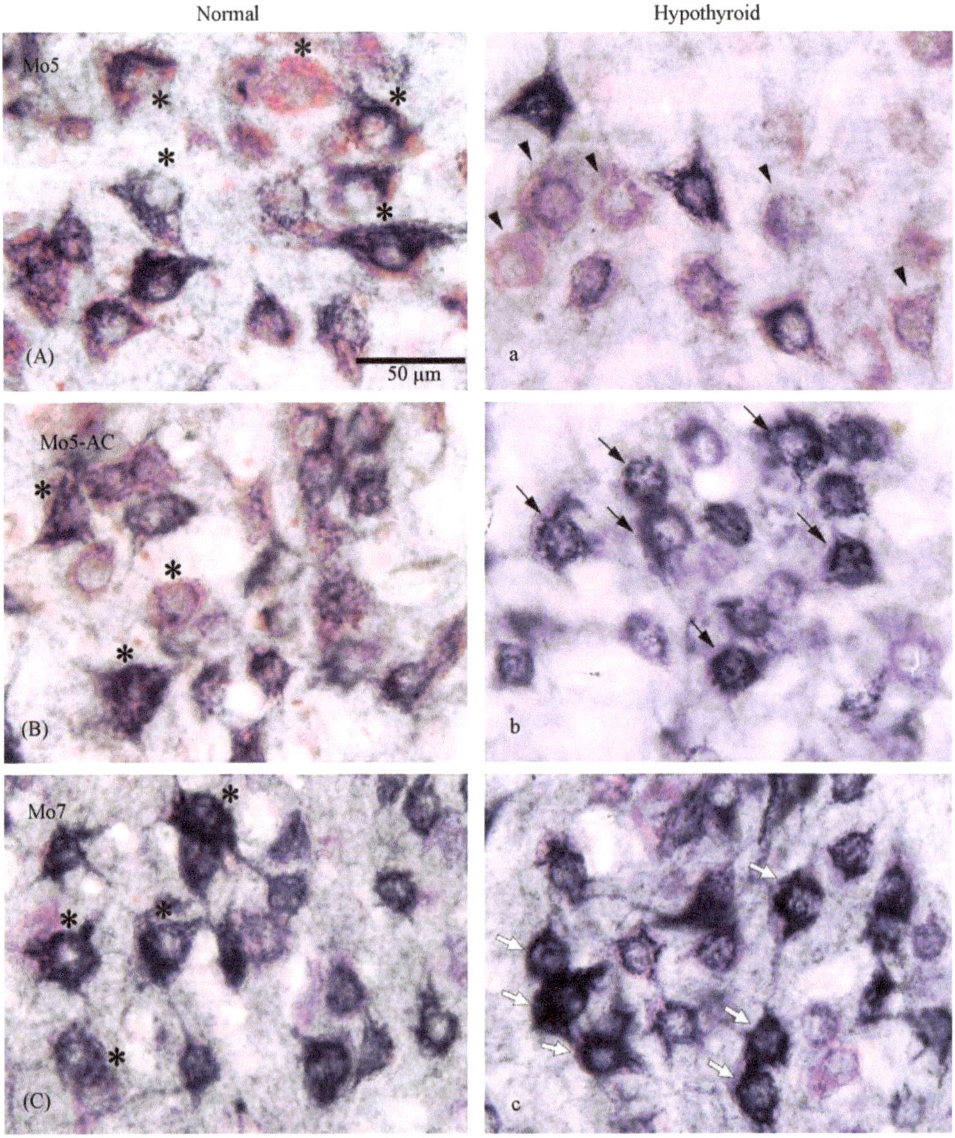

Fig. 7. High-power photomicrographs showing different CGRP immunoreactive intensity in hypothyroid Mo5 nucleus with numerous weakly stained motoneurons (arrowheads, a), and with mostly strong CGRP immunolabeling in Mo5-AC (arrows, b) as well as in Mo7 (white arrows, c). The presence of large immunopositive motoneurons (asterisks) is more detectable in normal motor nuclei compared to their hypothyroid homologues

3.3.1 Trigeminal motor nucleus (Mo5)

Although, the number of positive CGRP neurons is gradually increased from strong to moderate and weak in both normal and hypothyroid Mo5 nucleus, the small immunopositive motoneurons had a large proportion (~70%) in hypothyroid pups compared to normal ones (less than 50%). This increase is especially significant for weakly labeled motoneurons ($P < 0.05$). In contrast, the number of the strong, moderate and weakly stained large motoneurons decreased considerably ($P < 0.01$, <0.001 and <0.01, respectively) in comparison with normal motoneurons (see Table 3 a,b and Fig. 7 A,a).

(a) Small motoneurons with diameter < 25μm and percentage of increase in hypothyroid pups

Ø < 25 μm	Mo5			Mo5-AC			Mo7		
CGRP-ir	Normal	Hypothyroid	(%)	Normal	Hypothyroid	(%)	Normal	Hypothyroid	(%)
Strong	304 ± 7.8	354 ± 4.7	14	12 ± 0.6	65 ± 4.4	82**	488 ± 8.5	812 ± 25.5	40*
Moderate	848 ± 22.0	878 ± 12.2	4	61 ± 3.5	111 ± 3.8	45*	1 019 ± 21.4	1161 ± 5.9	13
Weak	1015 ± 25.8	1467 ± 19.3	31*	68 ± 2.7	119 ± 3.2	43*	1 011 ± 20.6	1255 ± 5.9	20

(b) Large motoneurons with diameter > 25μm and percentage of decrease in hypothyroid pups

Ø > 25 μm	Mo5			Mo5-AC			Mo7		
CGRP-ir	Normal	Hypothyroid	(%)	Normal	Hypothyroid	(%)	Normal	Hypothyroid	(%)
Strong	333 ± 8.5	170 ± 2.3	49**	9 ± 0.6	9 ± .06	0	132 ± 17.5	118 ± 2.9	11
Moderate	921 ± 16.1	422 ± 5.9	54** *	52 ± 1.5	15 ± 1.0	71**	294 ± 25.1	171 ± 3.8	42**
Weak	1107 ± 28.2	661 ± 9.2	40**	59 ± 3.3	16 ± 1.2	73**	294 ± 27.5	184 ± 4.4	37**

(c) Percentage of decrease in number of small and large motoneurons devoid of CGRP in hypothyroid pups

Negative	Mo5			Mo5-AC			Mo7		
	Normal	Hypo-thyroid	(%)	Normal	Hypo-thyroid	(%)	Normal	Hypo-thyroid	(%)
Ø < 25 m	181 ± 3.90	131 ±1.33	28*	0	0	0	124 ± 2.9	72 ± 1.5	42**
Ø > 25 m	195 ± 3.2	64 ± 2.6	67***	0	0	0	33 ± 0.6	13 ± 0.3	64***

* P<0.05 ** P<0.01 *** P<0.001

Table 3. Total number (±S.E.) of CGRP immunolabeled motoneurons with different intensity in each nucleus

3.3.2 Trigeminal accessory nucleus (Mo5-AC)

Normal trigeminal accessory motor nucleus showed almost the same pattern of immunolabeling intensity as Mo5 with a proportion of 55% for small motoneurons and 45% for large motoneurons. In the hypothyroid rats, this pattern contained 90% of small immunopositive motoneurons (strong $P < 0.01$, and moderate and weak $P < 0.05$) versus 10% of large ones with a significant decrease in moderate and weak intensity ($P < 0.01$) (Table 3 a,b and Fig. 7 B,b).

3.3.3 Facial motor nucleus (Mo7)

In comparison with the trigeminal motor nucleus, nor mal facial motor nucleus showed many more small CGRPcontaining motoneurons (>70%) mostly with moderate and weak immunoreactivity. This proportion reached 85% in hypothyroid rats with a significant increase ($P < 0.05$) in the number of small and strongly immunolabeled cells. The proportion of large motoneurons (~20%) in normal weaned pups dropped to ~12% in hypothyroid pups with significant reduction in moderate and weakly labeled motoneurons ($P < 0.01$) (Table 3 a,b and. Fig 7 C,c).

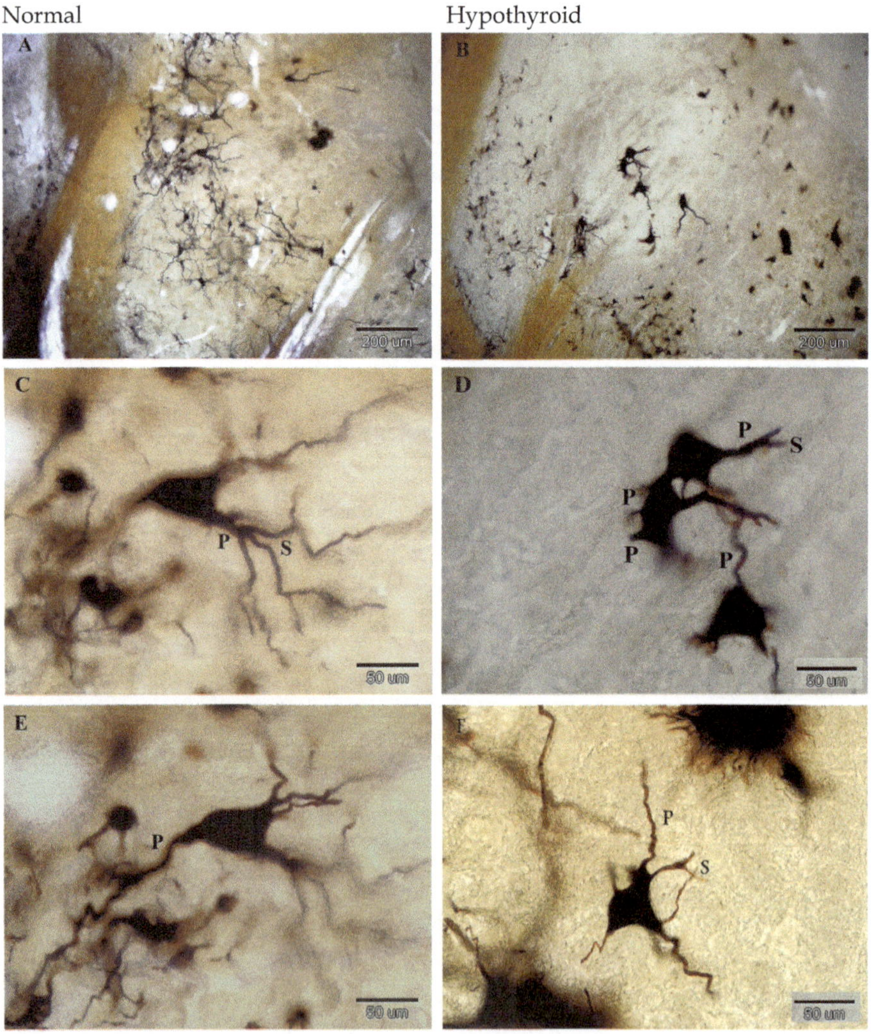

Fig. 8. Golgi staining sections from normal and hypothyroid 23 day old rat pups. Low magnification photomigrographs from Mo5 in normal (A) and hypothyroid (B) pups. Primary (P) and secondary (S) dendrites are shown.

3.3.4 Unlabeled motoneurons

In normal pups, about 7% of Mo5 motoneurons and about 5% of Mo7 motoneurons were devoid of CGRP immunos taining, while in the hypothyroid pups, this proportion shifted to 5 and 2%, respectively. In the hypothyroid Mo5, the number of small and large unlabeled neurons was reduced significantly ($P < 0.05$ and <0.001); however, Mo7 nucleus had a lower proportion of large motoneurons ($P < 0.001$) than the small ones ($P < 0.01$). It should be noted that both normal and hypothyroid Mo5-AC nucleus were devoid of unlabeled motoneurons (Table 3c). Nevertheless, no significant difference was observed in the total number of motoneurons in all experimental groups.

3.4 Golgi stained motoneurons

The results of cell measuring and counting the primary and secondary dendrites revealed that in hypothyroid pups beside the significant decrease in soma size in trigeminal large motoneurons (a 50% reduction in the number of 900-1200μm² motoneurons in PTU-treated group compared to controls, P<0.05), the number of secondary (3.8± 0.4 in PTU- treated compared to 4.3±0.5 in control group) - but not primary dendrites- showed a significant decrease comparing to normal group (4.1±0.3 vs 6.5±0.4 respectively, P<0.001).

4. Conclusion

In the present studies birth weights of hypothyroid animals were slightly lower than normal; this moderate retardation persisted until day 15, then hypothyroid animals stopped growing and clinically became cretinous. The premature profile of masseter muscle begins to appear around the pre-weaning time (day 15) in rats. To meet these muscle functional properties, 2 weeks after birth, the medium-sized labeled motoneurons appeared at the expense of a reduction in the number of small motoneurons. However, during the same period, the number of medium- sized motoneurons was more than 2-fold under the normal values and the quantity of small motoneurons was about 4- fold in hypothyroid pups.

During development hypothyroidism alters the patterns of masseter motoneurons morphology such as soma size, dendritic orientation and arborization pattern and also induces a severe delay in the size transition, which may affect the development and plasticity of oral feeding behavior. On the other hand, immunohistochemical studies in normal animals have shown that motoneurons supplying fast-twitch muscles show a higher level CGRP staining than motoneurons innervating muscles of slow twitch fiber type (Homonko & Theriault, 2000). A severe delay in the appearance of large fast-twitch jaw closing and jaw opening motoneurons due to congenital hypothyroidism suggests an intact thyroid and CGRP state are obligatory for the attainment of normal preadult oro-fascial masticatory profile.

5. References

Adams, G. R., McCue, S. A., Zeng, M., & Baldwin, K. M. (1999). Time course of myosin heavy chain transitions in neonatal rats: importance of innervation and thyroid state. *The American Journal of Physiology*, *276*(4 Pt 2), R954-961.

Agbulut, O., Noirez, P., Beaumont, F., & Butler-Browne, G. (2003). Myosin heavy chain isoforms in postnatal muscle development of mice. *Biology of the Cell / Under the Auspices of the European Cell Biology Organization*, *95*(6), 399-406.

d' Albis, A., Chanoine, C., Janmot, C., Mira, J. C., & Couteaux, R. (1990). Muscle-specific response to thyroid hormone of myosin isoform transitions during rat postnatal development. *European Journal of Biochemistry / FEBS*, *193*(1), 155-161.

d' Albis, A., Couteaux, R., Janmot, C., & Roulet, A. (1989). Specific programs of myosin expression in the postnatal development of rat muscles. *European Journal of Biochemistry / FEBS*, *183*(3), 583-590.

Bakels, R., Nijenhuis, M., Mast, L., & Kernell, D. (1998). Hypothyroidism in the rat results in decreased soleus motoneurone soma size. *Neuroscience Letters*, *254*(3), 149-152.

Barakat-Walter, I., & Riederer, B. M. (1996). Triiodothyronine and nerve growth factor are required to induce cytoplasmic dynein expression in rat dorsal root ganglion cultures. *Brain Research. Developmental Brain Research*, *96*(1-2), 109-119.

Barakat-Walter, I., Kraftsik, R., Kuntzer, T., Bogousslavsky, J., & Magistretti, P. (2000). Differential effect of thyroid hormone deficiency on the growth of calretinin-expressing neurons in rat spinal cord and dorsal root ganglia. *The Journal of Comparative Neurology*, *426*(4), 519-533.

Behzadi, G., & Ganji, F. (2005). Morphological alteration in oro-facial CGRP containing motoneurons due to congenital thyroid hypofunction. *Peptides*, *26*(8), 1486-1491. doi:10.1016/j.peptides.2005.03.053

Biesiada, E., Adams, P. M., Shanklin, D. R., Bloom, G. S., & Stein, S. A. (1996). Biology of the congenitally hypothyroid hyt/hyt mouse. *Advances in Neuroimmunology*, *6*(4), 309-346.

Blake, H. H., & Henning, S. J. (1985). Effect of propylthiouracil dose on serum thyroxine, growth, and weaning in young rats. *The American Journal of Physiology*, *248*(5 Pt 2), R524-530.

Blanco, C. E., Popper, P., & Micevych, P. (1997). alpha-CGRP mRNA levels in motoneurons innervating specific rat muscles. *Brain Research. Molecular Brain Research*, *44*(2), 253-261.

Buffelli, M., Pasino, E., & Cangiano, A. (2001). In vivo acetylcholine receptor expression induced by calcitonin gene-related peptide in rat soleus muscle. *Neuroscience*, *104*(2), 561-567.

Butler-Browne, G. S., Herlicoviez, D., & Whalen, R. G. (1984). Effects of hypothyroidism on myosin isozyme transitions in developing rat muscle. *FEBS Letters*, *166*(1), 71-75.

Butler-Browne, G. S., Prulière, G., Cambon, N., & Whalen, R. G. (1987). Influence of the dwarf mouse mutation on skeletal and cardiac myosin isoforms. Effect of one injection of thyroxine on skeletal and cardiac muscle phenotype. *The Journal of Biological Chemistry*, *262*(31), 15188-15193.

Copray, S., & Kernell, D. (2000). Neurotrophins and trk-receptors in adult rat spinal motoneurons: differences related to cell size but not to "slow/fast" specialization. *Neuroscience Letters*, *289*(3), 217-220.

Fernandez, H L, Chen, M., Nadelhaft, I, & Durr, J. A. (2003). Calcitonin gene-related peptides: their binding sites and receptor accessory proteins in adult mammalian skeletal muscles. *Neuroscience*, *119*(2), 335-345.

Fernandez, Hugo L., Ross, G. S., & Nadelhaft, Irving. (1999). Neurogenic calcitonin gene-related peptide: a neurotrophic factor in the maintenance of acetylcholinesterase molecular forms in adult skeletal muscles. *Brain Research, 844*(1-2), 83-97. doi:16/S0006-8993(99)01891-0

Gambke, B., Lyons, G. E., Haselgrove, J., Kelly, A. M., & Rubinstein, N. A. (1983). Thyroidal and neural control of myosin transitions during development of rat fast and slow muscles. *FEBS Letters, 156*(2), 335-339.

Green, J. R., Moore, C. A., Ruark, J. L., Rodda, P. R., Morvée, W. T., & VanWitzenburg, M. J. (1997). Development of chewing in children from 12 to 48 months: longitudinal study of EMG patterns. *Journal of Neurophysiology, 77*(5), 2704-2716.

Homonko, D. A., & Theriault, E. (2000). Downhill running preferentially increases CGRP in fast glycolytic muscle fibers. *Journal of Applied Physiology (Bethesda, Md.: 1985), 89*(5), 1928-1936.

Honma, S., Varathan, V., & Wakisaka, S. (2002). Postnatal development of synaptic inputs to rat masseter motoneurons. *Brain Research. Developmental Brain Research, 139*(1), 67-71.

Hughes, S. M., & Salinas, P. C. (1999). Control of muscle fibre and motoneuron diversification. *Current Opinion in Neurobiology, 9*(1), 54-64.

Ishihara, A, Naitoh, H., Araki, H., & Nishihira, Y. (1988). Soma size and oxidative enzyme activity of motoneurones supplying the fast twitch and slow twitch muscles in the rat. *Brain Research, 446*(1), 195-198.

Ishihara, Akihiko, Kawano, F., Okiura, T., Morimatsu, F., & Ohira, Y. (2005). Hyperbaric exposure with high oxygen concentration enhances oxidative capacity of neuromuscular units. *Neuroscience Research, 52*(2), 146-152. doi:10.1016/j.neures.2005.03.001

Kawagishi, S., Yoshino, K., Jones, T. E., Iwamoto, M., Arai, S., & Amano, N. (1992). Dopamine receptor antagonists increase markedly the quantity of retrograde transport of HRP in the rat masseteric motoneuron. *Brain Research, 585*(1-2), 196-204.

Kimura, I. (1998). Calcium-dependent desensitizing function of the postsynaptic neuronal-type nicotinic acetylcholine receptors at the neuromuscular junction. *Pharmacology & Therapeutics, 77*(3), 183-202.

Kragie, L., & Smiehorowski, R. (1993). Measures of skeletal muscle calcium channels and acetylcholine receptors in thyroidectomized rats. *Endocrine Research, 19*(2-3), 207-219.

Kubota, K., Narita, N., Ohkubo, K., Shibanai, S., Nagae, K., Kubota, M., Odagiri, N., et al. (1988). Morphological studies of the neuromuscular mechanism shifting from sucking to biting of mice. *Acta Anatomica, 133*(3), 200-208.

Maeda, N., Hanai, H., & Kumegawa, M. (1981a). Postnatal development of masticatory organs in rats II. Effects of hormones on the postnatal development of the M. masseter superficialis. *Anatomischer Anzeiger, 149*(5), 425-436.

Maeda, N., Hanai, H., & Kumegawa, M. (1981b). Postnatal development of masticatory organs in rats. III. Effects of mastication on the postnatal development of the M. masseter superficialis. *Anatomischer Anzeiger, 150*(4), 424-427.

Mesulam, M.-M. (1982). *Tracing neural connections with horseradish peroxidase*. Wiley.

Miyata, H., Sugiura, T., Wada, N., Kawai, Y., & Shigenaga, Y. (1996). Morphological changes in the masseter muscle and its motoneurons during postnatal development. *The Anatomical Record, 244*(4), 520-528. doi:10.1002/(SICI)1097-0185(199604)244:4<520::AID-AR10>3.0.CO;2-R

Mizuno, N., Konishi, A., & Sato, M. (1975). Localization of masticatory motoneurons in the cat and rat by means of retrograde axonal transport of horseradish peroxidase. *The Journal of Comparative Neurology, 164*(1), 105-115. doi:10.1002/cne.901640109

Munson, J. B., Foehring, R. C., Mendell, L. M., & Gordon, T. (1997). Fast-to-slow conversion following chronic low-frequency activation of medial gastrocnemius muscle in cats. II. Motoneuron properties. *Journal of Neurophysiology, 77*(5), 2605-2615.

Pette, D., & Staron, R. S. (2000). Myosin isoforms, muscle fiber types, and transitions. *Microscopy Research and Technique, 50*(6), 500-509. doi:10.1002/1097-0029(20000915)50:6<500::AID-JEMT7>3.0.CO;2-7

Popper, P., & Micevych, P. E. (1989). Localization of calcitonin gene-related peptide and its receptors in a striated muscle. *Brain Research, 496*(1-2), 180-186.

Ristanović, D., Milosević, N. T., & Stulić, V. (2006). Application of modified Sholl analysis to neuronal dendritic arborization of the cat spinal cord. *Journal of Neuroscience Methods, 158*(2), 212-218. doi:10.1016/j.jneumeth.2006.05.030

Roa, M., & Changeux, J. P. (1991). Characterization and developmental evolution of a high-affinity binding site for calcitonin gene-related peptide on chick skeletal muscle membrane. *Neuroscience, 41*(2-3), 563-570.

van Rossum, D., Hanisch, U. K., & Quirion, R. (1997). Neuroanatomical localization, pharmacological characterization and functions of CGRP, related peptides and their receptors. *Neuroscience and Biobehavioral Reviews, 21*(5), 649-678.

Rubinstein, N. A., Lyons, G. E., & Kelly, A. M. (1988). Hormonal control of myosin heavy chain genes during development of skeletal muscles. *Ciba Foundation Symposium, 138*, 35-51.

Saito, T., Ohnuki, Y., Yamane, A., & Saeki, Y. (2002). Effects of diet consistency on the myosin heavy chain mRNAs of rat masseter muscle during postnatal development. *Archives of Oral Biology, 47*(2), 109-115.

Sawin, S., Brodish, P., Carter, C. S., Stanton, M. E., & Lau, C. (1998). Development of cholinergic neurons in rat brain regions: dose-dependent effects of propylthiouracil-induced hypothyroidism. *Neurotoxicology and Teratology, 20*(6), 627-635.

Sickles, D. W., Oblak, T. G., & Scholer, J. (1987). Hyperthyroidism selectively increases oxidative metabolism of slow-oxidative motor units. *Experimental Neurology, 97*(1), 90-105.

Soukup, T., & Jirmanová, I. (2000). Regulation of myosin expression in developing and regenerating extrafusal and intrafusal muscle fibers with special emphasis on the role of thyroid hormones. *Physiological Research / Academia Scientiarum Bohemoslovaca, 49*(6), 617-633.

Stein, S. A., McIntire, D. D., Kirkpatrick, L. L., Adams, P. M., & Brady, S. T. (1991). Hypothyroidism selectively reduces the rate and amount of transport for specific SCb proteins in the hyt/hyt mouse optic nerve. *Journal of Neuroscience Research, 30*(1), 28-41. doi:10.1002/jnr.490300105

Sugasawa, K., & Mori, T. (1998). Effects of a soft diet and hypothyroidism on the oxidative capacity of the masseter muscle fibers of the young Japanese field vole Microtus montebelli. *Zoological Science, 15*(1), 97-102.

Terrado, J., Gerrikagoitia, I., Martinez-Millán, L., Pascual, F., Climent, S., Muniesa, P., & Sarasa, M. (1997). Expression of the genes for alpha-type and beta-type calcitonin gene-related peptide during postnatal rat brain development. *Neuroscience, 80*(3), 951-970.

Thompson, C. C., & Potter, G. B. (2000). Thyroid Hormone Action in Neural Development. *Cerebral Cortex, 10*(10), 939 -945. doi:10.1093/cercor/10.10.939

15

Thyroid-Stimulating Hormone Regulation and Transcription in Hypothyroidism

Koreaki Sugimoto[1] and Kouki Mori[2]
[1]*Department of Psychosomatic Medicine, Tohoku Fukushi University*
[2]*Department of Health Supervision, JR Sendai Hospital*
Japan

1. Introduction

Thyroid hormones play essential roles in mammalian life, especially in neurodevelopment (Porterfield & Hendrich, 1993). This fact is clearly shown in patients with neurological deficits from endemic cretinism, who reside in iodine-deficient areas (DeLong et at., 1985). In addition to neurological impairments, thyroid dysfunctions, such as hyperthyroidism and hypothyroidism, lead to a wide variety of clinical manifestations. Hypothyroidism is defined as deficient thyroid hormone action. It is caused most often by decreased thyroid hormone production, although in rare cases it is caused by reduced tissue responsiveness to or consumptive degradation of the hormone (Huang et al., 2000; Refetoff, Weiss, & Usala, 1993). There are two types of deficient thyroid hormone production: primary (thyroidal) hypothyroidism and central hypothyroidism. The former is commonly caused by iodine deficiency (DeLong et al., 1985) or chronic autoimmune thyroiditis, known as Hashimoto's thyroiditis (Dayan & Daniels, 1996). In iodine-sufficient areas, Hashimoto's thyroiditis is a major cause of primary hypothyroidism. The loss of functional follicles caused by intrathyroidal lymphocytic infiltration is attributable to impaired thyroid hormone production. Central hypothyroidism is due to reduced thyroid stimulation by thyroid-stimulating hormone (TSH) resulting from pituitary disease (secondary hypothyroidism) or hypothalamic disease (tertiary hypothyroidism) (Lania et al., 2008). Pituitary macroadenomas or radiotherapy of brain tumours and pituitary adenomas are frequently associated with insufficient TSH production in adults (Rose, 2001). In some cases of central hypothyroidism, abnormally glycosylated TSH with a reduced bioactivity is secreted (Faglia et al., 1979; Taylor & Weintraub, 1989). Because thyroid hormones negatively regulate pituitary TSH synthesis, decreased serum thyroid hormone concentrations lead to the stimulation of TSH production. Therefore, in primary hypothyroidism, serum TSH levels are increased, even at the stage of subclinical hypothyroidism (Fatourechi, 2009). By contrast, an increase in serum TSH is generally not observed in central hypothyroidism because of the impaired hypothalamic-pituitary-thyroid axis. Based on these observations, serum TSH serves as a useful indicator for the presence and the type of hypothyroidism. Therefore, measurements of TSH are quite useful in clinical practice (Ladenson et al., 2000).

2. Regulation of thyroid-stimulating hormone synthesis

TSH is produced in pituitary thyrotrophs and activates thyroid follicular cells by binding to the TSH receptor (Magner, 1990). This hormone promotes thyroid cell proliferation and thyroid hormone synthesis by inducing expression of thyroglobulin, thyroid peroxidase, sodium iodide symporter and type I iodothyronine deiodinase (D1) (Tang et al., 1995). TSH consists of an α and a β subunit (Shupnik et al., 1989). The α subunit is common to both TSH and gonadotropins. The β subunit is a prerequisite for the bioactivity of TSH. Both subunits are glycosylated posttranslationally, which is controlled by the thyrotropin-releasing hormone (TRH) and is essential for exerting sufficient hormonal bioactivity (Menezes-Ferreira et al., 1986; Taylor & Weintraub, 1989). In fact, abnormally glycosylated TSH with reduced bioactivity is found in some patients with central hypothyroidism (Faglia et al., 1979; Petersen et al., 1978).

TSH synthesis is largely dependent on serum thyroid hormone levels. Patients with primary hyperthyroidism or primary hypothyroidism consistently demonstrate suppressed or increased serum TSH levels, respectively (Ladenson et al., 2000). Clinically, serum TSH concentrations serve as a sensitive indicator of thyroid dysfunction since patients with abnormal thyroid function have altered serum TSH levels, even at a subclinical stage (Fatourechi, 2009). Thus, the measurement of serum TSH is routine for a thyroid evaluation in daily clinical practice. In addition to TSH production, the metabolic clearance rate of TSH is also influenced by serum thyroid hormone levels, i.e., increased in hyperthyroidism and decreased in hypothyroidism (Ridgway et al., 1974).

In contrast to the negative regulation of TSH production by thyroid hormones, the production is positively regulated by TRH. Mice devoid of the TRH gene exhibit hypothyroidism accompanied by low circulating TSH levels and reduced numbers of TSH-immunopositive cells in their pituitary glands (Yamada et al., 1997). In TRH and thyroid hormone receptor (TR) β-subunit double knockout mice, basal serum TSH levels are low, and hypothyroidism fails to increase serum TSH concentrations (Nikrodhanond et al., 2006). These studies have demonstrated the pivotal role of TRH in the regulation of TSH production.

Recent studies have demonstrated the presence of TSH receptors in the hypothalamus and pituitary folliculo-stellate cells (Crisanti et al., 2001; Prummel et al., 2000), suggesting short and ultra-short loop feedback regulation of TSH secretion (Prummel et al., 2004). However, their significance remains unknown.

3. Thyrotropin-releasing hormone as a positive regulator of thyroid-stimulating hormone production

TRH is synthesised in neurons located in the parvocellular part of the hypothalamic paraventricular nucleus (PVN) (Fekete & Lechan, 2007). These neurons project their axons to the median eminence where TRH is released into the portal vein, and the hormone subsequently reaches the anterior pituitary. The binding of TRH to its receptor activates phospholipase C and is followed by calcium mobilisation and protein kinase C (PKC) activation (Carr et al., 1991). However, recent studies suggest that cyclic adenosine monophosphate (cAMP) response element binding protein (CREB) rather than the calcium and PKC signalling pathways may play a central role in TRH-stimulated TSH synthesis (Hashimoto et al., 2000). In addition, the transcription factor Pit-1, which is pivotal in the differentiation of thyrotrophs, lactotrophs and somatotrophs (Andersen & Rosenfeld, 1994), induces a synergistic increase in TSHβ subunit gene transcription in the presence of CREB-binding protein (Hashimoto et al., 2000).

TRH synthesis is negatively regulated by thyroid hormones. In the brain, up to 80% of the triiodothyronine (T3) bound to nuclear TRs is locally generated through the conversion of thyroxine (T4) to T3 by the type 2 deiodinase (D2) (Crantz et al., 1982). Therefore, rather than T3, the amount of T4 in circulation is pivotal for the maintenance of adequate T3 levels in the brain. However, D2 is expressed in the tanycytes lining the third ventricle and in astrocytes, but not in neurons (Guadano-Ferraz et al., 1997; Tu et al., 1997). The T3 produced by tanycytes is the primary source of T3 in TRH neurons. In these neurons, the cellular uptake of T3 is mediated by monocarboxylate transporter 8 (MCT8) (Heuer & Visser, 2009). T3 binds to the TRs, of which there are three isoforms (TRα1, β1 and β2) in the brain (Cheng, 2005). Notably, TRβ2 is central in the suppression of TRH production since mice devoid of the TRβ2 gene exhibit increased TRH gene expression in the PVN (Abel et al., 2001). There are consensus sequences for thyroid hormone response element (TRE) half-sites (AGGTCA) in the TRH gene, which may be involved in the negative regulation of TRH gene expression by T3 (Wilber & Xu, 1998). The promotor region of the gene also contains a cAMP response element (CRE) that overlaps with a TRE (Wilber & Xu, 1998), which suggests that there is cross talk between the thyroid hormone and cAMP-dependent signalling pathways.

4. Triiodothyronine is a negative regulator of thyroid-stimulating hormone production

Transcription of the TSHα and β subunit genes is negatively regulated by T3 (Magner, 1990; Shupnik et al., 1989). Mice lacking the TRβ gene have been shown to exhibit inappropriate secretion of TSH (Abel et al., 1999; Weiss et al., 1997). By contrast, TSHβ subunit expression was not altered in mice devoid of the TRα gene (Wikstrom et al., 1998). Thus, a series of studies suggest a pivotal role for the TRβ isoforms, especially TRβ2, in T3-mediated TSH suppression. There is a TRE half-site-like sequence (GGGTCA) in the β subunit gene, and previous studies have suggested that it might act as a negative TRE in thyrotrophs (Carr et al., 1989). However, later studies demonstrated that this putative negative TRE was not required in TSH suppression (Matsushita et al., 2007). Instead, the transcription factor GATA2 interacts with Pit-1 and TR to play an essential role in both the T3-induced suppression and the TRH-induced potentiation of TSH expression (Matsushita et al., 2007; Nakano et al., 2004).

Approximately 50 to 60 % of T3 bound to TRs is locally produced by D2-mediated T4 to T3 conversion in the rat pituitary gland (Silva & Larsen, 1978). Human pituitary tissues also contain D2 (Itagaki et al., 1990). D2 inhibition by iopanoic acid results in an increase in rat serum TSH levels (Obregon et al., 1980), which indicates that D2-mediated T4 deiodination is the primary source of T3 in the pituitary. D2 activity is increased in hypothyroidism and is decreased in hyperthyroidism (Bianco et al., 2002). Thus, the intrapituitary T3 levels are carefully maintained by the fine-tuning of D2 activity.

5. Neuronal control of thyroid-stimulating hormone secretion (Fig. 1)

TSH secretion is indirectly controlled by neuronal afferents innervating hypothalamic TRH neurons. Adrenergic input from the C1-3 brainstem stimulates TRH synthesis in response to cold exposure (Arancibia et al., 1996; Arancibia et al., 1989). Catecholamine binding to α1 adrenergic receptors leads to CREB phosphorylation and subsequent activation of the TRH promoter (Thonberg et al., 2002). Adrenergic neurons that are in contact with the TRH neurons also contain cocaine- and amphetamine-regulated transcript (CART) and neuropeptide Y (NPY) (Wittmann et al., 2002, 2004). Previous studies have demonstrated that CART stimulates TRH synthesis, whereas NPY inhibits it (Fekete et al., 2000, 2001).

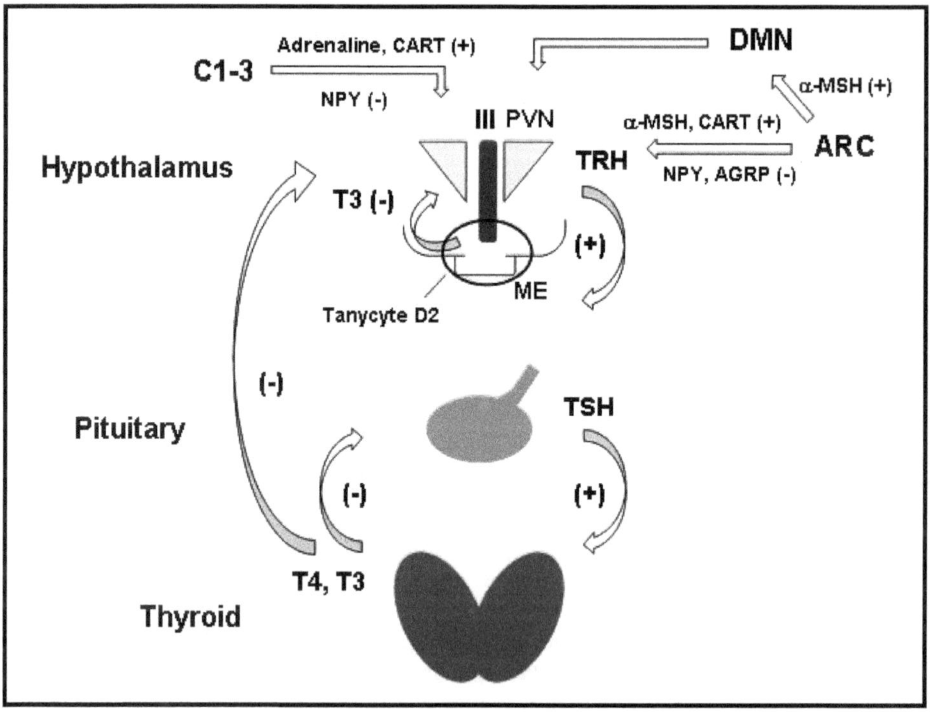

III, the third ventricle; AGRP, agouti-related protein; ARC, hypothalamic arcuate nucleus; C1-3, C1-3 adrenergic area of the brainstem; CART, cocaine- and amphetamine-regulated transcript; D2, type 2 iodothyronine deiodinase; DMN, hypothalamic dorsomedial nucleus; α-MSH, α-melanocyte stimulating hormone; ME, median eminence; NPY; neuropeptide Y; PVN, hypothalamic paraventricular nucleus; TRH, thyrotropin-releasing hormone; TSH, thyroid stimulating hormone.

Fig. 1. Regulatory mechanism of the hypothalamic-pituitary-thyroid axis.

Peptidergic input from the arcuate nucleus may mediate a fasting-induced decrease in TRH production (Lechan & Fekete, 2006). Leptin administration during fasting prevents the inhibition of TRH synthesis, suggesting its involvement in this process (Legradi et al., 1997). The arcuate nucleus also sends axon terminals containing NPY and agouti-related protein (AGRP) or α-melanocyte stimulating hormone (α-MSH) and CART to the TRH neurons and thus negatively or positively regulates TRH gene expression (Elias et al., 1998; Hahn et al.,

1998; Mizuno et al., 1998). Also, α-MSH-containing neurons innervate the hypothalamic dorsomedial nucleus (DMN), and the DMN subsequently projects to the TRH neurons in the PVN (Mihaly et al., 2001). Thus, there are two pathways to the TRH neurons: the direct arcuate-PVN and the indirect arcuate-DMN-PVN.

6. Drugs affecting thyroid-stimulating hormone secretion

Glucocorticoids can lower serum TSH concentrations through TRH suppression in the PVN (Alkemade et al., 2005; Wilber & Utiger, 1969). TRH neurons possess glucocorticoid receptors, and a response element to the hormone has been identified in the TRH gene (Cintra et al., 1990).

Dopamine can reduce TSH production and secretion through its binding to dopamine D2 receptors in the pituitary gland (Shupnik et al., 1986). Interestingly, it stimulates TRH secretion in the rat (Lewis et al., 1987), but this effect cannot override its inhibitory effect on the pituitary gland.

Somatostatin suppresses TSH secretion from the pituitary gland (Lamberts et al., 1989), and its analogues are therefore used for the treatment of TSH-producing adenomas (Beck-Peccoz et al., 1989).

In addition to drugs, several cytokines, such as interleukin-1β (IL-1β), IL-6 and tumour necrosis factor-α (TNFα), have been shown to inhibit TSH secretion (Bartalena et al., 1994; Pang et al., 1989). These cytokines can stimulate the D2 activity in pituitary cells (Baur et al., 2000), suggesting increased T4 to T3 conversion as one possible mechanism for the suppressed TSH production in cytokine-treated animals.

7. Quantitative analysis of thyroid-stimulating hormone transcription in hypothyroidism (Sugimoto et al., 2007)

TSH (thyrotropin) is the primary regulatory peptide for the synthesis and secretion of thyroid hormones, including T3 and T4. TRH secretion from the hypothalamus stimulates the release of TSH from the anterior lobe of the pituitary gland. TSH is then secreted into the blood to stimulate the release of T4, which is produced by the thyroid gland, and T3, which is produced by both the thyroid gland and by conversion of T4 in peripheral tissues. T3 has stronger biological effects than T4. This TRH–TSH–thyroid hormone (T3, T4) secretion relationship is called the hypothalamic–pituitary–thyroid axis (HPT axis), which operates on both short- and long-feedback mechanisms (O'Shea & Williams, 2002). The plasma levels of T3 and T4 are maintained by this mechanism.

Thyroid hormones are essential for maintaining many physiological functions, including metabolism, growth, and development. In hypothyroidism, TSH and TRH levels are elevated, owing to the lack of a suppressive action of the T3. Hypothyroidism in rats, induced by propylthiouracil (PTU) administration, is associated with high TSH mRNA expression, which is measured semiquantitatively by northern blotting or *in situ* hybridisation; however, these results varied widely from 3 to 22 times the level seen in control rats (Carr & Chin, 1988; Franklyn et al., 1987; Samuels et al., 1989; Shupnik & Ridgway, 1987; Steel et al., 1990; Taylor et al., 1990).

The LightCycler® system (Roche Applied Science, Switzerland) was developed for the quantitative analysis of gene expression by real-time polymerase chain reaction (PCR). It combines a thermocycler and a microvolume fluorimeter (Lyon, 2001) with the fluorescence-based assay requiring less manipulation than a basic PCR assay (Contini et al., 2005). Therefore, the LightCycler® is a highly sensitive quantitative method for the detection of RNA expression (Emrich et al., 2002; Schuster et al., 2004; Tan et al., 2004).

Posttranscriptional control of mRNA steady-state levels can occur at many steps after the synthesis of the initial heterogeneous nuclear RNA (hnRNA) transcript. hnRNA is therefore the primary transcript produced by RNA polymerase, which includes both the exonic and the intronic regions of the DNA. Transcriptional control of the mRNA occurs at the levels of hnRNA stability, splicing, polyadenylation, capping, methylation, editing, the nuclear-cytoplasmic transport of mature mRNA, and mRNA stability. Mature mRNA synthesised in the nucleus translocates into the cytoplasm, where it is stabilised, translated into protein, or degraded (Kren & Steer, 1996). The half-life of mRNA is comparatively longer than that of hnRNA, and changes in mRNA levels in the cell do not necessarily reflect the transcriptional level. It takes at least 0.5 h, and sometimes up to 2 h, for mRNA to accumulate to detectable levels after the start of transcription for most genes (Kren & Steer, 1996). A more reliable measure for evaluating the rate of transcription is hnRNA because of its short half-life of 15–30 min (Darnell, 1983), which makes it a valuable quantitative indicator of transcriptional activation.

In 2002, Johnson et al. (Johnson et al., 2002) reported a quantitative real-time reverse transcription (RT)-PCR analysis of prostaglandin endoperoxide H synthase hnRNA. Since then, several studies have successfully detected hnRNA expression using real-time PCR systems (Danzi et al., 2005; Ginsberg et al., 2006; Johnson et al., 2003; Kuroda et al., 2005; Li et al., 2005). However, only semiquantitative analyses of hnRNA have been reported for TSHβ gene transcription (Franklyn et al., 1987; Samuels et al., 1989; Shupnik & Ridgway, 1987; Taylor et al., 1990). In this study, we performed a quantitative analysis of TSHβ gene expression by real-time RT-PCR using the LightCycler® system. We present here the first quantitative demonstration of increased mRNA and hnRNA expression of TSHβ under a chronic condition of hypothyroidism in rats. This method for the detection of quantitative hnRNA is illustrated in **Fig. 2**.

7.1 Materials and methods

7.1.1 Animals and the induction of hypothyroidism

Adult male Wistar rats (Nippon Clea Inc., Shizuoka, Japan) weighing 280 g were allowed free access to food and water and were maintained on a 12 h light/12 h dark cycle (lights on 07:00–19:00 h). The rats were divided into two groups of four animals each: a hypothyroidism group and a control group. The rats were allowed free access to either 0.05% methimazole (MMI) in water (hypothyroid group) or water alone (controls). Fourteen days later, all rats were decapitated between 08:00 and 10:00 h, and blood was collected from their trunks to avoid contamination with the pituitary portal blood, which contains high TSH levels. The sample was collected into a tube containing ice-cold ethylenediaminetetraacetic acid (EDTA) and centrifuged at 1008×*g* for 30 min. Serum T3 and T4 levels were measured to assess the degree of hypothyroidism induced by MMI administration.

All animal experiments were conducted in accordance with the international standards for animal welfare from the National Institutes of Health Guide for the Care and Use of Laboratory Animals and the Animal Experiments Guidelines of the Institute for Animal Experimentation, Tohoku University Graduate School of Medicine.

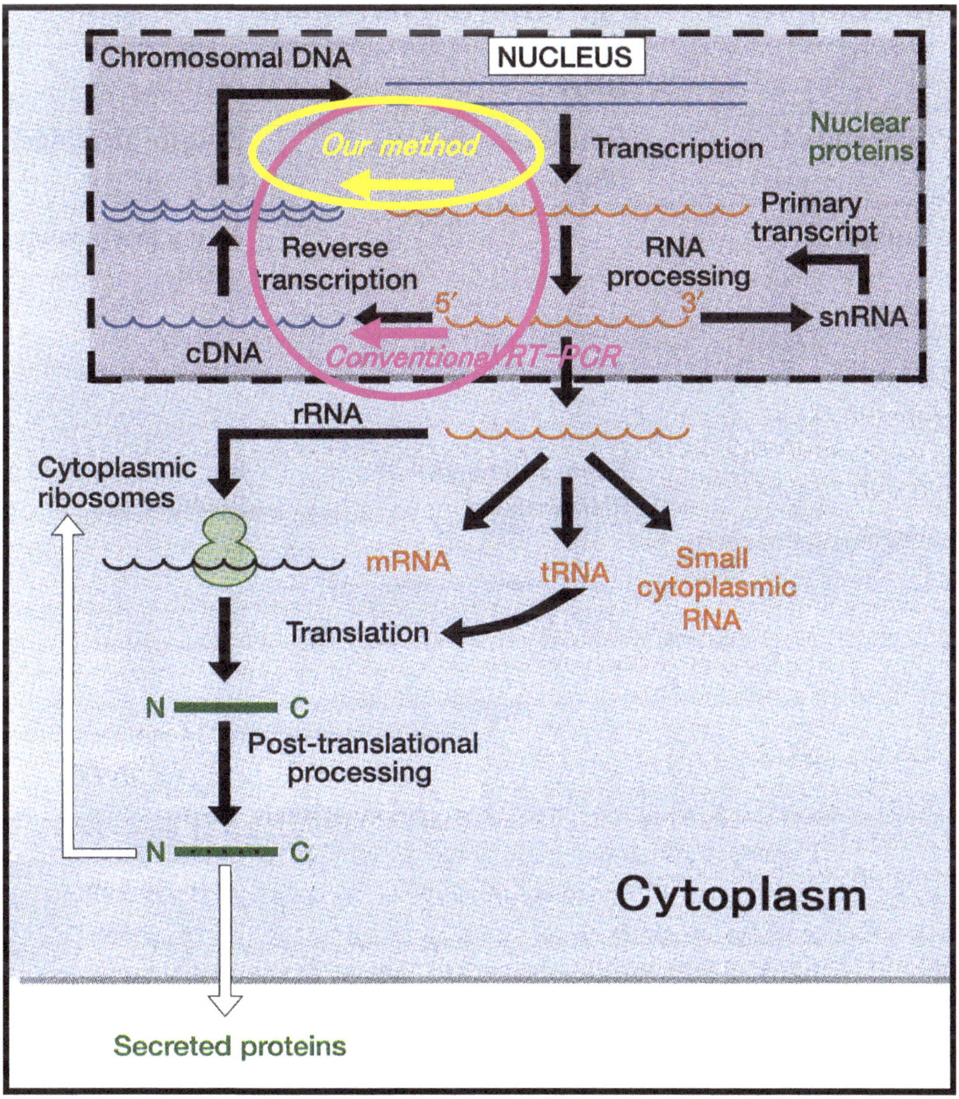

Real-time PCR was performed using the cDNA as a template, which was reverse transcribed from total RNA. The intron-specific primer pair was used to amplify hnRNA for primary transcript quantification. Figure modified from Strachan, T & Read, AP. (2004). DNA structure and gene expression, In: *Human Molecular Genetics 3rd*, pp15, Garland Science, ISBN 0-8153-4184-9, New York, USA.

Fig. 2. Our method for the detection of quantitative hnRNA.

7.1.2 Assay of serum T3 and T4 by EIA

Serum samples taken from the trunk blood were analysed for T3 and T4 levels by an Enzyme Immunoassay (EIA) kit (IMX Dynapac, Abbott Japan, Tokyo, Japan). The sensitivities of the assay were <15 ng/dl for T3 and 1.0 ug/dl for T4.

7.1.3 RNA isolation and reverse transcription for real-time PCR

Following decapitation, the rat brains were removed within 1 min. The pituitaries were dissected out, snap frozen in liquid nitrogen, homogenised and treated with a combination of Trizol and chloroform (Invitrogen, San Diego, CA) to extract total RNA (Guevremont et al., 2006). The RNA from the rat pituitary was purified using DNase I to remove genomic DNA, and the RNA concentration was determined by absorbance readings at 260 nm on a UV spectrophotometre (Bio-Rad, Hercules, CA). A total of 2 μg of RNA was reverse transcribed using the Omniscript Reverse Transcription (RT) kit (Qiagen, Hilden, Germany) with random hexamer primers. Refined cDNA was synthesised in a total volume of 20 ul, treated with RNase H and stored at −20°C until use.

The integrity of the RNA used for the cDNA preparations was tested by PCR amplification (using a thermal cycler) of the glyceraldehyde-3-phosphate dehydrogenase (GAPDH) housekeeping gene (primer sequences are listed in **Table 1**). After electrophoresis on 2% agarose gels, staining with ethidium bromide and visualisation by a UV light, the sizes of the PCR products were verified by comparing them against molecular weight markers.

	Forward primer 5′ – 3′	Reverse primer 5′ – 3′	Product size
TSHβ mRNA	ggcaaactgtttcttcccaa	gttggttttgacagcctcgt	210 bp
TSHβ hnRNA	gaccagtgatccagtcggtt	cgggctgtagaaaccaggta	447 bp
GAPDH mRNA	tgaacgggaagctcactgg	tccaccaccctgttgctgta	307 bp

Primers were designed using the computer programme Primer 3 Software (http://frodo.wi.mit.edu/cgibin/primer3/primer3_www.cgi).
All the produced sequences were checked for homology by the NCBI database BLASTn.

Table 1. Primer sequences for quantitative real-time RT-PCR.

7.1.4 Primer design and quantitative analysis by real-time PCR

TSHβ primers were designed to amplify two specific regions in the TSHβ RNA. To amplify mRNA, the exon-specific primer pair, which was designed to target sequences from exon 3, was used (**Table 1**). The intron-specific primer pair, which was designed to target sequences found in intron 1, was used to amplify hnRNA (**Table 1**). The amplified mRNA and hnRNA products were 210 and 447 bp, respectively. All RT-PCR assays were normalised against rat GAPDH using commercial PCR primers (Nihon Gene Research Laboratories) that amplify a 307 bp product (**Table 1**).

Quantification of the TSHβ mRNA and hnRNA was performed by real-time PCR using the LightCycler® system (Roche Diagnostics, Japan) with SYBR green detection of amplification products. PCR for all genes was performed in a final volume of 20 ul using the LC FastStart DNA Master SYBR Green I (Roche Molecular Biochemicals) with 2 ul of each primer at 0.5 M, 3 mM $MgCl_2$ and 2 ul of extracted cDNA, but without dimethyl sulfoxide (DMSO).

Table 2 shows the LightCycler® PCR amplification programmes. A single fluorescence reading for each sample was taken at the annealing step. Quantitative results were determined from the crossing point (CP), which marked the cycle when the fluorescence of a given sample significantly exceeded the baseline signal, and are expressed as a fractional cycle number. CP values plotted against known concentrations of TSHβ mRNA and hnRNA were used to obtain a standard curve. The TSHβ mRNA and hnRNA counts for

Gene		Programme for Real-time LightCycler			Melting curve		
		Denaturation	Annealing	Elongation			
TSHβ mRNA (cycles 45)	Temperature (°C)	95	62	72	95	62	96
	Incubation time (sec)	10	10	20	0	15	0
	Temperature transition rate (°C/sec)	20	20	20	20	20	0.1
TSHβ hnRNA (cycles 45)	Temperature (°C)	95	62	72	95	62	96
	Incubation time (sec)	10	10	20	0	15	0
	Temperature transition rate (°C/sec)	20	20	20	20	20	0.1
GAPDH mRNA (cycles 45)	Temperature (°C)	95	62	72	95	62	96
	Incubation time (sec)	10	10	20	0	15	0
	Temperature transition rate (°C/sec)	20	20	20	20	20	0.1

Table 2. LightCycler PCR amplification conditions.

a given rat sample were calculated by interpolation from this standard curve (Software LightCycler® 3.5). The melting point of each amplified product was calculated to check the PCR specificity (Fukushima et al., 2003), and transcription of each cDNA was quantified (**Fig. 3**).

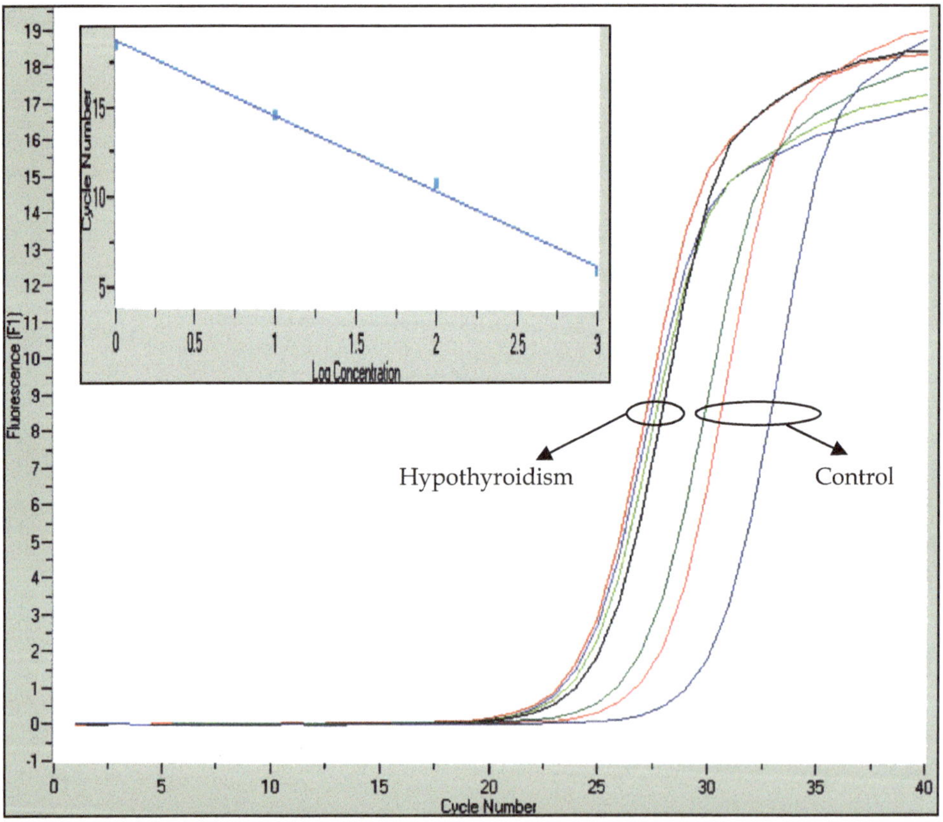

The horizontal and vertical axes show the PCR cycle number and the degree of fluorescence, respectively. In the hypothyroid rat group, the PCR amplification lines curve upward at lower PCR cycle numbers than those of the control group, indicating that the initial hnRNA content was higher in the hypothyroid rat group than in the control group.

Figure Inset: The unknown relative concentration of hnRNA can be calculated from the sample concentration (the horizontal axis; log X) and the cycle number (the vertical axis).

Fig. 3. Original graph from the LightCycler® 3.5 system for the quantification of TSHβ hnRNA.

7.1.5 Statistical analysis

All data are expressed as means ± S.D. T3 and T4 measurements and real-time PCR data were analysed for statistical significance using an unpaired *Student's t-test.* A *p*-value less than 0.01 was considered statistically significant difference.

7.2 Results

7.2.1 Serum T3 and T4 levels

The serum T3 and T4 levels for the hypothyroid rats and control rats are listed in **Table 3**. Oral administration of 0.05% MMI ad libitum was sufficient to induce hypothyroidism in rats. MMI administration resulted in a complete suppression of T3 levels.

	T3	T4
Hypothyroidism	n.d.*	1610 ± 1100*
Control	48.7 ± 2.1	6730 ± 210

Values are means ± SD. *p < 0.01 compared with the control group. Not detected (n.d.).

Table 3. Serum T3 and T4 levels (ng/dl).

7.2.2 Quantitative analysis of TSHβ mRNA and hnRNA by real-time PCR

TSH gene regulation at the transcriptional and posttranscriptional levels was evaluated by real-time RT-PCR to assess mRNA and hnRNA (mRNA precursor) expression. The total RNA extracts from pituitaries isolated from weight-matched rats were treated with DNase I to remove contaminating genomic DNA prior to RT-PCR. The TSHβ-specific primers were subsequently checked for their ability to amplify during PCR reactions in the thermal cycler using total RNA with or without DNase I treatment. Although a PCR product was created from the total RNA template in the absence of DNase I (**Fig. 4**), the presence of DNase I inhibited the reaction, and no product was produced (data not shown).

The TSHβ mRNA and hnRNA levels measured from real-time RT-PCR analysis were estimated relative to the values of GAPDH (the internal standard) and expressed as percentages of the control (**Fig. 5**). The expression levels of both TSHβ mRNA and hnRNA in hypothyroidism were approximately fourfold higher than the respective levels in control rats. The difference in CP between TSHβ mRNA and hnRNA was approximately 3–5 (**Fig. 3**), indicating that hnRNA expression was 8- to 32-fold lower than mRNA expression in chronically hypothyroid rats.

7.3 Discussion

The aim of this study was to detect hnRNA expression by quantitative real-time PCR analysis, and, in particular, the up-regulation of TSHβ gene transcription under the condition of hypothyroidism. Previous reports have shown a range of levels for the up-regulation of TSHβ mRNA (**Table 4**). Although these results were obtained under different experimental conditions, such as the length of PTU administration and the method of mRNA detection, our results confirmed a significant increase in TSHβ mRNA expression in hypothyroid rats.

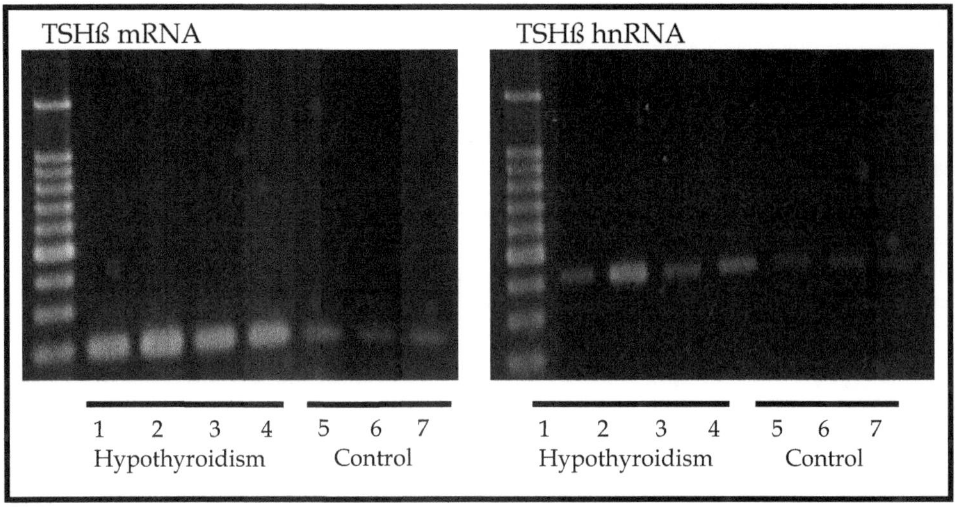

Both bands ofthe TSHβ mRNA and the hnRNA bands in the hypothyroid rats group looked were thicker than that those in the control group. The far left lanes show ladder is a DNA markerladder. After checking the size of the PCR ampliconslength by this ladder, we can forward proceed to the next step for a quantitative real-time PCR. Hypothyroid rats group: lanes 1-4. Control group: lanes 5-7.

Fig. 4. Detection of the RT-PCR amplicons for TSHβ mRNA and hnRNA by thermal cycler

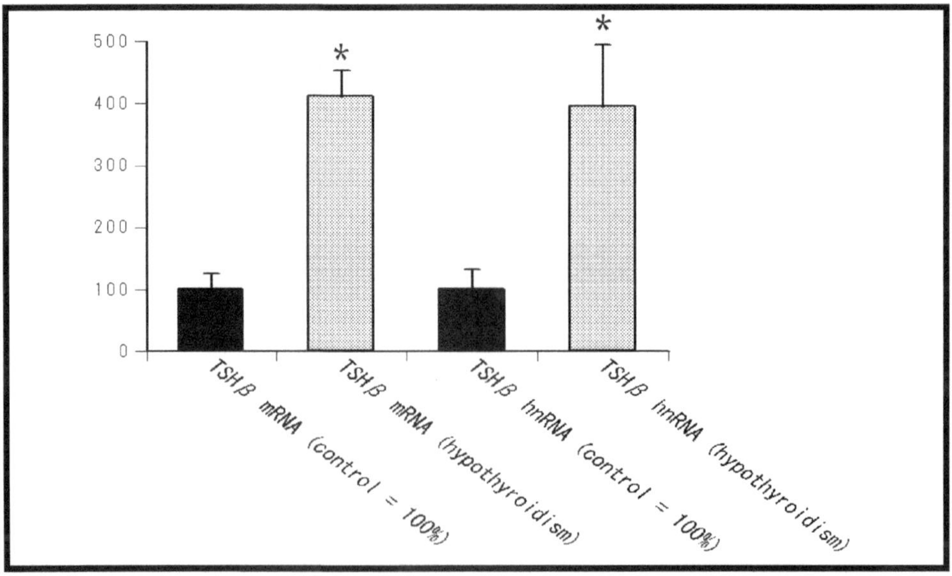

TSHβ mRNA and hnRNA levels in hypothyroid rats were approximately fourfold higher than those of the control rats. Control values were normalised to 100%. Data are expressed as means ± S.D. *$p < 0.01$ compared with the control group.

Fig. 5. Quantitative analysis of TSHβ mRNA and hnRNA levels in control and hypothyroid rats using a LightCycler® PCR system.

Most previous reports have used PTU to induce hypothyroidism (Franklyn et al., 1987; Samuels et al., 1989; Shupnik & Ridgway, 1987; Taylor et al., 1990). However, there is ample evidence that MMI should be used first as an antithyroid drug for Graves' disease (Ginsberg et al., 2006). In addition, some studies have shown that MMI is more effective than PTU at equivalent doses by reducing thyroid hormone levels more rapidly and achieving euthyroidism more quickly (Ginsberg et al., 2006). In this study, free access to a 0.05% MMI solution in drinking water for 2 weeks induced hypothyroidism in rats (**Table 3**). Because of its longer half-life, MMI can also be used as a single daily agent and is therefore more likely to be associated with patient compliance (Cooper, 1984, 1986). Most importantly, MMI may have a more favourable safety profile than PTU (Ginsberg et al., 2006).

Reference	Duration of PTU administration	TSHβ mRNA	Method
(Taylor et al., 1990)	2 weeks	4-fold up-regulation	*in situ* hybridisation
	4 weeks	16-fold up-regulation	
(Steel et al., 1990)		22-fold up-regulation	*in situ* hybridisation
(Samuels et al., 1989)	6 weeks	3-fold up-regulation	Northern blot analysis
(Carr & Chin, 1988)		6- to 8-fold up-regulation	Northern blot analysis
(Shupnik & Ridgway, 1987)	6 weeks	10-fold up-regulation	Northern blot analysis
(Franklyn et al., 1987)	3 weeks	10-fold up-regulation	Northern blot analysis
	10 weeks	20-fold up-regulation	

PTU administration; oral administration of 0.05% propylthiouracil in the drinking water

Table 4. Previous reports of semi-quantitative analysis of TSHβ mRNA expression in rat hypothyroidism.

In this study, we accurately measured the increased rate of TSH gene transcription in hypothyroid rats by detecting mRNA and hnRNA expression levels over time using the LightCycler® system. Our main recommendations for success with this system are as follows: (1) the extracted total RNA should be treated with DNase to ensure exclusion of genomic DNA and (2) degenerate oligonucleotide random primers should be used instead of the degenerate oligonucleotide dT primers that are more commonly used for mRNA detection.

The poly-A tail of a mature mRNA is immediately appended by poly-A polymerase at the final step of RNA processing. Oligonucleotide dT primers attach to the poly-A tail of the mRNA for cDNA synthesis until the RT reaction stops. Therefore, only the exonic regions of the DNA are reflected by RT-PCR when use of Oligonucleotide dT primers. However, in our experiments, we used a random hexamer primer, which attaches to DNA complementarily and randomly. When a hexamer primer attaches to any intronic region of the hnRNA, the RT reaction accurately makes cDNA, reflecting primary transcription. Using this cDNA containing intronic sequences as a template, we successfully amplified primary TSHβ transcripts with a TSHβ-specific intron primer.

The only difficulty in our method was dissecting tissues of the same size and location from the animals. In this study, we easily removed pituitary glands of the same size because the pituitary gland differentiates from a dual embryonic origin, unlike other nearby tissues (Kelberman et al., 2009), which allows the pituitary gland to be easily separated. However, in the case of continuous tissues, such as the hypothalamus, it may be difficult to dissect an area from the same location within the brain. If the dissected area dose not contain the target neurons, the internal gene of the area should show a relative increase.

The increased level of TSHβ mRNA was nearly equal to that of TSHβ hnRNA in hypothyroid rats. Since the transcriptional rate is often masked by the abundance of pre-existing mature mRNA, quantitative detection of hnRNA is important for the precise examination of transcriptional changes during an acute response. Therefore, the use of a quantitative real-time PCR method is beneficial for the analysis of genes with low expression levels, such as those genes that are undetectable when using an *in situ* hybridisation method.

In this report, we demonstrated for the first time that optimal conditions for real-time PCR enable the detection of TSHβ hnRNA expression levels in hypothyroid rats. In addition to its critical role in homeostasis, thyroid hormone can also regulate gene transcription in relation to various aspects of brain function (Refetoff et al., 1993), including synapse formation (Nicholson & Altman, 1972). Thus, our results are of particular importance for neuroendocrinological studies.

Finally, we determined the exact ratio for the up-regulation of TSHβ mRNA and hnRNA levels in hypothyroid rats using quantitative real-time PCR. Using this method, we can perform similar investigations on the transcription rates of other genes.

8. Conclusion

We have summarised TSH regulation (e.g., TSH secretion and synthesis), the HPT axis as a positive/negative regulator of TSH, the neuronal control of TSH, and drugs affecting TSH in hypothyroidism. We also described a method for the quantitative analysis of TSHβ hnRNA and mRNA expression using real-time PCR in induced hypothyroidism. Both the TSHβ mRNA and hnRNA expression levels in hypothyroidism induced by methimazole administration were increased approximately fourfold over the respective levels in control rats. Further, the level of TSHβ hnRNA expression was 8- to 32-fold lower than that of TSHβ mRNA in chronically hypothyroid rats. Using this method, we can perform similar investigations of the transcription rates for other genes.

9. Acknowledgement

This work was supported by a Grant-in-Aid for Exploratory Research (#22659380) from the Japan Society for the Promotion of Science.

10. References

Abel, E. D., Ahima, R. S., Boers, M. E., Elmquist, J. K., & Wondisford, F. E. (2001). Critical role for thyroid hormone receptor beta2 in the regulation of paraventricular thyrotropin-releasing hormone neurons. *The Journal of clinical investigation,* Vol.107, No.8, pp. 1017-1023, ISSN 0021-9738

Abel, E. D., Boers, M. E., Pazos-Moura, C., Moura, E., Kaulbach, H., Zakaria, M., Lowell, B., Radovick, S., Liberman, M. C., & Wondisford, F. (1999). Divergent roles for thyroid hormone receptor beta isoforms in the endocrine axis and auditory system. *The Journal of clinical investigation,* Vol.104, No.3, pp. 291-300, ISSN 0021-9738

Alkemade, A., Unmehopa, U. A., Wiersinga, W. M., Swaab, D. F., & Fliers, E. (2005). Glucocorticoids decrease thyrotropin-releasing hormone messenger ribonucleic acid expression in the paraventricular nucleus of the human hypothalamus. *The Journal of clinical endocrinology and metabolism,* Vol.90, No.1, pp. 323-327, ISSN 0021-972X

Andersen, B., & Rosenfeld, M. G. (1994). Pit-1 determines cell types during development of the anterior pituitary gland. A model for transcriptional regulation of cell phenotypes in mammalian organogenesis. *The Journal of biological chemistry,* Vol.269, No.47, pp. 29335-29338, ISSN 0021-9258

Arancibia, S., Rage, F., Astier, H., & Tapia-Arancibia, L. (1996). Neuroendocrine and autonomous mechanisms underlying thermoregulation in cold environment. *Neuroendocrinology,* Vol.64, No.4, pp. 257-267, ISSN 0028-3835

Arancibia, S., Tapia-Arancibia, L., Astier, H., & Assenmacher, I. (1989). Physiological evidence for alpha 1-adrenergic facilitatory control of the cold-induced TRH release in the rat, obtained by push-pull cannulation of the median eminence. *Neuroscience letters,* Vol.100, No.1-3, pp. 169-174, ISSN 0304-3940

Bartalena, L., Grasso, L., Brogioni, S., & Martino, E. (1994). Interleukin 6 effects on the pituitary-thyroid axis in the rat. *European journal of endocrinology / European Federation of Endocrine Societies,* Vol.131, No.3, pp. 302-306, ISSN 0804-4643

Baur, A., Bauer, K., Jarry, H., & Kohrle, J. (2000). Effects of proinflammatory cytokines on anterior pituitary 5'-deiodinase type I and type II. *The Journal of endocrinology,* Vol.167, No.3, pp. 505-515, ISSN 0022-0795

Beck-Peccoz, P., Mariotti, S., Guillausseau, P. J., Medri, G., Piscitelli, G., Bertoli, A., Barbarino, A., Rondena, M., Chanson, P., Pinchera, A., & et al. (1989). Treatment of hyperthyroidism due to inappropriate secretion of thyrotropin with the somatostatin analog SMS 201-995. *The Journal of clinical endocrinology and metabolism,* Vol.68, No.1, pp. 208-214, ISSN 0021-972X

Bianco, A. C., Salvatore, D., Gereben, B., Berry, M. J., & Larsen, P. R. (2002). Biochemistry, cellular and molecular biology, and physiological roles of the iodothyronine selenodeiodinases. *Endocrine reviews,* Vol.23, No.1, pp. 38-89, ISSN 0163-769X

Carr, F. E., Burnside, J., & Chin, W. W. (1989). Thyroid hormones regulate rat thyrotropin beta gene promoter activity expressed in GH3 cells. *Molecular endocrinology*, Vol.3, No.4, pp. 709-716, ISSN 0888-8809

Carr, F. E., & Chin, W. W. (1988). Differential thyroid hormone-regulated rat thyrotropin beta gene expression detected by blot hybridization. *Mol Endocrinol*, Vol.2, No.8, pp. 667-673, ISSN

Carr, F. E., Galloway, R. J., Reid, A. H., Kaseem, L. L., Dhillon, G., Fein, H. G., & Smallridge, R. C. (1991). Thyrotropin-releasing hormone regulation of thyrotropin beta-subunit gene expression involves intracellular calcium and protein kinase C. Biochemistry, Vol.30, No.15, pp. 3721-3728, ISSN 0006-2960

Cheng, S. Y. (2005). Thyroid hormone receptor mutations and disease: beyond thyroid hormone resistance. Trends in endocrinology and metabolism: TEM, Vol.16, No.4, pp. 176-182, ISSN 1043-2760

Cintra, A., Fuxe, K., Wikstrom, A. C., Visser, T., & Gustafsson, J. A. (1990). Evidence for thyrotropin-releasing hormone and glucocorticoid receptor-immunoreactive neurons in various preoptic and hypothalamic nuclei of the male rat. *Brain research*, Vol.506, No.1, pp. 139-144, ISSN 0006-8993

Contini, C., Seraceni, S., Cultrera, R., Incorvaia, C., Sebastiani, A., & Picot, S. (2005). Evaluation of a Real-time PCR-based assay using the lightcycler system for detection of Toxoplasma gondii bradyzoite genes in blood specimens from patients with toxoplasmic retinochoroiditis. *Int J Parasitol*, Vol.35, No.3, pp. 275-283, ISSN

Cooper, D. S. (1984). Antithyroid drugs. *N Engl J Med*, Vol.311, No.21, pp. 1353-1362, ISSN

Cooper, D. S. (1986). Which anti-thyroid drug? *Am J Med*, Vol.80, No.6, pp. 1165-1168, ISSN

Crantz, F. R., Silva, J. E., & Larsen, P. R. (1982). An analysis of the sources and quantity of 3,5,3'-triiodothyronine specifically bound to nuclear receptors in rat cerebral cortex and cerebellum. *Endocrinology*, Vol.110, No.2, pp. 367-375, ISSN 0013-7227

Crisanti, P., Omri, B., Hughes, E., Meduri, G., Hery, C., Clauser, E., Jacquemin, C., & Saunier, B. (2001). The expression of thyrotropin receptor in the brain. *Endocrinology*, Vol.142, No.2, pp. 812-822, ISSN 0013-7227

Danzi, S., Dubon, P., & Klein, I. (2005). Effect of serum triiodothyronine on regulation of cardiac gene expression: role of histone acetylation. *Am J Physiol Heart Circ Physiol*, Vol.289, No.4, pp. H1506-1511, ISSN

Darnell, J. E., Jr. (1983). The processing of RNA. *Sci Am*, Vol.249, No.4, pp. 90-100, ISSN

Dayan, C. M., & Daniels, G. H. (1996). Chronic autoimmune thyroiditis. *The New England journal of medicine*, Vol.335, No.2, pp. 99-107, ISSN 0028-4793

DeLong, G. R., Stanbury, J. B., & Fierro-Benitez, R. (1985). Neurological signs in congenital iodine-deficiency disorder (endemic cretinism). *Developmental medicine and child neurology*, Vol.27, No.3, pp. 317-324, ISSN 0012-1622

Elias, C. F., Lee, C., Kelly, J., Aschkenasi, C., Ahima, R. S., Couceyro, P. R., Kuhar, M. J., Saper, C. B., & Elmquist, J. K. (1998). Leptin activates hypothalamic CART neurons projecting to the spinal cord. *Neuron*, Vol.21, No.6, pp. 1375-1385, ISSN 0896-6273

Emrich, T., Chang, S. Y., Karl, G., Panzinger, B., & Santini, C. (2002). Quantitative detection of telomerase components by real-time, online RT-PCR analysis with the LightCycler. *Methods Mol Biol*, Vol.191, pp. 99-108, ISSN

Faglia, G., Bitensky, L., Pinchera, A., Ferrari, C., Paracchi, A., Beck-Peccoz, P., Ambrosi, B., & Spada, A. (1979). Thyrotropin secretion in patients with central hypothyroidism:

evidence for reduced biological activity of immunoreactive thyrotropin. *The Journal of clinical endocrinology and metabolism*, Vol.48, No.6, pp. 989-998, ISSN 0021-972X

Fatourechi, V. (2009). Subclinical hypothyroidism: an update for primary care physicians. *Mayo Clinic proceedings. Mayo Clinic*, Vol.84, No1, pp. 65-71, ISSN 1942-5546

Fekete, C., Kelly, J., Mihaly, E., Sarkar, S., Rand, W. M., Legradi, G., Emerson, C. H., & Lechan, R. M. (2001). Neuropeptide Y has a central inhibitory action on the hypothalamic-pituitary-thyroid axis. *Endocrinology*, Vol.142, No.6, pp. 2606-2613, ISSN

Fekete, C., & Lechan, R. M. (2007). Negative feedback regulation of hypophysiotropic thyrotropin-releasing hormone (TRH) synthesizing neurons: role of neuronal afferents and type 2 deiodinase. *Frontiers in neuroendocrinology*, Vol.28, No.2-3, pp. 97-114, ISSN 0091-3022

Fekete, C., Mihaly, E., Luo, L. G., Kelly, J., Clausen, J. T., Mao, Q., Rand, W. M., Moss, L. G., Kuhar, M., Emerson, C. H., Jackson, I. M., & Lechan, R. M. (2000). Association of cocaine- and amphetamine-regulated transcript-immunoreactive elements with thyrotropin-releasing hormone-synthesizing neurons in the hypothalamic paraventricular nucleus and its role in the regulation of the hypothalamic-pituitary-thyroid axis during fasting. *The Journal of neuroscience : the official journal of the Society for Neuroscience*, Vol.20, No.24, pp. 9224-9234, ISSN 1529-2401

Franklyn, J. A., Wood, D. F., Balfour, N. J., Ramsden, D. B., Docherty, K., Chin, W. W., & Sheppard, M. C. (1987). Effect of hypothyroidism and thyroid hormone replacement in vivo on pituitary cytoplasmic concentrations of thyrotropin-beta and alpha-subunit messenger ribonucleic acids. *Endocrinology*, Vol.120, No.6, pp. 2279-2288, ISSN

Fukushima, H., Tsunomori, Y., & Seki, R. (2003). Duplex real-time SYBR green PCR assays for detection of 17 species of food- or waterborne pathogens in stools. *J Clin Microbiol*, Vol.41, No.11, pp. 5134-5146, ISSN

Ginsberg, A. B., Frank, M. G., Francis, A. B., Rubin, B. A., O'Connor, K. A., & Spencer, R. L. (2006). Specific and time-dependent effects of glucocorticoid receptor agonist RU28362 on stress-induced pro-opiomelanocortin hnRNA, c-fos mRNA and zif268 mRNA in the pituitary. *J Neuroendocrinol*, Vol.18, No.2, pp. 129-138, ISSN

Guadano-Ferraz, A., Obregon, M. J., St Germain, D. L., & Bernal, J. (1997). The type 2 iodothyronine deiodinase is expressed primarily in glial cells in the neonatal rat brain. *Proceedings of the National Academy of Sciences of the United States of America*, Vol.94, No.19, pp. 10391-10396, ISSN 0027-8424

Guevremont, E., Brassard, J., Houde, A., Simard, C., & Trottier, Y. L. (2006). Development of an extraction and concentration procedure and comparison of RT-PCR primer systems for the detection of hepatitis A virus and norovirus GII in green onions. *J Virol Methods*, Vol.134, pp. 130-135, ISSN

Hahn, T. M., Breininger, J. F., Baskin, D. G., & Schwartz, M. W. (1998). Coexpression of Agrp and NPY in fasting-activated hypothalamic neurons. *Nature neuroscience*, Vol.1, No.4, pp. 271-272, ISSN 1097-6256

Hashimoto, K., Zanger, K., Hollenberg, A. N., Cohen, L. E., Radovick, S., & Wondisford, F. E. (2000). cAMP response element-binding protein-binding protein mediates thyrotropin-releasing hormone signaling on thyrotropin subunit genes. *The Journal of biological chemistry*, Vol.275, No.43, pp. 33365-33372, ISSN 0021-9258

Heuer, H., & Visser, T. J. (2009). Minireview: Pathophysiological importance of thyroid hormone transporters. *Endocrinology*, Vol.150, No.3, pp. 1078-1083, ISSN 1945-7170

Huang, S. A., Tu, H. M., Harney, J. W., Venihaki, M., Butte, A. J., Kozakewich, H. P., Fishman, S. J., & Larsen, P. R. (2000). Severe hypothyroidism caused by type 3 iodothyronine deiodinase in infantile hemangiomas. *The New England journal of medicine*, Vol.343, No.3, pp. 185-189, ISSN 0028-4793

Itagaki, Y., Yoshida, K., Ikeda, H., Kaise, K., Kaise, N., Yamamoto, M., Sakurada, T., & Yoshinaga, K. (1990). Thyroxine 5'-deiodinase in human anterior pituitary tumors. *The Journal of clinical endocrinology and metabolism*, Vol.71, No.2, pp. 340-344, ISSN 0021-972X

Johnson, R. F., Mitchell, C. M., Giles, W. B., Walters, W. A., & Zakar, T. (2002). The in vivo control of prostaglandin H synthase-2 messenger ribonucleic acid expression in the human amnion at parturition. *J Clin Endocrinol Metab*, Vol.87, No.6, pp. 2816-2823, ISSN

Johnson, R. F., Mitchell, C. M., Giles, W. B., Walters, W. A., & Zakar, T. (2003). The control of prostaglandin endoperoxide H-Synthase-2 expression in the human chorion laeve at term. *J Soc Gynecol Investig*, Vol.10, No.4, pp. 222-230, ISSN

Kelberman, D., Rizzoti, K., Lovell-Badge, R., Robinson, I. C., & Dattani, M. T. (2009). Genetic regulation of pituitary gland development in human and mouse. *Endocr Rev*, Vol.30, No.7, pp. 790-829, ISSN

Kren, B. T., & Steer, C. J. (1996). Posttranscriptional regulation of gene expression in liver regeneration: role of mRNA stability. *Faseb J*, Vol.10, No.5, pp. 559-573, ISSN

Kuroda, M., Oikawa, K., Yoshida, K., Takeuchi, A., Takeuchi, M., Usui, M., Umezawa, A., & Mukai, K. (2005). Effects of 3-methylcholanthrene on the transcriptional activity and mRNA accumulation of the oncogene hWAPL. *Cancer Lett*, Vol.221, No.1, pp. 21-28, ISSN

Ladenson, P. W., Singer, P. A., Ain, K. B., Bagchi, N., Bigos, S. T., Levy, E. G., Smith, S. A., Daniels, G. H., & Cohen, H. D. (2000). American Thyroid Association guidelines for detection of thyroid dysfunction. *Archives of internal medicine*, Vol.160, No.11, pp. 1573-1575, ISSN 0003-9926

Lamberts, S. W., Zuyderwijk, J., den Holder, F., van Koetsveld, P., & Hofland, L. (1989). Studies on the conditions determining the inhibitory effect of somatostatin on adrenocorticotropin, prolactin and thyrotropin release by cultured rat pituitary cells. *Neuroendocrinology*, Vol.50, No.1, pp. 44-50, ISSN 0028-3835

Lania, A., Persani, L., & Beck-Peccoz, P. (2008). Central hypothyroidism. *Pituitary*, Vol.11, No.2, pp. 181-186, ISSN 1386-341X

Lechan, R. M., & Fekete, C. (2006). The TRH neuron: a hypothalamic integrator of energy metabolism. *Progress in brain research*, Vol.153, pp. 209-235, ISSN 0079-6123.

Legradi, G., Emerson, C. H., Ahima, R. S., Flier, J. S., & Lechan, R. M. (1997). Leptin prevents fasting-induced suppression of prothyrotropin-releasing hormone messenger ribonucleic acid in neurons of the hypothalamic paraventricular nucleus. *Endocrinology*, Vol.138, No.6, pp. 2569-2576, ISSN 0013-7227

Lewis, B. M., Dieguez, C., Lewis, M. D., & Scanlon, M. F. (1987). Dopamine stimulates release of thyrotrophin-releasing hormone from perfused intact rat hypothalamus via hypothalamic D2-receptors. *The Journal of endocrinology*, Vol.115, No.3, pp. 419-424, ISSN 0022-0795

Li, G. J., Zhao, Q., & Zheng, W. (2005). Alteration at translational but not transcriptional level of transferrin receptor expression following manganese exposure at the blood-CSF barrier in vitro. *Toxicol Appl Pharmacol*, Vol.205, No.2, pp. 188-200, ISSN

Lyon, E. (2001). Mutation detection using fluorescent hybridization probes and melting curve analysis. *Expert Rev Mol Diagn*, Vol.1, No.1, pp. 92-101, ISSN

Magner, J. A. (1990). Thyroid-stimulating hormone: biosynthesis, cell biology, and bioactivity. *Endocrine reviews*, Vol.11, No.2, pp. 354-385, ISSN 0163-769X

Matsushita, A., Sasaki, S., Kashiwabara, Y., Nagayama, K., Ohba, K., Iwaki, H., Misawa, H., Ishizuka, K., & Nakamura, H. (2007). Essential role of GATA2 in the negative regulation of thyrotropin beta gene by thyroid hormone and its receptors. *Molecular endocrinology*, Vol.21, No.4, pp. 865-884, ISSN 0888-8809

Menezes-Ferreira, M. M., Petrick, P. A., & Weintraub, B. D. (1986). Regulation of thyrotropin (TSH) bioactivity by TSH-releasing hormone and thyroid hormone. *Endocrinology*, Vol.118, No.5, pp. 2125-2130, ISSN 0013-7227

Mihaly, E., Fekete, C., Legradi, G., & Lechan, R. M. (2001). Hypothalamic dorsomedial nucleus neurons innervate thyrotropin-releasing hormone-synthesizing neurons in the paraventricular nucleus. *Brain research*, Vol.891, No.1-2, pp. 20-31, ISSN 0006-8993

Mizuno, T. M., Kleopoulos, S. P., Bergen, H. T., Roberts, J. L., Priest, C. A., & Mobbs, C. V. (1998). Hypothalamic pro-opiomelanocortin mRNA is reduced by fasting and [corrected] in ob/ob and db/db mice, but is stimulated by leptin. *Diabetes*, Vol.47, No.2, pp. 294-297, ISSN 0012-1797

Nakano, K., Matsushita, A., Sasaki, S., Misawa, H., Nishiyama, K., Kashiwabara, Y., & Nakamura, H. (2004). Thyroid-hormone-dependent negative regulation of thyrotropin beta gene by thyroid hormone receptors: study with a new experimental system using CV1 cells. *The Biochemical journal*, Vol.378, No.2, pp. 549-557, ISSN 1470-8728

Nicholson, J. L., & Altman, J. (1972). Synaptogenesis in the rat cerebellum: effects of early hypo- and hyperthyroidism. *Science*, Vol.176, No.34, pp. 530-532, ISSN

Nikrodhanond, A. A., Ortiga-Carvalho, T. M., Shibusawa, N., Hashimoto, K., Liao, X. H., Refetoff, S., Yamada, M., Mori, M., & Wondisford, F. E. (2006). Dominant role of thyrotropin-releasing hormone in the hypothalamic-pituitary-thyroid axis. *The Journal of biological chemistry*, Vol.281, No.8, pp. 5000-5007, ISSN 0021-9258

O'Shea, P. J., & Williams, G. R. (2002). Insight into the physiological actions of thyroid hormone receptors from genetically modified mice. *J Endocrinol*, Vol.175, No.3, pp. 553-570, ISSN

Obregon, M. J., Pascual, A., Mallol, J., Morreale de Escobar, G., & Escobar del Rey, F. (1980). Evidence against a major role of L-thyroxine at the pituitary level: studies in rats treated with iopanoic acid (telepaque). *Endocrinology*, Vol.106, No.6, pp. 1827-1836, ISSN 0013-7227

Pang, X. P., Hershman, J. M., Mirell, C. J., & Pekary, A. E. (1989). Impairment of hypothalamic-pituitary-thyroid function in rats treated with human recombinant tumor necrosis factor-alpha (cachectin). *Endocrinology*, Vol.125, No.1, pp. 76-84, ISSN 0013-7227

Petersen, V. B., McGregor, A. M., Belchetz, P. E., Elkeles, R. S., & Hall, R. (1978). The secretion of thyrotrophin with impaired biological activity in patients with hypothalamic-pituitary disease. *Clinical endocrinology*, Vol.8, No.5, pp. 397-402, ISSN 0300-0664

Porterfield, S. P., & Hendrich, C. E. (1993). The role of thyroid hormones in prenatal and neonatal neurological development--current perspectives. *Endocrine reviews*, Vol.14, No.1, pp. 94-106, ISSN 0163-769X

Prummel, M. F., Brokken, L. J., Meduri, G., Misrahi, M., Bakker, O., & Wiersinga, W. M. (2000). Expression of the thyroid-stimulating hormone receptor in the folliculo-stellate cells of the human anterior pituitary. *The Journal of clinical endocrinology and metabolism*, Vol.85, No.11, pp. 4347-4353, ISSN 0021-972X

Prummel, M. F., Brokken, L. J., & Wiersinga, W. M. (2004). Ultra short-loop feedback control of thyrotropin secretion. Thyroid : official journal of the American Thyroid Association, Vol.14, No.10, pp. 825-829, ISSN 1050-7256

Refetoff, S., Weiss, R. E., & Usala, S. J. (1993). The syndromes of resistance to thyroid hormone. *Endocr Rev*, Vol.14, No.3, pp. 348-399, ISSN 0163-769X

Ridgway, E. C., Weintraub, B. D., & Maloof, F. (1974). Metabolic clearance and production rates of human thyrotropin. *The Journal of clinical investigation*, Vol.53, No.3, pp. 895-903, ISSN 0021-9738

Rose, S. R. (2001). Cranial irradiation and central hypothyroidism. *Trends in endocrinology and metabolism: TEM*, Vo.12, No.3, pp. 97-104, ISSN 1043-2760

Samuels, M. H., Wierman, M. E., Wang, C., & Ridgway, E. C. (1989). The effect of altered thyroid status on pituitary hormone messenger ribonucleic acid concentrations in the rat. *Endocrinology*, Vol.124, No.5, pp. 2277-2282, ISSN

Schuster, R., Max, N., Mann, B., Heufelder, K., Thilo, F., Grone, J., Rokos, F., Buhr, H. J., Thiel, E., & Keilholz, U. (2004). Quantitative real-time RT-PCR for detection of disseminated tumor cells in peripheral blood of patients with colorectal cancer using different mRNA markers. *Int J Cancer*, Vol.108, No.2, pp. 219-227, ISSN

Shupnik, M. A., Greenspan, S. L., & Ridgway, E. C. (1986). Transcriptional regulation of thyrotropin subunit genes by thyrotropin-releasing hormone and dopamine in pituitary cell culture. *The Journal of biological chemistry*, Vol.261, No.27, pp. 12675-12679, ISSN 0021-9258

Shupnik, M. A., & Ridgway, E. C. (1987). Thyroid hormone control of thyrotropin gene expression in rat anterior pituitary cells. *Endocrinology*, Vol.121, No.2, pp. 619-624, ISSN

Shupnik, M. A., Ridgway, E. C., & Chin, W. W. (1989). Molecular biology of thyrotropin. *Endocrine reviews*, Vol.10, No.4, pp. 459-475, ISSN 0163-769X

Silva, J. E., & Larsen, P. R. (1978). Contributions of plasma triiodothyronine and local thyroxine monodeiodination to triiodothyronine to nuclear triiodothyronine receptor saturation in pituitary, liver, and kidney of hypothyroid rats. Further evidence relating saturation of pituitary nuclear triiodothyronine receptors and the acute inhibition of thyroid-stimulating hormone release. *The Journal of clinical investigation*, Vol.61, No.5, pp. 1247-1259, ISSN 0021-9738

Steel, J. H., O'Halloran, D. J., Jones, P. M., Van Noorden, S., Chin, W. W., Bloom, S. R., & Polak, J. M. (1990). Combined use of immunocytochemistry and in situ hybridization to study beta thyroid-stimulating hormone gene expression in pituitaries of hypothyroid rats. *Mol Cell Probes*, Vol.4, No.5, pp. 385-396, ISSN

Sugimoto, K., Mori, K., Uchida, K., Kobayashi, D., & Itoi, K. (2007). Quantitative analysis of thyroid-stimulating hormone messenger RNA and heterogeneous nuclear RNA in hypothyroid rats. *Brain Res Bull*, Vol.74, No.1-3, pp. 142-146, ISSN

Tan, B. H., Lim, E. A., Liaw, J. C., Seah, S. G., & Yap, E. P. (2004). Diagnostic value of real-time capillary thermal cycler in virus detection. *Expert Rev Mol Diagn*, Vol.4, No.2, pp. 219-230, ISSN

Tang, K. T., Braverman, L. E., & DeVito, W. J. (1995). Tumor necrosis factor-alpha and interferon-gamma modulate gene expression of type I 5'-deiodinase, thyroid peroxidase, and thyroglobulin in FRTL-5 rat thyroid cells. *Endocrinology*, Vol.136, No.3, pp. 881-888, ISSN 0013-7227

Taylor, T., & Weintraub, B. D. (1989). Altered thyrotropin (TSH) carbohydrate structures in hypothalamic hypothyroidism created by paraventricular nuclear lesions are corrected by in vivo TSH-releasing hormone administration. *Endocrinology*, Vol.125, No.4, pp. 2198-2203, ISSN 0013-7227

Taylor, T., Wondisford, F. E., Blaine, T., & Weintraub, B. D. (1990). The paraventricular nucleus of the hypothalamus has a major role in thyroid hormone feedback regulation of thyrotropin synthesis and secretion. *Endocrinology*, Vol.126, No.1, pp. 317-324, ISSN

Thonberg, H., Fredriksson, J. M., Nedergaard, J., & Cannon, B. (2002). A novel pathway for adrenergic stimulation of cAMP-response-element-binding protein (CREB) phosphorylation: mediation via alpha1-adrenoceptors and protein kinase C activation. *The Biochemical journal*, Vol.364, No.1, pp. 73-79, ISSN 0264-6021

Tu, H. M., Kim, S. W., Salvatore, D., Bartha, T., Legradi, G., Larsen, P. R., & Lechan, R. M. (1997). Regional distribution of type 2 thyroxine deiodinase messenger ribonucleic acid in rat hypothalamus and pituitary and its regulation by thyroid hormone. *Endocrinology*, Vol.138, No.8, pp. 3359-3368, ISSN 0013-7227

Weiss, R. E., Forrest, D., Pohlenz, J., Cua, K., Curran, T., & Refetoff, S. (1997). Thyrotropin regulation by thyroid hormone in thyroid hormone receptor beta-deficient mice. *Endocrinology*, Vol.138, No.9, pp. 3624-3629, ISSN 0013-7227

Wikstrom, L., Johansson, C., Salto, C., Barlow, C., Campos Barros, A., Baas, F., Forrest, D., Thoren, P., & Vennstrom, B. (1998). Abnormal heart rate and body temperature in mice lacking thyroid hormone receptor alpha 1. *The EMBO journal*, Vol.17, No.2, pp. 455-461, ISSN 0261-4189

Wilber, J. F., & Utiger, R. D. (1969). The effect of glucocorticoids on thyrotropin secretion. *The Journal of clinical investigation*, Vol.48, No.11, pp. 2096-2103, ISSN 0021-9738.

Wilber, J. F., & Xu, A. H. (1998). The thyrotropin-releasing hormone gene 1998: cloning, characterization, and transcriptional regulation in the central nervous system, heart, and testis. *Thyroid : official journal of the American Thyroid Association*, Vol.8, No.10, pp. 897-901, ISSN 1050-7256

Wittmann, G., Liposits, Z., Lechan, R. M., & Fekete, C. (2002). Medullary adrenergic neurons contribute to the neuropeptide Y-ergic innervation of hypophysiotropic thyrotropin-releasing hormone-synthesizing neurons in the rat. *Neuroscience letters*, Vol.324, No.1, pp. 69-73, ISSN 0304-3940

Wittmann, G., Liposits, Z., Lechan, R. M., & Fekete, C. (2004). Medullary adrenergic neurons contribute to the cocaine- and amphetamine-regulated transcript-immunoreactive innervation of thyrotropin-releasing hormone synthesizing neurons in the hypothalamic paraventricular nucleus. *Brain research*, Vol.1006, No.1, pp. 1-7, ISSN 0006-8993

Yamada, M., Saga, Y., Shibusawa, N., Hirato, J., Murakami, M., Iwasaki, T., Hashimoto, K., Satoh, T., Wakabayashi, K., Taketo, M. M., & Mori, M. (1997). Tertiary hypothyroidism and hyperglycemia in mice with targeted disruption of the thyrotropin-releasing hormone gene. *Proceedings of the National Academy of Sciences of the United States of America*, Vol.94, No.20, pp. 10862-10867, ISSN 0027-8424

16

A 3,3'-Diiodothyronine Sulfate Cross-Reactive Material (Compound W), a Potential Marker for Fetal Hypothyroidism

Sing-Yung Wu and William L. Green
University of California, Irvine, VA Medical Center, Long Beach, California, and University of Washington, Seattle, Washington
USA

1. Introduction

In developing mammals (including humans), a deficiency or excess of thyroid hormone (TH) in the developing brain during the fetal and neonatal periods can lead to morphological and functional abnormalities (Nunez et al., 1992; Pasquini & Adamo, 1994; Morreale de Escobar et al., 2004; Harakawa et al., 1989). The most severe form of hypothyroidism in human fetus and neonate is the syndrome of cretinism. Recent studies indicate that abnormalities in intelligence quotient (IQ) and other neuropsychological tests may be found in children of women with subclinical hypothyroidism during pregnancy (Haddow et al., 1999; Mitchell & Klein, 2004; Casey et al., 2005). Subtle health impairment and reduced socio-educational achievement are observed in young adults with congenital hypothyroidism identified by neonatal screening and subsequently treated (Leger et al., 2011). This suggests the inadequacy in the current strategy with neonatal screening - it may already be too late to secure normal neurological development. Studies of populations indicate that congenital hypothyroidism affects 1 in 3,000 to 4,000 newborns; twice as many females as males. A recent report showed that the incidence in the United States increased from ~ 1:4100 in 1987 to ~ 1:2400 in 2002 (Rastogi & LaFranchi, 2010; Harris & Pass, 2007). The causes for this change are not entirely clear even though the screening strategy may have contributed to the increase (Rastogi & LaFranchi, 2010).

2. Etiology of congenital hypothyroidism

Most cases of congenital hypothyroidism are sporadic. But an estimated 15 to 20 percent of cases are inherited including mutations in the *DUOX2, PAX8, SLC5A5(NIS), SLC26A4(PDS), TG, TPO, DEHAL1, TSHB*, and *TSHR* genes (Table 1; Rastogi & LaFranchi, 2010; Grasberger & Refetoff, 2011). Many inherited cases are autosomal recessive but those with a mutation in the *PAX8* gene or certain *TSHR* gene mutations have an autosomal dominant pattern of inheritance. Another possible cause of fetal hypothyroidism is anti-thyroid medication treatment for maternal hyperthyroidism during pregnancy (Rastogi & LaFranchi, 2010; Rovet et al., 1999; Mirabella et al., 2000; Vanmiddlesworth et al., 2011). In severe iodine-deficient regions, the prevalence of cretinism can reach 10% of the local population; WHO estimates indicate a prevalence in the millions worldwide (World Health Organization [WHO], 2004; WHO et al., 2007).

Category	Etiology	Mechanism	Note
Thyroid Failure	Developmental Anomaly	Dysgenesis	98% unknown; others associated genetic mutation: TTF, NKX2.1, NKX2.5, PAX-8
	Impaired production	Mutations on TH synthesis	NIS**, Peroxidase (DUOX2, DUOXA2), Pendred syndrome, Tg, Iodotyrosine deiodinase (DEHAL1, SECISBP2)
	TSH Binding	Receptor defect	
	TSH Signaling	G-protein	
Secondary Hypothyroidism	TSH Recetor	TSH β	
	TRH	Synthetic defect	PSIS**, Hypothalamic lesion
		Resistance	Receptor mutation
	Pituitary development/ function	Deficient transcription factors	HESX1, LHX3, LhX4, PIT1, PROP1 gene mutations
Peripheral Tissue	TH resistance	TSH β	
	Transporter	Abnormal TH transporter	MCT8 mutation
Transient	Antithyroid medication	Maternal Hyperthyroidism	
	Antibodies	Autoimmune	TSHR blocking antibody
	Iodine	Excess or deficient	Endemic goiter, a major world health problem
	Hepatic Hemangioma	Excess TH degradation	Type III deiodinase
Associate with other Abnormalities	Cleft palate		TTF-2 mutation
	Respiratory distress, Benign Chorea	Choreoathetosis	NKX2.1/TTF-1 mutation

** NIS: Sodium-iodide symporter; ** PSIS: pituitary stalk interruption syndrome

Table 1. Causes of Congenital Hypothyroidism

Concerns regarding fetal hypothyroidism and timely treatment warrant close monitoring of fetal thyroid status. One method, cordocentesis, is invasive and has a fetal loss rate of 0.5 to 1% (Daffos, 1989). Recently, ultrasonography has been utilized to assess the fetal thyroid gland (Harris & Pass, 2007; Polak & Van Vliet, 2010; Luton et al., 2005; Abuhamad et al., 1995; Ribault et al., 2009). Cordocentesis and serial ultrasonographic measurements are either invasive or laborious. The development of a convenient non-invasive means to monitor fetal thyroid function is definitely needed.

3. Alternate pathways of Iodothyronines

The alternate pathways of thyroid hormone metabolism include conjugation (sulfation or sulfonation, and glucuronidation of the phenolic hydroxy group) and, to a lesser extent, oxidative deamination of the alanine side-chain leading to the formation of the corresponding iodothyroacetates and ether link cleavage (Fig. 1; Wu et al., 2005).

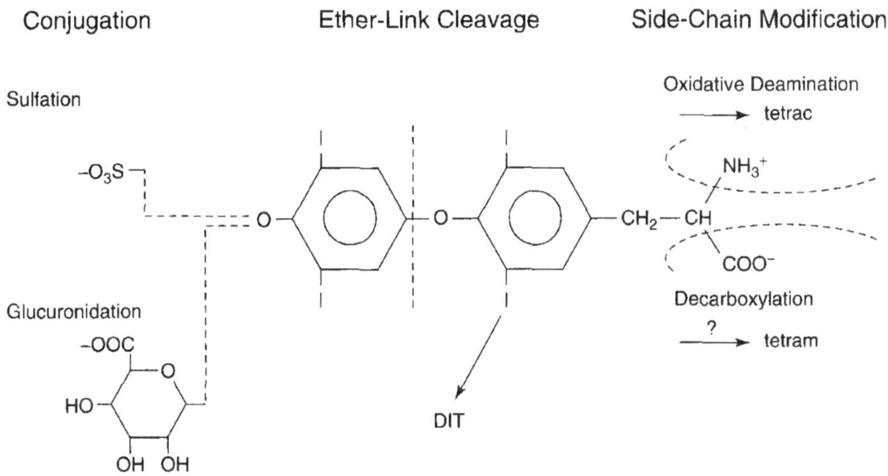

Fig. 1. Alternate pathways of thyroid hormone metabolism. The alternate pathways of thyroid hormone metabolism include conjugation (sulfation or sulfonation, and glucuronidation) and oxidative deamination of the alanine side-chain leading to the formation of the corresponding iodothyroacetates and ether link cleavage. DIT: diiodotyrosine; tetrac: tetraiodothyroacetic acid; tetram: tetraiodothyronamine.

Alternate pathways may serve as mechanisms for further regulation of the bioavailabilities of thyroid hormones in tissues, in addition to deiodination in various physiological and pathophysiological states. Sulfoconjugation of iodothyronines, for example, is an important pathway in developing mammals (Wu et al., 2005); and sulfated iodothyronines can also be deiodinated, even at a faster rate. Likewise, iodothyroacetates can be sulfated and further deiodinated. Iodothyronine glucuronides are rapidly excreted in the bile. Furthermore, sulfoconjugation and glucuronidation are not irreversible pathways for thyroid hormone metabolism. Glucuronides can be hydrolyzed in the intestine and reabsorbed, and sulfoconjugates can be desulfated in selective tissues, e.g. liver and brain, and become available to nuclear receptors, especially in fetuses where type I deiodinase (D1) activity is low. The *in vivo* occurrence of the decarboxylated metabolites of T_4 and T_3, 3,3′,5,5′-

tetraiodothyronamine (T_4AM), and 3,3'5-triiodothyronamine (T_3AM) have not been demonstrated (Leonard & Kohrle, 2000). However, recently, 3-monoiodothyronamine (3-monoam or 3-T_1AM) and thyronamine (T_0AM) have been identified in brain and other tissues in rodents (Scanlan et al., 2004); monoam was found to have rapid effect on reducing rectal temperature in mice and is a potent agonist of the G protein-coupled trace amine receptor TAR1 (Scanlan, 2009). A single dose of T_1AM administered to rodents induces a hypometabolic state that in certain ways resembles hibernation. Monoam may be derived from low iodinated iodothyronines by aromatic amino acid decarboxylase (Fig. 1 & 2), however, its role in developing mammals is not known.

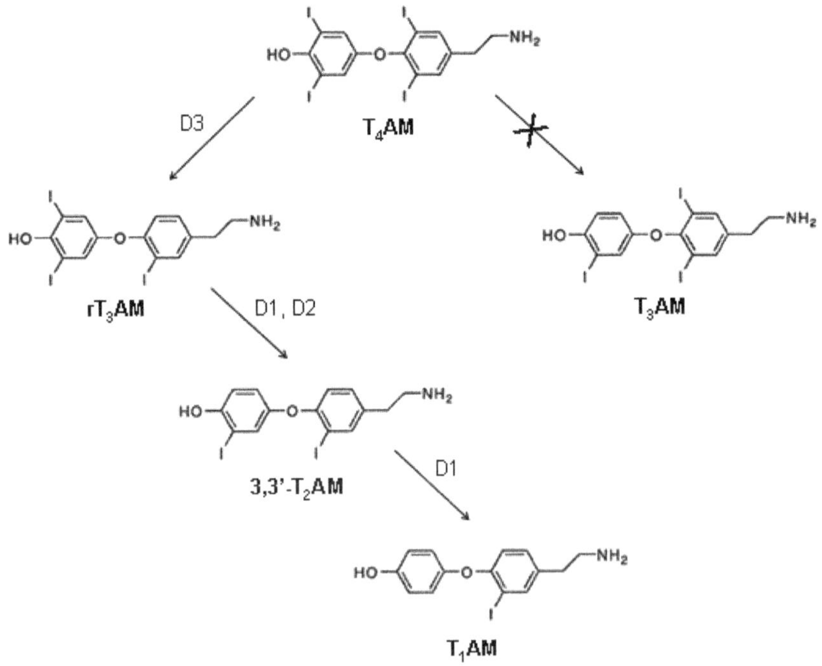

Fig. 2. Postulated T_1 AM (monoam) formation. T_4AM is not a substrate for type I or II deiodinase (D1 or D2) and cannot be deiodinated to T_3AM. However, T_4AM is readily deiodinated to rT_3AM by D3, and rT_3AM can be further deiodinated to ultimately provide T_1AM. This suggests a unique biosynthetic deiodination pathway for T_1AM starting from the decarboxylation products of either T_4 or rT_3.

4. Sulfoconjugation of Iodothyronines

Sulfoconjuation has been found to be a major pathway for thyroid hormone metabolism in mammalian fetuses (Fig. 1; Burrow et al., 1994; Wu et al., 2005; Simpson et al., 2005). The sulfation of thyroxine (T_4) and triiodothyronine (T_3) and their metabolites [reverse T_3 (rT_3) and 3,3'- diiodothyronine (T_2)] may accelerate their further degradation and excretion. The sulfation of T_4 completely blocks the outer-ring deiodination to T_3S. In addition, sulfated iodothyronines may serve as a reservoir for biologically active hormones such as T_3, which can be recovered from T_3S by sulfatases in selective tissues (Wu et al., 2005).

By far, T_2 is the preferred substrate for various mammalian sulfotransferases (SULTs). The purpose of rapid sulfation of T_2, as well as rT_3 in some tissues studied, is unknown. It is interesting that T_2 has been found to stimulate mitochondrial respiration in various rat tissues (Moreno et al., 1997) and rT_3 may play a role in regulating actin polymerization in brain cells (Leonard & Farwell, 1997). Also, sulfated T_2 is the preferred substrate for both human and rat arylsulfatase (ARS) in the microsomal fraction of liver and placenta (Wu et al., 2005). Thus, the possibility that these T_4 metabolites may play a physiological role in developing animals cannot be excluded.

5. Sulfoconjugation of Iodothyronines and their placental transfer in sheep

Before the onset of active synthesis and release of TH, iodothyronines detected in the fetus clearly are maternal in origin. This period is approximately the first 17 gestational days (d) in rats, 50d in sheep (Fig. 3) and 90d in humans.

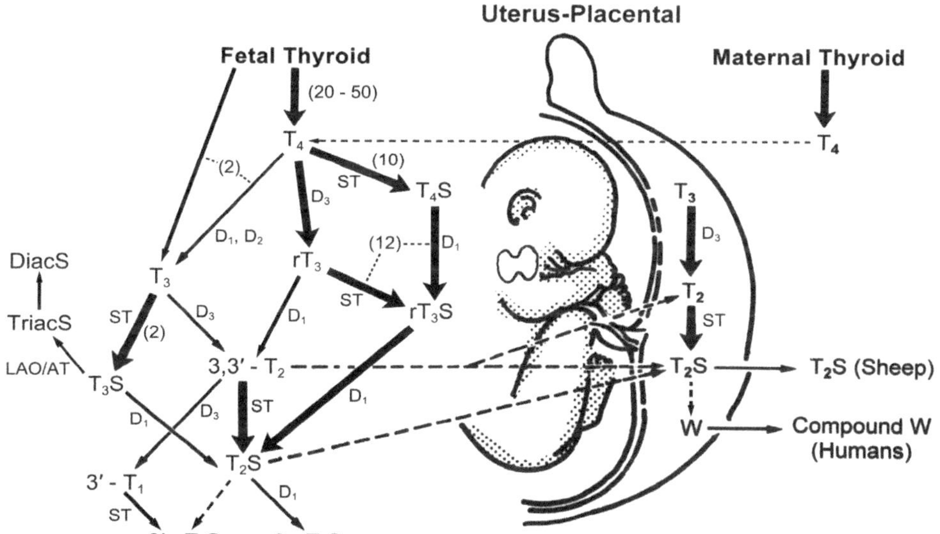

Fig. 3. Postulated metabolic pathways for ovine fetal thyroid hormones. D1, D2, and D3: type I, type II, and type III iodothyronine deiodinases; ST: iodothyronine sulfotransferases (SULT). LAO/AT: L-amino acid oxidase/aminotransferase; DiacS: sulfated 3,3'-diiodothyroacetic acid. Heavy solid lines indicate pathways that are more active in fetuses than in adults; thin solid lines, pathways that are less active in fetuses. The upper horizontal light dotted line depicts T_4 of maternal origin moving to the fetal compartment in the first trimester, before the fetal thyroid begins functioning. Other broken lines represent unconfirmed pathways. Numbers in parentheses indicate published production rates (μg/kg/d).

The proposed scheme for ovine fetal iodothyronine metabolism in late gestation (near term) depicts the production rates for sulfoconjugated thyroid hormone analogs (shown as numbers in parentheses along the thick arrows in Fig. 3). The high production rate (ug/kg/d) of T_4 sulfate (T_4S) reflects the activity of the sulfation pathway. The rT_3S production rate likely represents both sulfation of rT_3 and inner-ring deiodination of T_4S. This scheme shown in Fig. 3 also predicts 3,3'-T_2S is a major thyroid hormone metabolite in the fetus.

The transfer of TH and their metabolites may be a two-way street. We have shown high concentrations of sulfated iodothyronine analogs in human and ovine fetal serum. These include T_4S, T_3S, rT_3S, and 3,3'-T_2S (T_2S) (Wu et al., 2005). The high gradient between fetal and maternal serum concentrations of iodothyronine sulfates raises the possibility that there may be significant fetal to maternal transfer of iodothyronine sulfoconjugates. When the ovine fetus was infused with pharmacological amounts (0.46 μmoles) of T_3 or T_3S, significant fetal to maternal transfer of T_2S and T_3S occurred (Wu et al., 1995; Wu et al., 1999; Wu et al., 2006). It is noteworthy that significantly more T_3S than T_2S of fetal origin was recovered in maternal urine following the fetal infusion of either T_3 or T_3S.

Furthermore, maternal T_2S and T_3S levels were significantly higher after fetal T_3 than after T_3S infusion despite the fact that the mean fetal serum concentration of T_3S after fetal T_3S infusion was 20 times higher than following T_3 infusion (Wu et al., 1995). On the other hand, after fetal infusion of ^{125}I-T_3, without disturbing the fetal stable T_3 pool, a mean of 19% of infused radioactive dose was recovered in maternal urine in 4 h. T_2S, not T_3S, was identified as the major radioactive iodothyronine in fetal to maternal transfer; only minimal amounts of T_3S or T_3, were found (Wu et al., 2006).

We also assessed the contribution of fetal TH to the urinary T_2S and T_3S pool in ewes. Maternal urinary T_2S excretion (pmol/g creatinine) is significantly reduced by fetal thyroidectomy (Tx) but not by maternal Tx (Wu et al., 2001). Maternal urinary T_2S excretion correlated positively with fetal serum T_4 concentrations but not with maternal serum T_3 or T_4 levels (Wu et al., 2001). In view of a possible functional role of T_2 to stimulate mitochondrial respiration, the removal of T_2 from fetal compartment may be necessary for normal maturation of mammalian fetuses (Wu et al., 2005). Furthermore, recent study showed that ARSC, the only sulfatase that hydrolyzes iodothyronine sulfates, has a substrate preference for T_2 (Kester et al., 2002), which raises the possibility that T_2S could be readily reversed back to its precursor, an active iodothyronine. This would suggest a need for the fetus to remove T_2S from fetal compartment. Furthermore, in the sheep model, T_2S of fetal origin contributes significantly to maternal urinary T_2S excretion and may reflect fetal iodothyronine production.

6. The Evaluation a T_2S-crossreactive material (compound w) as a potential marker for fetal thyroid function

In humans, we found high levels of radioimmunoassayable T_2S in maternal serum (Wu et al., 1994) and urine (Wu et al., 1998). Levels increased with the progression of pregnancy and peaked before parturition. At delivery, a 20-fold increase in serum "T_2S" was found compared to non-pregnant women and "T_2S" levels returned to non-pregnant values in 7 to 10 days (Fig. 4 & 5). On closer examination, the radioimmunoassayable "T_2S" did not cochromatograph with synthetic T_2S by HPLC (Wu et al., 1994). The authentic T_2S was hydrolyzed by hot-acid digestion (Wu et al., 1994). Using this procedure, the recovery of T_2S-crossreactive material was near 82% in fetal and maternal serum (Fig. 6; Wu et al., 2007).

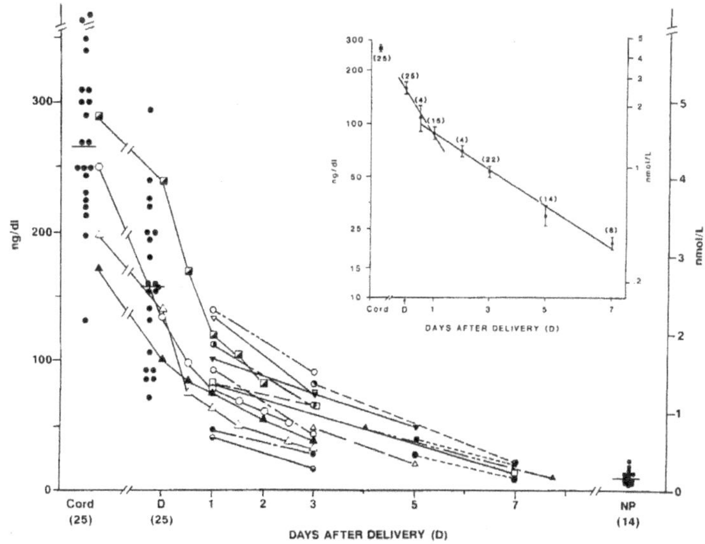

Fig. 4. Change of serum concentrations of compound W in cord and maternal serum. Compound W, expressed as ng/dl of T_2S, in newborns and maternal serum samples at the time of delivery (D). The connected lines represent serial measurements in the same patients (n = 18). T_2S concentrations also were measured in 14 nonpregnant women (NP) for comparison. The decrease in serum compound W concentrations after parturition is depicted in the semilog plot in the inset. The closed circles and vertical bars represent the mean ± SEM and (n) represents the total number of samples studied at each time period in a total of 35 patients.

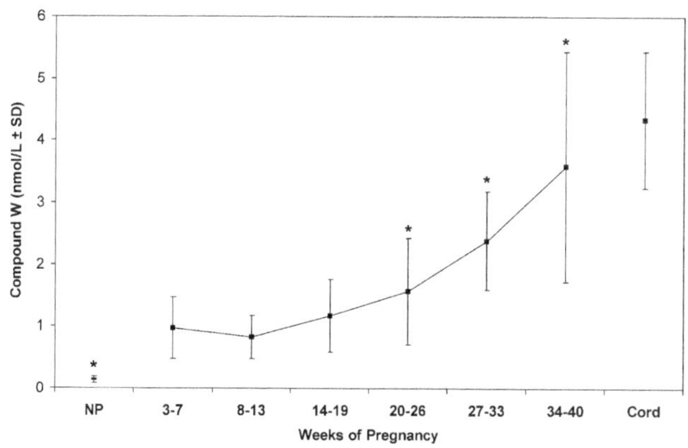

Fig. 5. Changes of compound W at different gestation periods. Normal values of T_2S-crossreactive material (compound W) in serum from pregnant women, nonpregnant women (NP), and newborns. Vertical bars are mean ± 1 SD. * $p < 0.05$ cf. 3-7 weeks pregnancy.

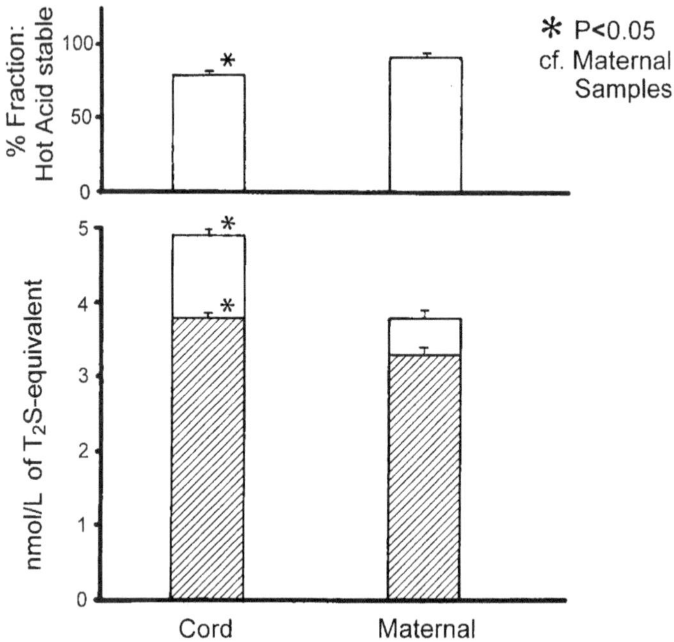

Fig. 6. Recovery of T_2S-crossreactive material following hot-acid treatment. Top: Percent of T_2S-crossreactive fraction that is hot-acid stable in cord (n = 6) and maternal (n = 12) serum samples.

The maternal and paired cord serum concentrations of T_2S-reactive material presented were adjusted by this percentage to obtain the hot-acid-resistant T_2S-equivalent activity, or the "corrected" value. Over 40 known synthetic thyroid hormone analogs were examined and none was found to be identical to the T_2S-like material in pregnant women's serum. Thus, the name Compound W was given. It is postulated that W is a side-chain modification of T_2S, which cross-reacts with T_2S antibody but is slightly more hydrophobic than T_2S. A possible candidate is N, N-dimethylated T_2S (Fig. 7; Wu et al., 2007).

To explore the possible origin of compound W, the serum concentrations of sulfated iodothyronines from cord arterial and venous samples were compared. There were no significant differences between the mean T_3S, T_4S, or rT_3S concentrations of arterial and venous serum samples. However, the venous T_2S-equivalent concentration was higher than arterial in seven of the paired samples and lower in two. The mean "corrected" W concentration in paired arterial/venous cord serum was found to be significantly higher in venous samples than in arterial samples (Wu et al., 2007). In addition, the mean of the maternal serum concentrations of T_2S-reactive material was significantly lower than that of the paired cord serum concentrations. The rapid disappearance of W from maternal serum immediately after delivery supports this hypothesis (Wu et al., 1994). A similar disappearance slope of serum W was also found in newborn infants (Chen et al., 2010). These findings support the postulation that W is produced in the placenta.

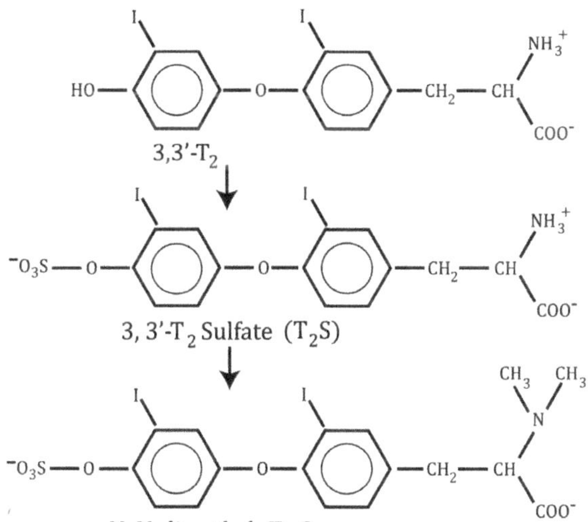

Fig. 7. Postulated pathway converting T_2S to N, N-methyl- T_2S. N, N-methyl- T_2S has the same physico-chemical characteristics on HPLC and reaction to T_2S-specific antibody.

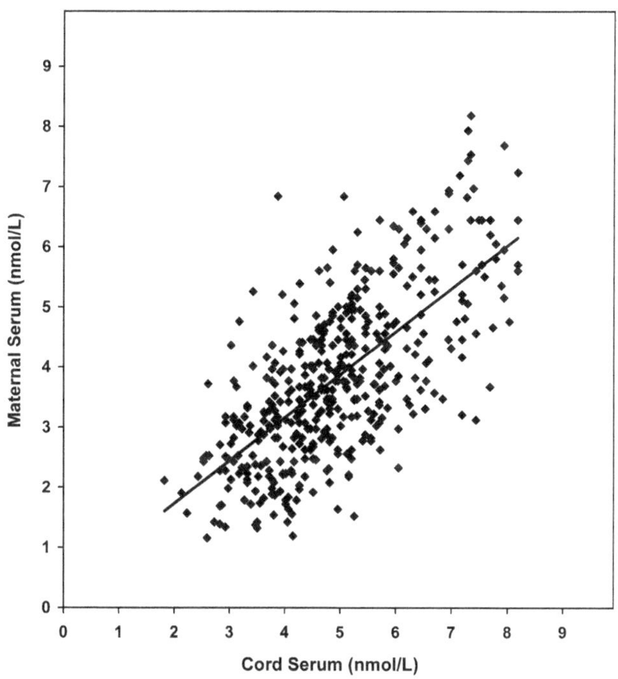

Fig. 8. Levels of T_2S-crossreactive material in paired maternal and cord serum at term. The solid line is the trend-line from lineal regression analysis for the correlation (n = 436, R = 0.686).

Prior studies suggest strongly that compound W is a metabolite of fetal thyroid hormone capable of transplacental fetal to maternal transfer (Wu et al., 2005; Wu et al., 1994; Cortelazzi et al., 1999; Wu et al., 2007). Both maternal and fetal compound W levels increase progressively during gestation with significant direct correlation (in both mothers and fetuses). Additionally, in 436 paired cord and maternal sera obtained at delivery, a highly significant positive correlation was observed between fetal and maternal compound W (Fig. 8). A significant positive correlation was also observed between serum levels of fetal compound W and fetal FT_4 and between maternal and fetal compound W (Fig. 9; Cortelazzi

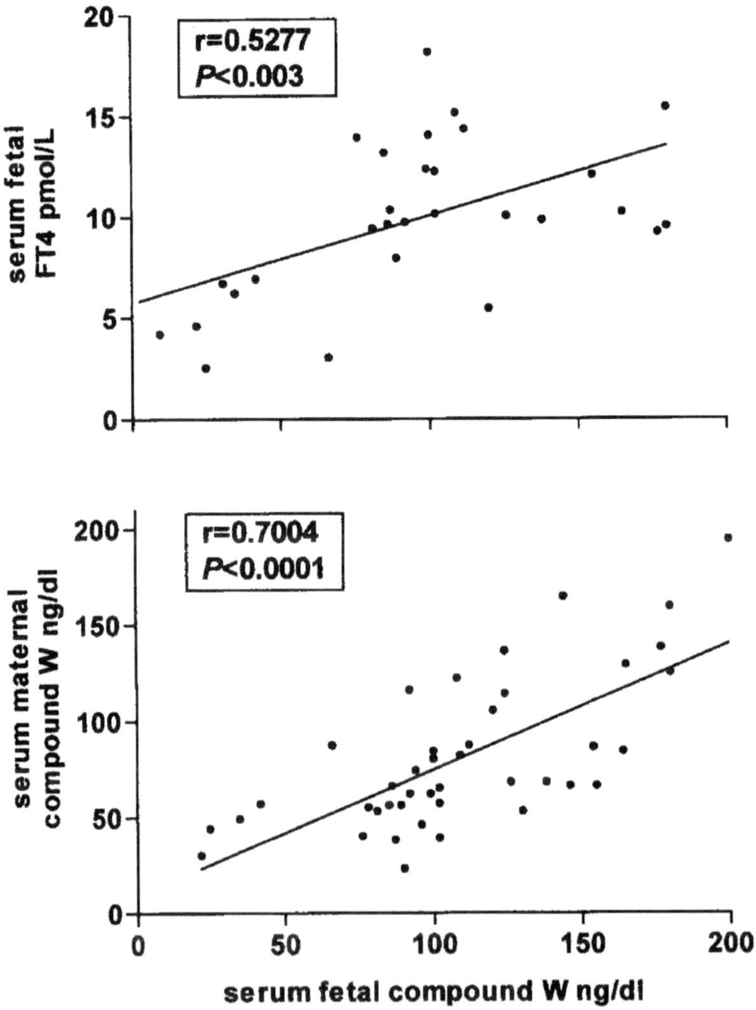

Fig. 9. Compound W levels in fetal serum: correlation with serum fetal FT4 (n=29) and maternal compound W (n=42). [Cortelazzi et al., 1999, reproduced with permission from European J. Endocrinology]

et al., 1999) whereas no correlation was observed between maternal serum compound W and maternal serum FT_4 in euthyroid or hyperthyroid women. Furthermore, maternal compound W levels seem to reflect the effects of drugs on fetal thyroid function (Cortelazzi et al., 1999). In women on propylthiouracil (PTU), maternal compound W levels were in the low normal range and did not show the usual increase with progression of gestation (Cortelazzi et al., 1999). The lack of progression in maternal compound W levels was confirmed in a recent study of 22 pregnant women treated with anti-thyroid medication (Fig. 10; Vanmiddlesworth et al., 2011). A significant increase in maternal compound W was observed when the PTU dose was decreased or discontinued.

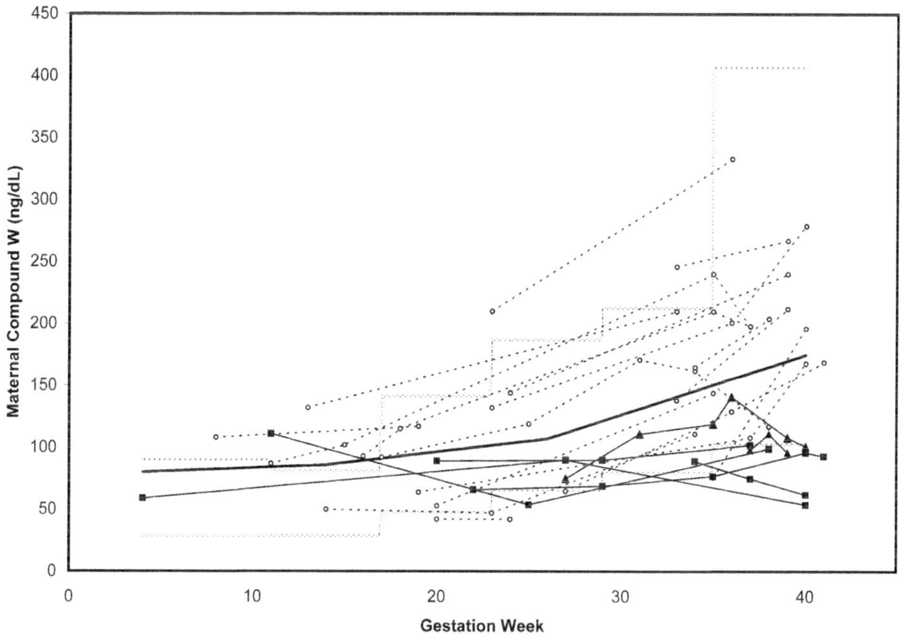

Fig. 10. Courses of compound W in serum of pregnant patients with hyperthyroidism receiving antithyroid therapy. Two or more points on dotted lines mark the course of compound W in each patient, and the thick continuous black line shows the marginal mean course. Thick gray lines represent the 10th (lower) and 90th (upper) percentiles. Square markers on solid lines indicate suppressed or nonprogressive serial measurements in 5 patients; triangular markers on solid lines denote 2 patients who had transient progression and then reduction below the 10th percentile at term.

Cortelazzi, et al. (Cortelazzi et al., 1999) suggest that abnormal thyroid function will be revealed by an absence of the normal rise of compound W during gestation. In comparison with relatively low incidence of congenital hypothyroidism in this population (Rastogi & LaFranchi, 2010; Harris & Pass, 2007), serial measurements of compound W in maternal serum can be considered a safe and practical test for the assessment of fetal thyroid function, particularly in hyperthyroid women treated with anti-thyroid drugs, whose fetuses can become hypothyroid due to the transplacental passage of the drug (Fig. 10; Vanmiddlesworth et al., 2011).

Further study is needed to include compound W levels in a greater number of hyperthyroid pregnant women treated with anti-thyroid medication or pregnant women with evidence of autoimmune thyroid illnesses, followed by long-term follow-up of psychomotor development in these seemingly euthyroid babies. Suppressed W levels may help to define the sub-group of children exposed to PTU in utero or born to mothers with autoimmune disease who have been shown to have an adverse cognitive outcome (Grasberger & Refetoff, 2011; Rovet et al., 1999; Mirabella et al., 2000; Mitchell & Klein, 2004; Casey et al., 2005).

7. Conclusion

Sulfoconjugation is a major metabolic pathway for thyroid hormone in developing mammals. The significant rise of sulfated iodothyronines in mammalian fetal compartments raises the possibility that significant fetal to maternal transfer of the conjugates may occur in late gestation as the fetal hypothalamic-pituitary-thyroid system becomes more mature. This transfer may be a novel mechanism to maintain low T_3 states or regulate serum T_2, a thermogenic hormone that is important for normal tissue maturity. The possibility that the transferred iodothyronine sulfate, especially T_2S and its metabolite, may serve as a marker of fetal thyroid function needs to be further explored.

8. References

Abuhamad, A.Z., Fisher, D.A., Warsof, S.L., et al. 1995. Antenatal diagnosis and treatment of fetal goitrous hypothyroidism: case report and review of the literature. *Ultrasound Obst Gynecol.* 6:368-371.

Burrow, G.N., Fisher, D.A., Larsen, P.R. 1994. Maternal and fetal thyroid function. *N Engl J Med.* 331:1072-1078.

Casey, B.M., Dashe, J.S., Wells, C.E., McIntire, D.D., Byrd, W., Leveno, K.J., Cunningham, F.G. 2005. Subclinical hypothyroidism and pregnancy outcomes. *Obstet Gynecol.* 105:239-245.

Chen, D.Z., Yu, H.Y., Bao, J.D., Xue, W., Fisher, D.A., Wu, S.Y. 2010. 3, 3′-diiodothyronine sulfate cross-reactive material (compound W) in human newborns. 14th International Thyroid Congress, Paris, September 11-16. #1017.

Cortelazzi, D., Morpurgo, P.S., Azmperini, P., Fisher, D.A., Beck-Peccoz, P., Wu, S.Y. 1999. Fetal Hypothyroidism: New diagnostic and therapeutic approaches. *Europ J Endocrinol.* 141:570-578.

Daffos, F. 1989. Fetal blood sampling. *Ann Rev Med.* 40:319-329.

Engler, D., Burger, A.G. 1984. The deiodination of the iodothyroninesand of their derivatives in man. *Endocr Rev.* 5:151–184.

Grasberger, H., Refetoff, S. 2011. Genetic causes of congenital hypothyroidism due to dyshormononogenesis. *Current Opin Pediat.* 23:421-428.

Haddow, J.E., Palomaki, G.E., Allan, W.C., Williams, J.R., Knight, G.J., Gagnon, J., O'Heir, C.E., Mitchell, M.L., Hermos, R.J., Waisbren, S.E., Faix, J.D., Klein, R.Z. 1999. Maternal thyroid deficiency during pregnancy and subsequent neuropsychological development of the child. *N Engl J Med.* 341:549-555.

Harakawa, S., Akazawa, S., Akazawa, M., Hashimoto, M., Yamashita, S., Izumi, M., Nagataki, S. 1989. Changes of serum thyroid hormone levels induce malformations on early embryogenesis in rats. *Acta Endocrinol.* 121:739-743

Harris, K.B., Pass, K.A. . 2007. Increase in congenital hypothyroidism in New York State and in the United States. *Mol Genet Metab.* 91(3):268–277.

Kester, M.H., Kaptein, E., van Dijk, C.H., Roest, T.J., Tibboel, D., Coughtrie, M.W., Visser, T.J. 2002. Characterization of iodothyronine sulfatase activities in human and rat liver and placenta. *Endocrinology.* 143:814-819.

Leger, J., Ecosse, E., Roussey, M., Lanoe, J.L., Larroque, B., and the French Hypothyroidism Study Group. 2011. Subtle health impairment and socioeducational attainment in young adult patients with congenital hypothyroidism diagnosed by neonatal screening: a longitudinal population-based cohort study. *J Clin Endocrinol Metab.* 96:1771-1782.

Leonard, J.L., Farwell, A. 1997. Thyroid hormone-regulated actin polymerization in brain. *Thyroid.* 7:147-151.

Leonard, J.L., Kohrle, J. 2000. Intracellular pathways of iodothyronine metabolism, In: Bravermen, L.E., Utiger, R.D. (eds), Werner and Ingbars, *The Thyroid: A Fundamental and Clinical Text*, 8th ed. JB Lippincott, New York, pp. 136–173.

Luton, D., Le Gac, I., Vuillard, E., et al. 2005. Management of Graves' disease during pregnancy: the key role of fetal thyroid gland monitoring. *J Clin Endocrinol Metab.* 90:6093-6098.

Mirabella, G., Feig, D., Astzalos, E., Perlman, K., Rovet, J.F. 2000. The effect of abnormal intrauterine thyroid hormone economies on infant cognitive abilities. *J Pediatr Endocrinol Metab.* 13:191-194.

Mitchell, M.L., Klein, R.Z. 2004. The sequelae of untreated maternal hypothyroidism. *Eur J Endocrinol.* 151 Suppl 3:U45-U48.

Moreno, M., Lanni, A., Lombardi, A., Goglia, F. 1997. How the thyroid controls metabolism in the rat: different roles for triiodothyronine and diiodothyronines. *J Physiol.* 505:529-538.

Morreale de Escobar, G., Obregon, M.J., Escobar del Rey, F. 2004. Role of thyroid hormone during early brain development. *Eur J Endocrinol.* 151:U25-U37.

Nunez, J., Couchie, D., Aniello, F., Bridoux, A.M. 1992. Thyroid hormone effects on neuronal differentiation during brain development. *Acta Medica Austriaca.* 19:36-39.

Pasquini, J.M., Adamo, A.M. 1994. Thyroid hormones and the central nervous system. *Develop Neurosci.* 16:1-8.

Polak, M., Van Vliet, G. 2010. Therapeutic approach of fetal thyroid disorder. *Hormone Research in Paediatrics.* 74:1-5.

Rastogi, M.V., LaFranchi, S.H. 2010. Congenital hypothyroidism, *Orphanet J Rare Dis.* 5:17.

Ribault, V., Castanet, M., Bertrand, A-M. et al. 2009. Experience with intraamniotic thyroxine treatment in nonimmune fetal goitrous hypothyroidism in 12 cases. *J Clin Endocrinol Metab.* 94:3731-3739.

Rovet, J., Mirabella, G., Arsenault, P., Myszak, M., Feig, D., Kelly, C. 1999. The effect of PTU exposure during pregnancy on infant cognitive development. A prospective study, Program of 72nd Annual Meeting of the Am Thyroid Assoc, Palm Beach, FL p. 33. (Abstract)

Scanlan, T.S., Suchland, K.L., Hart, M.E., Chiellini, G., Huang, Y., Kruzich, P.J., Frascarelli, S., Crossley, II D.A., Bunzow, J.R., Ronca-Testoni, S., Lin, E.T., Hatton, D., Zucchi, R., Grandy, D.K. 2004. 3-Iodothyronamine is an endogenous and rapid-acting derivative of thyroid hormone. *Nat Med.* 10:638–642.

Scanlan, T.S. 2009. 3-iodothyronamine (T1AM): A new player on the thyroid endocrine team? *Endocrinology* 150:1108-1111.

Simpson, J., Williams, F.L., Delahunty, C., van Toor, H., Wu, S.Y., Ogston, S.A., Visser, T.J., Hume, R. 2005. Scottish Preterm Thyroid Group Serum thyroid hormones in preterm infants and relationships to indices of severity of intercurrent illness. *J Clin Endocrinol Metab.* 90:1271-1279.

Vanmiddlesworth, L., Vanmiddlesworth, N.R., Egerman, R.S., Bush, A.J., Ramsey, R.D., Delmar, L.P., Ho, E.C., Wu, S.Y. 2011. Thyroid function and 3,3'-diiodothyronine sulfate cross-reactive substance (compound w) in maternal hyperthyroidism with antithyroid treatment. *Endocrine Pract.* 17:170-176.

WHO (ed.): Iodine status worldwide: WHO Global Database on Iodine Deficiency. Geneva: World Health Organization, 2004.

WHO, UNICEF, ICCIDD: Assessment of iodine deficiency disorders and monitoring their elimination: a guide for programme managers. Geneva: World Health Organization, 2007.

Wu, S.Y., Fisher, D.A., Huang, W.S., Kuo, S.W., Chen, W.L. 1998. The changes of urinary compound W concentrations in pregnant women. *Am J Obst-Gynecol.* 178:886-91.

Wu, S.Y., Green, W.L., Huang, W.S., Hays, M.T., Chopra, I. J. 2005. Alternate pathways of thyroid hormone metabolism. *Thyroid.* 15:945-960.

Wu, S.Y., Huang, W.S., Fisher, D.A. Florsheim W.H., Kashiwai K., Polk D.H. 2001. 3, 3'-diiodothyronine sulfate excretion in maternal urine reflects fetal thyroid function in sheep. *Pediat Res.* 50:358-364.

Wu, S.Y., Huang, W.S., Ho, E., Wu, E.S.C., Fisher, D.A. 2007. A 3,3'-diiodothyronine sulfate cross-reactive substance, compound W, in serum from pregnant women – a potential marker for fetal thyroid function. *Pediatr Res.* 61:307-312.

Wu, S.Y., Polk, D.H., Chen, W.L., Fisher, D.A., Huang, W.S., Yee, B. 1994. A 3, 3' – diiodothyronine-sulfate cross-reactive compound in serum from pregnant women. *J Clin Endocrinol Metab.* 78:1505-1509.

Wu, S.Y., Polk, D.H., Fisher, D.A., Huang, W.S., Reviczky, A., Chen, W.L. 1995. Identification of 3, 3' - T_2S as a fetal thyroid hormone derivative in maternal urine in sheep. *Am J Physiol.* 268 (Endocrinol Metab 31):E33-E39.

Wu, S.Y., Polk, D.H., Huang, W.S., Fisher, D.A. 1999. Fetal-to-maternal transfer of 3, 3', 5 - triiodothyronine sulfate and its metabolites in sheep. *Am J Physiol.* 268 (Endocrinol Metab 40):E915–E919.

Wu, S.Y., Polk, D.H., Huang, W.S., Green, W.L., Thai, B., Fisher, D.A. 2006. Fetal-to-maternal transfer of thyroid hormone metabolites in late gestation in sheep. *Pediatr Res.* 59: 102-106.

17

Structure and Function of the Circulatory System in Hypothyroid Patients

Jacek Drobnik
Laboratory of Connective Tissue Metabolism Department of General and Experimental Pathology Medical University of Lodz, Poland

1. Introduction

Hypothyroidism, thyroid gland hormone deficiency, is quite a common disease, affecting more women than men. Patients with an elevated risk of hypothyroidism comprise postpartum women, patients affected with autoimmune diseases as well as patients with autoimmune family history, primary pulmonary hypertension, Down's and Turner's syndromes. The main causes of congenital hypothyroidism are endemic iodine deficiency, agenesis or dysgenesis of the thyroid gland and impaired synthesis of the thyroid hormones. The causes of the primary hypothyroidism are autoimmune thyroiditis, injury by surgery, irradiation or drug side effects. Secondary hypothyroidism is caused by pituitary adenomas, adenoma treatment by surgery or radiotherapy, tumors of the suprasellar region, sarcoidosis or hemochromatosis.

Hypothyroid patients complain of cold intolerance, weight gain, constipation, dry skin, bradycardia, hoarseness and dementia (Roberts & Ladenson, 2004). However, thyroid hypofunction, and a consequent lower level of thyroid hormones in the blood, has also been observed in heart disease patients. In patients with acute myocardial infarction, both total and free levels of triiodotyronine were seen to be lower. Moreover, a transient decrease of tyroxine has been observed while the level of TSH was unchanged (Franklyn et al., 1984). Similar data was obtained on children who had undergone open heart surgery. In this case, decreased levels of free and total triiodothyronine, total thyroxine and TSH were observed; all of which, except TSH, remained depressed until the 5th to 8th days after surgery. These results support the statement that the pituitary-thyroid axis is suppressed in patients with open heart surgery (Mainwaring et al., 1994). According to the above data, a vicious circle is postulated (Klein & Ojaama, 2001; a); heart disease induces suppression of the thyroid gland function, which in turn, may influence the structure and function of the heart.

The heart is composed of several cell types: cardiomyocytes, fibroblasts / myofibroblasts, endothelial cells and smooth muscle cells of the blood vessels. Cardiomiocytes comprise more than 50% of the volume of the organ and exhibit contractile properties. Cardiac fibroblasts comprise as much as 67% of the cells in the heart of rats. The fibroblasts are responsible for the synthesis and catabolism of the extracellular matrix (collagen type I and III, elastin and laminin), influence the electrophysiological properties of cardiomyocytes as well as regulate myocyte growth and blood vessel formation in the heart (Krenning et al., 2010).

The cardiovascular system remains under the regulatory influence of thyroid hormones. Since dysfunction of the thyroid gland results in complex changes within the heart, the structure and function of the heart is disturbed in both hypothyroidism and hyperthyroidism. Hypothyroidism affects the electrophysiological, contractile and hemodynamic functions of the heart and is associated with disturbances of the heart's connective tissue stroma.

The effects of thyroid hormones on the circulatory system have both genomic and non-genomic bases. T_3, triiodothyronine (3, 5, 3'-triiodo-L-thyronine), the active thyroid hormone, is transported to the cardiomyocyte by a specific protein situated in the cell membrane (Everts et al. 1996) where it is then moved to the nucleus and bound by thyroid nuclear receptors: two α isoforms (TRα1, TRα2) and three β isoforms (TRβ1-TRβ3). Of these isoforms, TRα1 and TRβ1 bind 40% of the T_3 each, and the remaining 20% is bound by the TRβ2 receptor; TRα2 is unable to bind triiodothyronine. (Schwartz et.al., 1994; Kahaly & Dilmann, 2005). The receptor-hormone complex is bound to thyroid responsive elements (TRE) and, acting as gene regulator, may influence target gene expression (Brent et al., 1994). Several genes are upregulated by T_3: the α isoform of myosin heavy chains (Morkin et al., 1993), calcium activated ATPase (Dillman et al., 1990), β1 adrenergic receptor (Fazio et al.2004). The expression of other genes is inhibited by T_3: β isoform of myosin heavy chains or phospholamban (Fazio et al. 2004).

2. Electrophysiological function of heart

T_3 has been demonstrated to have a general regulatory effect on heart rate; bradycardia, a typical symptom of the patient with hypothyroidism, is related to a lowered level of triiodothyronine (T_3). In an isolated rat atrial neonatal myocyte model, T_3 was shown to increase the pacemaker rate mainly by elevation of the slope of spontaneous depolarization. Several ionic currents that may determine the pacemaker activity were considered as potential targets for the action of the thyroid hormones. The electrogenic Na^+-Ca^{2+} exchange current ($I_{Na/Ca}$) density was influenced by T_3 application. Thus, $I_{Na/Ca}$ alterations by thyroid hormone may change the slope of the spontaneous depolarization and modify the pacemaker rate (Sun et al., 2001).

The I_f current is defined as the current determining spontaneous diastolic depolarization and influence the activity of the heart pacemaker (Er et al, 2003). In vertebrates, proteins deriving from HCN genes form pores of the I_f current; three HCN isoforms have been found in the human heart : HCN1, HCN2 and HCN4. The experiments performed on neonatal rat ventricular cardiac myocytes showed that triiodothyronine (T_3) evoked a positive chronotropic effect on spontaneously beating myocytes. In myocytes with overexpression of the thyroid hormone receptor TRα1, increased beating activity linked with accelerated depolarization velocity and shortened action potential duration, as well as increased I_f current density and increased HCN2 and HCN4 transcripts and proteins were observed. The effect of thyroid hormones on CHN2 subunit expression is thought to be responsible for a positive chronotropic effect. The changes in both HCN2 and HCN4 gene expression seem not to be influenced by direct binding of thyroid hormone to the TREs in the promoter region of the two genes. On the other hand, in cells with TRβ1 overexpression, lower beating activities, inhibition of phase 4 depolarization and prolongation of the action potential were found. Reduced transcription of HCN4 was also obseved (Gassanow et al., 2009). Thus, the thyroid hormones would apper to be involved in regulation of the heart rate, and their low level could be responsible for bradycardia development.

In patients affected by hypothyroidism, atrioventricular blocks are rarely described. A complete atrioventricular block has been observed in a patient with severe hypothyroidism, complaining of bradycardia (15 beats/min), fatigue, dizziness and syncope (Schoenmakers et al. 2008). In another patient, bradycardia (44 beats/min) was caused by a 2:1 atrioventricular block with subclinical hypothyroidism (Nakayama et al., 2006). The blocks in two described patients were resolved after thyroxin supplementation. The functional blocks have been diagnosed.

Apart from bradycardia, the typical electrocardiographical changes in hypothyroid patients comprise prolongation of the PQ interval, reduced QRS complex voltage, elongation of the QT interval and flattening or inversion of the T wave. An acquired elongation of QT with a tendency toward ventricular arrhythmias has also been shown in many patients affected with hypothyroidism. The QT interval (Fig. 1) is the marker of ventricle repolarization. Prolongation of the QT is usually caused by prolongation of the action potential due to a reduction of repolarizing currents or elevation of the inward current (Antzelvitch, 2004). In patients with overt primary hypothyroidism, Galetta and coworkers (2008) highlighted the prolongation and increased dispersion of the QT interval, partial reduction of which was seen after replacement therapy. In addition, the reduction of heart rate variability parameters seen in the study suggests a sympato-vagal imbalance in hypothyroid patients. An increase of QT interval dispersion was also found in women with subclinical hypothyroidism. The differences of QTc (- QT dispersion corrected for heart rate) were normalized when TSH level (>10mIU/l) was lowered (Bakiner et al., 2008). The cardiomyocytes isolated from hypothyroid rats are characterized by a very long action potential duration compared with euthyroid cardiomyocytes, however application of T_3 reduces their action potential duration by 24% (Sun et al., 2000). The mechanism of QT prolongation in the hypothyroid subjects is not very well explained. However, prolongation of ventricular repolarisation is thought to be due to fibrous tissue accumulation in the heart and swelling due to excessive deposition of the osmotic compounds in the heart wall (Galetta et al., 2008).

Sun et al. (2000) postulate that both the genomic and non-genomic effects of the thyroid hormone (T_3) could be involved in the prolongation of action potential in the ventricular myocytes of hypothyroid rats. The genomic effects are involved with modulation of T_3-specific cardiac gene expression. I_{to} transient outward current density (Fig. 1) was decreased in the ventricular cardiomyocytes of hypothyroid rats compared to euthyroid cardiomyocytes; this effect is connected with reduced expression of KCND2 genes, which encode proteins of the voltage-dependent K^+ channel Kv4.2 (Nishiyama et al., 1998). The Kv4.2 and Kv4.3 gene products are molecular components determining the I_{to} current. I_{to} current is responsible for early repolarisation (phase 1) of action potential and is composed of the rapid form $I_{to,f}$ and slower form reffered as $I_{to,s}$. Le Bouter and coworkers (2003) found reduced transcription of several genes (KCNA5, KCNB1, KCND2 KCNK2) in hypothyroid mice while the expression of other genes was upregulated (KCNQ1, KCNE1); these genes encode the proteins of the voltage-gated K^+ channel proteins. The results were confirmed on the protein level and were linked with reductions of $I_{to,f}$ and delayed rectifying K^+ current (I_{kslow}) densities and elevation of slowly activating delayed rectifier (I_{ks}) density in cardiomyocytes isolated from hypothyroid mice. The thyroid hormone is thought to regulate the components of I_{to} on the transcriptional level (Shimoni & Severson, 1995). The reduction of I_{to} density could be partially responsible for prolongation of the action potential and QT interval elongation (Sun et al., 2000).

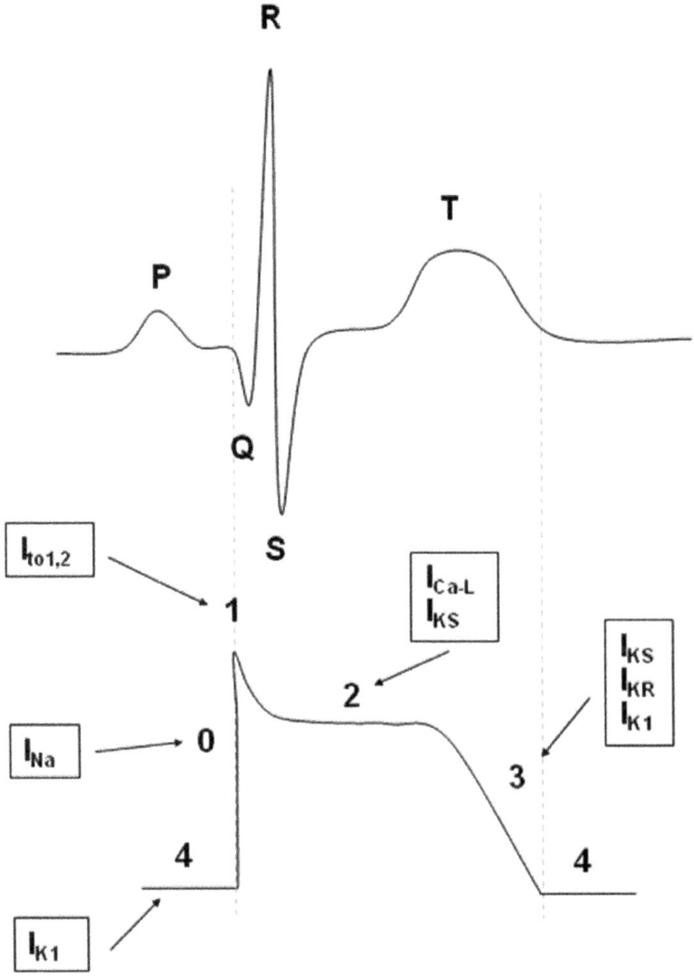

Fig. 1. The action potential of the cardiomyocyte (lower part) and surface electrocardiogram (upper part). The cardiomyocyte action potential is consisted of phases 0-4 and is generated by following currents: I_{Na} sodium current, I_{to} transient outward K^+ current, $I_{Ca\text{-}L}$ voltage-gated calcium current, I_{Ks} slowly activating delayed rectifier current, I_{Kr} rapidly activating K^+current, I_{K1} inward rectifier K^+ current.

Ionic characteristics however are not rapidly influenced by addition of T_3 to cardiomyocytes isolated from the hypothyroid rats, implying that changes in I_{to} current density are regulated at the transcriptional level (Sun et al., 2000). On the other hand, the rapid effect of T_3 treatment on the I_k current, the effects being seen in only 5-15 min, suggests a non-genomic influence of the thyroid hormone; transcription and translation processes need more time (Sun et al., 2000). Thus, different types of regulation have been noted for I_{to} and I_K (delayed rectifier): transcriptional and non-genomic regulation respectively. Non-genomic regulation was demonstrated also for the sodium channel and the I_{K1} channel: The action potential duration was shortened by T_3 application, which was linked with an increase of whole cell inward rectifier potassium current (I_{K1}; Sakaguchi et al. 1996). Application of T_3 elevated the burst activity of the sodium channel (Dudley & Baumgarten,1993).

A novel genetic link between inherited long QT interval and hypothyroidism has been proposed by Putrell and coworkers (2010). Mutations of the KCNQ1 and KCNE2 genes are related to long QT interval. hERC and KCNQ1, complexed with KCNE β, are the subunits of the voltage-gated potassium channels. They generate repolarisation currents I_{kr} and I_{ks}. I_{ks} is the slowly activated potassium current (generated by KCNQ1,-KCNE1 subunits) and I_{kr} is the rapidly activated potassium channel (generated by hERG-KCNE2 subunits). KCNQ1 mutations reduce ventricular muscle repolarisation capacity and prolong the QT interval. Furthermore, the KCNQ1-KCNE2 channel determines potassium influx to thyreocytes and correct accumulation of iodine ions. A mutation of KCNE could diminish the delivery of iodine ions to the thyreocytes, decreasing the substrate availability for thyroid hormone synthesis. Thus, two concomitant effects of KCNE dysfunction are observed: in the heart prolongation QT and possible arrhythmias, and in the thyroid gland inhibition of thyroid hormone synthesis and hypothyroidism formation. Hypothyroidism is associated by a molecular link with prolongation of QT (Purtell et al. 2010).

Life-threatening ventricular ectopic arrhythmias are rarely seen in hypothyroid patients (Schenck et al. 2006); additional factors triggering sustained or life-threatening ventricular arrhythmias are postulated (Galetta et al., 2008). Very few reports document ventricular arrhythmias in the course of hypothyroidism. The "torsade de pointes' (TdP) tachycardia was revealed in a few cases of women aged from 50 to 78 years affected with hypothyroidism with symptoms of hypometabolic crisis being commonly found. However, although different methods of treatment were applied, the authors stress that systematic therapy with thyroxine caused normalization of the electrocardiogram (Chojnowski et al. 2007, Shojaie & Eshraghian 2008, Schenck et al. 2006).

3. Heart contraction

Hypothyroidism causes a reduction of heart contractility, lowers the speed of myocardial relaxation (Jakab et al. 1994), decreases stroke volume, ventricular feeling and cardiac output. In hypothyroidism, the cardiac output is decreased by 30-50%. Thus, the hypodynamic status of the circulatory system can be diagnosed. In a hypothyroid subject while the expression of α isoform of myosin heavy chains (αMSH), sarcoplasmatic reticulum Ca^{2+} -ATPase (SERCa2) β1-adrenergic receptor genes is reduced due to a lowering of the triiodothyronine level (triiodothyronine is the factor which increases expression of these genes), the expression of β isoform of myosin heavy chains (βMSH) and phospholamban genes is increased.

Both transcript and protein levels of β–MSH (known as slow myosin) are elevated in experimental animals with induced hypothyroidism (Haddad et al., 2003). β–MSH demonstrates low ATPase activity and works more economically (Harris et al., 1994). However, higher ATPase activity with a faster heart myofiber shortening velocity can be found in α-MSH, known as fast myosin (VanBuren et al., 1995). Domination of β–MSH in rodents impairs both diastolic and systolic heart functions. (Dillman et al., 1989, Morkin, 1993). This phenomenon could be seen mainly in laboratory animals because the β–myosin heavy chain isoform comprises 95% of the myosin molecule in human (Gorza et al., 1984) and is not markedly influenced by changes of thyroid hormone level. In a hypothyroid patient with dilated cardiomyopathy, the cardiac output was reduced to 16% and the α-myosin heavy chain mRNA level was found to be low in biopsy samples. After 9-month therapy with thyroid hormone, not only was the cardiac output elevated to 37%, but the level of α-myosin heavy chain mRNA was also increased (Ladenson et al., 1992). Myofibrillar ATPase activity in the heart of thyreoidectomized rats was found to be lower (Dowell et al., 1994)

The β–adrenergic receptors in the heart remain under the positive regulatory influence of the thyroid hormone. In rats with experimentally-induced hypothyroidism, a decreased β-receptor number was found on cell membranes but the agonists' affinity to the receptors was not changed. Isoproterenol-induced activation of adenylate cyclase was reduced (Dowell et al., 1994). Novotny and coworkers (1999) confirmed the reduced number of β-receptors in hypothyroid rats. Moreover, the positive inotropic effect of isoproterenol was reduced. These results were contrasted by Ariogla and coworkers (2009), who noted a reduced effect of isoproterenol and noradrenalin on heart contractility in hypothyroid animals, but saw increased expression of β 2 and β 3 receptors with no change in expression of β 1 receptors.

In animals with hypothyroidism, reduced pressure dvelopment (dP/dt) was linked with decreased phosphorylation of cardiac troponin I (cTnI) in the heart. Moreover, mRNA of cardiac troponin I was increased 3 fold in hearts of hypothyroid rats but mRNA of slow skeletal troponin I was initialy elevated but later was decreased to undedectable level in animals with hypothyroidism. (Averyhart-Fullard et al., 1994).

The reduction of heart contractility due to overt hypothyroidism decreases stroke volume and ejection fraction. In hypothyroid patients, prolongation of the pre-ejection period and decrease of ventricular ejection period were observed, however these values were normalized after replacement therapy (Crowley 1977). Moreover, these phenomena, as well as bradycardia, decreases cardiac output in hypothyroid patients.

The changes of calcium concentration in the heart are regulated by calcium activated ATPase and phospholamban during both systole and diastole periods. Calcium-activated ATPase is responsible for the calcium influx to the endoplasmatic reticulum and, in this way, influences the myocardial relaxation velocity (Dillman et al., 1990, Kiss et al., 1994). Phosholamban was found to inhibit the activity of the calcium-activated ATPase (Kiss et al. 1994). Cardiac contractility was increased in phospholamban-deficient mice and the thyroid hormone treatment was not found to increase myocardium contractility (Kiss et al. 1998). Triodothyronin may determine the relaxation of the heart via regulation of gene expression through upregulation of calcium activated ATPase and downregulation of phospholamban. Thus, in hypothyroidism, the gene for calcium-activated ATPase expression is decreased but phospholamban gene expression is increased, which will affect the systo-diastolic function of the heart (Fazio et al. 2004). Impairment of the diastolic function in hypothyroidism patients by slow myocardial relaxation of the heart results in reduction of ventricular feeling. Furthermore, a decreased rate of active diastolic relaxation has been found in hypothyroid patients (Wieshammer et al., 1989). Echocardiographic studies of hypothyroid patients show the modifications of the acoustic properties and myocardial fiber velocity as well as regional myocardial deformations. Decreased intramyocardial contractility and the impairment of both the active and passive diastole phases have been observed (Di Bello et al., 2009). In women with subclinical hypothyroidism, magnetic resonance imaging revealed decreased end diastolic volume - preload and increased afterload causing impaired cardiac performance (Ripoli et al., 2005).

Exercise intolerance of the hypothyroid rats is related to decreased heart performance and increased total peripheral resistance. Lower blood flow to extensor muscles has been observed as well as reduced vasodilatator potential of isolated blood vessels (McAllister et al., 1995). Cardiac oxygen consumption measured by positron emission tomography is reduced in hypothyroid patients. This reduction is associated with decreased contractility and elevated total peripheral resistance (Bengel et al., 2000). Athea and coworkers (2007) investigated the effect of hypothyroidism on the cardiac energy metabolism. The maximal oxidative capacity of heart tissue was found to be markedly reduced, cytochrome oxidase and citrate synthase were inhibited and mitochondrial cardiolipin content was lower. Cardiolipin influences the activity of many inner membrane proteins and its amount increases in mitochondria with elevated metabolic rates. Utilization of 3 phospho-glycerol, malate and octanoate decreased in hypothyroid animals. Additionally, while the content or activity of creatine kinase is not changed, it was observed to have decreased efficacy in hypothyroid animals, leading to impairment of mitochondrial function. However, the mechanism of these changes remains to be elucidated. Expression of adenine nucleotide transferase is reduced in hypothyroidism. This effect is linked with impairment of mitochondrial permeability (Paradies et al., 1997; Chavez et al., 2008).

4. Connective tissue in the heart

The connective tissue of the heart remains under the regulatory influence of the thyroid hormones. Triiodothyronine increases the intracellular transport of amino acids, sugars and calcium and increases protein synthesis. However, interstitial fibrosis with excessive glycosaminoglycan accumulation was found on histological examination of a hypothyroid heart (Mohr-Kahaly et al. 1996). Additoinally, echocardiography showed changes of the heart structure in hypothyroid patients. The alterations could be the result of excessive accumulation of collagen, water retention or changes of the muscle fiber orientation (Monzani et al., 2001).

Ciulla and coworkers (2004) investigated the collagen content in the heart of hypothyroid patients with echocardiographical studies. The derived collagen volume fraction (dCVF% echocardiographical evaluation of the collagen content in the heart) was evaluated. Higher values of dCFV% were found in hypothyroid hearts, but echoreflectivity was normalized after thyroid hormone treatment. Experiments performed on rats with induced hypothyroidism by thyroidectomy or 4-methyl-2-thiouracil application demonstrated increased accumulation of collagen and glycosaminoglycans in the hearts of two groups with experimental hypothyreosis (Drobnik et al., 2009). Moreover, an increased level of hialuronic acid was found in hypothyroid rats in the heart and the hindlimb muscle (Wiig et al., 2000). An elevated level of hyaluronan was also noted in human fibroblasts cultured in conditions without thyroid hormones (Shishiba et al., 1988).

The mechanism of the observed changes remains a matter of debate. The elevation of the extracellular matrix in the hypothyroid heart is supposed to be related to a low level of thyroid hormones and reduced catabolism of extracellular compounds. Decreased hydroxyproline levels, the marker of collagen, were noticed in the urine and serum of hypothyroid subjects; these changes were normalized by replacement therapy. Additionally, decreased collagen degradation was confirmed in hypothyroid subjects by experiments with radiolabeled proline. Most importantly however, the final effect of the thyroid status would seem to be dependent on the target organ; increased collagen content was noted in both the skin and liver of the hypothyroid animals as well as a decreased collagen level in the bones (Kucharz, 1992). Previous results showed decreased collagen catabolism in hypothyroid animals, and this effect may explain the elevation of collagen level in the heart.

However, in primary hypothyroidism, a low level of the thyroid hormone is accompanied with an elevation of TSH, which is thought to influence the regulation of the connective tissue matrix in the heart. Although an increased number of cells was found in myofibroblast cultures isolated from newborn rat heart after TSH application, the level of collagen or glycosaminoglycans in the culture was unchanged; this elevation of myofibroblast number in TSH-treated cultures raises the question of whether a TSH-dependent effect could be responsible for connective tissue accumulation in the hypothyroid heart (Drobnik et al., 2009). Application of immunoglobulin from the sera of patients with Graves' disease increases collagen biosynthesis, which is explained by immunoglobulin binding to the TSH receptors (Kohn & Winand, 1975). Experimental outcomes prove that the TSH receptor transcript is present in the human heart (Koshiyama et al., 1996). TSH receptor transcripts and receptor immunoreactivity were found in fibroblasts of different origins (Daumiere et al., 2002; Feliciello et al., 1993). Collagen accumulation in the heart is responsible for the increased stiffness of the heart wall and may contribute to diastolic heart failure development.

Excessive glycosaminoglycan accumulation in the skin is linked with myxedema formation (Smith et al., 1989). Wiig and coworkers (2000) found increased interstitial fluid pressure in the skin and muscle in hypothyroid rats. Thus, accumulation of glycosaminoglycans and proteins in the interstitial space is supposed to increase the edema of the interstitium.

While pleural or pericardial effusions are noted in 10% to 30% of the adult hypothyroidism patients, this complication is rare in children (Martinez-Soto et al., 2010). The main symptoms of cardiac tamponade in hypothyroid patients are increased or normal heart rate (after pericardiocentesis, the tempo is slowed) distant heart sounds, enlarged jugular veins, low P valves, T valves and QRS complex in the electrocardiogram and massive pericardial effusion in echocardiography. The following mechanisms of the cardiac tamponade are possible: increased permeability in microcirculation, leakage of fluid with high protein concentration and disturbed lymphatic drainage. The cardiac tamponade is a rare complication of hypothyroidism because of the slow liquid accumulation and high distensibility of the pericardium (Lin et al., 2003).

5. Blood vessel

Low cardiac output and decreased blood pressure was noted in hypothyroid subjects however, increased total peripheral resistance was also noticed. On the other hand, diastolic hypertension was observed in 25% of the patients. Hypertension has been linked with increased systemic vascular resistance (Klein & Ojama, 2001; b). However, experimental hypertension could be reversed by hypothyroidism (Vargas et al., 1988).

The pressor response for vasoconstrictors and vasodilatators changes in the hypothyroid subject (Vargas et al., 2006). A reduced pressor response to noradrenalin has been proven in normotensive hypothyroid patients, suggesting a decreased sensitivity of blood vessels to noradrenalin, however, the response of blood vessels to noradrenalin become normal after thyroxin supplementation. Interestingly, in hypertensive hypothyroid patients, the sensitivity of blood vessel to noradrenalin was found to be normal (Bramnert et al., 1994). Similarly, aortic rings with an intact endothelium has been proven to demonstrate a reduced pressor response to phenylephrine (Pantes et al., 2006). The reduced sensitivity of blood vessels to $\alpha 1$ stimulators is thought to be due to a decreased number of $\alpha 1$-adrenoreceptors in tested samples (Vargas et al., 2006). Reduced arteries sensitivity to nitric oxide donors (sodium nitroprusside) has also been reported. Infusion of nitroprusside caused lower elevation of forearm blood flow in hypothyroid patients comparing with healthy subjects (Napoli et al., 2009). Moreover, both acetylcholine or histamine-induced vasodilatation was seen to be lower in hypothyroid rats but nitric oxide independent vasodilatation remained unchanged (Moreno et al., 2003).

Inhibited vasodilatation by endothelium dependent factors is thought to be responsible for the increased total peripheral vascular resistance seen in hypothyroid subjects (Vargas et al., 2006). Human smooth muscle cells are postulated to be targets for the thyroid hormones. The genomic and non-genomic mechanisms of thyroid hormones may well play a role in the regulation of smooth muscle cell contractility. However, the molecular targets are not known (Klein & Ojama, 2001; b). In hypothyroidism, a lower level of plasma renin concentration (Bouhnik et al., 1981) increased vasopressin level (Arnaout et al., 1992) and decreased concentration of atrial natriuretic peptide (Kohno et al., 1987) were observed.

Reduced activity of the thyroid gland was observed in subjects affected by hypertension. The inhibition of thyroid activity is supposed to be related to the thyroid-depressing factor found in the liver, spleen, kidney and plasma, which was released during hypertension development in rats. This thyroid-depressing factor reduces thyroid activity mainly by inhibiting the binding of ^{131}I and blocking thyrotropin-stimulated ^{131}I binding (Fregly & Threatte 1982; Vargas et al., 2006).

In hypothyroid patients elevation of total cholesterol, low-density lipoprotein (LDL) as well as the apo B levels was observed (Staub et al., 1992). These results could be explained by lowered number of LDL receptors. Thus, decreased level of mRNA for LDL receptor in the liver of hypothyroid rats was found; however this effect was reversed by thyroxine treatment (Staels et al., 1990). In hypothyroid women the LDL catabolism was decreased (Thompson et al., 1981). The genomic effects of the thyroid hormones on LDL receptor expression were proved (Bakker et al., 1998). The gene coding of the LDL receptor is positively regulated by thyroid hormones.

Patients affected with overt hypothyroidism are influenced by several risk factors of atherosclerosis: elevated levels of low-density lipoprotein, total cholesterol, diastolic hypertension and elevated coagulability. Higher prevalence of atherosclerotic changes in aorta and myocardial infarction in women with subclinical hypothyroidism was observed (Hak et al., 2000). On the other hand, the thyroid hormone supplementation could be responsible for exacerbation of the ischemic heart disease due to positive chronotropic and inotropic effects (Roberts and Ladenson 2004)

6. Summary

The paper shows that hypothyroidism is responsible for profound disturbances in the structure and function of the cardiovascular system. The symptoms of hypothyroidism comprise heart arrhythmias (bradycardia, atrioventricular block, tachycardia, torsade de points) and disturbances in myocardium contraction and relaxation, as well as decrease of oxygen consumption. Molecular mechanism of symptoms has been described. Decreased thyroid hormone content influences the mechanisms of the development of hypothyroidism symptoms through both genomic and non-genomic effects. Elevation of TSH is thought to be involved in some of the peripheral effects observed in rats with primary hypothyroidism. In patients with heart disease, hypothyroidism should be considered as a possible cause.

7. Acknowledgements

The author is grateful to Mrs Teresa Staszewska for her excellent technical assistance.

8. References

Antzelvitch, Ch. (2004). Drug induced Channelopathies. In: Zipes DP and Jalife J (ed.), *Cardiac Electrophysiology From Cell to Bedside,* Elsevier, Philadelphia , pp. 151 -157, .

Arioglu, E., Guner, S., Ozakca, I., Altan, VM. & Ozcelikay, AT. (2009). The changes in beta-adrenoeceptor-mediated cardiac function in experimental hypothyroidism the possible contribution of cardiac beta3 adrenoceptors. *Mol Cell Biochem* 335:59-66.

Arnaout, MA., Awidi, AS., El-Najdawi, AM., Khateeb, MS. & Ajlouni, KM. (1992). Arginine-vasopressin and endothelium-associated proteins in thyroid disease. *Acta Endocrinol*, 126:399-403.

Athea,Y., Garnier, A., Fortin, D., Bahi, L., Veksler, V. & Ventura-Clapier, R. (2007). Mitochondrial and energetic cardiac phenotype in hypothyroid rat. Relevance to heart failure. *Eur J Physiol*, 455:431-442.

Averyhart-Fullard, V., Fraker, L.D., Murphy, A.M. & Solaro, R.J. (1994). Differential regulation of slow-skeletal and cardiac troponin I mRNA during development and by thyroid hormone in rat heart. *J Mol Cell Cardiol*, 26:609-616.

Bakiner, O., Ertorer, ME., Haydardedeoglu, FE., Bozkirli, E., Tutuncu, NB., Demirag & NG. (2008). Subclinical hypothyroidism is characterized by increased QT interval dispersion among woman. *Med Princ Pract* , 17(5):390-394.

Bakker, O., Hudig, F., Meijssen, S. & Wiersinga, WM. (1998). Effects of triiodothyronine and amiodarone on the promoter of the human LDL receptor gene. *Biochem Biophys Res Comun*, 249:517-521.

Bengel, FM., Nekkola, SG., Ibrahim, T., Weniger, C., Ziegles, S. & Schwaiger, M. (2000). Effect of thyroid hormones on cardiac function geometry and oxidative metabolism assessed noninvasively by positron emission tomography and magnetic resonance imaging. *J Clin Endocrinol Metab*, 85:1822-1827.

Bouhnik, J., Galen, FX., Brown, H. & Zavaleta, J. (1981). The renin-angiotensin system in thyroidectomised rats. *Endocrinology*, 108:647-650.

Bramnet, M., Hallengren, B., Lecerof, H., Werner, R. & Manhem, P. (1994) Decreased blood pressure response to infused noradrenaline in normotensive as compared to hypertensive patients with primary hypothyroidism. *Clin Endocrinol*, 40:317-321.

Brent, GA. (1994). The molecular basis of thyroid hormone action.*N Engl J Med*, 331:847-853.

Ciulla, MM., Paliotti, R., Cortelazzi, D., Tortora, G., Barelli, MV., Buonamici, V., Magrini, F. & Beck-Peccoz, P. (2004). Effects of thyroid hormones on cardiac structure: A tissue characterization study in patients with thyroid disorders before and after treatment. *Thyroid*, 11:613-620.

Chavez, C., Zazueta, N., Garcia, E., Martinez-Abundis, E., Pavon, N. & Hernandez-Esquivel, L. (2008). Titration of cardiolipin by either 10-N-nonyl acridine orange or acridine orange sensitizes the adenine nucleotide carrier to permeability transition. *J Bioenergetics Biomembranes*, 40:77-84.

Chojnowski, K., Bielec, A., Czarkowski, M., Dmowska-Chalaba, J., Kochanowski, J. & Wąsowska, A. (2007). Repeated ventricular „torsade de pointes" tachycardia and cardiogenic shock in the course of hypothyroidism. *Cardiology*, J 14:198-201.

Crowley, W.F., Ridgway, E.C., Bough E.W., Francis G.S., Daniels G.H., Kourides I.A., Myers G.S. & Maloof F. (1977). Noninvasive evaluation of cardiac function in hypothyroidism. Response to gradual thyroxine replacement. *N Engl J Med*, 296:1-6.

Daumiere, C., Ludgate, M., Costagiola, S. & Many, M.C. (2002). Evidence for thyrotropin receptor immunoreactivity in pretibial connective tissue from patients with thyroid-associated dermopaty. *Eu. J Endocrinol*, 146, 35-38.

Di Bello, V., Talini, E., Grazia, M., Donne, D., Aghini-Lombardi, F.,Monzani, F., La Carrubba, S., Canterin, F.A., Dini, F.L.,Di Salvo, G., Carerj, S. & Marzilli, M. (2009). New echocardiographic techniques in evaluation of left ventricular mechanics in subclinical thyroid dysfunction. *Echocardiography*, 26:711-719, 2009.

Dillman,WH. (1989). Diabetes and thyroid hormones induced changes in cardiac function and their molecular basis. *Annu Rev Med*, 40:373-394.

Dillman, WH. (1990). Biochemical basis of thyroid hormones action in the heart. *Am J Med* ,88:626-630.

Dowell, RT., Atkins, FL. & Lore, S. (1994). Beta adrenergic receptors, adenylate cyclase activation and myofibril enzyme activity in hypothyroid rats. *Am J Physiol*, 266:H2527-H2534.

Drobnik, J., Ciosek, J., Stempniak, B., Słotwińska, D., Żukowska, D., Marczyński, A., Tosik, D., Bartel, H., Dąbrowski, R. & Szczepanowska, A. (2009). Experimental hypothyroidism increases collagen and glycosaminoglycans content in the heart. *J Physiol Pharmacol*, 60(3):57-62.

Dudley, S.C. & Baumgarten, CM. (1993). Bursting of cardiac sodium channels after acute exposure to 3, 5, 3′-triiodo-L-thyronine. *Circ Res*, 73:301-313.

Er, F., Larbig, R., Ludwig, A., Biel, M., Hofmann, F., Beuckelmann, D.J. & Hoppe, U.C. (2003). Dominant-negative supression of HCN channels markedly reduces the native pacemaker current I(f) and undermines spontaneous beating of neonatal cardiomyocytes. *Circulation*, 107:485-489.

Everts, ME., Verhoeven, FA., Bezstarosti, K., Moenngs, E.P., Hennemann, G., Visser, T.G. & Lamers, IM. (1996). Uptake of thyroid hormone in neonatal rat cardiac myocytes. *Endocrinology*, 137:4235-4242.

Fazio, S., Palmieri, EA., Lombardi, G. & Biondi, B. (2004). Effects of thyroid hormone on the cardiovascular system. *Recent Prog Horm Res* 59:31-50.

Feliciello, A., Porcellini, A., Ciulo, I., Bonavolonta, G., Averdimento, E.V. & Fenzi, G. (1993). Expression of thyrotropin-receptor mRNA in healthy and Graves disease retro-orbital tissue. *Lancet*, 342: 337-338.

Franklyn, JA., Gammage, MD., Raymsden, DB. & Sheppard, MC. (1984). Thyroid status in patients with acute myocardial infarction. *Clin Sci*, 67:585-590.

Fregly, MJ. & Threatte, RM. (1982) Renal-thyroid interrelationship in normotensive and hypertensive rats. *Life Sci*, 30:589-599.

Galetta, F., Franzoni, F., Fallahi, P., Tocchini, L., Braccini, L., Santoro, G. & Antonelli A. (2008). Changes in heart rate variability and QT dispersion in patients with overt hypothyroidism. *Eur J Endocrinol*, 158:85-90.

Gassanov, N., Er, F., Endres-Becker, J., Wolny, M., Schramm, Ch., Hoppe, UC. (2009). Regulation of cardiac If current via thyroid receptors alpha 1 and beta1. *Eur J Physiol*, 458:1061-1068.

Gorza, L., Mercadier, JJ., Schwartz, K., Thornel, LE., Sartore, S. & Schiaffino, S. (1984). Myosin types in the human heart: an immunofluorescence study of normal and hypertrophied atrial and ventricular myocardium. *Circ Res*, 54:694-702.

Haddad, F., Bodell, PW., Qin, AX., Giger, JM. & Baldw KM. (2003). Role of antisense RNA in coordinating cardiac myosin heavy chain gene switching. *J Biol Chem*, 278:37132-37138.

Hak, E., Pols, H.A., Visser, T.J., Dexhage, H.A., Hofman, A. & Witteman J.C. (2000). Subclinical hypothyroidism is an independent risk factor for atherosclerosis and myocardial infarction in elderly women: the Rotterdam study. *Ann Int Med*, 132:270278.

Harris, D.E., Work, S.S., Wright, R.K., Alpert, N.R. & Warshaw, D.M. Smooth, cardiac and skeletal muscle myosin force and motion generation assessed by cross-bridge mechanical interactions in vitro. *J Muscle Res Cell Motil*, 15:11-19, 1994

Jakab, G., Kiss, E., Kranias, E.G. & Edes, I. (1994). Effect of thyroids status on basal phosphorylationof cardiac myofibrillar phosphoproteins in rats. *Cardioscience,* 5:19-24.

Kahaly, G.J. & Dilmann, W.H. (2005). Thyroid hormone action in the heart. *Endocrine Reviews,* 26:704-728.

Kiss, E., Jakab, G. & Kranias, E.G. (1994). Thyroid hormone induced alteration in phospholamban protein expression: regulatory effects on sarcoplasmic reticulum Ca2+ transport and myocardial relaxation *Circ Res,* 75:245-251.

Kiss, E., Brittsan, A.G., Edes, I., Grupp, I.L. & Kranias, E.G. (1998). Thyroid hormone induced alterations in phospholamban deficient mouse hearts *Circ Res,* 83:608-613.

Klein, I. & Ojaama, K. (2001; a). Thyroid hormone – targeting the heart. *Endocrinology,* 142:11-12.

Klein, I. & Ojama, K. (2001; b). Thyroid hormone. Targeting the vascular smooth muscle cells. *Circ Res,* 88:260-261.

Kohn, L.D. & Winand R.J. (1975). Structure of exophtalmos-producing factor derived from thyrothropin pepsin digestion. *J Biol Chem,* 250:6503-6508.

Kohno, M., Murakawa, K., Yasunary, K., Nishizawa, Y., Morii, H. & Takeda T. (1987). Circulating atrial natriuretic peptides in hyperthyroidism and hypothyroidism. *Am J Med* 83:648-652.

Koshiyama, H., Sellitti, D.F., Akamiyu, T., Doi, S.Q., Takeuchi, Z., Inoue, D., Sakaguchi, H., Takemura, G., Sato, Y., Takatsu, Y. & nakao K. (1996). Cardiomyopathy associated with Graves disease. *Clin Endocrinol (Oxf)* 45 111 – 116.

Krenning, G., Zeisberg, E.M. & Kalluri R. (2010).The origin of fibroblasts and mechanism of cardiac fibrosis. *J Cell Physiol,* 225:631-637.

Kucharz, E. (1992) Hormonal regulation of collagen metabolism. In: *The collagens: Biochemistry and pathophysiology.* Springer-Verlag, Berlin, Heidelberg, New York, London, Paris, Tokyo, Hong Kong, Barcelona, Budapest, pp. 87-107.

Ladenson, P.W., Sherman, S.I., Baughman, K.I., Ray, P.E. & Feldman, A.M. (1992) Reversible alterations in myocardial gene expression in a young man with dilated cardiomyopaty and hypothyroidism. *Proc Natl Acad Sci USA,* 89:5251-5255.

Le Bouter, S., Demolombe, S., Chambellan, A., Bellocq, Ch, Aimond, F. Toumaniantz, G., Lande, G., Siavoshian, S., Baro, I., Pond, A.L., Nerbonne, J.M., Leger, J.J., Escande, D. & Charpentier, F. (2003) Microarray analysis reveals complex remodeling of cardiac ion channel expression with altered thyroid status. *Circ Rres,* 92:234-242.

Lin, T.Ch., Jen, Ch., Lin, T.K., Chen, Ch.W., Chen, B.Ch. & Lin, Ch.L. (2003). Mith cardiac tamponade. *Jap Heart J,* 44:447-450.

Mainwaring, R.D., Lamberti, J.J., Carter, T.L. & Nelson JC. (1994). Reduction in triiodothyronine levels following modified Fontan procedure. *J Cardiac Surg,* 9:322-331.

Martinez-Soto, T., Deal, C., Stephyre, D., Truwssell, R., Boutin, C., Djemli, A. & Ho I. (2010). Pericardial effusion in severe hypothyroidism in children. *J Pediatr Endocrinol Metab,* 23:1165-1168.

McAllister, R.M., Delp, M.D. & Loughlin, M.H. (1995). Thyroid status and exercise tolerance. Cardiovascular and metabolic consideration. *Sport Med,* 20:189-198.

Mohr-Kahaly, S., Kahaly, G., Meyer, J. (1996). Cardiovascular effects of thyroid hormones. Z. *Kardiol*, 85(Suppl 6):219-231.

Monzani, F., Di Bello, V., Caraccio, N., Bertini, A., Giorgi, D., Giusti, C., Ferrannini, E. (2001). Effect of levothyroxine on cardiac function and structure in subclinical hypothyroidism: a double blind placebo-controlled study. *J Clin Endocrinol Metab*, 86 (3): 1110-1115.

Moreno, J.M., Wangensteen, R., Sainz J., Rodriguez-Gomez, I., Camorro, V., Osuna, A. & Vargas F. (2003). Role of endothelium-derrived relaxing factors in the renal response to vasoactive agents in hypothyroid rats. *Am J Physiol*, 285:E182-E188.

Morkin, E. (1993). Regulation of myosin heavy chains in the heart. *Circulation*, 87:1451-1460.

Nakayama, Y., Ohno, M., Yonemura, S., Uozumi, H., Kobayakama, N., Fukushima, K., Takeuchi, H. & Aoyagi T. (2006). A case of transient 2:1 atrioventricular block, resolved by thyroxine supplementation for subclinical hypothyroidism. *PACE*, 29:106-108.

Napoli,R., Guardasole, V.,Zarra, E., D'Anna, C., Sena, A., Lupowi, G.A., Oliviero, U., Matarazzo, M., Lupowi, G. & Sacca, L. (2009). Impaired endothelial and nonendothelial-mediated vasodilatation in patients with acute or chronic hypothyroidism. *Clin Endocrinol (Oxf)*, 72:107-111.

Nishiyama, A., Kambe, F., Kamiya, K., Seo, H. & Toyama, J. (1998). Effects of thyroid status on expression of voltage-gated potassium channels in left ventricle. *Cardiovasc Res*, 40:343-351.

Novotny, I., Bourova, L., Malkova, D., Svoboda, P. & Kolar, F. (1999). G-proteins beta-adrenoreceptors and beta-adrenergic responsiveness in immature and adult rat ventricular myocardium, influence of hypo- and hyperthyroidism. *J Mol Cell Cardiol*, 31:761-772, 1999.

Pantes, C., Mourousis, C., Katramadou, M., Saranteas, T., Maurouzis, I., Karageorgiu, H., Tesseromatis, C., Kostopanagioyou, G., Asimacopoulos, P. & Cokkinos, D.V. (2006) Decreased vascular reactivity to alpha 1 adrenergic stimulation in the presence of hypothyroid state: a part of adaptative response? *Int Angiol*, 25:216-220.

Paradies, G., Ruggiero, F.M., Petrosillo, G. & Quagliariello, E. (1997). Alteretions in carnitine-acylcarnitine translocase activity and in phospholipid composition in heart mitochondria from hypothyroid rats. *Biochim Biophys Acta* , 1362:193-200.

Purtell, K., Roepke, T.K. & Abbott WG. (2010). Cardiac arrhythmia and thyroid dysfunction: A novel genetic link. *Intern J Biochem Cell Biol* 42:1767-1770.

Ripoli, A., Pingitore, A., Favilli, B., Bottoni, A., Turchi, S., Osman, N.F., De Marchi, D., Lombardi, M., Labbate, A. & Iervasi, G. (2005). Does subclinical hypothyroidism affect cardiac pump performance? Evidence from a magnetic resonance imaging study. *J Am Coll Cardiol*, 45:439-445.

Roberts, C.G.P. & Ladenson, P.W. (2004). Hypothyroidism. *Lancet*, 363:739-803.

Sakaguchi, Y., Cui, G. & Sen, L. (1996). Acute effects of thyroid hormone on inward rectifier potassium channel currents in guinea pig ventricular myocytes. *Endocrinology*, 137:4744-4751.

Schenck, J.B., Rizvi, A.A. & Lin, T. (2006). Severe primary hypothyroidism manifesting with torsades de pointes. *Am J Med Sci*, 331:154-156.

Schoenmakers, N., de Graff, W.E. & Peters, R.H.J. (2008). Hypothyroidism as the cause of atrioventricular block in an elderly patient. *Neth Heart J* 16:57-59.

Schwartz, H.L., Lazar, M.A. & Oppenheimer JH. (1994). Widespread distribution of immunoreactive thyroid hormone β2 receptor (TRβ2) in the nuclei of extrapituitary rat tissues. *J Biol Chem*, 269:24777-24782.

Shimoni, Y.C. & Severson, D.L. (1995). Thyroid status and potassium currents in rat ventricular myocytes. *Am J Physiol Heart Circ Physiol*, 268:H576-H583.

Shishiba, Y., Yanagishita, M. & Hascall, V.C. (1988). Effect of thyroid hormone deficiency on proteoglycan synthesis by human skin fibroblasts cultures. *Connect Tissue Res*, 17:119-135.

Shojaie, M. & Eshraghian, A. (2008). Primary hypothyroidism presenting with Torsade de pointes type tachycardia: a case report. *Cases J*, I:298:1-4, 2008.

Smith, T.J., Bahn. R.S. & Gorman CA. (1989). Connective tissue, glycosaminoglycans and diseases of the thyroid. *Endocr Rev*, 10:366-391.

Staels, B., Van Tol, A., Chan, L., Will, G., Verhoeven, G. & Auwerx J. (1990). Alterations in thyroid status modulate apolipoprotein, hepatic triglyceride lipase and low density lipoprotein receptor in rats. *Endocrinology*, 127:1144-1152.

Staub, J.J., Althaus, B.U., Engler, H., Ryff, A.S., Trabucco, P., Marguardt, K., Burckhardt, D., Girard, I. & Weintraub, B.D. (1992). Spectrum of subclinical and overt hypothyroidism: effect on thyrotropin prolactin and thyroid reserve and metabolic impact on peripheral target tissues. *Am J Med*, 92:631-642, 1992

Sun, Z.H., Ojamaa, K., Coetzee, W.A., Artman, M. & Klein I. (2000) Effects of thyroid hormone on action potential and repolarising currents in rat ventricular myocytes. *Am J Physiol Endocrinol Metab*, 278:E302-E307.

Sun, Z.H., Ojamaa, K., Nakamura, T.Y., Artman, M., Klein, I. & Coetzee WA. (2001). Thyroid hormone increased pacemaker activity in rat neonatal atrial myocytes. *J Mol Cell Cardiol*, 33:811-824.

Thompson, G.R., Soutar, A.K., Spengel, F.A., Jadhaw, A., Gavigan, S.J. & Myant NB. (1981) Defects of receptor mediated low density lipoprotein catabolism in homozygous familial hypercholesterolemia and hypothyroidism in vivo. *Proc Natl Acad Sci USA*, 78:2591-2595.

VanBuren, P., Harris, D.E., Alpert, N.R., Warshaw, D.M. (1995). Cardiac V1 and V3 myosins differ in their hydrolitic and mechanical activities in vitro. *Circ Res*, 77:439-444.

Vargas, F., Garcia del Rio, C., Luna, J.D., Haro, J.M. & Osorio, C. (1988). Studies on thyroid activityin deoxycorticosterone-salt and Goldblatt two-kidney one-clip hypertensive rats. *Acta Endocrinologica*, 118:22-30.

Vargas, F., Moreno, J.M., Rodriguez-Gomez, I., Wangensteen, R., Osuna, A., Alvarez-Guerra, M. & Garcia-Estan, J. (2006) Vascular and renal function in experimental thyroid disorders. *Eur J Endocrinol*, 154:197-212.

Wieshammer, S., Keck, F.S., Waizinger, J., Henze, E., Loos, K., Hombach, V. & Pfeiffer, E.F. (1989). Acute hypothyroidism slows the rate of left ventricular diastolic relaxation. *Can J Physiol Pharmacol*, 67:1007-1010.

Wiig, H., Reed, K.R. & Tenstad, O. (2000). Interstinal fluid pressure composition of intestitium, and interstitial exclusion of albumin hypothyroid rats. *Am J Physiol Heart Circ Physiol*, 278:H1627-H1639.

18

The Clinical Spectrum of Thyrotropin Receptor Gene (*TSHR*) Mutations

Yardena Tenenbaum-Rakover
Ha'Emek Medical Center, Afula and The Ruth & Rappoprt Faculty of Medicine, Technion, Haifa, Israel

1. Introduction

Resistance to thyrotropin (RTSH) is a condition in which thyroid cells show reduced sensitivity to TSH. This condition is characterized by elevated serum TSH concentration, a normal or hypoplastic thyroid gland and normal to very low levels of thyroid hormones. Loss-of-function mutations in the TSH receptor gene (*TSHR*) lead to RTSH syndrome, presenting with either congenital hypothyroidism (CH) or subclinical hypothyroidism (Beck-Peccoz et al., 2006; Refetoff, 2003).

CH occurs in about 1 in 3500 live births. Thyroid dysgenesis is responsible for 75% of these cases, dyshormonogenesis for 15%, central hypothyroidism for 5%, and 5% are due to other causes (Grüters et al., 2003; Kratzsch & Pulzer, 2008). Most cases of CH due to thyroid dysgenesis occur sporadically, but 2% of the patients are familial (Castanet et al., 2000, 2001). Dyshormonogenesis is commonly recessively inherited (Park & Chatterjee, 2005). Genes associated with thyroid gland dysgenesis include *TITF1*, *TITF2* and *PAX8* (De Felice & Di Lauro, 2004; Gillam & Kopp, 2001(a); Park & Chatterjee, 2005). Thyroid dyshormonogenesis is caused by genes that are involved in thyroid hormone synthesis including thyroperoxidase (*TPO*), thyroglobulin (*TG*), sodium iodide symporter (*NIS*), pendrin (*PDS*), dual oxidase 2 (*DUOX2*) and its maturation factor (*DUOXA2*), and dehalogenase (*DEHAL1*) (Gillam & Kopp, 2001(b); Grasberger & Refetoff, 2010). Loss-of-function mutations in *TSHR* lead to a spectrum of phenotypes, depending on the mutation's location and severity (Biebermann et al., 2010; De Felice & Di Lauro, 2004). The first report in 1968 of RTSH was of an 8-year-old boy with cretinism in whom the thyroid gland was small in a ^{99m}TC scan and radioiodine uptake was normal (Stanbury et al., 1968). It was only in 1995 that the cause for RTSH syndrome in that case was shown to be a mutation in *TSHR* (Sunthornthepvarakul et al., 1995). Since the first report of CH caused by a *TSHR* mutation, several cases of loss-of-function mutations of *TSHR* have been reported: most are missense mutations, but deletions and insertions have been identified as well (see http: www.hgmd.cf.ac.uk/ac/gene.php?gene=TSHR and OMIM#275200) (Abramowicz et al., 1997; Alberti et al., 2002; Biebermann et al., 1997, 2010; Bretones et al., 2001; Camilot et al., 2005; Cangul et al., 2010; Clifton-Bligh et al., 1997; De Marco et al., 2009; de Roux et al., 1996; Fricke-Otto et al., 2005; Gagne et al., 1998; Grasberger et al., 2007; Jeziorowska et al., 2006; Jordan et al., 2003; Kanda et al., 2006; Nagashima et al., 2001; Narumi et al., 2009; Narumi et al., 2011; Park et al., 2004;

Richter-Unruh et al., 2004; Rubio et al., 2008; Russo et al., 2000; Sriphrapradang et al., 2011; Sunthornthepvarakul et al., 1995; Sura-Trueba et al.,2009; Tenenbaum-Rakover et al., 2009; Tiosano et al., 1999; Tonacchera et al., 2000, 2001, 2004; Tsunekawa et al., 2006; Wonerow et al., 2001) (Table 1, Fig 1).

2. TSHR: Structure and function

TSH controls thyroid function upon its interaction with the G-protein-coupled TSHR. The family of G-protein-coupled receptors (GPCRs) shares seven transmembrane segments connected by three extracellular and three intracellular loops (ECL and ICL, respectively). Together with the receptors for glycoprotein hormones LH/HCG and FSH, TSHR has a long N-terminal domain that is involved in recognition and binding of the ligand. The *TSHR* gene located on chromosome 14q31 was cloned in 1989 (Libert et al., 1989). It encodes a protein with a large N-terminal ligand-binding extracellular domain, a hepta-helical transmembrane domain and an intracellular domain. The extracellular domain is encoded by the first nine exons and part of exon 10, whereas the transmembrane and intracellular domains are encoded entirely by exon 10. The protein consists of 744 amino acids and the N-terminal ectodomain consists of 398 amino acids composed of eight leucine-rich repeat motifs (Szkudlinski et al., 2002; Van Durme et al., 2006). Similar to other GPCRs, TSHR shares a common mode of intracellular signaling, stimulating the exchange of GDP for GTP on the Gα subunit (Gsα) and phosphoinositol (IP) turnover through Gq coupling. TSH binding to TSHR on the basolateral membrane of the thyroid follicular cells leads to stimulation of secondary-messenger pathways involving these two main pathways: Gs/cAMP, which mediates hormone secretion, thyroid cell growth and differentiation and iodide uptake, and IP/Ca^{+2}, which regulates thyroid hormone synthesis by stimulating iodide organification (Dumont et al., 1992; Vassart & Dumont, 1992; Wonerow et al., 2001). Mutations in *TSHR* result in either gain or loss of receptor function.

3. Gain-of-function mutations in *TSHR*

Germline gain-of-function mutations result in non-autoimmune hyperthyroidism, whereas somatic mutations that constitutively activate *TSHR* result in toxic thyroid nodules. Hyperthyroidism caused by germline mutations in *TSHR* exhibits autosomal dominant inheritance. The mutations are located mainly in exon 10, which encodes the transmembrane region and intracellular tail that constitutively activate TSHR. The phenotype of these patients is characterized by hyperthyroidism with the presence of goiter but the absence of ophtolmopathy, and a lack of thyroid autoantibodies as well as of lymphocytic infiltration in thyroid histology (Van Sande et al., 1995). The clinical spectrum of phenotypes is variable and onset can occur anywhere from birth to adulthood. The presence of either congenital or adulthood-onset hyperthyroidism, multinodular goiter (MNG) and follicular carcinoma has been reported in the same family (Karges et al., 2005). To date, more then 55 germline gain-of-function mutations have been reported, about 14 of them sporadic and the others with familial occurrence (http: www.hgmd.cf.ac.uk/ac/gene.php?gene=TSHR) (Akcurin et al., 2008; Davies et al., 2005; Farid et al., 2000; Führer et al., 1997(b); Holzapfel et al., 1997; Karges et al., 2005; Khoo et al., 1999; Tonacchera et al., 1996; Van Sande et al., 1995). Hyperthyroidism in affected individuals is often resistant to the conventional treatment used in Graves' disease, and either radiotherapy or total thyroidectomy is required.

Autonomous benign and malignant toxic thyroid nodules have been shown to result from a variety of somatic mutations leading to constitutive activation of *TSHR* and affecting cell proliferation and cell function. Somatic *TSHR* mutations commonly occur in the transmembrane and ECL domains, but hot spots are the sixth transmembrane domain and the third ICL where the receptor interacts with G-proteins. Toxic adenoma due to TSHR-activating mutations may occur in infancy (Kohn et al., 2009) or even *in utero* (Kopp et al., 1997) (OMIM#2603372) (Davies et al., 2005; Führer et al., 1997(a); Kohn et al., 2009). To date, about 25 different somatic TSHR-activating mutations have been reported manifesting with toxic adenoma, MNG and toxic thyroid carcinoma.

4. Loss-of-function mutations in *TSHR*

About 50 different loss-of-function mutations have been described in *TSHR* (Table 1). Affected individuals are either homozygous, compound heterozygous or heterozygous. The degree of insensitivity to TSH depends on the type and location of the *TSHR* mutation; more severe loss of TSHR function manifests as CH, whereas mild mutations present with euthyroid hyperthyrotropinemia or subclinical hypothyroidism. When both alleles carry mutated receptors with complete lack of function, the result is severe hypothyroidism, commonly presenting at birth, whereas carriers of a mutation on one allele present with compensated hyperthyrotropinemia. The thyroid gland is hypoplastic or invisible in a ^{99m}TC scan; however, in ultasonographic imaging, the gland is shown to be in a normal position and commonly of small size. *TSHR* mutations are distributed all along the receptor. Mutations located in the binding domain result in reduced binding capacity or decreased membrane expression of the receptor. The third ECL and the seventh intracellular domain of *TSHR* are hot spots for gain-of-function mutations, but some inactivating mutations have been identified in this domain as well (Alberti et al., 2002; Grasberger et al., 2007; Tiosano et al., 1999) (Fig. 1).

4.1 Prevalence of loss-of-function mutations

The exact prevalence of inactivating *TSHR* mutations is not known. A prevalence of 4.3% biallelic *TSHR* mutations was found among 134 Japanese infants with CH (Narumi et al., 2009). Among 38 children with non-autoimmune subclinical hypothyroidism, 11 (29%) were carriers of *TSHR* mutations (Nicoletti et al., 2009). A prevalence of 12% *TSHR* mutations was shown in 42 subjects with non-autoimmune isolated hyperthyrotropinemia in Italy; all were with familial occurrence (Tonacchera et al., 2004). Camilot et al. (2005) identified 13 patients with heterozygous mutations (11%) out of 116 pediatric patients with asymptomatic euthyroid hyperthyrotropinemia. A rate of 0.6% for carriers of W546X-mutated *TSHR* was identified in Welsh euthyroid individuals (Jordan et al., 2003). We found up to 2.4% carriers of two known mutations in a highly consanguineous population in the northern region of Israel (Tenebaum-Rakover et al., 2009). Moreover, the coexistence of two different novel mutations of *TSHR* in each of two separate clans has been shown (Sriphrapradang et al., 2011). In view of these data, it may be speculated that the occurrence of inactivating *TSHR* mutations in certain populations is not so rare, and therefore screening for *TSHR* mutations is indicated in cases with non-autoimmune subclinical hypothyroidism in those populations.

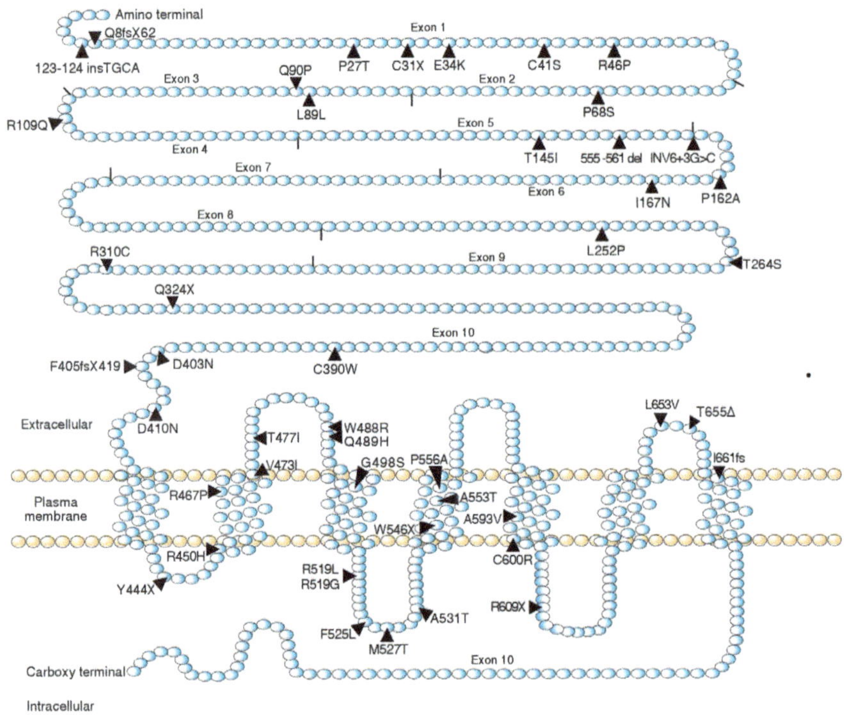

Fig. 1. Scheme of TSHR with known loss-of-function mutations

4.2 Clinical characteristics

Loss-of-function mutations manifest with a variable clinical spectrum of phenotypes. Severe uncompensated RTSH presents with CH, partially compensated RTSH manifests with subclinical hypothyroidism, and fully compensated RTSH presents with euthyroid hyperthyrotropinemia or even normal thyroid function. The diagnosis of TSHR defect is based on the absence of thyroid antibodies, a lack of goiter, measurable serum thyroglobulin, and familial occurrence of hyperthyrotropinemia or hypothyroidism. CH is commonly detected by TSH-based neonatal screening but may missed by total T_4 (TT_4)-based screening since, in many cases, TT_4 levels are within the normal range at birth (Table 1). The degree of CH is variable and depends on the genotype. Severe forms manifest as overt CH (Bretones et al., 2001; Gagne et al., 1998; Jeziorowska et al., 2006; Park et al., 2004; Tonacchera et al., 2000), moderate forms as hypothyroidism identified by neonatal screening without clinical symptoms of hypothyroidism (Abramowicz et al., 1997; Jordan et al., 2003), and mild forms present with hyperthyrotropinemia and normal thyroid hormones (de Roux et al., 1996; Nagashima et al., 2001; Narumi et al., 2009; Tenenbaum-Rakover et al., 2009). Gagne et al. (1998) described a case of CH with persistent neonatal jaundice, myxedematous facies, large fontanelle and absence of ossification centers of the knee on x-rays, indicating severe prenatal deficiency of thyroid hormone. Most of the described cases of CH are detected by neonatal screening with elevated TSH and normal TT_4 levels, but without any clinical symptoms or signs of hypothyroidism (de Roux et al., 1996; Tenenbaum-Rakover et al., 2009). Nevertheless, L-T_4 therapy is initiated in most cases to prevent future consequences of untreated CH. At the age of 2 to 3 years, when L-T_4 is withdrawn, thyroid hormones remain low in the severe mutations (Abramowicz et al., 1997; Biebermann et al., 1997; Tonacchera et al., 2000); however in milder mutations, despite extremely elevated TSH, thyroid hormone levels are normal, indicating compensated hypothyroidism (Clifton-Bligh et al., 1997; Tenenbaum-Rakover et al., 2009). ^{99m}TC scan commonly reveals a normal or hypoplastic gland but in some cases, an absence of thyroid gland has been demonstrated, suggesting thyroid agenesis (Table 1). The presence of detectable thyroglobulin as well as the demonstration of a thyroid gland in the normal position in ultrasonographic imaging exclude thyroid agenesis and indicate a diagnosis of RTSH. In a few reports, an enlarged thyroid gland has been described (de Roux et al., 1996; Grasberger et al., 2007). Inactivating *TSHR* mutations at older ages present with either subclinical hypothyroidism or euthyroid hyperthyrotropinemia without thyroid autoantibodies. The affected patients are commonly identified by routine laboratory tests and are asymptomatic. Most of the described cases are heterozygous for *TSHR* mutations, but biallelic mutations have been reported as well (Kanda et al., 2006; Russo et al., 2000; Sriphrapradang et al., 2011; Tenenbaum-Rakover et al., 2009; Tonacchera et al., 2001, 2007).

4.3 Mechanism of loss-of-function mutations

The mechanism leading to loss-of-function of TSHR includes abnormal binding affinity, abnormal receptor synthesis, accelerated degradation, defective receptor targeting to the cell membrane and abnormal signal transduction (Tao, 2006). Mutations may exert their activity by causing protein misfolding, misassembly or aberrant oligomerization. Loss-of-function mutations are located all along the TSHR (Biebermann et al., 2010) (Fig 1). The function of TSHR is assessed *in vitro* by cAMP response, IP accumulation, TSH binding and cell-surface expression of the mutated receptor. The analysis is performed with COS-7 cells transfected with the mutant receptor. Each mutation has a different effect on binding capacity, membrane expression and cAMP and IP accumulation, depending on its type and location along the *TSHR*. In *in-vitro* studies, it has been shown that *TSHR* mutations differ in their effect on the Gs and Gq pathways, which may lead to more severe loss of one pathway compared to the other (Claus et al., 2005). The third ECL represents an important domain for intermolecular TSHR signal transduction and single amino acids play different roles in receptor folding and cAMP and IP signaling (Claus et al., 2005). We identified a biallelic L653V mutation located in the third ECL in three sisters presenting with marked hyperthyrotropinemia and increased thyroid radioiodine uptake (Grasberger et al., 2007). Normal ligand binding, slightly reduced cell expression and mildly reduced basal and stimulated cAMP accumulation with markedly reduced IP formation were found in *in-vitro* studies using transfected COS-7 cells. These *in-vitro* findings explained the phenotype of the affected subjects manifesting compensated hyperthyrotropinemia concomitant with increased iodide uptake, and this was the first report to provide *in-vivo* evidence of the important role of the IP/Ca^{+2} pathway in the regulation of thyroid hormone synthesis. Narumi et al. (2011) recently reported two patients with CH and high iodide uptake harboring biallelic *TSHR* mutations (R450H+T145I in one and R450H+I166fs in the other), supporting our previous findings. They termed this apparently discrepant phenotype nonclassic TSH resistance.

Type of mutations		Phenotype	US	99mTC- scan	TSH (mIU/l)	TT_4 (µg/dl)	FT_4 (nmol/l)	Age*	Treatment	Reference
123-124 insTGCA	wt	SCH	NA	NA	NA	NA	NA	NA	NA	Camilot et al., 2005
Q8fsX62	wt	SCH	Normal	NA	6.6	NA	7.5	13 y	Yes	Tonacchera et al., 2007
P27T	wt	SCH	NA	NA	NA	NA	NA	NA	NA	Camilot et al., 2005
C31X	wt	SCH	Hypoplasia	NA	8.3		NA	NA	Yes	Nicoletti et al., 2009
E34K	wt	CH	NA	NA	NA	NA	NA	NA	NA	Camilot et al., 2005
C41S	F525L	CH	NA	Normal	129	NA	22	19 d	No	de Roux et al., 1996
C41S	wt	SCH	Normal	Normal	4.7-12.8	NA	19.3	30 d	NA	Alberti et al., 2002; Camilot et al., 2005
R46P	wt	SCH	NA	NA	NA	NA	NA	NA	NA	Camilot et al., 2005
P68S	wt	SCH	Normal	Normal	Slightly elevated	NA	Normal	Variable	No	Tenenbaum-Rakover et al., 2009
L89L+Q90P	P264S	CH	Normal	Low trapping	72	11.5	NA	3 w	Yes	Sriphrapradang et al., 2011
R109Q	wt	SCH	NA	NA	NA	NA	NA	NA	NA	Camilot et al., 2005
R109Q	W546X	CH	Normal	Normal	92	NA	10	8 w	Yes	Clifton-Bligh et al., 1997
555-561del	wt	SCH	NA	NA	6.5	NA	NA	NA	NA	Camilot et al., 2005
IVS6+3G>C	T655Δ	CH	Hypoplasia	Absent	1390	NA	<2.5	15 d	Yes	Gagne et al., 1998
P162A	P162A	CH, CH, SCH	NA	Normal	89, 99, 13.4	NA	12,NA, 10.7	14,NA, 47 y	Yes,NA,No	de Roux et al., 1996; Camilot et al., 2005; Tonacchera et al., 2004
P162A	wt	SCH	Normal	NA	3.8-8.6	NA	8.8	38 y	Yes	Tonacchera et al., 2007; Camilot et al., 2005
P162A	I167N	CH	NA	Normal	47	9.2		16 d	Yes	Sunthornthepvarakul et al., 1995
P162A	C600R	SCH	Hypoplasia	Normal	46	NA	13.4	25 y		Alberti et al., 2002
L252P	wt	SCH	Normal	NA	8.6	NA	12.7	34 y	NA	Tonacchera et al., 2004; Camilot et al., 2005
R310C	R310C	SCH	Normal	Normal	6.8	NA	14.2	63 y	Yes	Russo et al., 2000
Q324X	D410N	CH	NA	Slightly enlarged	44	NA	20	13 d	Yes	de Roux et al., 1996
C390W	F405 fsX419	CH	Hypoplasia	NA	89	6.0	8.2	Newborn	Yes	Biebermann et al., 1997
D403N	wt	SCH	NA	NA	NA	NA	NA	NA	NA	Camilot et al., 2005
C390W	W546X	SCH	NA	Slightly enlarged	34	NA	12.9	55 d	Yes	de Roux et al., 1996

Type of mutations		Phenotype	US	99mTC- scan	TSH (mIU/l)	TT_4 (µg/dl)	FT_4 (nmol/l)	Age*	Treatment	Reference
D410N	wt	SCH	Normal	NA	8.7	NA	12	31 y	Yes	Tonacchera et al., 2007
Y444X	Y444X	CH	Hypoplasia	Hypoplasia	68	NA	8.4	7 y	Yes	Jeziorowska et al., 2006
R450H	T145I	CH	NA	High ^{125}-I uptake	53.8	NA	7.7	Newborn	Yes	Narumi et al., 2011
R450H	G498S	CH	Hypoplasia	Normal	66.8	NA	8.8	12.9	Yes	Nagashima et al., 2001
R450H	V473I	SCH	Normal	NA	12.8	NA	15.5	NA	NA	Tsunekawa et al., 2006
R450H	R519C	SCH	NA	NA	22.9	8.4	NA	NA	NA	Tsunekawa et al., 2006
R450H	R519G	SCH	NA	NA	38.1	8.9	NA	NA	NA	Tsunekawa et al., 2006
R450H	I661fs	CH	Normal	High ^{125}-I uptake	178	NA	3.9	Newborn	Yes	Narumi et al., 2011
L467P	wt	SCH	Normal	Low uptake	9.6	NA	14	5 y	NA	Alberti et al., 2002
T477I	T477I	CH	Hypoplasia	Hypoplasia	NA	NA	<unde-tectable	22 y	Yes	Tonacchera et al., 2000
W488R	wt	SCH	NA, Normal	NA	NA	NA	NA	NA	NA	Camilot et al., 2005; De Marco et al., 2009
Q489H	Q489H	CH	Absent	Absent	180		1	Newborn	Yes	Sura-Trueba et al., 2009
M527T	wt	SCH	NA	NA	NA	NA	NA	NA	NA	Camilot et al., 2005
A531T	A531T	CH	Normal	NA	33	NA	16.8	NA	NA	Cangul et al., 2010
W546X	W546X	CH	Normal	Absent	126	NA	7	Newborn	Yes	Jordan et al., 2003
A553T	A553T	CH	Hypoplasia	Absent	>130	1.2	4.8	4 d	Yes	Abramowicz et al., 1997; Cangul et al., 2010
A553T	W546X	CH	Hypoplasia	Absent	160	1.4		Newborn	Yes	Park et al., 2004
P556A	P556A	CH	Absent	Absent	>100	NA	5.2	3 m	Yes	Cangul et al., 2010
A593V	A593V	SCH, CH	Normal	NA	18.9-33	7.0	NA	7 y, Newborn	Yes	Fricke-Otto et al., 2005
R609X	R609X	CH	Hypoplasia	Absent	>100	NA	1.2-7.0	Newborn	Yes	Tiosano et al.,1999; Richter-Unruh et al., 2004
L653V	L653V	CH+ SCH	Slightly enlarged	High ^{131}-I uptake	53	NA	Normal	10 y	No	Grasberger et al., 2007
T655Δ	wt	SCH	Normal	Normal	14.9	NA	14.1	23 d	NA	Alberti et al., 2002

* At diagnosis; NA, not available; CH, congenital hypothyroidism, SCH, sub-clinical hypothyroidism; y, years; w, weeks; d, days; wt, wild type; US, ultrasonographic imaging

Table 1. Summary of the *TSHR* loss-of-function mutations

4.4 Heterozygosity for loss-of-function mutations

Heterozygous subjects carrying loss-of-function mutations in *TSHR* are commonly mildly affected, presenting with euthyroid hyperthyrotropinemia but with variable expressivity (Camilot et al., 2005; Sriphrapradang et al., 2011; Tenenbaum-Rakover et al., 2009). Heterozygotes are typically diagnosed with slightly increased TSH but normal free T_4 (FT_4) levels. At least one case of neonatal hypothyroidism has been reported as well (Camilot et al., 2005). In *in-vitro* models expressing the combination of wild-type and mutated *TSHR*, it has been shown that basal and TSH-stimulated cAMP production are reduced compared to cells transfected with wild-type receptor, albeit less severely than in biallelic mutations. These *in-vitro* studies are consistent with the dominant-negative effect of the mutated receptor on the activity of the wild type and explain the mild phenotype of the carriers (Calebiro et al., 2005; Tenenbaum-Rakover et al., 2009). The dominant-negative effect of the mutated receptor may result in reduction of cAMP accumulation, as well as reduced membrane cell-surface expression of the receptor and retention in intracellular compartments (Calebiro et al., 2005).

5. Genotype-phenotype association

The phenotype of the affected subjects correlates with the severity of the mutation, which is dependent on its location and type, and whether it is mono- or biallelic. Most of the described cases reveal a direct association between the severity of the mutation and the phenotype, which is reflected by the extent of increase in TSH and decrease in FT_4 levels. The more severe mutations manifest in infancy with persistent CH, while the mild monoallelic mutations manifest as asymptomatic mild hyperthyrotropinemia. We identified 33 subjects carrying two novel *TSHR* gene mutations (P68S and L653V) in a large consanguineous kindred occurring as homozygous L653V (5 subjects), heterozygous P68S (4 subjects), heterozygous L653V (20 subjects), and compound heterozygous L653V/P68S (4 subjects). Our finding in a large cohort of affected members enabled us to assess the genotype-phenotype association. All homozygotes and compound heterozygotes presented with compensated RTSH, 9 out of 24 heterozygotes showed mild hyperthyrotropinemia and the others had normal TSH values. The clinical results were supported by *in-vitro* studies in which the L653V-mutated *TSHR* resulted in more severely impaired signal transduction than the other genotype combinations. However, large variability was found to exist between affected members. Among those with the homozygous L653V mutation, one child had CH and the other four, aged 3 to 20 years, had markedly elevated TSH, but FT_4 levels were within the normal range; among the heterozygous members for the two different mutations, variable hyperthyrotropinemia was observed, with a few of the affected subjects showing normal thyroid function (Tenenbaum-Rakover et al., 2009).

6. Outcome

Despite several reports of patients affected with *TSHR* mutations, there are limited data on the long-term outcome of this condition. In subjects with *TSHR* mutations, it has been shown that TSH levels remain stable and they do not develop hypothyroidism; in contrast, in autoimmune thyroid disease (AITD), overt hypothyroidism commonly develops over the years. In our abovementioned large cohort of affected family members, cross-sectional analysis showed neither a decrease nor an increase in TSH levels with age, suggesting stable compensated RTSH with an appropriately adjusted set point of pituitary-thyroid feedback (Tenenbaum-Rakover et al., 2009). In contrast to subclinical hypothyroidism in the context of AITD, the thyroidal compensation in mild to moderate RTSH is expected to be clinically stable with no progression toward true hypothyroidism or spontaneous regression toward normal TSH levels. Patients with homozygous or compound heterozygous mutations who are detected in infancy by neonatal screening to have CH may have normal FT_4 levels despite elevated TSH levels after L-T_4 withdrawal and in these patients, L-T_4 replacement may not be needed. In contrast, development of overt hypothyroidism at the age of 15 years was shown in a patient homozygous for the R540H mutation who presented with compensated hypothyroidism in infancy (Mizuno et al., 2009), but not in an additional four subjects with the same genotype after long-term follow-up. Asymptomatic heterozygotes for *TSHR* mutations have normal or slightly elevated TSH levels with negative thyroid antibodies (Camilot et al., 2005). However, coexistence of thyroid autoantibodies has been reported in some cases of compensated RTSH, leading to overt hypothyroidism (Tonacchera et al., 2001). It is possible that carriers of *TSHR* mutations are at increased risk for AITD. TSHR is involved in AITD, TSH-stimulating autoantibodies in Graves' disease and TSH-blocking antibodies in Hashimoto thyroiditis. Therefore, it has been speculated that modification of TSH structure by the mutated receptor may lead to AITD (Tonacchera et al., 2001). Fluctuation of TSH levels from slightly above normal to normal values have been observed in some cases by us and others (Tenenbaum-Rakover et al., 2009; Tonacchera et al., 2001). In view of the variability in outcome among affected individuals, careful long-term follow-up is recommended.

7. Treatment

The question of whether to treat patients with *TSHR* mutations with L-T_4 is a matter of debate (Utiger, 1995). In cases with loss-of-function mutations in *TSHR* presenting with CH, early initiation of L-T_4 therapy is recommended to prevent late-effect consequences of hypothyroidism as in other etiologies of CH. However, withdrawal of L-T_4 at the age of 2 to 3 years revealed transient hypothyroidism in some cases, putting the need for lifelong replacement therapy into question (Alberti et al., 2002; Tenenbaum-Rakover et al., 2009). Euthyroid hyperthyrotropinemia caused by *TSHR* mutations with mild to moderate loss of function maintains stable compensated RTSH and may not necessitate thyroid hormone replacement. Moreover, most patients with RTSH do not present with symptoms of hypothyroidism or with biochemical parameters of uncompensated hypothyroidism, such as elevated CPK and liver enzymes and hyperlipidemia (Tenenbaum-Rakover et al., 2009). The presence of normal FT_4 levels argues against the need for replacement treatment, especially when inadvertent overtreatment, producing subclinical hyperthyroidism, can have undesirable effects (Samuels et al., 2008). In our long experience, no clinical benefit has been observed with L-T_4 therapy. Contrasting with this approach, it has been shown that some subjects with RTSH have a slight decrease in FT_4 levels compared to controls, although remaining within the normal range, which may point to subclinical hypothyroidism in these affected patients. In addition, the possibility of secondary pituitary enlargement in patients with extreme hyperthyrotropinemia may support L-T_4 replacement therapy. In view of the variability of phenotypes in different types of mutations, as well as between individuals with the same genotypes, it is recommended that careful follow-up and cautious administration of L-T_4 be considered based on individual thyroid hormone levels in the clinical context.

8. Differential diagnosis

The diagnostic work-up of RTSH should exclude *PAX8* mutations, which are characterized by thyroid dysgenesis associated with kidney abnormalities (Grüters et al., 2003; Park & Chatterjee, 2005), and mutations in guanine nucleotide binding subunit 1 (*GNAS1*), which encodes Gsα subunit and causes pseudohypoparathyroidism (PHP) type Ia. The latter inactivating mutations in Gsα lead to a syndrome of resistance to multiple hormones, including TSH (Mantovani et al., 2002). Another form of RTSH is an autosomal dominantly inherited disease characterized by euthyroid hyperthyrotropinemia, for which the specific gene has not yet been identified. This condition has been linked to a locus on chromosome 15q25.3-26.1 (Grasberger et al., 2005(b)). In many of the cases with clinical characteristics of RTSH, no mutations have been found in *TSHR*, suggesting that additional genes are involved in RTSH syndrome (Xie et al., 1997). Bigenic defects in thyroid-synthesis pathways have been recently described. Coexistence of mutations in *TPO* (Sriphrapradang et al., 2011) and *GNAS* (Lado-Abeal et al., 2011), in addition to mutations in *TSHR*, has been reported in the same individuals. In those reports, the coexistence of mutated *TPO* and *TSHR* in the same individuals belonging to the same kindred did not aggravate the severity of the RTSH phenotype (Sriphrapradang et al., 2011); similar observations were made for the presence of a monoallelic *TSHR* mutation coexisting with a *GNAS* mutation (Lado-Abeal et al., 2011). It is therefore suggested that in cases where *TSHR* mutations do not explain the phenotype, additional genes that are involved in thyroid hormone synthesis be screened. RTSH must be differentiated from AITD (Ross, 2000), the most common cause of subclinical hypothyroidism in the adult population. The presence of autoantibodies as well as a typical hypoechogenic pattern of the thyroid in ultasonographic imaging support the diagnosis of AITD. This is important from a clinical standpoint since in RTSH, hyperthyrotropinemia is almost always stable while in AITD, hypothyroidism develops with time in about 30% of the cases.

9. Conclusion

To date, about 50 different *TSHR* mutations have been reported presenting with a spectrum of phenotypes ranging from overt CH to mild euthyroid hyperthyrotropinemia. Subjects with euthyroid hyperthyrotropinemia commonly have stable TSH levels and do not develop overt hypothyroidism with time. The phenotype correlates with the genotype as the latter is reflected by the severity of hyperthyrotropinemia and the decrease in FT_4 levels. Screening for *TSHR* mutations should be considered in individuals with apparent non-autoimmune subclinical hypothyroidism. In view of the variability in phenotypes and in outcome among individuals in this condition, careful long-term follow-up is recommended and replacement therapy should be considered on an individual basis according to thyroid hormone levels in the clinical context.

10. Acknowledgments

Thanks to Camille Vainstein for professional language editing, to Dr. Zaki Kraiem for fruitful discussion and to Dr. Morad Khayat for useful assistance.

11. References

Abramowicz, M.J.; Duprez, L.; Parma, J.; Vassart, G. & Heinrichs, C. (1997). Familial congenital hypothyroidism due to inactivating mutation of the thyrotropin receptor causing profound hypoplasia of the thyroid gland. *The Journal of Clinical Investigation*, Vol.99, No. 12, (June 1997), pp. 3018-3024, ISSN 0021-9738

Akcurin, S.; Turkkahraman, D.; Tysoe, C.; Ellard, S.; De Leener, A.; Vassart, G. & Costagliola, S. (2008). A family with a novel TSH receptor activating germline mutation (p.Ala485Val). *European Journal of Pediatrics,* Vol.167, No.11, (November 2008), pp. 1231-1237, ISSN 0340-6199

Alberti, L.; Proverbio, M.C.; Costagliola, S.; Romoli, R.; Boldrighini, B.; Vigone, M.C.; Weber, G.; Chiumello, G.; Beck-Peccoz, P. & Persani, L. (2002). Germline mutations of TSH receptor gene as cause of nonautoimmune subclinical hypothyroidism. *Journal of Clinical Endocrinology and Metabolism,* Vol.87, No.6, (June 2002), pp. 2549-2555, ISSN 0021-972X

Beck-Peccoz, P.; Persani, L.; Calebiro, D.; Bonomi, M.; Mannavola, D. & Campi, I. (2006). Syndromes of hormone resistance in the hypothalamic-pituitary-thyroid axis. *Best Practice & Research: Clinical Endocrinology & Metabolism,* Vol.20, No.4, (December 2006), pp. 529-546, ISSN 1521-690X

Biebermann, H.; Schöneberg, T.; Krude, H.; Schultz, G.; Gudermann, T. & Grüters, A. (1997). Mutations of the human thyrotropin receptor gene causing thyroid hypoplasia and persistant congenital hypothyroidism. *Journal of Clinical Endocrinology and Metabolism*, Vol.82, No.10, (October 1997), pp. 3471-3480, ISSN 0021-972X

Biebermann, H.; Winkler, F. & Kleinau, G. (2010). Genetic defects, thyroid growth and malfunctions of the TSHR in pediatric patients. *Frontiers in Bioscience*, Vol.15, No.3, (June 2010), pp. 913-933, ISSN 1093-9946

Bretones, P.; Duprez, L.; Parma, J.; David, M.; Vassart, G. & Rodien, P. (2001). A familial case of congenital hypothyroidism caused by a homozygous mutation of the thyrotropin receptor gene. *Thyroid*, Vol.11, No.10, (October 2001), pp. 977-980, ISSN 1557-9077

Calebiro, D.; de Filippis, T.; Lucchi, S.; Covino, C.; Panigone, S.; Beck-Peccoz, P.; Dunlap, D. & Persani, L. (2005). Intracellular entrapment of wild-type TSH receptor by oligomerization with mutants linked to dominant TSH resistance. *Human Molecular Genetics*, Vol.14, No.20, (October 2005), pp. 2991-3002, ISSN 0964-6906

Camilot, M.; Teofoli, F.; Gandini, A.; Franceschi, R.; Rapa, A.; Corrias, A.; Bona, G.; Radetti, G. & Tato, L. (2005). Thyrotropin receptor gene mutations and TSH resistance:

variable expressivity in the heterozygotes. *Clinical Endocrinology*, Vol.63, No.2, (August 2005), pp. 146-151, ISSN 1365-2265

Cangul, H.; Morgan, N.V.; Forman, J.R.; Saglam, H.; Aycan, Z.; Yakut, T.; Gulten, T.; Tarim, O.; Bober, E.; Cesur, Y.; Kirby, G.A.; Pasha, S.; Karkucak, M.; Eren, E.; Cetinkaya, S.; Bas, V.; Demir, K.; Yuca, S.A.; Meyer, E.; Kendall, M.; Hogler, W.; Barrett, T.G. & Maher, E.R. (2010). Novel TSHR mutations in consanguineous families with congenital nongoitrous hypothyroidism. *Clinical Endocrinology*, Vol.73, No.5, (November 2010), pp. 671-677, ISSN 1365-2265

Castanet, M.; Lyonnet, S.; Bonaiti-Pellie, C.; Polak, M.; Czernichow, P. & Leger J. (2000). Familial forms of thyroid dysgenesis among infants with congenital hypothyroidism. *New England Journal of Medicine*, Vol.343, No.6, (August 2000), pp. 441-442, ISSN 0028-4793

Castanet, M.; Polak, M.; Bonaiti-Pellie, C.; Lyonnet, S.; Czernichow, P. & Leger, J. (2001). Nineteen years of national screening for congenital hypothyroidism: familial cases with thyroid dysgenesis suggest the involvement of genetic factors. *Journal of Clinical Endocrinology and Metabolism*, Vol.86, No.5, (May 2001), pp. 2009-2014, ISSN 0021-972X

Claus, M.; Jaeschke, H.; Kleinau, G.; Neumann, S.; Krause, G. & Paschke, R. (2005). A hydrophobic cluster in the center of the third extracellular loop is important for thyrotropin receptor signaling. *Endocrinology*, Vol.146, No.12, (December 2005), pp. 5197-5203, ISSN 0013-7227

Clifton-Bligh, R.J.; Gregory, J.W.; Ludgate, M.; John, R.; Persani, L.; Asteria, C.; Beck-Peccoz, P. & Chatterjee, V.K.K. (1997). Two novel mutations in the thyrotropin (TSH) receptor gene in a child with resistance to TSH. *Journal of Clinical Endocrinology and Metabolism*, Vol.82, No.4, (April 1997), pp. 1094-1100, ISSN 0021-972X

Davies, T.F.; Ando, T.; Lin, R.Y.; Tomer, Y. & Latif, R.J. (2005). Thyrotropin receptor-associated diseases: from adenomata to Graves disease. *The Journal of Clinical Investigation*, Vol.115, No.8, (August 2005), pp. 1972-1983, ISSN 0021-9738

De Felice, M. & Di Lauro, R. (2004). Thyroid development and its disorders: genetics and molecular mechanisms. *Endocrine Reviews*, Vol.25, No.5, (October 2004), pp. 722-746, ISSN 0163-769X

De Marco, G.; Agretti, P.; Camilot, M.; Teofoli, F.; Tatò, L.; Vitti, P.; Pinchera, A. & Tonacchera, M. (2009). Functional studies of new TSH receptor (TSHr) mutations identified in patients affected by hypothyroidism or isolated hyperthyrotrophinaemia. *Clinical Endocrinology*, Vol.70, No.2, (February 2009), pp. 335-338, ISSN 1365-2265

de Roux, N.; Misrahi, M.; Brouner, R.; Houang, M.; Carel, J.C.; Granier, M.; Le Bouc, Y.; Ghinea, N.; Boumedienne, A.; Toublanc, J.E. & Milgrom, E. (1996). Four families with loss of function mutations of the thyrotropin receptor. *Journal of Clinical Endocrinology and Metabolism*, Vol.81, No.12 (December 1996), pp. 4229-4235, ISSN 0021-972X

Dumont, J.E.; Lamy, F.; Roger, P. & Maenhaut, C. (1992). Physiological and pathological regulation of thyroid cell proliferation and differentiation by thyrotropin and other factors. *Physiological Reviews*, Vol.72, No.3, (July 1992), pp. 667-697, ISSN 0031-9333

Farid, N.R.; Kascur, V. & Balazs, C. (2000). The human thyrotropin receptor is highly mutable: a review of gain-of-function mutations. *European Journal of Endocrinology*, Vol.143, No.1, (July 2000), pp. 25-30, ISSN 0804-4643

Fricke-Otto, S.; Pfarr, N.; Mühlenberg, R. & Pohlenz, J. (2005). Mild congenital primary hypothyroidism in a Turkish family caused by a homozygous missense thyrotropin receptor (TSHR) gene mutation (A593 V). *Experimental and Clinical Endocrinology & Diabetes*, Vol.113, No.10, (December 2005), pp. 582-585, ISSN 0947-7349

Führer, D.; Holzapfel, H.P.; Wonerow, P.; Scherbaum, W.A. & Paschke, R. (1997a). Somatic mutations in the thyrotropin receptor gene and not in the Gs alpha protein gene in 31 toxic thyroid nodules. *Journal of Clinical Endocrinology and Metabolism*, Vol.82, No.11, (November 1997), pp. 3885-3891, ISSN 0021-972X

Führer, D.; Wonerow, P.; Willgerodt, H. & Paschke, R. (1997b). Identification of a new thyrotropin receptor germline mutation (Leu629Phe) in a family with neonatal onset of autosomal dominant nonautoimmune hyperthyroidism. *Journal of Clinical Endocrinology and Metabolism*, Vol.82, No.12, (December 1997), pp. 4234-4238, ISSN 0021-972X

Gagne, N.; Parma, J.; Deal, C.; Vassart, G. & van Vliet, G. (1998). Apparent congenital athyreosis contrasting with normal plasma thyroglobulin levels and associated with inactivating mutations in the thyrotropin receptor gene: are athyreosis and ectopic thyroid distinct entities? *Journal of Clinical Endocrinology and Metabolism*, Vol.83, No.5, (May 1998), pp. 1771-1775, ISSN 0021-972X

Gillam, M.P. & Kopp, P. (2001a). Genetic regulation of thyroid development. *Current Opinion in Pediatrics*, Vol.13, No.4, (August 2001), pp. 358-363, ISSN 1040-8703

Gillam, M.P. & Kopp, P. (2001b). Genetic defects in thyroid hormone synthesis. *Current Opinion in Pediatrics*, Vol.13, No.4, (August 2001), pp. 364-372, ISSN 1040-8703

Grasberger, H. & Refetoff, S. (2010). Congenital defects of thyroid hormone synthesis. In: *Genetic Diagnosis of Endocrine Disorders*, R.E. Weiss, S. Refetoff, (Eds.), 1st ed., 87-95, Academic Press, ISBN 012-374-430X, Burlington, Massachusetts, USA

Grasberger, H.; Mimouni-Bloch, A.; Vantyghem, M.C.; van Vliet, G.; Abramowicz, M.; Metzger, D.L.; Abdullatif, H.; Rydlewski, C.; Macchia, P.E.; Scherberg, N.H.; van Sande, J.; Mimouni, M.; Weiss, R.E.; Vassart, G. & Refetoff, S. (2005a). Autosomal dominant resistance to thyrotropin as a distinct entity in five multigenerational kindreds: clinical characterization and exclusion of candidate loci. *Journal of Clinical Endocrinology and Metabolism*, Vol.90, No.7, (July 2005), pp. 4025-4034, ISSN 0021-972X

Grasberger, H.; Vaxillaire, M.; Pannain, S.; Beck, J.C.; Mimouni-Bloch, A.; Vatin, V.; Vassart, G.; Froguel, P. & Refetoff, S. (2005b). Identification of a locus for nongoitrous congenital hypothyroidism on chromosome 15q25.3-26.1. *Human Genetics*, Vol.118, No.3-4, (December 2005), pp. 348-355, ISSN 0340-6717

Grasberger, H.; Van Sande, J.; Hag-Dahood Mahameed, A.; Tenenbaum-Rakover, Y. & Refetoff, S. (2007). A familial TSH receptor mutation provides in vivo evidence that the inositol phosphates/Ca^{2+} cascade mediates TSH action on thyroid hormone synthesis. *Journal of Clinical Endocrinology and Metabolism*, Vol.92, No.7, (July 2007), pp. 2816-2820, ISSN 0021-972X

Grüters, A.; Biebermann, H. & Krude, H. (2003). Neonatal thyroid disorders. *Hormone Research*, Vol.59, Suppl.1, (January 2003), pp. 24-29, ISSN 0301-0163

Holzapfel, H.P.; Wonerow, P.; von Petrykowski, W.; Henschen, M.; Scherbaum, W.A. & Paschke, R. (1997). Sporadic congenital hyperthyroidism due to a spontaneous germline mutation in the thyrotropin receptor gene. *Journal of Clinical Endocrinology and Metabolism*, Vol.82, No.11, (November 1997), pp. 3879-3884, ISSN 0021-972X

Jeziorowska, A.; Pniewska-Siark, B.; Brzeziańska, E.; Pastuszak-Lewandoska, D. & Lewiński, A. (2006). A novel mutation in the thyrotropin (thyroid-stimulating hormone) receptor gene in a case of congenital hypothyroidism. *Thyroid*, Vol.16, No.12, (December 2006), pp. 1303-1309, ISSN 1557-9077

Jordan, N.; Williams, N.; Gregory, J.W.; Evans, C.; Owen, M. & Ludgate, M. (2003). The W546X mutation of the thyrotropin receptor gene: potential major contributor to thyroid dysfunction in a Caucasian population. *Journal of Clinical Endocrinology and Metabolism*, Vol.88, No.3, (March 2003), pp. 1002-1005, ISSN 0021-972X

Kanda, K.; Mizuno, H.; Sugiyama, Y.; Imamine, H.; Togari, H. & Onigata, K. (2006). Clinical significance of heterozygous carriers associated with compensated hypothyroidism in R450H.; a common inactivating mutation of the thyrotropin receptor gene in Japanese. *Endocrine*, Vol.30, No.3, (December 2006), pp. 383-388, ISSN 0969-711X

Karges, B.; Krause, G.; Homoki, J.; Debatin, K.M.; de Roux, N. & Karges, W. (2005). TSH receptor mutation V509A causes familial hyperthyroidism by release of interhelical constraints between transmembrane helices TMH3 and TMH5. *Journal of Endocrinology*, Vol.186, No.2, (August 2005), pp. 377-385, ISSN 0022-0795

Khoo, D.H.; Parma, J.; Rajasoorya, C.; Ho, S.C. & Vassart, G. (1999). A germline mutation of the thyrotropin receptor gene associated with thyrotoxicosis and mitral valve prolapse in a Chinese family. *Journal of Clinical Endocrinology and Metabolism*, Vol.84, No.4, (April 1999), pp. 1459-1462, ISSN 0021-972X

Kohn, B.; Grasberger, H.; Lam, L.L.; Ferrara, A.M. & Refetoff, S. (2009). A somatic gain-of-function mutation in the thyrotropin receptor gene producing a toxic adenoma in an infant. *Thyroid*, Vol.19, No.2, (February, 2009), pp. 187-191, ISSN 1557-9077

Kopp, P.; Muirhead, S.; Jourdain, N.; Gu, W.X.; Jameson, J.L. & Rodd, C. (1997). Congenital hyperthyroidism caused by a solitary toxic adenoma harboring a novel somatic mutation (serine281-->isoleucine) in the extracellular domain of the thyrotropin receptor. *The Journal of Clinical Investigation*, Vol.100, No.6, (September 1997), pp. 1634-1639, ISSN 0021-9738

Kratzsch, J. & Pulzer, F. (2008). Thyroid gland development and defects. *Best Practice & Research: Clinical Endocrinology & Metabolism*, Vol.22, No.1, (February 2008), pp. 57-75, ISSN 1521-690X

Lado-Abeal, J.; Castro-Piedras, I.; Palos-Paz, F.; Labarta-Aizpún, J.I. & Albero-Gamboa, R. (2011). A family with congenital hypothyroidism caused by a combination of loss-of-function mutations in the thyrotropin receptor and adenylate cyclase-stimulating G alpha-protein subunit genes. *Thyroid*, Vol.21, No.2, (February 2011), pp. 103-109, ISSN 1557-9077

Libert, F.; Lefort, A.; Gerard, C.; Parmentier, M.; Perret, J.; Ludgate, M.; Dumont, J.E. & Vassart, G. (1989). Cloning, sequencing and expression of the human thyrotropin

(TSH) receptor: evidence for binding of autoantibodies. *Biochemical and Biophysical Research Communications,* Vol.165, No.3, (December 1989), pp. 1250-1255, ISSN 0006-291X

Mantovani, G.; Ballare, E.; Giammona, E.; Beck-Peccoz, P. & Spada, A. (2002). The gsalpha gene: predominant maternal origin of transcription in human thyroid gland and gonads. *Journal of Clinical Endocrinology and Metabolism,* Vol.87, No.10, (October 2002), pp. 4736-4740, ISSN 0021-972X

Mizuno, H.; Kanda, K.; Sugiyama, Y.; Imamine, H.; Ito, T.; Kato, I.; Togari, H.; Kamoda, T. & Onigata, K. (2009). Longitudinal evaluation of patients with a homozygous R450H mutation of the TSH receptor gene. *Hormone Research,* Vol.71, No.6, (June 2009), pp. 318-323, ISSN 0301-0163

Nagashima, T.; Murakami, M.; Onigata, K.; Morimura, T.; Nagashima, K.; Mori, M. & Morikawa, A. (2001). Novel inactivating missense mutations in the thyrotropin receptor gene in Japanese children with resistance to thyrotropin. *Thyroid,* Vol.11, No.6, (June 2001), pp. 551-559, ISSN 1557-9077

Narumi, S.; Muroya, K.; Abe, Y.; Yasui, M.; Asakura, Y.; Adachi, M. & Hasegawa, T. (2009). TSHR mutations as a cause of congenital hypothyroidism in Japan: a population-based genetic epidemiology study. *Journal of Clinical Endocrinology and Metabolism,* Vol.94, No.4, (April 2009), pp. 1317-1323, ISSN 0021-972X

Narumi, S.; Nagasaki, K.; Ishii, T.; Muroya, K.; Asakura, Y.; Adachi, M. & Hasegawa, T. (2011). Nonclassic TSH resistance: TSHR mutation carriers with discrepantly high thyroidal iodine uptake. *Journal of Clinical Endocrinology and Metabolism* [Epub ahead of print] (June 2011), ISSN 0021-972X

Nicoletti, A.; Bal, M.; De Marco, G.; Baldazzi, L.; Agretti, P.; Menabò, S.; Ballarini, E.; Cicognani, A.; Tonacchera, M. & Cassio, A. (2009). Thyrotropin-stimulating hormone receptor gene analysis in pediatric patients with non-autoimmune subclinical hypothyroidism. *Journal of Clinical Endocrinology and Metabolism,* Vol.94, No.11, (November 2009), pp. 4187-4194, ISSN 0021-972X

Park, S.M. & Chatterjee, V.K. (2005). Genetics of congenital hypothyroidism. *Journal of Medical Genetics,* Vol.42, No.5, (May 2005), pp. 379-389, ISSN 0022-2593

Park, S.M.; Clifton-Bligh, R.J.; Betts, P. & Chatterjee, V.K. (2004). Congenital hypothyroidism and apparent athyreosis with compound heterozygosity or compensated hypothyroidism with probable hemizygosity for inactivating mutations of the TSH receptor. *Clinical Endocrinology,* Vol.60, No.2, (February 2004), pp. 220-227, ISSN 1365-2265

Refetoff, S. (2003). Resistance to thyrotropin. *Journal of Endocrinological Investigation,* Vol.26, No.8, (August 2003), pp. 770-779, ISSN 0391-4097

Richter-Unruh, A.; Hauffa, B.P.; Pfarr, N. & Pohlenz, J. (2004). Congenital primary hypothyroidism in a Turkish family caused by a homozygous nonsense mutation (R609X) in the thyrotropin receptor gene *Thyroid,* Vol.14, No.11, (November 2004), pp. 971-974, ISSN 1557-9077

Ross, D.S. (2000). Subclinical hypothyroidism. In: *Werner and Ingbar's the Thyroid: a Fundamental and Clinical Text,* L.E. Braverman, R.D. Utiger, (Eds.), 8th ed., 467–473,

Lippincott Williams & Wilkins, ISBN 978-078-1750-47-9, Philadelphia, Pennsylvania, USA

Rubio, I.G.; Galrao, A.L.; Pardo, V.; Knobel, M.; Possato, R.F.; Camargo, R.R.; Ferreira, M.A.; Kanamura, C.T.; Gomes, S.A. & Medeiros-Neto, G. (2008). A molecular analysis and long-term follow-up of two siblings with severe congenital hypothyroidism carrying the IVS30+1G>T intronic thyroglobulin mutation. *Arquivos Brasileiros de Endocrinologia & Metabologia*, Vol.52, No.8, (November 2008), pp. 1337-1344, ISSN 0004-2730

Russo, D.; Betterle, C.; Arturi, F.; Chiefari, E.; Girelli, M.E. & Filetti, S. (2000). A novel mutation in the thyrotropin (TSH) receptor gene causing loss of TSH binding but constitutive receptor activation in a family with resistance to TSH. *Journal of Clinical Endocrinology and Metabolism*, Vol.85, No.11, (November 2000), pp. 4238-4242, ISSN 0021-972X

Samuels, M.H.; Schuff, K.G.; Carlson, N.E.; Carello, P.; Janowsky, J.S. (2008). Health status, mood, and cognition in experimentally induced subclinical thyrotoxicosis. *Journal of Clinical Endocrinology and Metabolism*, Vol.93, No.5, (May 2008), pp. 1730-1736, ISSN 0021-972X

Sriphrapradang, C.; Tenenbaum-Rakover, Y.; Weiss, M.; Barkoff, M.S.; Admoni, O.; Kawthar, D.; Caltabiano, G.; Pardo, L.; Dumitrescu, A.M. & Refetoff, S. (2011). The coexistence of a novel inactivating mutant thyrotropin receptor allele with two thyroid peroxidase mutations: a genotype-phenotype correlation. *Journal of Clinical Endocrinology and Metabolism*, Vol.96, No.6, (June 2011), pp. E1001-E1006, ISSN 0021-972X

Stanbury, J.B.; Rocmans, P.; Buhler, U.K. & Ochi, Y. (1968). Congenital hypothyroidism with impaired thyroid response to thyrotropin. *New England Journal of Medicine*, Vol.279, No.21, (November 1968), pp. 1132-1136, ISSN 0028-4793

Sunthornthepvarakul, T.; Gottschalk, M.E.; Hayashi, Y. & Refetoff, S. (1995). Resistance to thyrotropin caused by mutations in the thyrotropin-receptor gene. *New England Journal of Medicine*, Vol.332, No.3, (January 1995), pp. 155-160, ISSN 0028-4793

Sura-Trueba, S.; Aumas, C.; Carre, A.; Durif, S.; Leger, J.; Polak, M. & de Roux, N. (2009). An inactivating mutation within the first extracellular loop of the thyrotropin receptor impedes normal posttranslational maturation of the extracellular domain. *Endocrinology*, Vol.150, No.2, (February 2009), pp. 1043-1050, ISSN 0013-7227

Szkudlinski, M.W.; Fremont, V.; Ronin, C. & Weintraub, B.D. (2002). Thyroid-stimulating hormone and thyroid-stimulating hormone receptor structure-function relationships. *Physiological Reviews*, Vol.82, No.2, (April 2002), pp. 473-502, ISSN 0031-9333

Tao, Y.X. (2006). Inactivating mutations of G protein-coupled receptors and diseases: structure-function insights and therapeutic implications. *Pharmacology & Therapeutics*, Vol.111, No.3, (September 2006), pp. 949–973, ISSN 0163-7258

Tenenbaum-Rakover, Y.; Grasberger, H.; Mamanasiri, S.; Ringkananont, U.; Montanelli, L.; Barkoff, M.S.; Dahood, A.M. & Refetoff, S. (2009). Loss-of-function mutations in the thyrotropin receptor gene as a major determinant of hyperthyrotropinemia in a consanguineous community. *Journal of Clinical Endocrinology and Metabolism*, Vol.94, No.5, (May 2009), pp. 1706-1712, ISSN 0021-972X

Tiosano, D.; Pannain, S.; Vassart, G.; Parma, J.; Gershoni-Baruch, R.; Mandel, H.; Lotan, R.; Zaharan, Y.; Pery, M.; Weiss, R.E.; Refetoff, S. & Hochberg, Z. (1999). The hypothyroidism in an inbred kindred with congenital thyroid hormone and glucocorticoid deficiency is due to a mutation producing a truncated thyrotropin receptor. *Thyroid*, Vol.9, No.9, (September 1999), pp. 887-894, ISSN 1557-9077

Tonacchera, M.; Van Sande, J.; Cetani, F.; Swillens, S.; Schvartz, C.; Winiszewski, P.; Portmann, L.; Dumont, J.E.; Vassart, G. & Parma, J. (1996). Functional characteristics of three new germline mutations of the thyrotropin receptor gene causing autosomal dominant toxic thyroid hyperplasia. *Journal of Clinical Endocrinology and Metabolism*, Vol.81, No.2, (February 1996), pp. 547-554, ISSN 0021-972X

Tonacchera, M.; Agretti, P.; Pinchera, A.; Rosellini, V.; Perri, A.; Collecchi, P.; Vitti, P. & Chiovato, L. (2000). Congenital hypothyroidism with impaired thyroid response to thyrotropin (TSH) and absent circulating thyroglobulin: evidence for a new inactivating mutation of the TSH receptor gene. Journal of Clinical Endocrinology and Metabolism, Vol.85, No.3, (March 2000), pp. 1001-1008, ISSN 0021-972X

Tonacchera, M.; Agretti, P.; De Marco, G.; Perri, A.; Pinchera, A.; Vitti, P. & Chiovato, L. (2001). Thyroid resistance to TSH complicated by autoimmune thyroiditis. *Journal of Clinical Endocrinology and Metabolism*, Vol.86, No.9, (September 2001), pp. 4543-4546, ISSN 0021-972X

Tonacchera, M.; Perri, A.; De Marco, G.; Agretti, P.; Banco, M.E.; Di Cosmo, C.; Grasso, L.; Vitti, P.; Chiovato, L. & Pinchera, A. (2004). Low prevalence of thyrotropin receptor mutations in a large series of subjects with sporadic and familial nonautoimmune subclinical hypothyroidism. *Journal of Clinical Endocrinology and Metabolism*, Vol.89, No.11, (November 2004), pp. 5787-5793, ISSN 0021-972X

Tonacchera, M.; Di Cosmo, C.; De Marco, G.; Agretti, P.; Banco, M.; Perri, A.; Gianetti, E.; Montanelli, L.; Vitti, P. & Pinchera, A. (2007). Identification of TSH receptor mutations in three families with resistance to TSH. *Clinical Endocrinology*, Vol.67, No.5, (November 2007), pp. 712-718, ISSN 1365-2265

Tsunekawa, K.; Onigata, K.; Morimura, T.; Kasahara, T.; Nishiyama, S.; Kamoda, T.; Mori, M.; Morikawa, A. & Murakami, M. (2006). Identification and functional analysis of novel inactivating thyrotropin receptor mutations in patients with thyrotropin resistance. *Thyroid*, Vol.16, No.5, (May 2006), pp. 471-479, ISSN 1557-9077

Utiger, R.D. (1995). Thyrotropin-receptor mutations and thyroid dysfunction. *New England Journal of Medicine*, Vol.332, No.4, (January 1995), pp. 183-185, ISSN 0028-4793

Van Durme, J.; Horn, F.; Costagliola, S.; Vriend, G. & Vassart, G. (2006). GRIS: glycoprotein-hormone receptor information system. *Molecular Endocrinology*, Vol.20, No.9, (September 2006), pp. 2247-2255, ISSN 0888-8809

Van Sande, J.; Parma, J.; Tonacchera, M.; Swillens, S.; Dumont, J. & Vassart, G. (1995). Somatic and germline mutations of the TSH receptor gene in thyroid diseases. *Journal of Clinical Endocrinology and Metabolism*, Vol.80, No.9, (September 1995), pp. 2577-2585, ISSN 0021-972X

Vassart, G. & Dumont, J.E. (1992). The thyrotropin receptor and the regulation of thyrocyte function and growth. *Endocrine Reviews,* Vol.13, No.3, (August 1992), pp. 596-611, ISSN 0163-769X

Wonerow, P.; Neumann, S.; Gudermann, T. & Paschke, R. (2001). Thyrotropin receptor mutations as a tool to understand thyrotropin receptor action. *Journal of Molecular Medicine,* Vol.79, No.12, (December 2001), pp. 707-721, ISSN 0946-2716

Xie, J.; Pannain, S.; Pohlenz, J.; Weiss, R.E.; Moltz, K.; Morlot, M.; Asteria, C.; Persani, L.; Beck-Peccoz, P.; Parma, J.; Vassart, G. & Refetoff, S. (1997). Resistance to thyrotropin (TSH) in three families is not associated with mutations in the TSH receptor or TSH. *Journal of Clinical Endocrinology and Metabolism,* Vol.82, No.12, (December 1997), pp. 3933-3940, ISSN 0021-972X

19

Spirometry in Patients with Clinical and Subclinical Hypothyroidism

Gulfidan Cakmak
Haseki Training and Research Hospital, Istanbul, Turkey

1. Introduction

Hypothyroidism is defined as a clinical state resulting from insufficient secretion of thyroid hormone from thyroid gland due to some structural or/and functional impairments in thyroid hormone production (Kek PC et al., 2003, Dashe JS & Cunningham FG., 2001). Hypothyroidism effects all of the organ systems. Main clinical findings are fatigue, weakness, dryness and coarseness of the skin, cold intolerance, swelling of the extremities, hair loss, lack of concentration and memory, constipation, weight gain without loss of appetite, dyspnea, hoarseness of speech, menorrhagia, paraesthesia, hearing disorders, diffuse alopecia, bradycardia, delayed relaxation of tendon reflexes, carpal tunnel syndrome and serous cavitary effusions (Kek PC et al., 2003). All of these signs and symptoms recover after replacement of thyroid hormone (Larsen PR & Davies TF, 2003, Fatourechi V., 2001).). Subclinical hypothyroidism reflects the earliest stage of thyroid dysfunction with subjects having normal or decreased fT_4, normal fT_3 and decreased TSH levels. Since diagnosis depends on laboratory values, theoretically, no symptoms or signs are expected but yet patients may suffer from somnolence, weakness and fatigue (Kek PC et al., 2003).

In the English literature there exsists several studies revealing the effect of clinical hypothyroidism on respiratory and cardiovascular systems but we were not able to find any comparative effect of subclinical hypothyroidism on these systems. In this study we evaluated the respiratory function in subclinical hypothyroidism as well as comparing the results with clinical hypothyroidism and healthy control groups. Our aim was to determine if respiratory function was effected in subclinical hypothyroidism by using simple spirometry.

2. Materials and methods

Two hundred and sixty-seven subjects were enrolled in the study. None of the participants had a history of smoking, any respiratory illness or any other systemic pathology affecting the respiratory system. The patients did not suffer from goitre disturbing the respiratory function. The body mass indices (BMI) of all of the participants were under 30 kg/m^2. Following the approval of the local ethics committee written informed consent was obtained from all of the participants.

Serum fT_3, fT_4 levels were assessed by Chemiluminescent Competitive Enzyme Immunoassay method with Immulite 2000 of BIODPC. Serum TSH analysis was performed by Enzyme Chemiluminescent Immunometric Assay method with the same analyser. Normal range for TSH was <4.0 uIU/ml, 1.57-4.71 ng/ml for fT_3, and 0.8-1.8 ng/ml for fT_4. If the patients' serum fT_3 level was between 1.57-4.71 ng/ml, fT_4 was between 0.8-1.8 ng/ml and TSH level was >4.0 uIU/ml, they were included in the subclinical hypothyroidism group. On the other hand, if their serum levels of fT_3 was <1.57 ng/ml, fT_4<0.8 ng/ml and TSH was >4.0 uIU/ml; they were included in the clinical hypothyroidism group. The control group consisted of subjects having normal fT_3, fT_4 and TSH values.

Spirometric analysis was performed with Jaeger Master Scobe (version 4.5). All respiratory parameters including FVC, FVC %, FEV_1, FEV_1 %, FEV_1/FVC, FEF_{25-75}, FEF_{25-75} %, PEF, PEF % were assessed.

The mean and standard deviation of parametric values were assessed with Students'-t test and ANOVA. Chi-square test was used when assessing the percentages of the groups and Pearson correlation was used to compare the groups. P<0.05 was considered as significant.

3. Results

Among 120 patients enrolled into the study with subclinical hypothroidism, 114 of them were women and 6 were men while there were 86 women and 3 male patients with clinical hypothyroidism. Control group consisted of 51 women and 9 men. The mean age of the patients was 43±13 years and 41±13 years with subclinical hypothyroidism and clinical hypothyroidism, respectively. The mean age was 41±12 years in the control group. There was not a significant difference between groups regarding age (Table 1).

		Subclinical hypothyroidism (n=120)	Clinical hypothyroidism (n=87)	Control group (n=60)
Age/years		43.68±13.31	41.97±13.22	41.45±11.98
Gender	F	114	84	51
	M	6	3	9

Table 1. Demographic features of the participants

Serum fT_3, fT_4 and TSH values and spirometric parameters of the groups are shown at Table 2 and 3, respectively. Spirometric values were the lowest in the clinical hypothyroidism group while it was higher in subclinical hypothyroidism and the highest in the control group.

	Subclinical hypothyroidism (n=120)	Clinical hypothyroidism (n=87)	Control group (n=60)
fT_3 (ng/ml)	2,82±0,76	1,65±0,85	3,12±1.01
fT_4(ng/dl)	1,06±0,16	0,52±0,22	1,17±0,23
TSH(uIU/m)	10,19±6,22	74,17±140,78	1,60±1,07

Table 2. Thyroid function values of the participants

The comparison between clinical hypothyroidism and control group demonstrated that all of the spirometric parameters were higher in control group;but only the differences among FVC, FVC %, FEV_1, FEF_{25-75} reached statistical significance

($p<0.05$); the others were not statistically significant.

According to the comparison between subclinical hypothyroidism and control group, spirometric parameters were higher in the control group and lower in patients with subclinical hypothyroidism and there was a statistical significant difference regarding FVC, FVC %, FEV_1 and FEF_{25-75} ($p<0.05$).

Statistically significant positive correlation was found between FT_4 and FVC % in patients with subclinical hypothyroidism (r=0.198, p=0.030).

	Subclinical hypothyroidism (n=120)	Clinical hypothyroidism (n=87)	Control group (n=60)
FVC(ml)	3284±574*	3218±767*	3565±806
FVC %	109±18*	105±19*	115±15
FEV_1(ml)	2661±529*	2614±623*	2866±706
FEV_1 %	103±16	100±21	106±14
FEV_1/FVC	80±9	80±7	78±6
FEF_{25-75}(ml)	4716±1415*	4534±1470*	9034±13162
FEF_{25-75} %	81±22	79±26	81±20
PEF(ml)	4966±1413	4940±1337	5374±1932
PEF %	77±20	77±21	80±21

Table 3. Spirometry parameters of the participants

There was a positive correlation between fT_3 and FEF_{25-75} (r=0.484, p=0.0001), FEF_{25-75} % (r=0.490, p=0.0001), PEF (r=0.419, p=0.0001) and PEF% (r=0.432, p=0.0001) in the clinical hypothyroidism group. There was also a positive correlation between fT_4 and FEF_{25-75} (r=0.211, p=0.05), FVC (r=0.251, p=0.019) and FVC% (r=0.248, p=0.021). On the other hand, there was a negative correlation between TSH and FVC% (r= -0.249, p=0.02).

4. Conclusion

Hypothyroidism and subclinical hypothyroidism is a clinical disorder occuring frequently in community. Literature research reveals many studies regarding the effects of clinical hypothyroidism on respiratory and cardiovascular systems. But there exists no study concerning the effect of subclinical hypothyroidism on respiratory system nor there exists any study comparing healthy subjects to clinical hypothyroid patients in terms of respiratory function tests. Therefore we aimed to assess the respiratory function of patients with subclinical hypothyroidism in comparison with clinical hypothyroidism and healthy subjects.

The incidence of primary hypothyroidism is 2% in women and 0.2% in men. Hypothyroidism effects all of the organ systems (Kek PC et al., 2003, Larsen PR & Davies TF, 2003). The clinical presentation of thyroid hormone deficiency alters from one person to another depending on the duration, cause and the degree of deficiency. The decrease in both expiratory and inspiratory muscle strength (Siafakas NM et al., 1992), alveolar hypoventilation due to depression of hypoxic and hypercapnoeic ventilatory drives (Kahaly GJ, 2000) and decrease in maximal breathing and diffusing capacity (Zwillich CW et al., 1975) are evident in patients with hypothyroidism. These impairments are reversible with hormone replacement therapy. Respiratory infections are more common than healthy people (Harrison RN & Tattersfield AE., 1984, Krishnan R et al., 1984). Obstructive sleep apnea syndrome is common in severe hypothyroidism but it is reversible with restoration of a euthyroid state (Larsen PR & Davies TF, 2003). The prominent features like somnolence, apathy and lethargy may also recover with replacement therapy (Krishnan R et al., 1984, Jameson JL & Weetman AP, 2001). Muscle strength measurement and sleep investigation is not routine analysis in these patients, so simple spirometric evaluation is preferred. Thus, we used only spirometric measurements in our study since this method is easier, more available and cheaper than other respiratory function tests.

Siafakas et al. found a significant decrease in the strength of inspiratory and expiratory muscles in patients with clinical hypothyroidism. In the mentioned study, vital capacity (VC), forced vital capacity (FVC), forced vital capacity one second (FEV_1), FEV_1/FVC were significantly lower in patients with clinical hypothyroidism compared to healtly controls. In our study, the patients with clinical hypothyroidism had significantly lower spirometric parameters such as vital capacity (VC), forced vital capacity (FVC), forced vital capacity in one second (FEV_1), FEV_1/FVC, peak expiratory flow (PEF) and forced expiratory flow 25-75 (FEF 25-75) than control group.

Subclinical hypothyroidism reflects the earliest stage of thyroid dysfunction. Chronical autoimmune thyroiditis, subacute thyroiditis, thyroidectomy, radioactive iodine treatment, insufficient thyroid hormone replacement therapy may be the cause of subclinical hypothyroidism. The rate of progression to clinical hypothyroidism from subclinical hypothyroidism is about 7,8 %-17,8 %. Initiating therapy doesn't change the natural course of the illness, but it prevents the progression of clinical hypothyroidism (Biondi B et al., 2002, Surks MI & Ocampo E., 1996).

Subclinical hypothyroidism is a common phenomenon seen more often in women with increasing age. The prevalance in women is 6-8 % and 3 % in men (Kek PC et al., 2003, Surks MI & Ocampo E., 2004). In our study 114 female and 6 male patients had subclinical hypothyroidism. Theoretically no symptoms or findings are expected in subclinical hypothyroidism. On the contrary, almost all of our patients suffered from at least one or more of the symptoms like fatigue, weakness and somnolence. This situation revealed that clinical findings also associated to spirometric abnormalities. Fatigue is observed in subclinical hypothyroidism because of muscle dysfunction. Diagnosis depends on laboratory evaluation. (Kahaly GJ, 2000, Biondi B et al., 2002, Biondi B et al., 2002).

The effect of subclinical hypothyroidism on several organ systems are well known, whereas the effect on respiratory system is not fully understood (Col NF et al., 2004, Beyer IW et al., 1998). The study we designed led us to the conclusion that the measurements of spirometric variables are higher in subclinical hypothyroidism than in clinical hypothyroidism but lower than healthy subjects reaching statistical significance.

In conclusion it is possible to claim that respiratory system is effected in subclinical hypothyroidism. Since subclinical hypothyroidism is common in general population, the patients at high risk who had clinical signs and symptoms may be screened with simple spirometry.

5. References

Beyer IW, Karmali R & Demester MR. (1998). Muscle dysfunction in subclinical hypothyroidism. *J Clin Endocrinol Metab,* May; 83, 50, 1823.

Biondi B, Palmieri EA & Lombardi G. (2002). Effects of subclinical thyroid dysfunction on the heart. *Ann Intern Med,* Dec 3, 137, 11, 904-914.

Biondi B, Palmieri FA & Lombardi G. (2002). Subclinical hypothyroidism and cardiac function. *Thyroid,* Jun, 12, 6, 505-510.

Col NF, Sarks MI & Daniels GH. (2004). Subclinical thyroid disease: Clinical applications. *JAMA,* Apr 7, 291, 13, 1562.

Dashe JS & Cunningham FG. (2001). Subclinical hypothyroidism. *N Engl J Med,* Dec 20, 345, 25, 1855.

Fatourechi V. (2001). Subclinical thyroid disease. *Mayo Clin Proc,* Apr, 76, 4, 413-417.

Harrison R.N & Tattersfield A.E. (1984). Airway response to inhaled salbutamol in hyperthyroid and hypothyroid patients before and after treatment. *Thoraks,* 39, 34-39.

Jameson JL, Weetman AP. (2001). Diseases of thyroid gland, In: *Harrison's Internal Medicine,* Braunwald E, Fauci AJ, Kasper DL, Hauser SL, Longo DL, Jameson JL, 2060-2084, 15th ed, New York: McGraw-Hill.

Kahaly GJ(2000) Cardiovascular and atherogenic aspects of subclinical hypothyroidism, *Thyroid,*Aug,10,8,665-679.

Kek PC, Ho SC& Khoo DH. (2003). Subclinical thyroid disease. *Singapore Med J,* 44, 11 595-600.

Krishnan R, Peter HA & Sarkis SD. (1984). Obstructive Sleep Apnea in Hypothyroidism. *Annuals of Internal Medicine,* 101, 491-494.

Larsen PR & Davies TF. (2003). Hypothyroidsm and thyroiditis, In: *Williams Textbook of Endocrinology,* Larsen PR, Kronenberg HM, Melmed S, Polonsky KS, 423-456, 10th ed. Saunders.

Siafakas NM, Salesiotou V& Filaditaki V. (1992) Respiratory muscle strength in hypothyroidism. *Chest,*J ul, 102,1, 189-194.

Surks MI & Ocampo E. (1996). Subclinical thyroid disaese. *Am J Med. Feb,* 100, 2, 217-223.

Surks MI, Ortiz E & Danniels GH. (2004). Subclinical thyroid disease: Scientific review and guidelines for diagnosis and management. *JAMA,* Jan 14, 291, 2, 228-238.

Zwillich CW, Pierson PJ & Hofeldt FD. (1975). Ventilatory control in myxedema and hypothyroidism. *N Eng J Med,* Mar, 27, 292, 13, 662-665.

20

Cognitive Function in Elderly with Subclinical Hypothyroidism

Lilia Cárdenas-Ibarra, Jesús Zacarías Villarreal-Pérez
and Abraham Antonio Vázquez-García
*Endocrinology service, and Geriatric service,
University Hospital, School of Medicine, Autonomous University of Nuevo Leon
México*

1. Introduction

Overt thyroid disease often involves mood disorders and cognitive impairment in adults. But at the subclinical level a relationship has been difficult to establish. Some authors regard thyroid stimulant hormone small elevation in the elderly as part of aging. However, there is a body of studies that demonstrate the impact of SH in target tissues; vg, ejection fraction and lipid profile alterations; thus many experts recommend comprehensive treatment, adjusting it to the patient´s specific context, age, comorbidities etc. However, regarding cognitive and mood problems there is still controversy. There are studies concluding no association between SH, cognition or depression but these used insensitive instruments to measure cognition and depression, or they had some other methodological bias. There are also cross-sectional and case studies showing an association with newly-developed more sensitive instruments. Subclinical hypothyroidism, cognitive impairment and depression occur more often in old age. Population aging increases SH, cognitive impairment, and depression prevalence and this will be a health burthen for patients, their families, and society; thus measures to minimize it is urgent in developing countries, where a high increase in the elderly population is expected. Indeed Heathcare polices everywhere must strive for mind and physical well-being. We will review instruments to screen and score different spheres of cognitive function in the geriatric or general practitioner´s office, and assess the available evidence, and aspects that need further investigation.

2. Definitions

1. Subclinical hypothyroidism (SH) is defined as an elevated serum thyroid stimulant hormone (TSH) level ≥ 4.0 mUI/L with free thyroxine (FT4) within normal range, with or without symptoms.
2. Cognition impairment: refers to decrease ability in mental activities to acquire, store, retrieve and use information. People with mild cognitive impairment are able to perform basic everyday activities, but present mental decline (forgetfulness, confusion, inattention etc) noticeable by themselves, their relatives, or test. While in dementia the performing of everyday activities are also deteriorated.

3. Depression is a long lasting sadness accompanied by loss of interest in activities; even activities the subject finds enjoyable. It can affect mental activity, behavior, and general well-being.

3. Subclinical hypothyroidism

3.1 Prevalence and risk factors for SH

SH comprises the largest fraction of TSH elevation. SH predominates in women, and its prevalence increases with age. In the United States, the percent of individuals with TSH over 4.5 mIU/L raises to 14% after 70 years of age [Hollowell et al 2002]. But a study [Hoogendoorn et al 2006] in Netherlands reported 4.4% of adult population with TSH over 4.0 mU/L; it also reported a decrease in the mean TSH by age (Figure 1). In Spain, a study reported a prevalence of hypothyroidism (TSH >6.7 mUI/L) of 11% in 60-69 age group population [Sender Palacios et al, 2004]. In Cuba, [Hernandez-Perera et al 2005] reported that 5.3% of population older than 59 years had a serum TSH >5.6 mU/L. The prevalence estimates have varied depending on the population studied and the criteria used to define it.

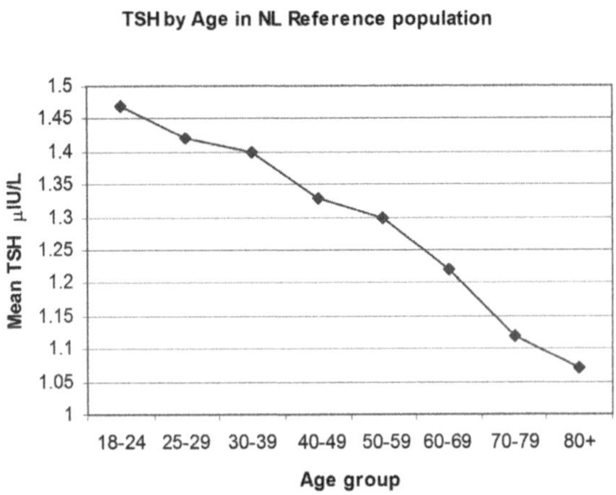

Fig. 1. TSH µIU/L by Age Adapted from Hoogendoorn et al 2006

Besides age and gender, genetics is among the population factors that inflict variation to prevalence estimates, accounting for almost 65% thyroidal phenotype [Samollow et al 2004, Peeters RP 2009]. Also, the amount of dietary iodine has to be considered. Its deficiency translates into endemic goiter, congenital hypothyroidism and other thyroidal dysfunction [Jameson & Weetman, 2005]. Sustained implementation of iodinated salt has been successful in abating simple goiter and cretinism [Basil S Hetzel 2004]. In Mexico City, Martinez et al [1999] reported 11% of subjects 55 and older with TSH higher than 5.6 µIU/L; however, in Monterrey Mexico, a region formally known for endemic goiter, 27.3% of geriatric outpatients had TSH >4.5 µIU/L [Cárdenas-Ibarra et al 2008]. The unexpectedly high frequency was confirmed by a population study [Cárdenas-Ibarra et al 2011a]. Another interesting observation of this study was a non significant difference of prevalence by gender, suggesting that advancing age decreases the gender gap of SH prevalence. The inhabitants of this region tend to ingest rather large quantities of iodinated salt (the only one available for a half century now) owing to the very hot weather that characterized this region. According with iodine sufficiency is the region low goiter prevalence (Cárdenas-Ibarra et al 2011a) and that 93.4% of congenital hypothyroidism is due to thyroid dysgenesis and 6% dyshormogenesis (Vela-Amieva et al 2003). Albeit, urinary iodine excretion was not measured. NHANES III [Hollowell et al 2002] reported an increase in mean TSH with age (see Figure 2) and also significantly higher TSH concentrations in persons with high iodine excretion (>500 μg/g creatinine) than in persons with normal iodine excretion (50–500 μg/g creatinine) ($P < .02$). Moreover, in a borderline sufficient iodine intake prevalence of overt hypothyroidism was 0.4% and subclinical 4.0%. In this study decreasing TSH serum levels with age were also observed [Hoogendoorn et al 2006] (Fig 1). Thyroid malfunction may come from an excess of iodine intake by a direct inhibitory effect to the thyroidal gland or by eliciting autoimmunity [Teng et al 2006]. Impairment in thyroid function changes directly with thyroid autoimmunity; but high urinary iodine excretion predicted an increase of TSH and antithyroperoxidase antibodies one month later [Karmisholt & Laurberg 2008]. Surveillance of dietary iodine is recommended.

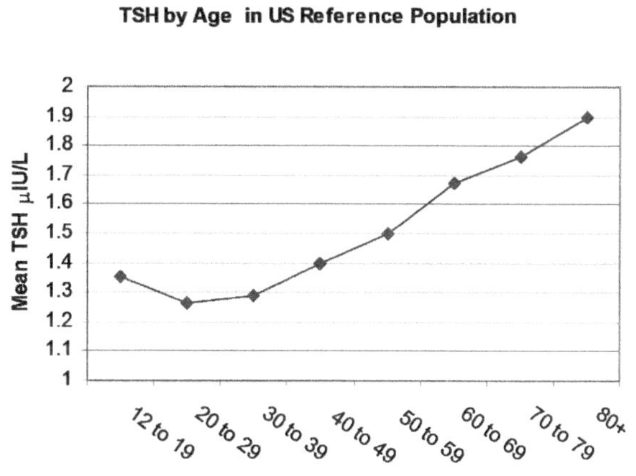

Fig. 2. TSH μIU/L by Age Adapted from Hollowell et al 2002

3.2 Clinical aspects of SH in the old

Thyroxine regulates the metabolism of all cells, rendering multisystem unspecific symptoms. Diagnosis of hypothyroidism in the elderly is specially challenging, since it develops very insidiously and symptoms usually go unnoticed [VermaA & Hasan 2009]. Even when symptoms are noted, they are confused with other health problems or are disregarded because they are thought to be part of aging. A questionnaire assessing hypothyroidism somatic symptoms was not able to predict abnormal TSH levels [Cárdenas-Ibarra et al 2011a]. See Table 1. In general, in symptom comparison among groups [Canaris et al 2004], subclinical hypothyroidism versus euthyroidism can show significant differences. These researchers reported a positive but weak association between the proportion of symptoms reported by the patients and progression of thyroid failure. Single or grouped symptoms are of little value at the individual level in just one consultation; thus most often SH is regarded as asymptomatic.

It is not until the patient is on levothyroxine that he/she notices improvement, such as less body aches, and not running out of energy. However, other symptoms such as weight change, puffy eyes, or hoarse voice take longer too reverse, if they do. Other functions such as cognition and mood symptoms can be reliably measured through validated instruments, but memory and depression complaints can not discriminate SH from euthyroidism. Mental slowing and depression are among the early hypothyroidism symptoms. Screening thyroid function in the elderly can save a lot of time, permit the implementation of appropriate measures, and avoid anguish to the patients and their families.

Symptom	Sensitivity	Especificity
Doesn't sweat	0.28	0.76
Deep voice	0.31	0.70
Paresthesia	0.64	0.47
Dry skin	0.56	0.59
Constipation	0.51	0.65
Can't lose weight	0.49	0.76
Slow to move	0.36	0.76
Rough skin	0.35	0.74
Puffy eyes	0.47	0.78
Cold intolerance	0.31	0.78

Cárdenas-Ibarra et al 2011a

Table 1. Symptoms on subjects with and without SH

3.3 Brain and thyroidal hormones

The availability of active thyroid hormone in adult brain results from the balance of its activation and inactivation [Kester et al 2004]. The selenoenzyme, type 2 iodothyronine deiodinase, removes an outer ring iodine atom from the thyroxine to generate thriiodothyronine, the active hormone. The type 3 iodothyronine deiodinase removes an iner ring iodine to inactivate the hormone. Brain protection from thriiodothyronine swings is attained by coordinating the expression of type 2 and 3 deiodinases. This is, expression of type 2 increases while type 3 decreases in low thyroxine; the opposite occurs with excess thyroxine. The monocarboxylate transporter-8 is a thyroid hormone specific transporter protein that crosses the blood-brain barrier. It is expressed in all brain locations involved in negative thyrotrophic releasing hormone feedback.

The hypothalamus-pituitary-thyroid axis is controlled by thyroid receptor beta 2 isoform, which is expressed solely in the hypothalamus and anterior pituitary, and is specific for thriiodothyronine [Abel et al 1999]. Low level of hypothalamic triiodothyronine elevates TSH. Thyroid hormone receptor studies on mutant mice report that the behavior of mice, lacking receptor beta, brings to mind the attention-deficit-hyperactivity disorder. The mice lacking TR alpha respond poorly to fear conditioning, showing poor memory, high anxiety, and inhibition of exploratory behavior. [Williams 2008]

Triiodothyronine deficiency prevents proper glucose uptake in neurons and decreases brain perfusion impairing processes of cognition and mood [Kinuya et al 1999]. Functional Magnetic resonance imaging revealed load effect of blood oxygen level dependent on the response in regions of interest in the frontal cortex (working memory), absent in subjects with SH, but present after six months of levothyroxine and improved performance in n-back task [Zhu et al 2006]. Hage &Azar 2011 review concluded that thyroid hormone supplements might help in the clinical response to antidepressive drugs. It seems sensible to screen for thyroidal problems in patients with depression that do not respond to treatment.

3.4 Normal thyroidal aging changes

Morphologic changes are reduction of follicle and colloidal content; but the individual remains clinical healthy. In iodine plentiful regions, age and thyroid stimulant hormone are positively related, while free thyroxine does not show a significant change with age. Anti-thyroeroxidase antibodies increase with age 8.5% in the 20-29 year age group to 22.3% in the 70-79 year age group; but antibodies are related to disease rather than senescence. [Hollowell et al 2002]. In borderline sufficient iodine, THS decreases while free thyroxine increases with age and antithyroperoxidase antibodies show insignificant changes. Atzmon et al [2009] reported that remarkably old individuals had high serum TSH levels, and that their offspring also had higher TSH values than age-matched controls, but this might not be extrapolable to other populations.

There is decreased production and release of TSH which produces 25% less production of thyroxine, but the serum level of thyroxine does not decrease due to underactive peripheral diiodinase type 2 function; also, the level of rT3 is positively age-related [Marioti et al 1993]. Hence the level of free Triiodothyronine decreases, but free thyroxine remains unchanged [Latrofa & Pinchera 2005]. There is no data of hypothalamic Triiodothyronine turnover to mantain adequate glucose uptake and brain perfusion in old age.

4. Cognition

Cognition comes from the Latin word *cognoscere*, meaning "to know". Cognition refers to mental activities to acquire, store, retrieve and use information. The mental processes most tested to evaluate cognition decline are: orientation (time, place, person), memory (code and retrieval), visuospatial (perception and memory), attention (speed and discrimination), language (denomination, fluency, comprehension, read & write), and executive function (concept, association, praxis) [Albert et al 1988].

4.1 Instruments to measure cognition and mood

The screening instruments most used to measure one or more of the above cognitive processes in general or geriatric clinical settings are:

- Mood: "Geriatric Depression Scale" (GDS) Yesavage validated for screening; it is widely use in English and Spanish-speaking population [Yesavage 1986]. The Hospital Anxiety and Depression Scale (HADS) is a self-assessment scale for English speaking educated outpatients. [Zigmond & Snaith 1983]; Beck Depression Inventory is a self - administrated 21 close-ended questionnaire [Beck 1961 in Jorde et al 2006].

- Mini-Mental-State-Examination (MMSE); low sensitivity in mild cognitive impairment; low specificity in subjects with less than middle schooling [Crum et al 1993].
- Katz's "Activities of daily-living" (Katz) useful for detecting dependence [Katz et al 1970].
- Lawton's "Instrumental activities of daily-living" (LW) tests subject's functionality. It has been used to screen for dementia [Lawton et al 1969].
- Dementia Rating Scale (DRS). Its application requires specialized personnel [APA 1994].
- Brief Neuropsychological Batteries; best options for screening (a paramedic can be trained to apply them):
  - ADAS-COG, (Alzheimer's Disease Assessment Scale-Cognitive) developed in educated Anglo population. Assesses orientation, memory, language, praxis, and executive function [Kolibas E et al 2000].
  - NEUROPSI: it assesses orientation, attention, memory: coding (verbal and visuospacial) dilayed memory (verbal and visuoespacial), language, and executive function. It was validated and standardized in Latin-American population; it is also useful in illiterate subjects [Ostrosky et al 1999].
- Evaluation of just one mental process saves times but the partial information can be misleading and many still need specialized personnel to apply it. [Begin et al 2008] For attention: paced auditory serial addition task, Stroop test, concept shifting, digit spans backward; for memory: Wechsler memory scale, facial memory test, selective reminding test, word learning task. Praxis clock drawing, Rey_Osterrieth complex figure, etc.

4.2 Cognitive function in elderly

Advancing age is the first risk factor for dementia, although dementia is not part of normal aging. There is a cognitive continuum disease that can be differentiated from normal although mild cognitive impaiment overlaps with both normal and disease [Petersen 2004]. Mood disorders are also overrepresented in the elderly, mainly depression: a long lasting feeling of sadness, hopeless, helpless, worthless, and aversion. Depression can affect mental activity, behavior and physical well-being. Cognitive function is affected by depression through interference in attention, memory (coding and retrieval), and decision taking.

In absence of overt disease, a decline of cognitive performance is seen in aging. The decline is associated to brain age changes: less glucose utilization, long-term potentiation and paired-pulse facilitation, protein expression, neurotransmitter levels and trophic changes. But it is not known if the above changes produce or are a product of alterations in the old brain. Freeman et al 2009 in a proteomic study in an animal model demostrated that changes in hippocampal proteom were related to cognitive performance. They also indicated the relevance of comparing old subjects sub grouped by cognitive level; they found that 9 hippocampal proteins were related with cognitive status. Only one was detected when comparing old with young animals.

A study [Cárdenas-Ibarra et al 2006] in a randomly selected sample of 142 geriatric outpatients to determine the frequency of impaired cognition by Mini-mental test examination found that 74.5% of subjects did not completed basic schooling, thus MMSE scores above 20 instead of 26 were considered normal. Still, impaired cognition was found in 59% vs 20% of those with partial vs full basic schooling (X^2=4.52, gl=1,$p<0.05$). The proportion of subjects with normal cognition decreased by age; in the over 80 y/o than in the 60-69 y/o, 27.3% vs 66.6% respectively (X^2=15.3, gl=6,$p<0.05$). Disadvantaged scores for GDS and LW were among CI and dementia ($p<0.05$, ANOVA); and Katz only to dementia ($p<0.05$, ANOVA) concluded that 31.7% were known dementia cases; another 24% had a new diagnosis of impaired cognition.

Ostrosky et al [Ardila et al 2000] used NEUROPSI in elderly urban population to describe normal cognitive decline in relation to education. They measured cognition in 806 subjects, of these 56.8% were over 50 years old. They reported different relationship patterns among education and specific cognitive domain; for example parallelism for copying a figure task, protection for word recall, confluence upwards for digits backwards, confluence downwards for semantic verbal fluency. they also found that healthy illiterate subjects showed no significant age decline in the domains of orientation, digits backward, language (repetition, naming, comprehension), and motor functions (hand position imitation, and alternating movement). Age changes are affected by education. Among the illiterate, peak performance is reached at an older age than subjects with formal education. Performance by age group and schooling on orientation, attention, coding, language motor function and memory subscales are shown in figure 3.

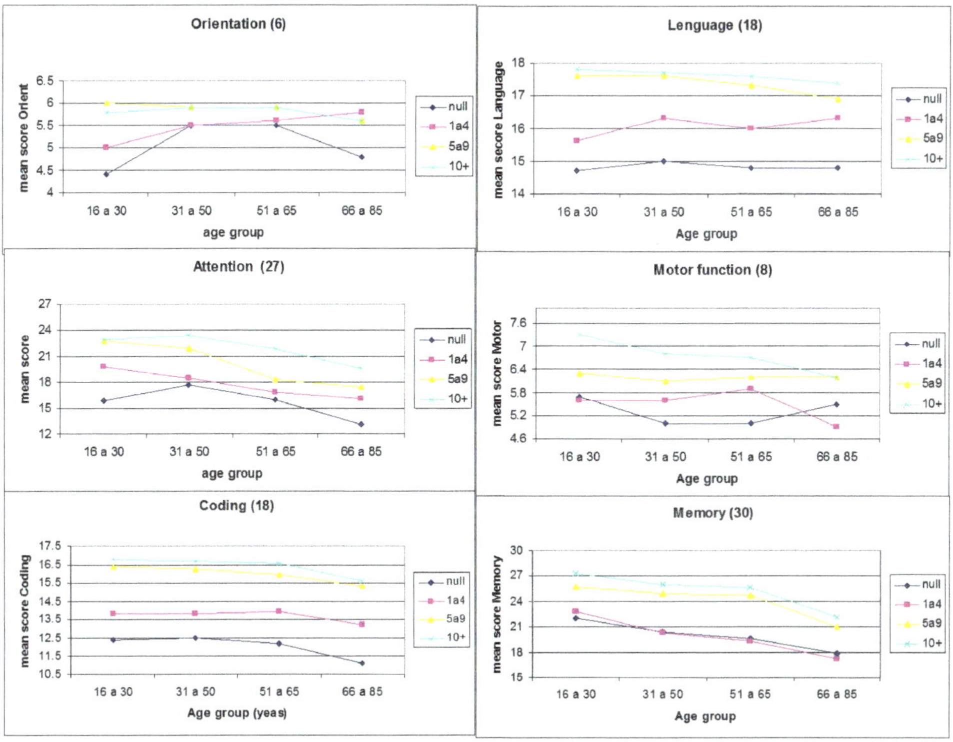

Adapted from ref Ardila et al 2000 Max. Score in brackets

Fig. 3. Mean scores of Six Mental Processes by Age and Schooling

In agreement with cognitive preservation notion, a study in open elderly rural population found that about 12% of the subjects scored higher than normal ranges for age and schooling supplied in the NEUROPSI manual (Figure 4), confirming that lucidity can be present in advancing age with little or no formal education [Cárdenas-Ibarra et al 2011].

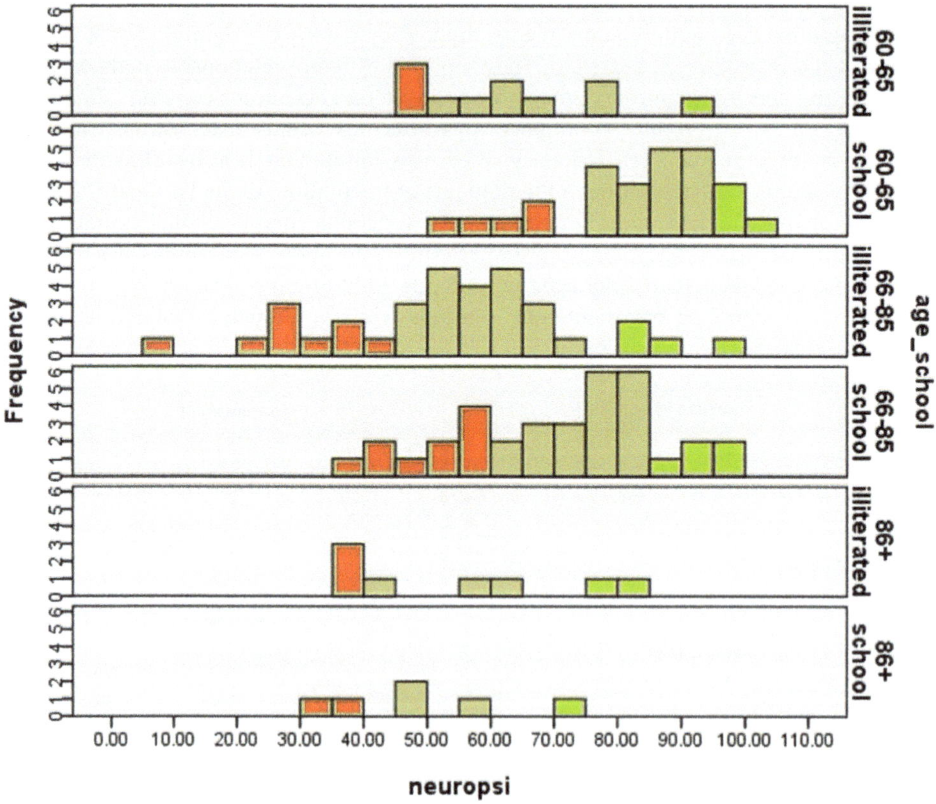

Cognitive scores: Red=Impaired, Amber=normal, Green=excel

Cárdenas-Ibarra et al 2011b

Fig. 4. Distribution of Rural Eldery's Neuropsi Score

5. Thyroidal status and cognitive function

Elderly people have the highest risk for thyroidal dysfunction as well as cognitive and mood disorders. Depression and memory complaints are excessively often in old age. In fact, depression is among the early symptoms of hypothyroidism; and memory loss relates to the level and length of thyroidal deficiency. Overall intellect is irreversibly affected in the developing brain as seen in congenital hypothyroidism.

The importance of thyroxine in the developing brain is well documented; the inability to focus and mood disturbances in the hyperthyroidal sate. Also in overt hypothyroidism lack of concentration, slow thinking and depression are described. In fact, it has been identified among the reversible causes of dementia [Jamerson & Weetman 2005]. But, Roberts et al [Roberts et al 2006] did not find association; neither did Gussekloo et al [Gussekloo et al 2004]] in a cohort of aging subjects. But the cognitive assessment instrument they used was the Mini-Mental-State-Examination, which is not sensible for mildly impaired cognitive function; including LW and Katz in the cognitive assessment did not increase sensitivity for dysfunction not reaching dementia. However, Gussekloo et al also reported that low free T3 was associated with rapid cognitive decline. These conflicting results demand studies with adequate assessments and well defined study groups.

A cross-sectional study [Cárdenas-Ibarra et al 2008] was set to compare the frequency of thyroid stimulating hormone (TSH) >4.5 mUI/L level in 33 randomly selected geriatric outpatients without dementia versus 101 dementia cases (DSM-IV-R). High TSH was found in nine (27.3%, CI: 12.1- 42.5%) and thirty (29.7%, CI: 20.8-38.6%), respectively. It is worth mentioning that 76.7% were subclinical hypothyroidism; i.e., free thyroxin was in normal range. However, average free thyroxine levels in patients with a high TSH were significantly lower than those with a normal TSH; the free thyroxine level of most of the subclinical hypothyroidism cases were in the lower half in contrast with the Gaussian distribution of free thyroxine in those with TSH in normal range. McDermott et al [McDermott & Ridway 2001] conclude that many of subclinical hypothyroidism cases require treatment. Monzani et al [Monzani et al 1993] and Lauberg et al [Laurberg et al 2005] point out that in the presence of depression and/or cognitive decline, thyroid supplementation will improve symptoms. From the perspective of quality of life and patient care; even a modest cognitive improvement is highly desirable [Steverson 1990].

Treatment is only being recommended for patients with low range thyroxin levels; while the presence of cognitive decline, not reaching level of dementia, in subclinical hypothyroidism must be addressed in other studies to assess it potential benefit.

To circumvent MMSE sensibility, specificity, language and cultural bias, we turn to NEUROPSI, an abovementioned instrument. We found it easy to apply and calculated a Cronbach's alpha of 0.86 denoting it as a reliable instrument [Cardenas-Ibarra et al 2011b and 2011c]. NEUROPSI was used to describe the cognitive function of the elderly in a rural open population study. These results are being submitted for publication. Our team is committed to a project with an open population to determine the local overt and subclinical hypothyroidism prevalence in urban elderly. To identify enough elderly subjects with SH, besides the population section, additionally a convenient sample of elderly visiting hospital patients with unknown thyroidal status were invited to be tested. Subjects with known thyroidal problems were excluded, subjects with known dementia, arrhythmia, kidney, lung, heart severe dysfunction or cancer were also excluded. Thus, subjects identified as having subclinical hypothyroidism were invited to a clinical trial [Cárdenas-Ibarra et al 2008b] with parallel control random assignment to test thyroxine versus placebo; which has not ended yet. Meanwhile, with the baseline data comparison was made between 37 subjects with SH and 39 controls (normal thyroid function) who were age and schooling matched. Impaired cognition in subjects with SH was almost double of that found in controls, in who the prevalence of impaired cognition was as expected. These results have only been discussed in a congress [Cárdenas-Ibarra et al 2011d]

A lower global cognitive status has been reported in hypothyroidism, specifically: attention, memory, word fluency, and psychomotor and visuospatial processes. Mixed results are reported for specific domains even in those with positive association. Moreover, improvement of cognitive impairement after levothyroxine replacement in elderly with SH has been reproted. Bono et al [Bono et al 2004] reported better verbal fluency after 6 moths with levothyroxine treatment. Enhanced elevating memory was reported by Monzani et al [Monzani et al 1993]. Enhanced working memory was noted after six months of thyroxine supplementation [Zhu et al 2006]. Improved response to antidepressants with levothyroxine has been documented in subjects with SH [Hage&Azar 2011]

Data on the extent of dysfunction reversibility for cognitive processes is lacking. Much work needs to be done to standardize cognitive results for comparison and uniform protocols to get homogenous groups on thyroidal function (including and excluding criteria). Long survival without cognitive enjoyment of being is pointless. The goal now is quality of life. Since the cognitive processes are central to well-being, its preservation is as important as a healthy body.

Cognitive labeling must be avoided; nevertheless timely repeated cognitive evaluation must be pursued to detect early decline and risks. Along with protocols to overcome cardiovascular risk and other preventable health problems, cognitive assessment by trained personnel to apply a neuropsychologically validated, reliable, and culturally compatible instrument must be performed. Interpretation and recommendations should be made by neuropsychologist or gerontologist consultants.

6. Acknowledgement

Our thanks go to Sergio Lozano-Rodriguez, M.D. for his help in reviewing the chapter; to Javier Ramos-Cardenas MD, and Macarena del Rosario Sifuentes-Martinez MD for their help at the rural communities; to Psychologist Xochitl A Ortiz Jimenez for her advice in instruments to measure cognitive function. And finaly to the Endocrinology Laboratory team, QCB Gloria Alejandra Jasso de la Peña y QCB Ramón Valdez-Leal.

7. References

Abel ED, Boers ME, Pazos-Moura C, Moura E, Kaulbach H, Zakaria M, Lowell B, Radovick S, Liberman MC, & Wondisford F. Divergent roles for thyroid hormone receptor beta isoforms in the endocrine axis and auditory system. J Clin Invest 1999; 104: 291–300.

Albert MS & Heaton R 1988. Intelligence testing. In Albert MS & Moss MB (Eds), Geriatric neuropsychology New York. The Guildford Press. pp10-32.

American Psychiatric Association, 1994. Diagnostic and Statistical Manual, 4th Ed APA Press, Washington DC.

Ardila A, Ostrosky-Solis F, Rosselli M, & Gomez C. Age-related cognitive decline during normal aging: The complex effect of education. Archives of Clinical Neuropsychology 2000; 15:495-514.

Atzmon G, Barzilai N, Hollowell JG, Surks MI & Gabriely I. Extreme longevity is associated with increased serum thyrotropin. J Clin Endocrinol Metab 94:1251-1254.

Begin ME, Langlois MF,Lorrain D, & Cunnane SC. Thyoid function and cognition during aging. Current gerontology and geriatrics research 2008; 2008:1-11.

BonoG, Fancellu R, Blandini F, Santoro G, & Mauri M. Cognitive and affective startus in mild hypothyroidism and interactions with L-thyroxine treatment. 2004; 1

Canaris GJ, Manowitz NR, Mayor G & Ridgway ECh. The Colorado Thyroid Disease Prevalence Study. *Arch Intern Med. 2000;160:526-534*

Cárdenas-Ibarra L, Villarreal-Perez JZ, & Salinas-Martinez R. Capacidad Cognitiva en Pacientes Ancianos de un Servicio Geriátrico Ambulatorio en Monterrey, México. Medicina Universitaria 2006; 8:84-87.

Cárdenas-Ibarra L, Solano Velazquez JA, Salinas –Martinez R, Aspera-Ledezma TD, Sifuentes-Martinez MR, & Villarreal-Perez JZ. Cross-sectional Observations of thyroid function in Geriatric Mexican Outpatients with and without dementia. Arch Gerontol Geriatr 2008a, 46:173-180.

Cárdenas-Ibarra L, Mellado-Urbina PA, Turner-Llaguno AL, Montemayor-Alatorre A, Ramos-Cárdenas J, Lira-Castillo JC, Gutierrez Herrera RF, & Villarreal-Pérez JZ. Prevalence and risk factors for Hypothyroidism in Elderly Urban Population. (to be published 2011a)

Cárdenas-Ibarra L, Ramirez-Navarro A, Ramos-Cárdenas J, Sifuentes_Martínez MR, Vázquez-García AA, & Villarreal-Perez JZ. Cognitive score distribution among elders of a rural population. (to be publish 2011b).

Cárdenas-Ibarra L, Ramos-Cárdenas J, Ramirez_Navarro EA, Nava-Aleman A, Sifuentes-Martinez MR, Ortiz-Jimenez XA, Saucedo Martinez D, & Villarreal-Perez JZ. Semantic verbal fluency in rural Elderly at Northeastern Mexico. (2011c)

Cardenas-Ibarra L, Sepulveda-Morelos H, Mellado-Urbina PA, Turner-Llaguno AL, Montemayor-Alatorre A, Ramos_Cardenas J, Lira-Castillo JC, Gutierrez-Herrera RF, & Villarreal-Perez JZ. Cognitive function of elderly subjects with and without subclinical hypothyroidism. Cell Symposia: Metabolism & Aging Conference March 27– 9, 2011d Cape code MA.

Cárdenas-Ibarra L, Mellado-Urbina PA, Turner-Llaguno AL, Montemayor-Alatorre A, Ramos-Cárdenas J, Lira-Castillo JC, Gutierrez Herrera RF, Vázquez-García AA, & Villarreal-Pérez JZ. Subclinical Hypothyroidism and Mind in the Elderly. ClinicalTrails.gov: NCT00921050, 2008b.

Crum RM, Anthony JC, Bassett SS, & Folstein MF. Population-based norms for the Mini-Mental State Examination by age and educational level. JAMA 1993; 269(18): 2386–2391.

Freeman WM, VanGuilder HD,Bennett C, & Sonntag WE. Cognitive performance and age-related changes in hippocampal proteome. Neuroscience 2009:159:183-195.

Gussekloo, J, Van Exel E, de Craen AJM, Meinders AE, Frölich M, & Westendorp RGJ. Thyroid status, disability and cognitive function, and survival in old age. Jama, 2004. 292:2591-9.

Hage MP, & Azar ST, The link between thyroid function and depression. Journal of thyroid research accepted 26 sep 2011.

Hatzel BS. The Nature and Magnitude of the Iodine Deficiency Disorders (IDD) In *Towards the Global Elimination Of Brain Damage Due to Iodine Deficiency*. Editors: Delange F., Dunn JT., Ling J., Mannar V. and Pandav Ch. Delhi Oxford University Press CALCUTTA 2004 http://www.iccidd.org iccidd.server295.com/media/Hetzel%20book/hetzel-a-frontpage.pdf

Hernández-Perera A, López-González LE, Hernández-Perera A, & Mesa-Santamarina A. Hipotiroidismo subclínico en el anciano ambulatorio. Rev Biomed 2007;18:162-166.

Hollowell JG, Steahling NW, Flanders WD, Hannon WH, Gunter EW, Spencer CA & Braverman LE. Serum TSH, thyroxin and Thyroid Antibodies in the US Population (1988 to 1994): National Health and Nutrition Examination Survey. J Clin Endocrinol Metab, 2002; 87:489-499.

Hoogendoorn EH, Hermus AR, Vegt FD, Ross HA, Verbeek ALM, Kiemeney LALM, Swinkels DW, Sweep FCG, & Heijer MD. Thyroid Function and Prevalence of Anti-Thyroperoxidase antibodies in a population with borderline sufficient iodine intake: Influences of Age and sex. Clinical Chemistry 2006, 52:104-111.

Jameson JL & Weetman AP, 2005. Disorders of the thyroid gland. In Kasper, Braunwald, Fauci, Hauser, Longo and Jameson (Eds). *Harrison's Principles of Internal Medicine.* New York: McGraw-Hill, pg 2104 - 2126.

Jorde R, Waterloo K, Storhaug H, Nyrnes A, Sundsfjord J, &Jenssen TG. Neuropsychological function and symptoms in subjects with subclinical hypothyroidism and the effect of thyroxine treatment. J Clin Endocrinol Metab 2006;91:145-153.

Karmisholt J & Laurberg P. Serum TSH and serum thyroidperoxidase antibody fluctuate in parallel and high urinary iodine excretion predicts subsequent thyroid failure in a 1-year study of patients with untreated subclinical hypothyroidism. European Journal of Endocrinology 2008;158:209-215.

Katz S. Downs TD, Cash HR, & Grotz RC. Progress in the development of the index of ADL, Gerontologist 1970; 10:20-30.

Kester MH, Martinez de Mena R, Obregon MJ, Marinkovic D, Howatson A, Visser TJ, Hume R, & Morreale de Escobar G. Iodothyronine levels in the human developing brain: major regulatory roles of iodothyronine deiodinases in different areas. J Clin Endocrinol Metab 2004; 89: 3117–3128.

Kinuya S, Michigishi T, Tonami N, Aburano T, Tsuji S, & Hashimoto T. Reversible cerebral hypoperfusion observed with Tc-99m HMPAO SPECT in reversible dementia caused by hypothyroidism. Clin Nucl Med. 1999 Sep;24(9):666-8

Kolibas E, KorinkovaV,.Novotny V, Vajdickova K, & HunakovaD. ADAS-cog (Alzheimer´s Disease Assessment Scale-cognitive-subscale) validation of the Slovak version. Bratisl Lek Listy 2000; 101:598-602.

Latrofa F & Pinchera A. Aging and the thyroid. Hot Thyroidology 2005. www.hotthyroidology.com

Laurberg P, Andersen S, Pedersen I B & Carlé A. Hypothyroidism in the elderly: pathophysiology, diagnosis and treatment. Drugs Aging 2005; 22:23-38.

Lawton MP, & Brody EM. Assessment of older people: Self-maintaining and instrumental activities of daily living. The Gerontologist 1969; 9: 179-186.

Maritti S, Barbesino G, Caturegli P, Bartalena L, Sansoni P, Fagnoni F, Monti D, Fagiolo U, Franceschi C & Pinchera A. Complex Alterations of thyroid function in healthy centenarians. J Clin Endocrinol Metab 77:1130-1134.

Martinez Lara E, Morales Yepez HA, Sandoval Pacheco R, & Lopez Hernandez CM. Prevalencia de hipotiroidismo en pacientes mayors de 55 años en la consulta de geriatria del Horpital Central Militar. Rev Sanid Milit Mex 1999; 53:105-108.

McDermott MT & Ridgway EC. Subclinical hypothyroidism is mild failure and should be treated. J Clin Endocrinol Metab, 2001; 86:3585- 4590

Monzani F, Del Guerra P, Caraccio N, Prunetti CA, Pucci E, Luisi M & Baschieri L. Subclinical hypothyroidism: neurobehavioral features and beneficial effect of l-thyroxin treatment. Clin Investig, 1993; 71:367-71.

Ostrosky F, Ardila A & Rosselli M. "Neuropsi". A brief neuropsychological test battery in Spanish with norms by age and educational level. Journal of the International Neuropsychological Society. 1999; 5:413-433.

Peeters RP. Thyroid function and longevity New insights into an old dilema. J Clin Endocrinol metab 2009, 94:4658-4660.

Petersen RC. Mild cognitive impairment as diagnostic entity. Journal of Internal Medicine 2004;256:183-194.

Roberts LM, Pattison H, Roalfe A, Franklin J, Wilson S, Hobbs R, & Parle JV. Is subclinical thyroid dysfunction in the elderly associated with depression or cognitive dysfunction? Ann Intern Med 2006; 145:573-581.

Samollow PB, Pérez G, Kammerer CM, Finegold D, Zwartjes PW, Havill LM, Comuzzie AG, Mahaney MC, Göring HH, Blangero J, Foley TP, & Barmada MM. Genetic and Environmental Influences of Thyroid Hormone Variation in Mexican Americans. J Clin Endocrinol Metab, 2004; 89:3276-84.

Sender Palacios MJ, Vernet Vernet M, Pérez López S, Faro Colomel M, Rojas Blanc M & Pallisa Gabriel L. Enfermedad funcional tiroidea en la población de edad avanzada. Atención primaria, 2004;34:192-7.

Stevenson JP. Family stress related to home care of Alzheimer's disease patients and implications for support. J Neurosci Nurs, 1990; 22:179-88

Teng W, Shan Z, Teng X, Guan H, Li Y, Teng D, Jin Y, Yu X, Fan C, Chong W, Yang F, Dai H, Yu Y, Li J, Chen Y, Zhao D, Shi X, Hu F, Mao J, Gu X, Yang R, Tong Y,WangW, Gao T & Li C. Effect of iodine intake on thyroid diseases in China. New England Journal of Medicine 2006;354:2783–2793.

Vela-Amieva M, Gamboa-Cardiel S, Pérez-Andrade ME, Ortiz-Cortés J, Gonzalez-Contreras CR, Ortega-Velazquez V. Epidemiología del hipotiroidismo congénito en México. Salud Publica Mex 2004;46:141-148.

Verma A. & Hasan T. Clinical Geriatrics Thyroid disorders in older people. Reviews in Clinical Gerontology 2009;19: 193-206

Williams GR. Neurodevelopmental and Neurophysiological Actions of Thyroid Hormone. Journal of Neuroendocrinology 20:784–794.

Yesavage: The use of Rating Depression Series in the Elderly, en Poon (ed.):*Clínical Memory Assessment of Older Adults*, American Psychological Association, 1986

Zhu DF, Wang ZX, Zhang DR, Pan ZL, He S, H eu XP, Chen XCh & Zhou JN. fMRI revealed neural substrate for reversible working memory dysfunction in subclinical hypothyroidism. Brain 2006;129:2923-2930.

Zigmond AS & Snaith RP The hospital anxiety and depression scale . Acta Psychiatr Scand. 1983;67:361-370.

Permissions

The contributors of this book come from diverse backgrounds, making this book a truly international effort. This book will bring forth new frontiers with its revolutionizing research information and detailed analysis of the nascent developments around the world.

We would like to thank Drahomira Springer, for lending her expertise to make the book truly unique. She has played a crucial role in the development of this book. Without her invaluable contribution this book wouldn't have been possible. She has made vital efforts to compile up to date information on the varied aspects of this subject to make this book a valuable addition to the collection of many professionals and students.

This book was conceptualized with the vision of imparting up-to-date information and advanced data in this field. To ensure the same, a matchless editorial board was set up. Every individual on the board went through rigorous rounds of assessment to prove their worth. After which they invested a large part of their time researching and compiling the most relevant data for our readers. Conferences and sessions were held from time to time between the editorial board and the contributing authors to present the data in the most comprehensible form. The editorial team has worked tirelessly to provide valuable and valid information to help people across the globe.

Every chapter published in this book has been scrutinized by our experts. Their significance has been extensively debated. The topics covered herein carry significant findings which will fuel the growth of the discipline. They may even be implemented as practical applications or may be referred to as a beginning point for another development. Chapters in this book were first published by InTech; hereby published with permission under the Creative Commons Attribution License or equivalent.

The editorial board has been involved in producing this book since its inception. They have spent rigorous hours researching and exploring the diverse topics which have resulted in the successful publishing of this book. They have passed on their knowledge of decades through this book. To expedite this challenging task, the publisher supported the team at every step. A small team of assistant editors was also appointed to further simplify the editing procedure and attain best results for the readers.

Our editorial team has been hand-picked from every corner of the world. Their multi-ethnicity adds dynamic inputs to the discussions which result in innovative outcomes. These outcomes are then further discussed with the researchers and contributors who give their valuable feedback and opinion regarding the same. The feedback is then collaborated with the researches and they are edited in a comprehensive manner to aid the understanding of the subject.

Apart from the editorial board, the designing team has also invested a significant amount of their time in understanding the subject and creating the most relevant covers. They scrutinized every image to scout for the most suitable representation of the subject and create an appropriate cover for the book.

The publishing team has been involved in this book since its early stages. They were actively engaged in every process, be it collecting the data, connecting with the contributors or procuring relevant information. The team has been an ardent support to the editorial, designing and production team. Their endless efforts to recruit the best for this project, has resulted in the accomplishment of this book. They are a veteran in the field of academics and their pool of knowledge is as vast as their experience in printing. Their expertise and guidance has proved useful at every step. Their uncompromising quality standards have made this book an exceptional effort. Their encouragement from time to time has been an inspiration for everyone.

The publisher and the editorial board hope that this book will prove to be a valuable piece of knowledge for researchers, students, practitioners and scholars across the globe.

List of Contributors

Ahmed S. BaHammam
University Sleep Disorders Center, King Saud University, Riyadh, Saudi Arabia

Suhaila E. Al-Jawder
University Sleep Disorders Center, King Saud University, Riyadh, Saudi Arabia
Department of Medicine, Salmaniya Medical Complex, Manama, Kingdom of Bahrain

J. Coria Mariela, V. Carmona Yamila, B. Oliveros Liliana and S. Giménez Maria
Instituto Multidisciplinario de Investigaciones, Biológicas-CONICET, San Luis Universidad Nacional de San Luis, Argentina

P. de Gortari, E. Alvarez-Salas, M. Morales-Mulia and V. Alcántara-Alonso
Dirección de Investigaciones en Neurociencias /Instituto Nacional de Psiquiatría Ramón de la Fuente M., México

Jandee Lee and Woong Youn Chung
Department of Surgery,Yonsei Univeristy College of Medicine, South Korea

Kallistheni Farmaki
General Hospital of Corinth, Greece

Antonio Mancini, Sebastiano Raimondo and Chantal Di Segni
Department of Internal Medicine, Catholic University of the Sacred Heart, Rome, Italy

Elena Giacchi
Center for Study and Research on Natural Fertility Regulation, Catholic University of the Sacred Heart, Rome, Italy

Andrea Silvestrini and Elisabetta Meucci
Institute of Biochemistry and Clinical Biochemistry, Catholic University of the Sacred Heart, Rome, Italy

Hande Turker and Nilgun Cengiz
Ondokuzmayis University, School Of Medicine, Department of Neurology, Samsun, Turkey

Cuneyt Turker
Gazi State Hospital, Clinic of Internal Medicine, Samsun, Turkey

Hamiyet Yılmaz
Aydin State Hospital, Department of Endocrinology and Metabolism, Turkey

Barış Pamuk
Bozyaka Training and Research Hospital, Department of Internal Medicine, Turkey

Derun Taner Ertugrul
Kecioren Training and Research Hospital, Department of Internal Medicine, Turkey

Erdem Yaşar
Acıpayam State Hospital, Department of Anaesthesia, Turkey

Irena Kostic
University of Kragujevac, Serbia
University of Udine Medical School, Dip. di Scienze Mediche e Biologiche, Italy

Francesco Curcio
University of Udine Medical School, Dip. di Scienze Mediche e Biologiche, Italy
University of Udine Teaching Hospital, Santa Maria della Misericordia, Dip. di Medicina di Laboratorio, Italy

Jack R. Wall and Bernard Champion
Department of Medicine, the University of Sydney, Nepean Hospital, Penrith, New South Wales, Australia

Valentine V. Fadeyev and Galina A. Melnichenko
I.M. Sechenov First Moscow State Medical University, Department of Endocrinology, Russia
Federal Endocrinological Research Centre, Russia

Tatyana Morgunova
I.M. Sechenov First Moscow State Medical University, Department of Endocrinology, Russia

Otakar Kraft
Clinic of Nuclear Medicine, University Hospital Ostrava, Ostrava, Czech Republic
Faculty of Medicine, University of Ostrava, Ostrava, Czech Republic

Chao-Jung Tsao and Yin-Hsun Feng
Chi-Mei Medical Center, Taiwan

Farzaneh Ganji
Department of Biology, Faculty of Science, Golestan University, Gorgan, Iran

Koreaki Sugimoto
Department of Psychosomatic Medicine, Tohoku Fukushi University, Japan

Kouki Mori
Department of Health Supervision, JR Sendai Hospital, Japan

Sing-Yung Wu and William L. Green
University of California, Irvine, VA Medical Center, Long Beach, California
University of Washington, Seattle, Washington, USA

Jacek Drobnik
Laboratory of Connective Tissue Metabolism, Department of General and Experimental Pathology Medical University of Lodz, Poland

Yardena Tenenbaum-Rakover
Ha'Emek Medical Center, Afula and the Ruth & Rappoprt Faculty of Medicine, Technion, Haifa, Israel

Gulfidan Cakmak
Haseki Training and Research Hospital, Istanbul, Turkey

Lilia Cárdenas-Ibarra, Jesús Zacarías Villarreal-Pérez and Abraham Antonio Vázquez-García
Endocrinology service, and Geriatric service, University Hospital, School of Medicine, Autonomous University of Nuevo Leon, México